Nursing Today

Transition and Trends

REVISED REPRINT

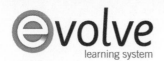 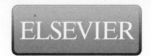
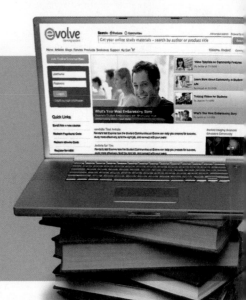

Nursing Today

Transition and Trends

Seventh Edition
Revised Reprint

JoAnn Zerwekh, MSN, EdD, RN
Executive Director
Nursing Education Consultants
Ingram, Texas;
Nursing Faculty–Online Campus
University of Phoenix
Phoenix, Arizona

Ashley Zerwekh Garneau, PhD, RN
Nursing Faculty
GateWay Community College
Phoenix, Arizona

ELSEVIER
SAUNDERS

3251 Riverport Lane
St. Louis, Missouri 63043

NURSING TODAY: TRANSITION AND TRENDS   ISBN: 978-0-323-24101-4
Copyright © 2014, 2012, 2009, 2006, 2003, 2000, 1997, 1994 by Saunders, an imprint of Elsevier Inc.

No part of this publication may be reproduced or transmitted in any form or by any means, electronic or mechanical, including photocopying, recording, or any information storage and retrieval system, without permission in writing from the publisher. Details on how to seek permission, further information about the Publisher's permissions policies and our arrangements with organizations such as the Copyright Clearance Center and the Copyright Licensing Agency, can be found at our website: www.elsevier.com/permissions.

This book and the individual contributions contained in it are protected under copyright by the Publisher (other than as may be noted herein).

Notices

Knowledge and best practice in this field are constantly changing. As new research and experience broaden our understanding, changes in research methods, professional practices, or medical treatment may become necessary.

Practitioners and researchers must always rely on their own experience and knowledge in evaluating and using any information, methods, compounds, or experiments described herein. In using such information or methods they should be mindful of their own safety and the safety of others, including parties for whom they have a professional responsibility.

With respect to any drug or pharmaceutical products identified, readers are advised to check the most current information provided (i) on procedures featured or (ii) by the manufacturer of each product to be administered, to verify the recommended dose or formula, the method and duration of administration, and contraindications. It is the responsibility of practitioners, relying on their own experience and knowledge of their patients, to make diagnoses, to determine dosages and the best treatment for each individual patient, and to take all appropriate safety precautions.

To the fullest extent of the law, neither the Publisher nor the authors, contributors, or editors, assume any liability for any injury and/or damage to persons or property as a matter of products liability, negligence or otherwise, or from any use or operation of any methods, products, instructions, or ideas contained in the material herein.

Library of Congress Cataloging-in-Publication Data

Nursing today : transition and trends / [edited by] JoAnn Zerwekh, Ashley Zerwekh Garneau.—7th ed. revised reprint
        p.   ;   cm.
    Includes bibliographical references and index.
    ISBN 978-0-323-24101-4 (pbk. : alk. paper)
    1. Nursing—Vocational guidance.   2. Nursing—Social aspects.   I. Zerwekh, JoAnn Graham.   II. Garneau, Ashley Zerwekh.
    [DNLM: 1. Nursing.   2. Vocational Guidance. WY 16]
    RT82.N874 2011
    610.7306′9—dc22

                                                                                    2011005796

Executive Publisher: Darlene Como
Acquisitions Editor: Maureen Iannuzzi
Senior Developmental Editor: Robin Levin Richman
Publishing Services Manager: Deborah Vogel
Project Manager: Brandilyn Tidwell
Designer: Amy Buxton

Printed in the United States of America

Last digit is the print number: 9 8 7 6 5 4 3 2 1

Working together to grow
libraries in developing countries

www.elsevier.com | www.bookaid.org | www.sabre.org

ELSEVIER   BOOK AID International   Sabre Foundation

Contributors

Susan Lynne Ahrens, RN, PhD
Associate Faculty, Graduate Nursing Programs
Indiana University–Purdue University Fort Wayne
Fort Wayne, Indiana
Chapter 25: Workplace Issues

Tim J. Bristol, PhD, RN, CNE
Consultant
Nursing Education Consultants
Ingram, Texas;
Faculty
Nursing Education–Graduate Program
Walden University
Minneapolis, Minnesota
Chapter 21: Cultural and Spiritual Awareness

Jo Carol Claborn, MS, RN
Executive Director
Nursing Education Consultants
Ingram, Texas
*Chapter 5: NCLEX-RN® Examination and the New
    Graduate*

Sharon Decker, PhD, RN, ACNS-BC, ANEF
Professor and Covenant Health System Endowed
    Chair in Simulation and Nursing Education
Director of the F. Marie Hall SimLife Center
Director of TTUHSC Quality Enhancement
Texas Tech University Health Sciences Center
Lubbock, Texas
*Chapter 2: Personal Management: Time and
    Self-Care Strategies*

Michael L. Evans, PhD, RN, NEA-BC, FAAN
Maxine Clark and Bob Fox Dean and Professor
Goldfarb School of Nursing
Barnes-Jewish College
St. Louis, Missouri
Chapter 17: Political Action in Nursing

Ashley Zerwekh Garneau, PhD, RN
Nursing Faculty
GateWay Community College
Phoenix, Arizona
*Chapter 3: Mentorship, Preceptorship, and
    Nurse Residency Programs*
Chapter 8: Nursing Theory

Ruth I. Hansten, RN, MBA, PhD, FACHE
Principal, Hansten Healthcare PLLC
Ludlow, Washington
Chapter 14: Delegation in the Clinical Setting

Judy Irvin, RN, JD
National Surgical Hospitals
Mesa, Arizona
Chapter 20: Legal Issues

Marilynn Jackson, RN, PhD, CHTP, CCA
Intuitive Options
Parma, Idaho
Chapter 14: Delegation in the Clinical Setting

Mary Mackenburg-Mohn, RN, PhD, CNP
Program Director/Associate Professor
Acute Care Pediatric Nurse Practitioner Program
Brandman University School of Nursing and
    Health Professions
Irvine, California
Chapter 24: Using Nursing Research in Practice

Peter Melenovich, MS, RN, CCRN-CSC, CNE
Nursing Faculty
GateWay Community College
Phoenix, Arizona
Chapter 19: Ethical Issues

Mary Ellen Murray, PhD, RN
Associate Professor
Associate Dean, Academic Affairs
School of Nursing
University of Wisconsin–Madison
Madison, Wisconsin
*Chapter 16: Economics of the Health Care Delivery
    System*

Theresa M. Pape, PhD, RN, CNOR
Associate Professor
College of Nursing
Texas Woman's University
Denton, Texas
Chapter 22: Quality Patient Care

Cheryl D. Parker, MSN, PhD, RN
Contributing Faculty
Nursing
Walden University
Minneapolis, Minnesota
Chapter 23: Nursing Informatics

Jessica Maack Rangel, MS, RN
Director of Patient Safety and Customer Relations
Texas Health Harris Methodist Hospital
Fort Worth, Texas
Chapter 11: Building Nursing Management Skills

Catherine Rosser, EdD, CNA-BC, RN
Undergraduate Program Director
Louise Herrington School of Nursing
Baylor University
Dallas, Texas
Chapter 11: Building Nursing Management Skills

Margi Schultz, PhD, RN, CNE, PLNC
Director, Nursing Division
GateWay Community College
Phoenix, Arizona
*Chapter 9: Image of Nursing: Influences of the
    Present*

Susan Sportsman, RN, PhD
Dean, College of Health Sciences and Human
    Services
Midwestern State University
Wichita Falls, Texas
*Chapter 15: The Health Care Organization and
    Patterns of Nursing Care Delivery*

Gayle P. Varnell, PhD, APRN, CPNP-PC
Associate Professor and Assistant Dean for
    Advanced Practice
College of Nursing and Health Sciences
The University of Texas at Tyler
Tyler, Texas
Chapter 7: Nursing Education

Joann Wilcox, RN, MSN, LNC
Director, Education
Creative Training Solutions
Kansas City, Kansas;
Health Sciences/Nursing–Online Faculty
University of Phoenix
Phoenix, Arizona
*Chapter 10: Challenges of Nursing Management
    and Leadership*
*Chapter 18: Collective Bargaining: Traditional
    (Union) and Nontraditional Approaches*

JoAnn Zerwekh, MSN, EdD, RN
Executive Director
Nursing Education Consultants
Ingram, Texas;
Nursing Faculty–Online Campus
University of Phoenix
Phoenix, Arizona
Chapter 1: Role Transitions
Chapter 4: Employment Considerations:
  Opportunities, Resumes, and Interviewing
Chapter 6: Historical Perspectives: Influences on the
  Present
Chapter 12: Effective Communication and Team
  Building
Chapter 13: Conflict Management
Chapter 23: Nursing Informatics
Chapter 26: Emergency Preparedness

Tyler Zerwekh, MPH, DrPH
Environmental Health Services Bureau, Deputy
  Administrator
Memphis and Shelby County Health Department
Memphis, Tennessee
Chapter 26: Emergency Preparedness

Reviewers

Marie H. Ahrens, MS, RN
School of Nursing
University of Tulsa
Tulsa, Oklahoma

Carol C. Annesser, RN, MSN, BC, CNE
Mercy College of Northwest Ohio
Toledo, Ohio

Margaret E. Barnes, RN, MSN
School of Nursing
Indiana Wesleyan University
Marion, Indiana

Jo Ann Brooks, PhD, RN, FAAN, FCCP
Clarion Health
Indianapolis, Indiana

Margaret Dean, MSN, RN, CS-BC, GNP-BC
School of Nursing
School of Medicine Faculty
Texas Tech University Health Sciences Center
Lubbock, Texas

Joyce Foresman-Capuzzi, BSN, RN, CEN, CPN, CTRN, CCRN, CPEN, SANE-A, EMT-P
Lankenau Hospital
Wynnewood, Pennsylvania

Joellen W. Hawkins, RN, PhD, WHNP-BC, FAAN, FAANP, NAP
William F. Connell School of Nursing
Boston College;
Nursing Department
Simmons College
Chestnut Hill, Massachusetts

Kimberly O. Lacey, DNSc, MSN, BSN, RN
Department of Nursing
Southern Connecticut State University
New Haven, Connecticut

Kathy J. Morris, DNP, APRN, FNP-C, FAANP
College of Nursing
University of Nebraska Medical Center
Omaha, Nebraska

Laura C. Parker, MSN, RN, CCRN
County College of Morris
Randolph, New Jersey

Gerry Walker, DHEd, MSN, RN
Park University
Parkville, Missouri

Polly Gerber Zimmermann, RN, MS, MBA, CEN, FAEN
Harry S. Truman College
Chicago, Illinois

Preface

Nursing Today: Transition and Trends evolved out of the authors' experiences with the nursing student in his or her final semester and the student's transition into the realities of nursing practice. With the changes in health care and the practice of nursing, there is even more emphasis on the importance of assisting the new graduate to transition from education to practice. Nursing education and the transition process are experiencing a tremendous impact from changes in the health care delivery system. We have responded to these changes by adding information in areas that nursing faculty specifically requested. In this updated seventh edition, we would like to provide you with several new features that we feel are vital to the success of our future generation of nurses!

We have continued to provide the graduate nurse with information on nursing informatics and management. We have continued the increased focus on the use of information technology for the transitioning graduate by including information on point of care electronic documentation. We have expanded on nursing management by adding a section on evidence-based protocols and interventions for the new graduate nurse to effectively manage and lead in the healthcare setting along with updated "hands-off" communication reporting tools recommended by the Joint Commisssion.Chapters related to current issues in health care, such as Ethical Issues, Legal Issues, Collective Bargaining: Traditional (Union) and Nontraditional Approaches, and The Health Care Organization and Patterns of Nursing Care Delivery have been expanded. We have also combined chapter information to make topics easier to find and to make for easier reading with less repetition. We kept the same easy reading style to present timely information, along with updated information on the NCLEX-RN® Detailed Test Plan and sample images of the new alternate-format test items appearing on the NCLEX-RN®. One of our goals with this book is to provide the graduating nurse with practical guidelines that can be implemented in his or her transition from nursing student to effective nursing practice at entry level. For this reason, we have provided useful information on nurse residency programs for the new graduate nurse and use of peer mentoring programs as a capstone course for the senior nursing student in the Mentorship, Preceptorship, and Nurse Residency Programs chapter. An additional feature of this book includes online resources and relevant websites for each chapter. This new element aligns to today's technologically-driven classroom and clinical setting. We have outlined recommendations from the 2010 Institute of Medicine report regarding requiring all new graduate nurses to complete a nurse residency program following completion from a pre-licensure program. In addition, the NCLEX-RN chapter has been updated to reflect the *2013 NCLEX-RN Detailed Test Plan* with weighted percentages for the four levels of client needs.

The classic findings and experience of Marlene Kramer and her research on reality shock, as well as Patricia Benner's work on performance characteristics of beginning and expert nurses, continue to impact the need for transition courses in the school curriculum. These courses focus on trends and issues to assist the new graduate to be better prepared to practice nursing in today's world. With the increased demands and realities of the health care system, it is necessary for the new graduate to rapidly make the transition to an independent role. We have written this book to be used in these transition-type courses, as well as by individual students to assist them in anticipating encounters in a rapidly changing, technologically oriented work environment.

We have revised and updated each chapter regarding the changes in the health care delivery system. To illustrate this, genetics and genomics has been included in the Ethical Issues chapter, discussion highlighting the emergence of formal unions and professional nursing organizations has been updated under Collective Bargaining, and information related to delivering patient-centered care has been expanded in The Health Care Organization and Patterns of Nursing Care Delivery chapter. Some of the lengthy tables and figures have been moved to Evolve Resources as to keep the material intact and make for easier reading. We have maintained the cartoons drawn by C.J. Miller, RN. We feel they add a smile and perhaps make the difficult information a little easier. Each chapter begins with student objectives and a quote as an introduction to the content of the chapter. Within each chapter, there is a practical application of the concepts discussed. Critical Thinking boxes in the text highlight information to facilitate the critical thinking process. Using a question approach, material is presented in a logical, easy-to-read manner. There are also opportunities to respond to thought-provoking questions and student exercises to facilitate self-evaluation.

The student is given an overall view of the nursing profession from historical events that influenced nursing to the present day image, as well as the legal, ethical, political, and on-the-job issues confronting today's nurse. Communication in the workplace, time management, how to write an effective resume, interviewing tips, employee benefits, and self-care strategies are among the sound career advancement tools provided.

FOR NURSING FACULTY

Our key goal in developing this book has been timely information that is applicable to current practice and fun to read. An Instructor's Manual, which is web-based, is available from the publisher to assist faculty in planning and promoting a positive transition experience. This valuable website contains suggestions for classroom and clinically based student activities.

At the request of nursing faculty using our book, we have provided a secure, updated web-based Test Bank with detailed rationales included on higher-order level test questions and text page references indicating where the correct answer can be obtained in the chapter has been provided for all test items. Additional alternate-format test items have also been added to the Test Bank. We have included accompanying textbook appendixes and have expanded the content within Evolve, which supports the textbook. The Evolve website will continue to provide updated information as new trends and issues affect the practice of nursing.

Please consult your local Elsevier representative for more details.

JoAnn Zerwekh
Ashley Zerwekh Garneau

Acknowledgments

The success of previous editions of this book is due to the contributions and efforts of our chapter contributors, who provided their expertise and knowledge, and to our book reviewers, for their insight and suggestions on pertinent issues in nursing practice. This new edition is no exception. We thank the staff at Elsevier for their assistance and guidance during the revision of the seventh edition: Maureen Iannuzzi, Senior Nursing Editor, and Robin Levin Richman, Senior Developmental Editor. We would also like to extend our gratitude to Brandi Tidwell for monitoring the production of this book to ensure the book's delivery on schedule.

I would like to thank my children, Tyler and Ashley (my new co-author!!); their spouses (Cassi Zerwekh and Brian Garneau) and my grandchildren (Maddie Zerwekh and Ben Garneau) for putting a smile on my face and getting me to step away from the computer during those challenging times in the revision process.

Finally we thank our spouses John Masog and Brian Garneau for their unending support, patience, and sense of humor during the revision of the seventh edition. We appreciate your willingness in completing the additional "honey-do" lists we managed to compile for you while we were entrenched in the book revision. We love you all!

Contents

UNIT IV: NURSING MANAGEMENT

UNIT V: CURRENT ISSUES IN HEALTH CARE

16 Economics of the Health Care Delivery System, 335

17 Political Action in Nursing, 355

18 Collective Bargaining: Traditional (Union) and Nontraditional Approaches, 374

19 Ethical Issues, 395

20 Legal Issues, 422

UNIT VI: CONTEMPORARY NURSING PRACTICE

21 Cultural and Spiritual Awareness, 466

22 Quality Patient Care, 480

23 Nursing Informatics, 511

CHAPTER **1**

Role Transitions

JoAnn Zerwekh, MSN, EdD, RN

If only dreams and reality were not so far apart.
—Miguel de Cervantes

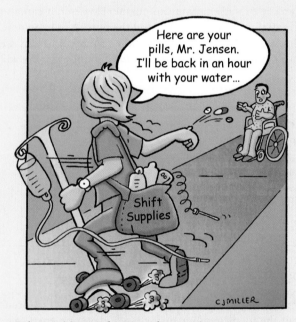

Role transition can be a complex experience.

After completing this chapter, you should be able to:

- Discuss the concept of transitions.

- Identify the characteristics of reality shock.

- Compare and contrast the phases of reality shock.

- Identify times in your life when you have experienced a reality shock or role transition.

- Describe methods to promote a successful transition.

*W*elcome to the profession of nursing! This book is written for nursing students who are in the midst of transitions in their life. As a new student, you are beginning the transition to becoming indoctrinated into nursing, and sometimes it is not an easy transition. For those of you who are in the middle of nursing school, do you wonder if life even exists outside of nursing school? To the student who will soon graduate, hang on; you are almost there! For whatever transition period you are encountering, our goal is to help make your life easier during this period of personal and professional adjustment into nursing. We have designed this book to help you keep your feet on the ground and your head out of the clouds as well as to boost your spirits when the going gets rough.

As you thumb through this book, you will notice that there are cartoons and critical thinking questions that encourage your participation. Do not be alarmed; we know you have been over-loaded with "critical thinking" during nursing school! These critical thinking questions are not meant to be graded; instead, their purpose is to encourage you to begin thinking about your transition, either into nursing school or into practice, and to guide you through the book in a practical, participative manner. Our intention is to add a little humor here and there while giving information on topics we feel will affect your transition. We want you to be informed about the controversial issues affecting nursing today. After all, the future of nursing rests with **you!**

Are you ready to begin? Then let's start with the real stuff. You are beginning to experience transitions—for some of you, just getting into nursing school has been a long struggle—and you are there! For others, you can see the light at the end of the tunnel, as graduation becomes a reality. Nursing is one of the most rewarding professions you can pursue. However, it can also be one of the most frustrating. As with marriage, raising children, and the pursuit of happiness, there are ups and downs. We seldom find the world or our specific situation the exact way we thought it would or should be. Often your fantasy of what nursing *should* be is not what you will find nursing to be.

> You will cry, but you will also laugh.
> You will share with people their darkest hours of pain and suffering, but
> You will also share with them their hope, healing, and recovery.
> You will be there as life begins and ends.
> You will experience great challenges that lead to success.
> You will experience failure and disappointment.
> You will never cease to be amazed at the resilience of the human body and spirit.

TRANSITIONS

What Are Transitions?

Transitions are passages or changes from one situation, condition, or state to another that occur over time. They have been classified into the following four major types: developmental (e.g., becoming a parent, midlife crisis), situational (e.g., graduating from a nursing program, career change, divorce), health/illness (e.g., dealing with a chronic illness), and organizational (e.g., change in leadership, new staffing patterns) (Schumacher and Meleis, 1994).

> Transitions are complex processes, and a lot of transitions occur at the same time.

What Are Important Factors Influencing Transitions?

Understanding the transition experience from the perspective of the person who is experiencing it is important because the meaning of the experience may be positive, negative, or neutral and the expectation may or may not be realistic. The transition may be desired (e.g., passing the NCLEX Exam) or undesirable (e.g., the death of a family member, after which you have to assume a new role in your family).

> Often, when you know what to expect, the stress associated with the change or transition is reduced.

Another factor in the transition process is the new level of knowledge and skill required, as well as the availability of needed resources within the environment. Dealing with new knowledge and skills can be challenging and stressful, and can lead to a variety of different emotions (Box 1-1). This will resolve as your confidence grows and you have more understanding of the concept of how to "think like a nurse."

Transitions are a part of life and certainly a part of nursing. Although the following discussions on role transition and reality shock focus on the graduate nurse experience, there are many applicable points for the new student as well. As you learn more about transitions, reality shock, and the graduate nurse experience, think about how this information may also apply to your transition experience into and through nursing school (Critical Thinking Box 1-1).

Looking back, what transitions have you experienced? What transitions are occurring in your life now? Has your entry into, as well as progress through, nursing school caused transitions in your personal life? Has your anticipated job search caused transitions in your professional as well as personal life?

BOX 1-1	Stresses Reported by New Graduates*

1. Not feeling confident and competent
2. Making mistakes because of increased workload and responsibilities
3. Encountering new situations, surroundings, and procedures
4. Inconsistent preceptors
5. Getting to know the staff
6. Encounters with unhappy nurses and other personnel
7. Short staffing
8. Staff nurses who were unwilling to help

From Oermann MH, Garvin MF: Stresses and challenges for new graduates in hospitals, *Nurse Educ Today* 22:225, 2002.
* Listed in order of frequency.

CRITICAL THINKING BOX 1-1

What is your greatest concern about your transition? Is it personal or work transitions because you are a student nurse, or is it your transition from school to practice?

Transitions in Nursing

The paradox of nursing will become obvious to you early in your nursing career. This realization may occur during nursing school, but it frequently becomes most obvious during the first 6 months of your first job.

Health care organizations are very concerned about your transition experience and job satisfaction during that first 6 months of employment. Have you been hearing about "evidence-based practice?" Well, it is working for you now! During the first 6 months of employment, new graduates need a period of time to develop their skills in a supportive environment. Employee retention and job satisfaction are key issues with the hospital; confidence in performing skills and procedures, peer and preceptor relationships, and dependence versus independence are key graduate nurse issues driving this research. The well-being of the graduate nurse and the ability to deliver quality nursing care during the transition period has sparked research to validate the need for special considerations of the graduate nurse experiencing transition (Casey et al, 2004; Godinez et al, 1999; Lavoie-Tremblay et al, 2002; Steinmiller et al, 2003). With identification of the basic problems encountered by new graduates during this first 6 months, there is a concerted effort to begin to meet the special needs of the graduate nurse (Evidence-Based Practice Box 1-1).

The role-transition process that occurs on entry into nursing school and the process from student to graduate nurse do not take place automatically. Having the optimal experience during role transition requires a great deal of attention, planning, and determination on your part. How you perceive and handle the transition will determine how well you progress through the process. It is important that you keep a positive attitude. The challenges and rewards of clinicals, tests, and work situations will cause your emotions to go up and down, but that is okay. It is expected, and you will be able to deal with it effectively. It is important that you keep a positive attitude. The wide range of emotions experienced during the transition process can often affect your *emotional and physical well-being;* check out the discussion of self-care strategies in Chapter 2.

So, let's get started. Reality shock is often one of the first hurdles of transition to conquer in your new role as a graduate nurse or registered nurse (RN or Real Nurse ☺).

REALITY SHOCK

What Is Reality Shock?

Reality shock is a term often used to describe the reaction experienced when one moves into the work force after several years of educational preparation. The recent graduate is caught in the situation of moving from a familiar, comfortable educational environment into a new role in the work force in which the expectations are not clearly defined or may not even be realistic. For example, as a student you were taught to consider the patient in a holistic framework, but in practice you often do not have the time to consider the psychosocial or teaching needs of the patient, even though they must be attended to and documented.

The recent graduate in the workplace is expected to be a capable, competent nurse. That sounds fine. However, sometimes there is a hidden expectation that graduate nurses should function as though they have 5 years of nursing experience. Time management skills, along with the increasing acuity level of patients, are common problems for the new graduate. This situation may leave you with feelings of powerlessness, depression, and insecurity because of an apparent

BOX 1-1   EVIDENCE-BASED PRACTICE

Role Transition: Think Like a Nurse

PRACTICE ISSUE

Students report that when they first entered their nursing courses they were unaware of the complexity of thinking and problem solving that occurs in the clinical setting. They often are unable to "think on their feet" and change a planned way of doing something based on what is happening with a specific patient at any given moment. Research supports the finding that the beginning nursing graduate continues to have difficulty making clinical judgments (i.e., thinking like a nurse). Graduates with baccalaureate degrees in nursing were interviewed three times in 9 months to determine their perceptions of how they learned to think like nurses.

IMPLICATIONS FOR NURSING PRACTICE

Clinical Judgments—Thinking Like a Nurse

- Nursing students and new graduates are often unaware of the level of responsibility required of nurses and lack confidence in their ability to make clinical judgments.
- The process of learning to think like a nurse is characterized by building confidence, accepting responsibility, adapting to changing relations with others, and thinking more critically.
- Multiple clinical experiences, support from faculty and experienced nurses, and sharing experiences with peers were critical in the transition from student nurse to beginning practitioner.
- Nursing education must assist nursing students to engage with patients and act on a responsible vision for excellent care of those patients and with a deep concern for the patients' and families' well-being. Clinical reasoning must arise from this engaged, concerned stance.

Considering This Information:

What characteristics have you observed in staff members who effectively "think like a nurse?" How can you begin to incorporate these aspects into your practice?

Reference for the Evidence

Etheridge SA: Learning to think like a nurse: stories from new nurse graduates, *J Contin Educ Nurs* 38(1):24-30, 2007.
Tanner CA: Thinking like a nurse: a research-based model of clinical judgment in nursing, *J Nurs Educ* 45(6), 2006. Retrieved from *www.ahn.mnsu.edu/nursing/facultyformsandinfo/thinkinglikeanurse.pdf.*

lack of effectiveness in the work environment. There are positive ways to deal with the problems. You are not alone! Reality shock is not unique to nursing. It is present in many professions as graduates move from the world of academia to the world of work and begin to adjust to the expectations and values of the work force.

What Are the Phases of Reality Shock?

Kramer (1974) described the phases of reality shock as they apply to nursing (Table 1-1).

Although she identified this process in 1974, these phases remain the basis for understanding the implications of reality shock and successfully progressing through the process. In our current world of nursing, we are still dealing with this same process. Adjustments begin to take place as the graduate nurse adapts to the reality of the practice of nursing. The first phase of adjustment is the honeymoon phase (Figure 1-1). The recent graduate is thrilled with completing school and accepting a first job. Life is a "bed of roses" because everyone knows nursing school is much

TABLE 1-1   Phases of Reality Shock

HONEYMOON	SHOCK AND REJECTION	RECOVERY
Sees the world of nursing looking quite rosy	Has excessive mistrust	Beginning to have sense of humor (first sign)
Often fascinated with the thrill of "arriving" in the profession	Experiences increased concern over minor pains and illness	Decrease in tension
	Experiences decrease in energy and feels excessive fatigue	Increase in ability to be objective
	Feels like a failure and blames self for every mistake	
	Bands together and depends on people who hold the same values	
	Has a hypercritical attitude	
	Feels moral outrage	

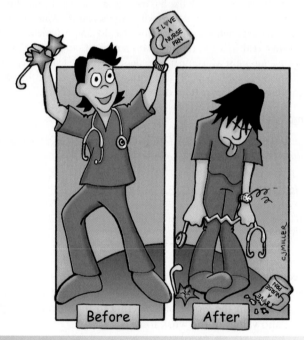

FIGURE 1-1

Reality shock. The honeymoon's over.

harder than nursing practice. There are no more concept care maps to create, no more nursing care plans to write, and no more burning the midnight oil for the next day's examination. No one is watching over your shoulder while you insert a catheter or administer an intravenous medication. You are not a "student" anymore; now you are a nurse! During this exciting phase, your perception of the situation may feel unreal and distorted, and you may not be able to understand the overall picture.

HONEYMOON PHASE
I just can't believe how wonderful everything is! Imagine getting a paycheck—money, at last! It's all great. Really, it is.

The honeymoon phase is frequently short-lived as the graduate begins to identify the conflicts between the way she or he was taught and the reality of what is done. Every graduate nurse will have a unique way of coping with the situations; however, some common responses have been identified. The graduate may cope with this conflict by withdrawing or rejecting the values learned during nursing school. This may mark the end of the honeymoon phase of transition. The phrase "going native" was used by Kramer and Schmalenberg (1977) to describe recent graduates as they begin to cope and identify with the reality of the situation by rejecting the values from nursing school and beginning to function as everyone else does.

SHOCK AND REJECTION PHASE
Mary was assigned 10 patients for the morning. There were numerous medications to be administered. It was difficult to carry all of the medication administration records to each room for patient identification. Because she "knew the patients" and because the other experienced nurses did not check identification, she decided she no longer needed to check a patient's identification before administering medication. Later in the day, she gave insulin to Mrs. James, a patient she "knew"; unfortunately, the insulin was for Mrs. Phillips, another patient she "knew."

With experiences such as this during transition, graduates may feel as though they have failed and begin to blame themselves for every mistake. They may also experience moral outrage at having been put in such a position. When the bad days begin to outnumber the good days, the graduate nurse may experience frustration, fatigue, and anger and may consequently develop a hypercritical attitude toward nursing. Some graduates become very disillusioned and drop out of nursing altogether. This is the period of shock and rejection.

I had just completed orientation in the hospital where I had wanted to work since I started nursing school. I immediately discovered that the care there was so bad that I did not want to be a part of it. At night, I went home very frustrated that the care I had given was not as I was taught to do it. I cried every night and hated to go to work in the morning. I did not like anyone with whom I was working. My stomach hurt, my head throbbed, and I had difficulty sleeping. It was hard not to work a double shift because I was worried about who would take care of those patients if I was not there.

A successfully managed transition period begins when the graduate nurse is able to evaluate the work situation objectively and predict the actions and reactions of the staff effectively. Prioritization, conflict management, time management, and support groups (peers, preceptors, and mentors) can make a significant difference in promoting a successfully managed transition period.

Nurturing the ability to see humor in a situation may be the first step. As the graduate begins to laugh at some of the situations encountered, the tension decreases and the perception increases. It is during this critical period of recovery that conflict resolution occurs. If this resolution occurs in a positive manner, it enables the graduate nurse to grow more fully as a person. This growth also enables the graduate to meet the work expectations to a greater degree and to see that she or he has the capacity to change a situation. If the conflict is resolved in a less-positive manner, however, the graduate's potential to learn and grow is limited.

Kramer (1974) described four groups of graduate nurses and the steps they took to resolve reality shock. The graduates who were considered to be most successful at adaptation were those who "made a lot of waves" within both their job setting and their professional organizations. Accordingly, they were not content with the present state of nursing but worked to effect a better system. This group of graduates was able to take worthwhile values learned during school and integrate them into the work setting. Often they returned to school—but not too quickly.

> RECOVERY PHASE
> I am really glad that I became a nurse. Sure, there are plenty of hassles, but the opportunities are there. Now that I am more confident of my skills, I am willing to take risks to improve patient care. Just last week my head nurse, who often says jokingly, "You're a thorn in my side," appointed me to the Nursing Standards Committee. I feel really good about this recognition.

Another group limited their involvement with nursing by just putting in the usual workday. Persons in this group seldom belonged to professional organizations and cited the following reasons for working: "to provide for my family," "to buy extra things for the house," and "to support myself." Typically, this group's negative approach to conflict resolution leads to burnout, during which time the conflict is turned inward, leading to constant griping and complaining about the work setting.

> I was so happy, at first. Gee, I was able to buy my son all those toys he wanted. But things here always seem to be the same—too many patients, not enough help. I get so upset with the staff, especially the nursing assistants, and the care that is given to patients. I wonder whether I will ever get the opportunity to practice nursing as I was taught. Well, I'll hang on until my husband finishes graduate school; then I'll quit this awful job!

Another group of graduates seemed to have found their niche and were content within the hospital setting. However, their positive attitude toward the job did not extend to nursing as a profession; in fact, it was the opposite. Rather than leave the organization during conflict, these "organization nurses" would change units or shifts—anything to avoid increasing demands for professional performance.

> During those first few months as I was just getting started, I sure had a tough time. It was difficult learning how to delegate tasks to the aides and practical nurses. But now that I have started working for Dr. Travis, everything is under my control. I just might go back to school someday.

The last group of graduates frequently changed jobs. After a short-lived career in hospital nursing, this group would pirouette off to graduate school, where they could "do something else in nursing" (meaning, "I can't nurse the way I've been taught, so I might as well teach others how to do things right"). Achieving a high profile in professional nursing organizations was common for these graduates, along with seeking a safer, more idealistically structured environment in which the values learned in school prevail.

> Finally, I got so frustrated with my head nurse that I just resigned. What did she expect from a recent graduate? I couldn't do everything! Cost containment; early discharge; no time for teaching; rush, rush, rush, all the time. Well, I've made up my mind to look into going back to school to further my career.

The job expectations of the hospital administration or the employing community agency and the educational preparation of the graduate nurse are not always the same. This discrepancy is considered to be the basis of reality shock. Relationships among the staff, nursing professionalism, job satisfaction, and employee alienation were studied by Roche and colleagues (2004), Casey and colleagues (2004), and Godinez and colleagues (1999). What is interesting is that the issues of reality shock and role transition described by Kramer in the early 1970s are still around. We (nurses) have entered the 21st century with many of the same issues we had in the 20th century. Much of this problem may be related to the fact that clinical instructors often focus on the needs of the patient rather than the needs of the student (Polifroni et al, 1995).

It might seem to you right now, after reading all of this information, that reality shock is a life-threatening situation. Be assured, it is not. You may, however, experience some physical and psychological symptoms in varying degrees of intensity. For example, you may feel stressed out or have headaches, insomnia, gastrointestinal upset, or a bout of post student blues. Just remember that it takes time to adjust to a new routine and that sometimes, even after you have gotten used to it, you still may feel overwhelmed, confused, or anxious. The good news is that there are various ways to get through this critical phase of your career while establishing a firm foundation for future professional growth and career mobility. Try the assessment exercise in Critical Thinking Box 1-2.

ROLE TRANSFORMATION

Remember when you first started nursing school? The war stories everybody told you? The changes that occurred in your family as a result of your starting nursing school? Are you in the midst of that now, or does it seem like a long time ago? Can you really believe where you are now and where you were when you first began nursing school, those first nursing courses, and

CRITICAL THINKING
BOX 1-2

REALITY SHOCK INVENTORY

All students, as well as new graduates, experience reality shock to some extent or another. The purpose of this exercise is to make you aware of how you feel about yourself and your particular life situation.

Directions: To evaluate your views and determine your self-evaluation of your particular life situation, respond to the statements with the appropriate number.

1 Strongly agree	4 Slightly disagree
2 Agree	5 Disagree
3 Slightly agree	6 Strongly disagree

1. I am still finding new challenges and interests in my work.
2. I think often about what I want from life.
3. My own personal future seems promising.
4. Nursing school and/or my work has brought stresses for which I was unprepared.
5. I would like the opportunity to start anew knowing what I know now.
6. I drink more than I should.
7. I often feel that I still belong in the place where I grew up.
8. Much of the time my mind is not as clear as it used to be.
9. I have no sense of regret concerning my major life decision of becoming a nurse.
10. My views on nursing are as positive as they ever were.
11. I have a strong sense of my own worth.
12. I am experiencing what would be called a crisis in my personal or work setting.
13. I cannot see myself as a nurse.
14. I must remain loyal to commitments even if they have not proven as rewarding as I had expected.
15. I wish I were different in many ways.
16. The way I present myself to the world is not the way I really am.
17. I often feel agitated or restless.
18. I have become more aware of my inadequacies and faults.
19. My sex life is as satisfactory as it has ever been.
20. I often think about students and/or friends who have dropped out of school or work.

To compute your score, reverse the number you assigned to statements 1, 3, 9, 10, 11, and 19. For example, 1 would become a 6, 2 would become a 5, 3 would become a 4, 4 would become a 3, 5 would become a 2, and 6 would become a 1. Total the number. The higher the score, the better your attitude. The range is 20 to 120.

Modified from White E: Doctoral dissertation, *Chronicle of Higher Education*, April 23, 1986, p 28. Reprinted with permission.

clinicals? It has taken a lot of work and sacrifice to get to where you are now. Believe it or not, you have already experienced a role transition—you successfully transitioned to a student nurse. Now, as you draw nearer to the successful completion of that experience, you are ready to embark on a new one. Take a minute to read the thoughts of one of your peers about her transition into nursing. I'm sure you will smile at her satire (Critical Thinking Box 1-3).

Give yourself a well-deserved pat on the back for what you have accomplished thus far. It is important to learn early in your practice of nursing to take time to reflect on your accomplishments. Now, back to the present. Let's look at the current role-transition process at hand, from student to graduate nurse RN (real nurse).

SURVIVAL TECHNIQUES FROM ONE WHO HAS SURVIVED

You finally did it; you have decided nursing is what you want to do for the rest of your life. After all, who would go through all this anguish if you only wanted to do this as a pastime? If you are taking this like everyone else, you are probably going to do this by trial and error, "war" stories, or by helpful hints from the nursing staff.

You need to prioritize your time. This is a familiar and much used term that you will hear often. It is also easier said than done. If you are single, you have an advantage—maybe. You can decide right now that single is "where it's at" and stay that way for the duration. Of course this means literally living the "single" life. There are no "dinners-for-two," no telephone conversations, no movies at the cinema (rarely any TV)—in other words, no physical contact with the opposite sex. I know you were not thinking about it anyway, but in case you are studying anatomy and physiology, and hormonal thoughts pervade your consciousness, dismiss them.

If you are married, I am not suggesting divorce, just abstinence. Hopefully, you kissed your spouse good-bye when you came to school for your first day of class because your next chance will be on your breaks or when you graduate.

If you happen to be a parent, do as I did. I put pictures of myself in all rooms of my house when I started to school so that kids would not forget me. My children, in return, helped me by plastering their faces in my fridge (they know I'll look there) or on my mirror (another sure spot). I have acquired a son-in-law, a daughter-in-law, and five grandchildren in the past 2½ years, and I usually do not recognize them if I run into them on the rare occasions when I go to the store for essentials (like food) or out to pay our utility bills. Christmas is fun, though, because each year I get to spend a few days getting to know the family again. But we all must wear name tags for the first day!

If your children are small, buy them the Fisher Price Kitchen and teach them how to "cook" nourishing "hot" cereal on the stove that does not heat up. For the infant, hang a TPN (hint: Total Parental Nutrition) of Similac with iron at 40 mL/hr that the baby can control by sound! Crying should do it! Instead of a needle, use a nipple …

Diapers—what would we do without those disposable diapers that stay dry for 2 weeks at a time? You can even buy the kind that you touch the waistband, and Mickey Mouse and his friends jump off to entertain your baby.

Some of you may feel guilty about not fixing those delicious meals your family once enjoyed. Do not! We get two "breaks" a year, and during that time, fix barrels of nourishing liquid (you can add a few veggies). When your family gets hungry, just take out enough to keep fluids and lytes balanced. Remind them that this is only going to last another year or two.

Have I covered everything? Oh I forgot dust. … Dust used to bother me, but not anymore. I use it to write notes to my 17-year-old, to let him know what time I am going to be in the house, so he will not mistake me for a burglar, and to say "I Love You."

On a serious note, each semester you will get regrouped with new classmates. They will become your family, your support group. You will form a chain, and everyone is a strong link. This is a group effort. These are people who will laugh with you and cry with you. You will form friendships that will last a lifetime. Take advantage of these opportunities.

On a closing note, do not listen to all the "war stories" that go around—just to the credible ones like mine!

From Beagle B: Survival techniques, *AD Clinical Care*, May/June, 1990, p 17. Reprinted with permission.

When Does the Role Transition to Graduate Nurse Begin?

Does the transition begin at graduation? No. It started when you began to move into the novice role while in your first nursing course (Table 1-2). According to Benner (1984, p 20):

> Beginners have no experience of the situation in which they are expected to perform. To get them into these situations and allow them to gain experience also necessary for skill development, they are taught about the situation in terms of objective attributes, such as weight, intake/output, temperature, blood pressure, pulse, and other objective, measurable parameters of a patient's conditions—features of the task world that can be recognized without situational experience.

TABLE 1-2 From Novice to Expert

STAGE	CHARACTERISTICS
NOVICE Nursing student Experienced nurse in a new setting	• No clinical experience in situation expected to perform • Needs rules to guide performance • Experiences difficulty in applying theoretical concepts to patient care
ADVANCED BEGINNER Last-semester nursing student Graduate nurse	• Demonstrates ability to deliver marginally acceptable care • Requires previous experience in an actual situation to recognize it • Begins to understand the principles that dictate nursing interventions • Continues to concentrate on the rules and takes in minimum information regarding a situation
COMPETENT 2-3 years' clinical experience	• Conscientious, deliberate planning • Begins to see nursing actions in light of patients' long-term plans • Demonstrates ability to cope with and manage different and unexpected situations that occur
PROFICIENT Nurse clinicians Nursing faculty	• Ability to recognize and understand the situation as a whole • Demonstrates ability to anticipate events in a given situation • Holistic understanding enhances decision making
EXPERT Advanced practice nurse clinicians and faculty	• Demonstrates an understanding of the situation and is able to focus on the specific area of the problem • Operates from an in-depth understanding of the total situation • Demonstrates highly skilled analytical ability in problem solving; performance becomes masterful

Modified from Brenner P: The Dreyfus Model of Skill Acquisition Applied to Nursing. In *From Novice to Expert, Commemorative Edition*, Menlo Park, CA, 2001, Addison-Wesley.

For example, the instructor gives the novice or student nurse specific directions on how to listen for bowel sounds. There are specific rules on how to guide their actions—rules that are very limited and fairly inflexible. Remember your first clinical nursing experiences? Your nursing instructor was your shadow for patient care. As nursing students enter a clinical area as novices, they have little understanding of the meaning and application of recently learned textbook terms and concepts. Students are not the only novices; any nurse may assume the novice role on entering a clinical setting in which he or she is not comfortable functioning or has no practical experience. Consider an experienced medical-surgical nurse who floats to the postpartum unit; she would be a little uncomfortable in that clinical setting.

By graduation, most nursing students are at the level of advanced beginner. According to Benner (1984, p 22):

Advanced beginners are ones who can demonstrate marginally accepted performance, ones who have coped with enough real situations to note (or to have pointed out to them by a mentor) the recurring meaningful situation components ...

To be able to recognize characteristics that can be identified only through experience is the signifying trait of the advanced beginner. Thus, when directed to perform the procedure of checking bowel sounds, the students at this level are learning how to discriminate bowel sounds and understand their meaning. They do not need to be told specifically how to perform the procedure.

Let's look at what you and your nursing instructors can do to promote your well-being and success during the role-transition experience. These activities reinforce your progress and movement along the continuum from advanced-beginner to competent nurse (see Table 1-2).

How Can I Prepare Myself for This Transition Process?

During the last semester of nursing school, it is very advantageous to have as much clinical experience as possible (Evidence-Based Practice Box 1-2). The most productive area for experience is a general medical-surgical unit. This will help you ground your assessment and communication skills, as well as help you to apply principles that are most often tested on the NCLEX Exam. This is also the area in which you will most likely be able to obtain some much needed experience with basic nursing skills.

No More "Mama Management." It is time to have your nursing instructor cut the umbilical cord and allow you to function more independently during the last semester of clinical experience.

More Realistic Patient-Care Assignments. Start taking care of increasing numbers of patients to help you with time management and work organization. Evaluate the nursing staff's assignments to determine what a realistic workload is for a recent graduate.

Clinical Hours That Represent Realistic Shift Hours. Obtain experience in receiving shift reports, closing charts, completing patient care, and communicating with the oncoming staff. As a recent graduate, you will be in for a rude awakening if you have never had the opportunity to work a full shift.

Perform Nursing Procedures Instead of Observing. Take an inventory of your nursing skills and be sure to have this available for potential employers, so they can see what skills you are familiar with. If there are nursing skills you lack or procedures you are uncomfortable with,

BOX 1-2 EVIDENCE-BASED PRACTICE

Role Transition

PRACTICE ISSUE

With the increased complexity of the health care environment, new graduates struggle with the transition into clinical practice. This matter is related to several issues: the shortened gap between taking NCLEX and being licensed, variable transition experiences, increased patient workload due to the nursing shortage, high job stress and turnover rates in new graduate RNs, and practice errors.

IMPLICATIONS FOR NURSING PRACTICE

- Transition experiences of new RNs vary across practice settings.
- New graduate RNs are more competent in patient care and less competent in clinical reasoning and recognizing limits and seeking help.
- During the first 3 months of practice, new RNs who had a primary preceptor practiced at higher competent levels.
- Without the assistance of preceptors, new RNs practiced at less competent levels during the 3 to 6 months of their initial phase of independent practice.
- New RNs with preparation for specialty practice in transition programs made fewer errors.
- Less competent and/or stressed new RNs made more practice errors.
- New RNs who had an internship experience were less likely to leave their current position within the next 6 months.

Considering This Information:

What can you do to ease your transition process?

References for the Evidence

Li S (2007): *The impact of transition experience on practice of newly licensed registered nurses*, Chicago. National Council State Boards of Nursing. Retrieved from *www.ncsbn.org/363.htm*.

NCSBN (2009): *Transition evidence grid*. Retrieved from *www.ncsbn.org/Evidence_Grid_2009.pdf*.

Rider L: Transition to professional practice in baccalaureate nursing: a multiple case study approach using the middle range theory of transition, 2009. Retrieved from ProQuest Dissertations & Theses.

take this opportunity while you are still in school to gain the experience. Identify your clinical objectives to meet your personal needs. Request opportunities to practice from your instructor and staff nurses. Casey and colleagues (2004) identified skills that were challenging for the graduate nurses in the first year of practice. These skills included code blues, chest tubes, intravenous skills, central lines, blood administration, and patient-controlled analgesia (PCA). Make an effort to gain experience in these areas while you are still in school; you will be more comfortable in your nursing care as a graduate.

More Truth About the Real Work-Setting Experience. Identify resource people with whom you can objectively discuss the dilemmas of the workplace. Talk to graduates: Ask them what they know now that they wish they had known the last semester of school.

Look for Opportunities to Problem-Solve and Practice Critical Thinking. No more "spoon feeding" from instructors who tell you what to do and how to do it. Now is the time to stand on your own two feet while there is still a backup—your instructor—available.

Request Constructive Feedback from Staff and Instructors. Stop avoiding evaluation and constructive criticism. Find out now how you can improve your nursing care. Evaluate your progress on a periodic basis. The consequences may be less severe now than later with your new employer.

Request Clinical Experience in an Area or Hospital of Interest. If you have some idea of where you would like to work, it is very beneficial to have some clinical experiences in that facility the last semester of school. This gives you the opportunity to become involved with staff nurses, identify workload on the unit, and evaluate resources and support people. It also gives the employing institution an opportunity to evaluate you—Are you someone that institution would like to have work for them?

> Attitude is the latitude between success and failure.

Think Positively! Be prepared for the reality of the workplace environment, including both its positives and negatives. You may have encountered by now the "ole' battle ax" who has a grudge against new nursing graduates.

> I do not know why you ever decided to be a nurse. Nobody respects you. It's all work, low pay. I guess as long as you've got a good back and strong legs, you'll make it. Boy, do you have a lot to learn! I wouldn't do it over again for anything!

When you find these nurses, tune them out and steer out of their way! They have their own agenda, and it does not include providing supportive assistance to you. Eventually, you will learn how to work with this type of individual (see Chapter 12), but for now, you should concentrate on identifying nurses who share your philosophy and are still smiling.

> Surround yourself with nurses who have a positive attitude and are supportive in your learning and growing transition.

Another way to keep a positive perspective is to focus on the good things that have happened during the shift rather than on the frustrating events. When you feel yourself climbing onto the proverbial "pity pot," ask yourself "Who's driving this bus?" and turn it around!

Anticipate small irritations and disappointments and keep them in perspective. Do not let them mushroom into major problems. Turn disappointments and unpleasant situations into learning experiences. Once you have encountered an unpleasant situation, the next time it occurs you will recognize it sooner, anticipate the chain of events, and be better able to handle it.

> Do not major in a minor activity.

Be Flexible! Procedures, policies, and nursing supervisors are not going to be the same as those you experienced in school. Be prepared to do things differently than you learned as a student. You do not have to give up all the values you learned in school, but you will need to reexamine them in light of the reality of the workplace setting.

School-Learned Ideal. Sit down with the patient before surgery, and provide preoperative teaching.

Workplace Reality. One of your home care patients is receiving daily wound care for an extensive burn. You receive a pager message that the patient has been scheduled for grafting in the outpatient surgery department and is to be a direct admit at 6 AM the next morning. You have two more home visits to make: one to hang an intravenous preparation of vancomycin and the other a new hospice admission, which you know will take considerable time.

Compromise. You delegate to one of the home care practical nurses to take the preoperative teaching and admission instructions to your patient. Later on, you make a telephone call to your preoperative patient and go over the preoperative care teaching information from the home care practical nurse. You make arrangements to meet this patient at home immediately after the grafting procedure is complete.

Get Organized! Does your personal life seem organized or chaotic, calm or frantic? Sit back and take a quick inventory of your personal life. How do you expect to get your professional life in order when your personal life is in turmoil? For some helpful tips on organizing your personal life, check out the personal management chapter (see Chapter 2).

Stay Healthy! Have you become a "couch potato" while in school? Are you too tired, or do you lack the time to exercise when you get home from work? Candy bars during breaks, pepperoni pizza at midnight, and Twinkies PRN? How have your eating habits changed during your time in school? Your routine should include exercise, relaxation, and good nutrition. Becoming aware of the negative habits that can have detrimental effects on your state of mind and overall physical health is important in developing a healthy lifestyle.

Find a Mentor! Negotiating this critical transition as you begin your nursing career should not be done in isolation. Evidence suggests that close support relationships, mentors, and preceptors are key, if not essential, ingredients in the career development of a successful, happy graduate (Casey et al, 2004; Roche et al, 2004). In addition to your family and close nursing school friends, it will be important to develop professional support relationships.

Find Other New Graduates! Frequently, several new graduates are hired at the same time. Some of them may even be your classmates. Find them and establish a peer support group. Sharing experiences and problems and knowing that someone else is experiencing the same feelings you are can be a great relief!

Have Some Fun! Do something that makes you feel good. This is life, not a funeral service! Nursing has opportunities for laughter and for sharing life's humorous events with patients and coworkers. Surround yourself with people and friends who are lighthearted and merry and who bring those feelings out in you. Remember, the return of humor is one of the first signs of a healthy role transition. Loosen up a little bit. Go ahead, have some fun! Check out the information in Chapter 3 for more on selection of mentors and preceptors.

Know What to Expect! Plan ahead. Plan your employment interviews; ask to talk to nurses on the units and find out how nursing care is delivered in the institution. The length of orientation, staffing patterns, opportunity for internship, areas where positions are open, and resources for new graduates are all important to establish prior to employment. This helps you know what to expect when you go to work. Work satisfaction is a positive predictor of a successful role transition during the first year (Roche, 2004). Know what is expected of you on your work unit. How can you expect to do a job correctly if you do not know what the expectations are? Learn the "rules of the road" early. This may be in the hospital, doctor's office, or community setting. While still in school, you may find it helpful to interview nurse managers to determine their perspectives on the role of the graduate nurse during her first 6 months of employment. This will give you a base of reference when you interview for your first job. How do you measure up to some of the common expectations nurse managers may be looking for in a graduate nurse?

Are you:
- Excited and sincere about nursing?
- Open-minded and willing to learn new ideas and skills?
- Comfortable with your basic nursing skills?
- Able to keep a good sense of humor?
- Receptive to constructive criticism?
- Able to express your thoughts and feelings?
- Able to evaluate your performance and request assistance?
- Comfortable talking with your patients regarding their individual needs?

What Is the Future of Role Transition? At the August 2008 annual meeting of the National Council of State Boards of Nursing (NCSBN), the Practice and Education Committee reported "there was adequate evidence to support a regulatory model for transitioning new graduates to practice" (NCSBN, 2008a, p 259). The committee noted that the need for a transition regulatory model has grown from the changes occurring in health care over the past 20 years, not from deficiencies in nursing education and/or unrealistic expectations of the workplace. In the report from the committee to the NCSBN, the goal for the transition to practice regulatory model is "to promote public safety by supporting newly licensed nurses in their critical entry and progression into practice" (NCSBN, 2008b, p 262). In 2009, the NCSBN finalized the design of an evidence-based "transition to practice" regulatory model (Figure 1-2) that includes modules on communication and teamwork, patient-centered care, evidence-based practice, quality improvement, and informatics. Because of individual state's rights, the NCSBN encourages states to adopt this model; however, they do not have the authority to mandate adoption of the model. What is happening in your state regarding the transition to practice model?

The transition to practice model recommends a 6-month internship followed by 6 months of continued support. In order for the transition process to be effective, it should occur across all settings and at all education levels. This would include both the RN and the LPN/LVN. To promote safer nursing practice through a regulatory transition period, practice, education and regulation, all must work together on the development of a model that will effectively support the new nurse in his or her transition to safe practice (NCSBN, 2009a).

CONCLUSION

What will be the direction for role transition of graduate nurses? Will your state adopt the "transition to practice" regulatory model? How will preceptors be selected and will they be credentialed? As you progress through the chapters in this book, you will find references to the Institute of Medicine (IOM), The Joint Commission (TJC), and other health care resources concerned with the safety of patients, the reduction of errors, and the economic impact of errors, retention

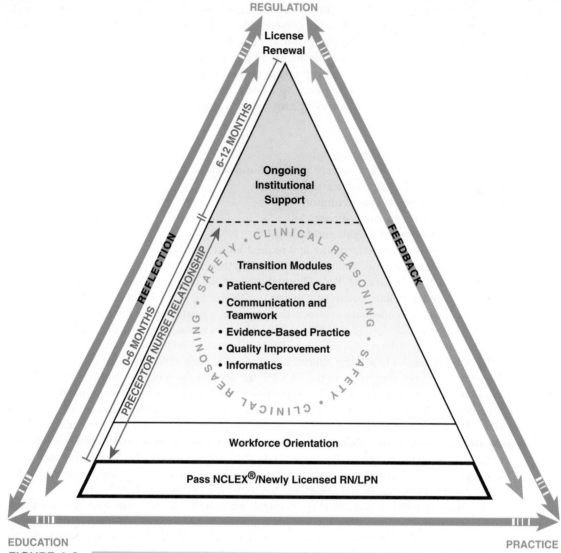

FIGURE 1-2

Transition to Practice Model.

of nurses, and cost of health care. These are key players and important considerations in the new nurse's transition to safe nursing practice.

As you progress through your own personal transition into nursing practice, the "rules of the road" for transition can be likened to traffic signs (Figure 1-3). Check out the following signs that will help you to direct your transition experience. Figure 1-4 gives additional advice from graduates who have successfully made the transition.

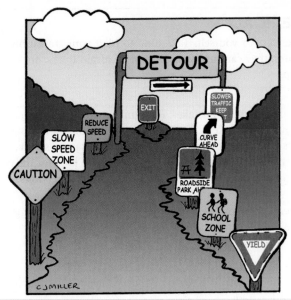

FIGURE 1-3

"Rules of the road" for transition.

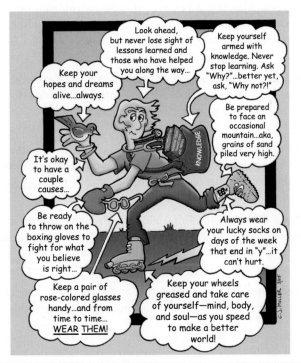

FIGURE 1-4

Advice for the new grad.

RULES OF THE ROAD

 Stop. Take care of yourself. Take time to plan your transition. Get involved with other recent graduates; they can help you. Do not be afraid to ask questions, and do not be afraid to ask for help.

 Detour. You will make mistakes. Recognize them, learn from them, and put them in the past as you move forward. Regardless of how well you plan for change, there are always detours ahead. Detours take you on an alternate route. They can be scenic, swampy, or desolate, or they can bog you down in heavy traffic. Do not forget to look for the positive aspects—the detour may open your eyes to new horizons and new career directions.

 Curve Ahead. Get your personal life in order. Anticipate changes in your schedule. Be adaptable, because the transition process is not predictable.

 Yield. You do not always have to be right. Consider alternatives and make compromises within your value system.

 Resume Speed. Maintain a positive attitude. As you gain experience, you will become better organized and begin to really enjoy nursing. Be aware; sometimes as you resume speed, you may be experiencing another role transition as your career moves in a different direction.

 Exit. Pay attention to your road signs; do not take an exit you do not really want. Before you exit your job, critically evaluate the job situation. "Look before you leap" by making sure the change will improve your work situation.

 Slow Traffic, Keep Right. You may be more comfortable in the slower traffic lane with respect to your career direction. Take all the time you need; it is okay for each person to travel at a different speed. Do not get run over in the fast lane.

 School Zone. Plan for continuing education, whether it is an advanced degree program or one to maintain your clinical skills or license. Allow yourself sufficient time in your new job before you jump back into the role of full-time student.

 Slow Speed Zone. Take time to get organized before you resume full speed! Have a daily organizational sheet that fits your needs and works for you both in your job and your personal life.

Caution. Do not commit to anything with which you are not professionally or personally comfortable. Think before you act. Do not react. Do not panic. If in doubt, check with another nurse.

Roadside Park Ahead. Take a break, whether it is 15 minutes or 30 minutes a day to indulge yourself—or a week to do something you really want to do.

Look for the humor in each day and take time to laugh. You will be surprised by how good it makes you feel!

BIBLIOGRAPHY

Benner P: *From novice to expert*, Menlo Park, Calif, 1984, Addison-Wesley; Commemorative edition, Upper Saddle River, NJ, 2001, Prentice-Hall.

Casey K et al: The graduate nurse experience, *JONA* 34(6):303-311, 2004.

Godinez G et al: Role transition from graduate to staff nurse: a qualitative analysis, *J Nurse Staff Dev* 15:97-110, 1999.

Kramer M: *Reality shock*, St. Louis, 1974, Mosby.

Kramer M, Schmalenberg C: *Path to biculturalism*, Rockville, Md, 1977, Aspen.

Lavoie-Tremblay M et al: How to facilitate the orientation of new nurses into the workplace, *J Nurse Staff Dev* 18(2):80-85, 2002.

National Council of State Boards of Nursing (NCSBN) (2008a): *2008 business book. Report from Transitions to Practice Committee,* pp 259-295. Annual meeting, Nashville, Tenn, 2008. Retrieved from *www.ncsbn.org/2008_BusinessBook_Section2.pdf.*

NCSBN (2008b): *NCSBN transition to practice report.* Retrieved from *www.ncsbn.org/388.htm.*

NCSBN (2008c): *Transition to practice: promoting public safety: the fact sheet.* Retrieved from *www.ncsbn.org/Transition_factsheet_final.pdf.*

NCSBN (2009a): *Goals of NCSBN's transition to practice model.* Retrieved from *www.ncsbn.org/TransitiontoPractice_goals_042409.pdf.*

NCSBN (2009b): *NCSBN's transition to practice model: frequently asked questions.* Retrieved from *www.ncsbn.org/TransitiontoPractice_whitepaper_FAQs.pdf.*

NCSBN (2009c): *Transition evidence grid.* Retrieved from *www.ncsbn.org/Evidence_Grid_2009.pdf.*

Polifroni C et al: Activities and interaction of baccalaureate nursing students in clinical practice, *J Prof Nurs* 11:161-169, 1995.

Roche J, Lamoureux E, Teehan T: A partnership between nursing education and practice, *JONA* 34(1):26-32, 2004.

Schumacher KL, Meleis AI: Transitions: a central concept in nursing, *Image* 26:119-127, 1994.

Spector N (2008): *Toward an evidence-based regulatory model for transitioning new nurses to practice.* Retrieved from *www.ncsbn.org/Pages_from_Leader-to-Leader_FALL08.pdf.*

Steinmiller E, Levonian C, Lengetti E: Rx for success, *Am J Nurs* 103(11):64A-66A, 2003.

Additional resources are available online at *http://evolve.elsevier.com/Zerwekh/nsgtoday/.*

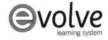

CHAPTER 2

Personal Management: Time and Self-Care Strategies

Sharon Decker, PhD, RN, ACNS-BC, ANEF

> *Gain control of your time, and you will gain control of your life.*
> —ANONYMOUS

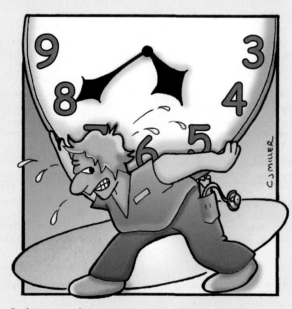

Is time managing you, or are you managing time?

After completing this chapter, you should be able to:

- Identify your individual time style and personal time-management strategies.

- Discuss strategies that increase organizational skills and personal priority setting.

- Describe early signs of burnout and how it affects nurses.

- Discuss the importance of caring for yourself.

- Identify strategies for self-care.

*T*here are so many activities that individuals need to accomplish at any one time that deciding "how to get it all done" and "what to do when" is a daily challenge—one that can sometimes be overwhelming. Nursing school complicates the daily routine. This relentless competition for our attention is described by the term *timelock* (Keyes, 1991).

MANAGING YOUR TIME

Regrettably, there is no way to alter the minutes in an hour or the hours in a day. Although we cannot create more actual time, we can alter how we use the time we have available.

Lack of organizational and time-management skills have been identified by employers of new graduates as areas in which the new nurse frequently needs the most improvement and assistance. The methods and strategies identified by time-management experts can help you cope with timelock.

This section introduces you to the principles of effective time management. You will learn how to gain control of your time, increase your organizational skills, and reduce time waste. Also, you will learn strategies for using those newly acquired hours to achieve your personal and professional goals.

Balance Is the Key

Making time to meet your individual, family, and professional needs and goals is vital to your overall success. If you neglect your health maintenance needs, completing school may be jeopardized. Integrating the principles of time management into your daily life can help you achieve both your personal and professional goals.

What Are Your Biological Rhythms, and How Do You Use Them?

Individuals have different biorhythms that affect their energy levels during the day and can even vary from season to season. Rest and sleep are essential for optimal health and emotional and physical responsiveness.

> Whenever possible, schedule difficult activities at your high-energy times.

When possible, get 8 solid hours of sleep. Maintaining a regular sleep-wake rhythm (circadian rhythm) with adequate hours of sleep has both physiological and psychological restorative effects. Disruption of this rhythm causes chronic fatigue and decreases one's coping abilities and performance. Factors affecting rest and sleep include anxiety, work schedules, diet, and the use of alcohol and nicotine.

Fatigue, which can lead to impaired decision making, can occur with changes in the circadian rhythm and sleep deprivation. Physiological, psychological, and emotional problems have also been correlated to sleep deprivation; these include ischemic disease, increased peptic ulcers, indigestion, increased susceptibility to viral and bacterial infections, weight gain, sleep disturbances, and mood disorders. Therefore, if situations occur that interfere with your normal circadian rhythm, it is important to take measures to prevent these possible complications. Self-care tips to prevent complications caused by interferences in the normal circadian rhythm are presented in Box 2-1. Try these strategies, tossing out those that do not work for you.

> Engage in a relaxing activity 1 hour before going to bed; for example, take a warm bath, read an interesting novel, or learn to initiate progressive relaxation techniques.

BOX 2-1   Self-Care Tips for When Circadian Rhythms Are Disrupted

- Reserve the bedroom for sleeping.
- Avoid watching television or using the computer while in bed.
- Leave your stressors at the door and pamper yourself just before sleeping by reading; stretching; meditating; or taking a warm, scented bath.
- Establish and maintain a bedtime routine.
- Decrease noise or create "white noise" in the bedroom.
- Turn off the telephone.
- Sleep with earplugs.
- Use a bedroom fan.
- Darken and cool down your sleeping environment.
- Use eye shields.
- Maintain a diet high in protein and low in carbohydrates to support your immune system.

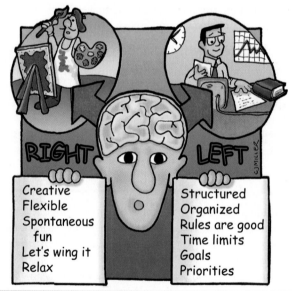

FIGURE 2-1

Are you right- or left-brain–dominant?

What Is Meant by Right- and Left-Brain Dominance, and Where Is My Brain?

People think about and manage time differently, depending on their characteristic brain dominance—left, right, or both (Figure 2-1).

Left-brain–dominant people process information and approach time in a linear, sequential manner. Their thinking structures time by minutes and hours. They tend to schedule activities in time segments and carry them out in an ordered sequence. Left-brain–dominant people like to know the rules and play by them. They are usually able to meet their goals, but if this behavior is carried to an extreme, the individual is in danger of overwork at the expense of creative, artistic, and relaxing activities.

Right-brain–dominant people resist rules and schedules. They prefer looking at a project as a whole and completing it in their own way and time. These are creative, flexible thinkers. However, if their behaviors are taken to an extreme, they can fail to meet needed completion times, which can induce guilt.

Some people are neither left-brain–dominant nor right-brain–dominant; hence they are more mixed in their behaviors. In fact, everyone uses both sides of the brain to some extent, thus tapping into the benefits of the brain's full capacities. The use of lists and calendars engages the left brain, whereas techniques such as the use of colored folders and whimsical office supplies help individuals to use right-brain holistic thinking to solve problems.

Which Are You?

(Check out The Brain-Dominance Questionnaire at *www.scs.sk.ca/cyber/present/brain.htm*.)
- I am left-brain–dominant.
- I am right-brain–dominant.
- I am left-brain–dominant and right-brain–dominant.

In addition to assessing your own dominant time style, it is helpful to be aware of the time styles of the people with whom you live and work. Heaping rigid rules on a right-brain–dominant person will lead to increased resistance and frustration for everyone. Better to assign them clean-up of the kitchen or utility room to be completed by a specific time and inform them of the consequences of it not being done. It would be appropriate to have some right-brain–dominant persons on the recruitment and retention committee and some left-brain–dominant persons on the policy and procedures committee.

Knowing your time style can help you maximize your strengths and modify your weaknesses. Individual time styles can be modified, but it is wasted energy to fight or work against natural inclination. Once you are aware of your time style, you can begin to create more time for what you want and need to do by increasing your organizational skills.

How Can I Manage My Physical Environment?

A place for everything and everything in its place.

Organizing and maintaining your physical environment at home, school, and work can dramatically reduce hours of time and the emotional frustration associated with "looking for stuff" (Figure 2-2).

At home, set up a specific work area for such things as school supplies, papers, and books. A separate area or corner should be established where you can pay bills, send letters, order take-out food, and take care of other household chores. When studying or working on major projects, find a space that provides a comfortable, but not too cozy area. This space should have adequate lighting and be as free from distractions as possible. If you are studying, break your time into 50-minute segments followed by 10-minute breaks. Prior to beginning each study session, gather the appropriate tools—textbooks, paper, pens, highlighters, laptop, smartphone or handheld device, and reference material—to avoid wasting time once you begin your work.

Start an ongoing list of "Things to Do." It feels so good to cross off the task as you complete it.

If you don't already have a file folder, then start one immediately. If you can't keep up with the magazine and journal articles or if you don't have time to put your notes together, then file them. Get to them when you can.

Post a large calendar on the refrigerator door. It is a great way to keep track of a busy family's schedule. Assign each person to write down his or her meetings, practices, and other activities in a different colored ink.

Keep a shopping list posted on your refrigerator. When you run out of something, write it down right away. Extra trips to the grocery store for forgotten items will be eliminated, and your cabinets will be kept fully stocked.

Don't spend a lot of time in card shops searching for birthday and anniversary cards. Keep a supply of attractive blank cards on hand for those last-minute greetings to be made, or buy a bunch of greeting cards and keep them in a letter holder with dividers indicating the month and day that cards should be mailed.

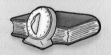

Set a food timer or alarm clock, and make time for yourself. Tell the children that this is your time to read, watch television, and relax.

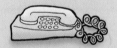

Neighborhood teenagers are often willing to run errands, mow lawns, wash cars, or clean house. Call on them.

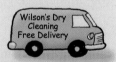

Check to see whether your cleaners, drug store, or grocer has free delivery, and then use it.

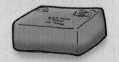

Do your shopping by mail, television, or telephone. Make use of the numerous catalogs that are around; get on a mailing list, and buy from your armchair or by watching Home Shopping on television or finding it on the Internet.

Learn to say "No." Remember that "No" is a complete sentence! It's so easy to get involved in too many activities. Set priorities, and do just one to two activities that please you, then say "No" to the rest.

FIGURE 2-2

Ten suggestions for organizing yourself.

Compartmentalize. Place pens, notebooks, your smartphone or handheld device, or other reference materials in a designated holder or in a specific compartment of your backpack for quick access.

Color-Code. Do this for your files, keys, and whatever you can. Office supply stores are good sources of color-coded items. For example, color-coding keys with a plastic cover enables you to immediately pick out your car key, house key, or locker key.

Convenience. Move and keep frequently used items nearest to where they are used.

Declutter the Clutter. At work, as well as at home, regularly clear your study and work areas.

What About All the Paperwork—How Can I Manage It? Handling each piece of paper only one time is a great time-saver. Whenever possible, spend 30 seconds filing an important paper in the appropriate folder. This technique can save you time when you need the information again. Following are five ways to deal with paper: Read each piece of paper then:

- File it.
- Forward it.
- Respond to it—on the same sheet if possible.
- Delegate it.
- Discard it.

What About Managing the Telephone?

Polite comments at the beginning and end of a telephone conversation are necessary to maintain positive interpersonal communications. However, when time limits are necessary, focus the conversation on the business at hand. Some possible phrases to move things along include "How can I help you?" or "I called to …" To end the conversation, summarize the actions to be followed through: "I understand. I am to find out about … and get back to you by the end of the week. Thanks for calling." Professional courtesy demands that you turn off your cellular phone while at work, in the classroom, during clinical rotation, and while attending a workshop.

Allocate a specific time during the day for business- or school-related telephone calls. Plan these calls by writing key points that need to be discussed during the conversation. If you need to leave a message, provide enough detail, with the time and date, and a time when the individual can contact you. When making a call: (1) introduce yourself and your business or relationship to the individual, (2) relax—speak as if the individual is sitting in the room beside you, (3) smile—smiling will modify the tone of your voice, (4) keep the conversation short and to the point, and (5) summarize the conversation, review any action items, and thank the individual for his or her time.

Having conversations to maintain friendships, to touch base with a relative, to relax yourself, to vent your emotions, or to serve similar social purposes can be combined with routine housekeeping duties. Who has not swept the floor, put away dishes, sorted mail, or cleaned out a drawer while chatting with a friend?

One time-management principle is, "Don't agonize. Organize!"

What About All That E-Mail?

Restrict work- or school-related e-mail to one account with another account designated for personal communication. Turn off the notification chime and set aside a specific time during the day to read and answer your e-mail instead of answering each one as it arrives. This could be the first task in the morning while you are enjoying your coffee. Do not let e-mail pile up in your Inbox. Read it, answer it, and, if important, transfer it to a designated folder. Activate the junk e-mail function of your computer or read the subject line, determine whether a message is "junk" and delete it without even taking the time to read it. Your e-mail program may have parameters that allow you to designate specific messages to be sent directly into a special file. This helps move information out of the Inbox and keeps you organized. Spend some time investigating your e-mail program. Look at all of the functions and find out what the program can do. Use your e-mail program to your best advantage—it can become your best friend in terms of helping you organize your messages in folders. Specific tips for effective use of e-mail are provided in Box 2-2.

When communicating with your instructor by e-mail, be sure that you include your class number or title in the subject line. Many instructors manage their e-mail by sorting messages according to class, so a standardized subject line saves your instructor time.

Use your delete key aggressively, and eliminate junk e-mail without reading it.

How Can I Manage My Time?

Time management is a skill and involves planning and practice. Multiple Time Management Worksheets are available to assist in completing a personal analysis of your time. For example, the website *Mind Tools Essential Skills for an Excellent Career*, at *www.mindtools.com/pages/main/newMN_HTE.htm*, provides multiple tools, worksheets, and strategies to assist in developing and refining time-management skills. Rutgers University has a Time Management Worksheet and instructions available at *www.rutgers.edu/osp/MoI/TimeManagement.pdf*.

Calendars are available to schedule to-do activities by the month, week, and day. You gain control of your life by completing a schedule (Table 2-1). Scheduling provides you with a method

---

BOX 2-2   Tips for Effective E-Mail

- Before committing—THINK.
- If it is in writing, you are accountable.
- E-mail is not necessarily confidential.
- Use that "SUBJECT" line.
- Proofread before you send.
- Follow the same principles of courtesy as you expect in face-to-face communication.
- Respect other's time and bandwidth.
- Keep flaming responses under control.
- Send responses to appropriate individuals only.
- Be brief and always close with a farewell.

TABLE 2-1 Weekly Personal Calendar				
MONDAY	TUESDAY	WEDNESDAY	THURSDAY	FRIDAY
Cleaners 9 AM workout	Pick up health insurance forms 3:30 PM carpool	4 PM workout	4-7 PM professional organization meeting	9 AM workout

CRITICAL THINKING BOX 2-1

Develop your time calendar—will it be a week-at-a-glance or a month-at-a-glance? Think about what works the best for you.

to allocate time for specific tasks and is a constant reminder of your tasks, due dates, and deadlines. Schedule only what can realistically be accomplished and leave extra time before and after every major activity. Tasks, meetings, and travel can take longer than anticipated, so give yourself some time to transition from one project to another. Schedule personal time in your calendar. If someone wants to meet with you during this time, just say, "I'm sorry; I've got an important appointment. When would be another convenient time?" Or ask, "Could we meet tomorrow afternoon?" Color-code your appointments according to priorities or specific roles to stimulate the right side of your brain.

Leave white space (nothing) in your schedule so you will have time for yourself and family, or schedule uninterruptible time for both.

At the beginning of each week, review the week's activities to avoid unexpected "surprises." Over-scheduling of more tasks than any human being can do in a single day inevitably leads to frustration. Build in some flexibility. It will not always be possible to follow your exact schedule. However, when you do get "derailed," having a plan will help you get back on track with a minimum of time and effort (Critical Thinking Box 2-1).

Strategy: Leave some extra time before and after every major event to allow for transition.

MANAGING TASKS

How Do I Deal with Procrastination?

Everyone procrastinates, especially when a task is unpleasant, overwhelming, or cannot be done perfectly. Procrastination can lead to last-minute rushes that cause unnecessary stress. The time spent stressing about doing something takes more time than actually doing it! The anticipation itself can also be worse than the actuality, draining your energy and accomplishment. Here are some tips for getting started.

Consider the Consequences

Ask yourself what will happen if you do something and what will happen if you do not do it. If there are no negative outcomes of not doing something, there is no point in spending time doing it. You can eliminate that activity!

> If something will happen because you don't do it, then, of course, you need to get started.

The Earlier, the Better

Most projects take longer than planned, and glitches happen; for example, coffee spills all over your study notes the night before the test, your computer crashes, or your dog eats your notes. To compensate for the inevitable delays and to avoid crises, start in advance and plan for your project to take three times longer than you think. Be realistic and use your common sense in scheduling this time frame.

> Schedule times to work on your project, and track your progress on a calendar.

"By the Inch, It's a Cinch." Break projects into small, manageable pieces; gather all the resources required to finish the project; and plan to do only the first step initially. For example, to study for a test, first collect all the related notes and books in one place. Next, review the subjects likely to be tested. If you are having difficulty getting started, plan to work on these steps for only 5 to 10 minutes. (Anybody can do just about anything for 5 to 10 minutes, eh?) Frequently, this will create enough momentum to get you going. When you have to stop, leave yourself a note regarding what the next steps should be. Here are some hints for effective studying.

- Study difficult subjects or concepts first.
- Study in short "chunks" of 50 minutes each.
- Take a brief 10-minute break after every 50 minutes of studying.
- Schedule study time when you are at your best.
- Use waiting times. (Compile and carry 3 × 5 note cards wherever you go. They should contain information you need to review and can be pulled out anywhere—even when you are standing in that long line at the checkout counter.)
- Keep a calendar for the semester that includes all of your assignments, tests, and papers. Use a different color for entering deadlines for each course.
- Make a weekly to-do list. Prioritize this list and cross off each task as you complete it.
- Before beginning a project, know what you are doing. Determine the goals, benefits, costs, and timetable for the endeavor. If you are working in a group, at the beginning of the project, make sure everyone understands his or her responsibilities. You should also designate someone to be in charge of organizing group meetings. Leave time during the project for unexpected delays and to revisit and modify your goals. Be flexible.

If you are taking an online or web-enhanced course, remember these courses take as much, if not more time, then traditional face-to-face classes. Here are some hints to assist with your time management related to online courses.

- Print the syllabus and place deadlines on your calendar prior to the first course meeting.
- Identify how to contact your instructor and schedule online office hours in your calendar.
- Schedule weekly times for logging into the class website.
- Schedule a time for class work and select a specific site.
- Develop collegial support groups.
- Be active in the course by participating appropriately in discussion groups.
- Establish an evidence-based file to download important articles (pdf format).
- Bookmark websites (but prior to bookmarking these; review the information—Don't assume all sites are up-to-date and evidence-based).
- There are a few online sites that offer online storage and retrieval of documents, files, and assignments. Check out the following link for more information on storing files via the Internet: www.dropbox.com.

Reward Yourself. Bribing yourself with a reward can help you get started and keep going: "If I concentrate well for 1 hour on reading the assigned chapter, then I can watch my favorite television show guilt-free." Often, the stress reduction that comes from working on the project that has been put off is a reward in itself! (Critical Thinking Box 2-2.)

Schedule a time for celebration and self-reward with all of your projects.

Avoid the Myth of Perfection. Many of us were brought up with the well-intentioned philosophy that "Anything worth doing is worth doing well." Unfortunately, this is often interpreted as "Anything worth doing is worth doing *perfectly*." The fear of not doing something well enough or perfectly also feeds the tendency to procrastinate.

Certainly, everyone needs to make the best effort possible, but not everything needs to be done perfectly. Consider what the expected standard is—not the standard of perfection possible—and how you can meet it with a minimum amount of time and effort. Effective procrastination (i.e., procrastination that is used appropriately) is recognizing when a task should be purposefully postponed. This technique is a conscious decision and is used when time is needed to accomplish a task with a higher priority. Priority setting, delegating tasks when possible, eliminating wasted time by avoiding excessive social telephone calls, breaking tasks into separate small steps, and establishing realistic short-term goals are some strategies for managing procrastination.

CRITICAL THINKING BOX 2-2   What do you do to reward yourself for a job done well?

BOX 2-3	Tips for Managing Time and Others

- Use an activity planner or calendar (paper copy or on your smartphone)—review it daily.
- Prioritize your activities.
- Make use of "mini" or waiting time periods.
- AVOID PERFECTIONISM.
- Take "mini" vacations throughout the day to refresh your brain.
- Minimize the time spent with individuals who constantly complain and criticize.
- Use assertive communication with individuals with whom you are having a problem.
- Develop rituals (such as changing clothes) when you get home that say "I'm off duty."
- Avoid always saying yes—before agreeing—take a deep breath—think about the real expectation of the project.
- Delegate when appropriate.
- Don't let your e-mail and the cell phone manage you and your time.

MANAGING OTHERS

Communicating and getting along with other people can be challenging. Most people are straightforward, supportive, and easy to be with. They add to your energy and ability to function effectively, and they contribute to your goal attainment. However, some individuals drain energy from you and jeopardize organizational accomplishment through their whining, criticizing, negative thinking, chronic lateness, poor crisis management, overdependency, aggression, and similar unproductive behaviors. Occasional exhibitions of such behavior in relation to a personal crisis can be understood. Even in the best of human relationships, conflict and extreme emotions are inevitable. However, when people use these behaviors as their everyday *modus operandi* (method of operating), they interfere with attainment of individual and organizational goals. To protect your time and achieve your goals, it may be necessary to limit your time with such individuals. Avoidance is one strategy. Learning to say "no" and practicing assertive communication can help as well. Chapters 12 and 13 provide assistance in learning these communication skills. Box 2-3 provides some hints for managing others.

What About Delegation and Time Management?

You do not have to handle everything personally. Use your delegation skills at home to identify tasks and activities that can be completed by others, leaving you more time to study and concentrate on important projects. The website, *Mind Tools: Essential Skills for an Excellent Career*, at *www.mindtools.com/pages/article/newLDR_98.htm*, provides multiple strategies related to delegation and a delegation worksheet to assist in determining whether a task can be delegated and to whom (see Chapter 14).

MANAGING YOUR GOALS

Goals are the incremental steps required to achieve long-term success. Personal and professional goals are critical to lifestyle management. Keeping your goals in mind enables you to plan and carry out activities that contribute to your goals and eliminate or reduce those that do not. Be realistic when setting your goals: allow enough time to complete them appropriately. Activities that contribute to goals are your high-payoff, high-priority activities; those that do not are low-payoff, low-priority activities. Your goals should be demanding enough that completion provides a feeling of satisfaction.

Many goal-directed activities need to be scheduled with completion times. This is sometimes called *deadlining* the to-do list; the use of the term *completion times* may seem less stress-producing than the use of *deadlines*. All kinds of calendars are available to schedule to-do activities by the month, week, and day. There are organizer notebooks and computerized organizers. It is also easy to make your own forms. Knowing your goals and priorities promotes flexible rescheduling, resulting in more effective time management and successful accomplishment.

Begin by Listing

It will be helpful to list all your goal-related activities on a master to-do list. Using all of the features of Microsoft Outlook by identifying tasks in the email and/or calendar program and setting up reminders will be helpful for both tasks that are listed and tasks based on emails received or sent (e.g., assignments). Another approach, which is also a useful learning exercise, is to record all your activities in a time log as they occur (e.g., record them every day for several days or a week). This will give you an overview of how you are using your time and provide a baseline for a to-do list. Either way, decide the order in which to do the activities in your list. You will have to decide the order in which your activities need to be completed—in other words, you will have to prioritize.

Cross out items on your to-do list, cards, and schedule as you do them. This will give you immediate, positive feedback—an instant reward for your efforts and progress. When the inevitable interruptions occur, scan the to-do list and reevaluate your priorities in relation to your remaining time.

Reward yourself as you cross out items on your to-do list.

Prioritize with the ABCD System

Others are constantly demanding your time and energy; therefore you need to establish priorities but also be flexible. Being flexible will allow you to change your priorities throughout the day as situations change. Additionally, as you work, always try to combine activities (multitask) or delegate tasks in an effort to manage your time appropriately.

Scan your to-do list and decide which are A, B, C, or D items (Box 2-4). The activities that are most closely related to your goals are the high-payoff ones; these are A priorities. Effective

BOX 2-4	Prioritization Using the ABCD System
A	Absolute (immediate priority)—do it now or as soon as possible
B	Better (as soon as possible)—necessary, but it can be done later
C	Can wait until later—or when you get around to it
D	Don't worry about it—let someone else take care of it

use of your time-management skills demands that you focus most of your energy on A-priority items. List these according to the urgency of the time limits. Train yourself to do the hardest task first. Attending to the most difficult activity first reduces the nagging, anxiety-provoking thought that you "should be doing ___ instead" and helps you make early progress in identifying, gaining control of, and possibly preventing additional problems. This is an example of the classic time-management principle known as Pareto's 80/20 Rule.

According to Pareto, an early 1900s economist, 20% of the effort produces 80% of the results. For example, spending 20% of your time studying the hardest course can produce 80% success. In your home, 80% of what needs cleaning is in the kitchen and bathroom; spend 20% of your cleaning time on these two rooms and 80% of the cleaning will be done. Likewise, 80% of your nursing care will be with 20% of your patients. This illustrates that there are proportionally greater results in concentrating at least 20% of your efforts on higher-payoff priorities. You will need to balance your priorities because it is impossible to achieve our best at all times.

The B items on your list also contribute to goal achievement; thus they are high-payoff items but generally less urgent than A times and can be delayed for a while. Eventually, many B items become A items, especially as completion times approach. It is also possible to "squeeze in" some B items in short periods of time—for instance, reading an article as you wait in a long line or "waste" time waiting for someone.

Items that do not substantially contribute to goals or do not have to be accomplished within a specific time frame are C items. These activities really can wait until you get around to them; they are things to be done when, or if, time permits. Of course, some C items become B or A priorities. However, many C items will fit the "nothing will happen if you do not do something" category and become D items. D items are those "nice to do" but not necessary. Some of these items could be classified as time wasters and can be ignored when you have limited time.

> Develop daily (or time) benchmarks that allow you to assess your daily progress in relation to the time spent on a specific project.

Keep It Going

Continuously review your lists, schedules, and outcomes, and reward yourself for achieving your goals. As you evaluate and revise accordingly, ask yourself: "Did I have a plan with priorities in writing?" "Was I doing high-payoff activities that pertain to my goals?" "Was I doing the right job at the right time?"

No one is perfect. Omissions and errors will occur, and these are good learning experiences. Do not waste time regretting failure or feeling guilty about what you did not do; consider these learning experiences of "what not to do" and opportunities for learning "what to do." Remind yourself that there is always time for important things and that if it is important enough, you will find the time to do it.

SELF-CARE STRATEGIES

I will use words which emanate power, strong words to guide me. My words today will be strong and powerful. I will choose words that convey a sense of mastery, competence, and ability: I can. I will. I am. I do …
—ROCHELLE LERNER, 1985

Role strain theory states demands and stress for one role takes time and energy away for our other roles. Research has demonstrated a direct link between (1) work stressors and family function, and (2) job satisfaction and turnover. Results demonstrated the higher the job satisfaction the lower the work-family conflict; the higher the spousal support the lower the work-family conflict; the higher the spousal support the higher the job satisfaction (Patel et al, 2008).

For nurses to effectively take care of their patients, they must first take care of themselves (Figure 2-3). As a nursing student or a new graduate, you need to make "taking care of yourself" a top priority. Many nurses do not practice the self-care strategies that would show them to handle the stress resulting from the work environment. The work environment will be demanding; you will be exposed to learning opportunities and be introduced to multiple professional responsibilities. How you perceive yourself and respond to these stressors often determines how effective you are as a nurse. The way you feel about yourself and respond will be influenced by your values, actions, successes, and failures.

Self-care, the practice of engaging in activities that promote a healthy lifestyle, is the foundation that will assist you in thriving in nursing instead of just surviving. Engaging in the practice

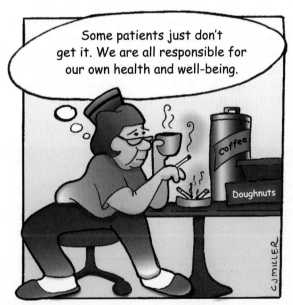

FIGURE 2-3
How do I take care of my physical self?

of self-care requires knowledge, motivation, time, and effort, but it is mandatory in your ability to manage stress. Self-care practices that decrease stress-related illness can be learned. Physical illnesses correlated to stress include cardiovascular problems, migraine headaches, irritable bowel syndrome, and muscle and joint pain. Mental health problems include unresolved anxiety, depression, and insomnia. Finally, stress and burnout among nursing personnel can contribute to organizational problems and attrition.

Is Burnout Inevitable for Nurses?

Much has been written about the concept of burnout in nurses. In early research, burnout was thought to be a problem within a nurse or a problem inherent in the nursing profession. However, the stressors in the current workplace caused by staffing shortages, along with an increase in patient acuity and the accelerated rate of change in the health care environment, have increased the potential for burnout among nurses. Nurses have learned to recognize and manage burnout related to caring too much for their patients. What nurses are currently struggling with is that they may be working in environments that are not congruent with their personal philosophies of nursing care.

Burnout associated with job stress can leave nurses vulnerable to depression, physical illness, and alcohol and drug abuse. Symptoms include a loss of energy, weariness, gloominess, dissatisfaction, increased illness, decreased efficiency, absenteeism, and self-doubt. Burnout typically progresses through five stages that are particularly notable within the work setting: an initial feeling of enthusiasm for the job, followed by a loss of enthusiasm, continuous deterioration, crisis, and finally devastation and the inability to work effectively. Box 2-5 lists early warning signs of burnout.

The increase in patient acuity, coupled with shortened hospital stays, is not compatible with the emphasis on high-quality, safe patient care and consumer satisfaction. These opposing philosophies create conflict for nurses and lead to burnout that is not as easily remedied as burnout caused by internal factors. Therefore, it is important to recognize clearly the mission of the hospital or corporation when you apply for your first job. Is their mission similar to yours? Will you be able to give the quality care that you want to deliver, or will you be required to compromise your values to fit into the system?

BOX 2-5   Early Warning Signs of Burnout

- Irritability
- Weight changes
- Frequent headaches and gastrointestinal disturbances
- Chronic fatigue
- Insomnia
- Depression
- Feeling of helplessness
- Negativity
- Cynicism
- Angry outbursts
- Self-criticism

There are many strategies designed to combat burnout, and many of them are detailed in this chapter. However, nurses need to determine whether their burnout is caused by internal or external factors. A nurse who neglects his or her own needs can develop feelings of low self-esteem and resentment. These feelings could affect the care you provide to others, Therefore, by taking care of yourself, you are ultimately able to provide better care for others. In some cases, it may be necessary for the nurse to relocate to a place of employment that is more in line with her or his personal belief system.

Empowerment and Self-Care

Learning about self-care is really about empowerment. The word *power* comes from the French word *pouvoir*, which means "to be able." To empower means to enable—enable self and others to reach their greatest potential for health and well-being. However, the concept of "enabling" is seen in a negative light because it refers to doing things for others that they can do for themselves. Actually, preventing friends and loved ones from dealing with the consequences of their behavior is very disempowering.

With empowerment comes a feeling of well-being and effectiveness. There are times and situations in our lives when we feel more or less powerful. Examples of occasions when one feels powerful or powerless are listed in Box 2-6. You may find as you read through these lists that there are some situations in your life in which you do feel powerful and some in which you do not. Self-assessment of our sense of well-being and self-esteem helps us to know where to begin. Because change is a constant, and all of us are in varying states of emotional, physical, and mental change at any given time, it is important to assess ourselves on a regular basis. As a matter of fact, knowing one's self is the very first step in learning to care for one's self. Empowerment in all spheres of our being is very important. Examine the Holistic Self-Assessment Tool (Critical Thinking Box 2-3), which includes measures of our emotional, mental, physical, social, spiritual, and choice potentials.

Emotional wholeness is about our ability to feel. The ability to express a wide range of emotions is indicative of good mental health. Nurses are often very good at helping their patients

BOX 2-6	Examples of Times When One Feels Powerless or Powerful
I FEEL POWERLESS WHEN	**I FEEL POWERFUL WHEN**
• I'm ignored.	• I'm energetic.
• I get assigned to a new hospital unit.	• I get positive feedback.
• I can't make a decision.	• I know I look good.
• I'm exhausted.	• I tell people I'm a nurse.
• I'm being evaluated by my instructor.	• I have clear goals for my career.
• I have no choices.	• I stick to decisions.
• I'm being controlled or manipulated.	• I speak out against injustice.
• I have pent-up anger.	• I allow myself to be selfish without feeling guilty.
• I don't think or react quickly.	• I tell a good joke.
• I don't speak loudly enough.	• I work with supportive people.
• I don't have control over my time.	• I'm told by a patient or family that I did a good job.

Adapted from Josefowitz N: *Paths to power*, Menlo Park, Calif, 1980, Addison-Wesley, p 7. Reprinted with permission.

HOLISTIC SELF-ASSESSMENT TOOL

Emotional Potential

I _____ push my thoughts and feelings out of conscious awareness (denial).
I feel I have to be in _____ control.
I am unable to express _____ basic feelings of sadness, joy, anger, and fear.
I see myself as a _____ victim.
I feel guilty and _____ ashamed a lot of the time.
I frequently take things _____ personally.

Social Potential

I _____ am overcommitted to the point of having no time for recreation.
I am unable to be honest _____ and open with others.
I am unable to admit _____ vulnerability to others.
I am attracted to needy _____ people.
I feel overwhelmingly _____ responsible for others' happiness.
My only friends are _____ nurses.

Physical Potential

I _____ neglect myself physically—overweight/underweight, lack of adequate rest and
   exercise.
I feel tired and lack _____ energy.
I am not interested in _____ sex.
I do not engage in _____ regular physical and dental check-ups.
I have seen a doctor in _____ the past 6 months for any of the following conditions:
   migraine headaches, backaches, gastrointestinal problems, hypertension, or cancer.
I am a workaholic—work _____ is all-important to me.

Spiritual Potential

I _____ see that events that occur in my life are controlled by external choices.
I find the world a _____ basically hostile place.
I lack a spiritual base _____ for working through daily problems.
I live in the past or _____ the future.
I have no sense of power _____ greater than myself.

Mental Potential

I _____ read mostly professional literature.
I spend most waking _____ hours obsessing over people, places, or things.
I am no longer able to _____ dream or fantasize about my future.
I can't remember much of _____ my childhood.
I can't see much change _____ happening for myself, either personally or
   professionally.

Choice Potential

I _____ have difficulty making decisions, I am prone to procrastination, and I am frequently
   late for personal and professional appointments.
I find it difficult to _____ say no.
I find myself unwilling _____ to take reasonable risks.
I find it difficult to _____ take responsibility for myself.

From Zerwekh J, Michaels B: Co-dependency: assessment and recovery, *Nurs Clin North Am* 24(1):109-120, 1989.

"feel" their feelings but often have a difficult time feeling and expressing their own. Nurses frequently neglect their physical health. We make certain that our patients receive excellent health education and discharge instructions and worry when they are noncompliant. As nurses, however, we do not always follow through when it comes to such things as physical examinations, mammograms, and dental health for ourselves. We work long hours and do not plan adequate time for physical recuperation.

Because our profession is such a demanding one, we often do not take the time to cultivate our social potential. When we do spend time with friends, it is because they "need" us. When we get together with friends who are also nurses, we spend the time together talking about work. Spiritual potential simply means that we have a daily awareness that there is something more to living than mere human existence. The lives of nurses with spiritual potential have meaning and direction.

The ability to know that we have choices in life is the final area of the assessment tool. Nurses without "choice power" see life as black-and-white, with little gray in the middle. Awareness of our choices eliminates the black-and-white extremes and enables us to act rather than react in situations. Nurses with choice power are able to make decisions, take risks, and feel good about it.

Remember to use this tool not only to assess the negatives in your life, but also to assess areas in which you are experiencing growth. You cannot survive nursing school, for example, without experiencing growth in all areas.

Suggested Strategies for Self-Care That Are Based on the Holistic Self-Assessment Tool. Not having life in a state of balance and not having a vision for the future often reflect a state of poor self-esteem. Nathaniel Branden (1992), often referred to as the "father of the self-esteem movement," has identified several factors found in individuals with healthy self-esteem. These include the following:

- A face, manner, and way of talking and moving that project the pleasure one takes in being alive.
- Ease in talking of accomplishments or shortcomings with directness and honesty.
- An attitude of openness to and curiosity about new ideas, new experiences, and new possibilities of life.
- Openness to criticism and comfortable about acknowledging mistakes because one's self-esteem is not tied to an image of perfection.
- An ability to enjoy the humorous aspects of life in one's self and others (Branden, 1992, p 43). The key to developing a healthy self-esteem is to become aware of the areas that need the most repair and to work on them. However, it is essential to maintain a sense of balance; going overboard in one or two areas is counterproductive. For example, a nurse who exercises five times a week, follows a healthy diet, and sleeps well but is emotionally numb and does not have a clear vision for her future is out of balance.

Am I Emotionally Healthy/Emotionally Intelligent? Being emotionally healthy means that you are aware of your feelings and are able to acknowledge them in a healthy way. In the best-selling book *Emotional Intelligence*, Goleman (1995) states that emotional intelligence consists of the following five domains: knowing one's emotions, managing emotions, motivating one's self, recognizing emotions in others, and handling relationships. It is certainly best when the basics of emotional intelligence are taught by parents who are good emotional coaches. However, it is never too late to learn.

Nurses who have good emotional health know when they are feeling fearful, angry, sad, ashamed, happy, guilty, or lonely, and they are able to distinguish these feelings. They have found appropriate ways to express their feelings without offending others. When feelings are not expressed or at least acknowledged, they frequently build up, which results in emotional binging. Sometimes our bodies take the brunt of unacknowledged feelings in the form of headaches, gastrointestinal problems, anxiety attacks, and so on.

Feelings or emotions are neither good nor bad. They are indications of some of our self-truths, our desires, and our needs. Critical Thinking Box 2-4 is an exercise to help access and acknowledge feelings.

What About Friends and Fun? How Do I Find the Time? An occupational hazard of nursing is over-committing, both personally and professionally. Nurses who do this frequently have difficulty in meeting their social potential.

Student nurses often say they do not engage in recreational activities because of the cost and that all their money goes toward living expenses. First, it is important to include some money in your monthly budget for fun. Depriving yourself of time for recreation on a regular basis may lead to impulsive recreational spending such as a shopping binge with credit cards or with money allotted for something else. Second, there are many pleasurable things to do and fun places to go that do not cost a lot of money. Several examples are found in Box 2-7.

Another social area in which many nurses have difficulty is forming relationships outside of nursing. If you spend all your free time with nurses, chances are that you will "talk shop." Nursing curricula are very science-intensive because there is so much to learn in such a short period of

---

CRITICAL THINKING
BOX 2-4

EXERCISE TO HELP ACCESS AND ACKNOWLEDGE FEELINGS

1. Turn your attention to how you are feeling. What part of your body feels what?
2. Acknowledge that this is how you are feeling, and give it a name. If you hear an inner criticism for feeling this way, just set it aside. Any feeling is acceptable.
3. Let yourself experience the sensations you are having. Separate acknowledging these feelings from having to do anything about them.
4. Ask yourself whether you want to express your feelings now or some other time. Do you want to take some other action now or later? Remind yourself that you have choices.

BOX 2-7   Some Pleasurable Activities

- Go on a picnic with friends.
- Invite friends over for a potluck dinner.
- Go to a movie.
- Plan celebrations after exams or completion of a project.
- Introduce yourself to three new people.
- Visit a museum.
- Call an old friend.
- Play with your children.
- "Borrow" someone else's children for play.
- Volunteer for a worthwhile project.
- Get involved in religious or spiritual activities.
- Spend some time people-watching.
- Take up a new hobby.
- Invite humor into your life.

time. Cultivate some friends who have a liberal arts or fine arts background. Choose friends who have different political opinions or come from a different part of town, a different culture, or a different socioeconomic class.

How Do I Take Care of My Physical Self? Nurses are great when it comes to patient education; it is one of the strengths of the nursing profession. Sometimes, though, we have difficulty applying this information to ourselves. Physically taking care of ourselves is extremely important. Our profession is both mentally and physically challenging. This physical self-care entails getting the proper nutrition, maintaining a healthy weight, obtaining adequate sleep, quitting smoking, limiting alcohol consumption to one drink daily, and exercising on a regular basis (Figure 2-4; Critical Thinking Box 2-5). Engaging in some form of relaxation will trigger the relaxation response which prevents chronic stress from harming your health (Stark et al, 2005). According to Kernan and Wheat (2008), health and learning are linked; optimal learning cannot be achieved unless the environment is supportive and promotes the development of effective learning skills. They identified mental health concerns (stress, anxiety), respiratory tract infections, interpersonal concerns, and sleep difficulties as the greatest threats to academic success.

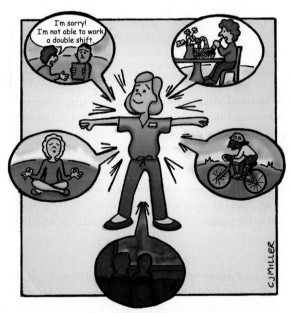

FIGURE 2-4

Learn to take care of yourself.

| **CRITICAL THINKING** BOX 2-5 | What am I doing that interferes with my health and well-being? |

Self-Care Activities

Physical Exercise. Incorporate 30 minutes or more of moderate-intensity physical activity, such as walking, into your schedule (preferably daily). A good exercise program is one that includes activities that foster aerobic activity, flexibility, and strength. A very important part of an exercise program is that it be a regular habit. To be effective, the program should take 3 to 6 hours a week. And it does not have to cost money. You do not need to belong to a gym or invest in exercise equipment. Aerobic activities include walking, jogging, swimming, bicycling, and dancing. Minimal fitness consists of raising your heart rate to 100 beats/min and keeping it there for 30 minutes. Other strategies to increase your physical activity could include the following:

- Park your car farther away from the entrance door.
- Use the stairs instead of the elevator whenever possible.
- Stretch during your breaks from homework or housework.
- Take your dog for a walk (or volunteer to walk someone else's pet).

Laughter. Seek 20 minutes of laughter every day. Laughing promotes deep breathing and releases neuropeptides that decrease stress and lower blood pressure. (Check out www.laughteryoga.org for inspiring thoughts and affirmations.)

Mental Exercise. Engage in some activity daily for at least 30 minutes that challenges your way of thinking. This activity will increase the number of connections between your brain cells (rewiring your brain). Activities that could promote brain function include:

- Take a walk in the park to stimulate all your senses.
- Try out a new restaurant.
- Listen to new music.
- Try puzzles or word games (see *www.sudokupuzz.com*).

Motivate Yourself. In the morning read an inspiring quote, listen to upbeat music, or do stretching exercises. Take time for a balanced breakfast and visualize your day. Take periodic breaks or switch activities throughout your day to maintain a high energy level. Tension can be released by simple stretching exercises and laughter.

> Alternate mental and physical tasks. This strategy includes taking periodic breaks from studying to engage in a short game of basketball or a short run with the vacuum cleaner.

Strategies to Foster My Spiritual Self: Does My Life Have Meaning? People who have a sense of spiritual well-being find their lives to be positive experiences, have relationships with a power greater than themselves, feel good about the future, and believe there is some real purpose in life. If we find that our lives lack meaning and our spiritual health is lacking, how do we go about finding spiritual well-being?

Daily prayer and meditation are very important in maintaining a spiritual self. M. Scott Peck (1978) states that the process of spiritual growth is an effortful and difficult one because it is conducted against a natural resistance, a natural inclination to keep things the way they were, to cling to the old maps and old ways of doing things, to take the easy path. Reading religious or philosophical material and studying the great religions are two examples of ways to foster spiritual growth.

In addition to reading what others have written about the subject, many people access their spiritual selves with the practice of meditation. Meditating allows us time to become quiet, heal our thoughts and bodies, and be grateful. The engagement of daily prayer or meditation allows for a time of self-reflection. Reflection, according to Johns (2004), is "being mindful of self"; it is the "window through which the practitioner can view and focus self within the context of a particular experience, in order to confront, understand and move toward resolving contradiction between one's vision and actual practice" (p 3). The conscious practice of reflection has been correlated to a heightened perception of self-awareness, self-empowerment (Teekman, 2000), enhanced self-confidence and empathy (Gustafsson and Fagerberg, 2004).

How Do I Increase My Mental Potential? Is it Okay to Daydream? Nursing students get considerable opportunity to exercise their mental potential while they are in nursing school. This activity, however, is primarily in the form of formal education. There are many other ways to exercise this potential. One of the first ways is to concentrate on removing negative thoughts or self-defeating beliefs from our minds. Here are some examples of statements that nursing students frequently make:

- "I must make *As* in nursing school."
- "I must have approval from everyone, and if I don't, I feel horrible and depressed."
- "If I fail at something, the results will be catastrophic."
- "Others must always treat me fairly."
- "If I'm not liked by everyone, I am a failure."
- "Because all my miseries are caused by others, I will have no control over my life until they change."

If you relate to any of these statements, you have some work to do on your belief system. You are setting yourself up for failure by having extremely high expectations of yourself. You are also giving other people power over your own destiny. Remember, you cannot change others. The only person you can change is yourself.

One way that we can change these internal beliefs is to learn how to give ourselves daily affirmations—or daydream a little (Figure 2-5). Simply put, affirmations are powerful, positive statements concerning the ways in which we would like to think, feel, and behave. Some examples are "I am a worthwhile person"; "I am human and capable of making mistakes"; and "I am able to freely express my emotions." Always begin affirmative statements with "I" rather than "you." This practice keeps the focus on self rather than others and encourages the development of inner self-worth.

The power of affirmation exercises lies in consistency—repetition encourages ultimate belief in what is being said. Begin each day with some affirmations. Try some of the examples in Box 2-8. These enable us to feel better about ourselves and consequently raise our self-esteem. Stand in front of a mirror and tell yourself that you are a special person and worthy of self-love and the love of others. Another suggestion is to record some positive affirmations on your telephone answering machine and call your telephone number in the middle of the day or when you are having a slump or attack of self-pity; hearing you own voice say you are okay can have a very positive effect. For example, "Hello—Glad you're having a great day, please leave a message" (Critical Thinking Box 2-6).

What Are My Choices, and How Do I Exercise Them? Many of us negotiate our way through life never realizing that we have many choices. We remain victims, waiting for life to happen, rather than taking a proactive stance. In his best-selling book *Seven Habits of Highly*

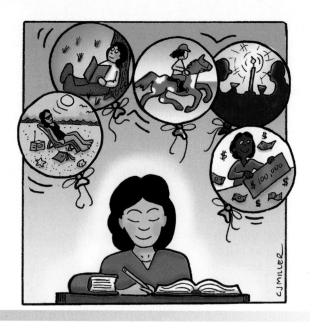

FIGURE 2-5

Daydream: Send up your brain balloons!

BOX 2-8	Affirmations

- I am a worthwhile person.
- I am a child of God.
- I am willing to accept love.
- I am willing to give love.
- I can openly express my feelings.
- I deserve love, peace, and serenity.
- I am capable of changing.
- I can take care of myself without feeling guilty.
- I can say no and not feel guilty.
- I am beautiful inside and out.
- I can be spontaneous and whimsical.
- I am human and capable of making mistakes.
- I can recognize shame and work through it.

- I forgive myself for hurting myself and others.
- I freely accept nurturing from others.
- I can be vulnerable with trusted others.
- I am peaceful with life.
- I am free to be the best me I can.
- I love and comfort myself in ways that are pleasing to me.
- I am automatically and joyfully focusing on the positive.
- I am giving myself permission to live, love, and laugh.
- I am creating and singing affirmations to create a joyful, abundant, fulfilling life.

CRITICAL THINKING BOX 2-6	What are some positive affirmations that work for you? How can you increase the effectiveness of these affirmations?

BOX 2-9	Examples of Reactive and Proactive Language

REACTIVE	PROACTIVE
There's nothing I can do.	Let's look at our alternatives.
That's just the way I am.	I can choose a different approach.
He makes me so mad.	I control my own feelings.
They won't allow that.	I can create an effective presentation.
I have to do that.	I will choose an appropriate response.
I can't.	I choose.
I must.	I prefer.
If only.	I will.

Effective People, Stephen Covey (1989; 2004) states that the very first habit we must develop is to be proactive. We stop thinking in black-and-white and come to realize that in every arena of our lives, we have choices about how to respond and react. Covey differentiates between people who are proactive and people who are reactive. Examples of proactive versus reactive language are included in Box 2-9. Pay attention to your own language patterns for the next few weeks. Are there times when you could say "I choose"? You can choose to respond to people and situations rather than react. Exercising our choice potential also entails that we act responsibly toward others. We recognize that other people have the right to choose for themselves and to be accountable for their own behavior.

CONCLUSION

Before we can act responsibly toward others, we must first act responsibly toward ourselves. This involves self-acceptance and self-love. In his book *Born for Love: Reflections on Loving,* Leo Buscaglia (1992) states this very eloquently:

> *Being who we are, people who feel good about themselves are not easily threatened by the future. They enthusiastically maintain a secure image whether everything is falling apart or going their way. They hold a firm base of personal assuredness and self-respect that remains constant. Though they are concerned about what others think of them, it is a healthy concern. They find external forces more challenging than threatening. Perhaps the greatest sign of maturity is to reach the point in life when we embrace ourselves—strengths and weaknesses alike—and acknowledge that we are all that we have; that we have a right to a happy and productive life and the power to change ourselves and our environment within realistic limitations. In short, we are, each of us, entitled to be who we are and become what we choose (p 177).*

When you get your personal life organized, you will become effective in getting priorities accomplished at home. When you get your school activities organized, you will study more effectively, be less stressed, and be able to prioritize more effectively. With these two areas organized, there will be more time for you to spend on yourself! You will find that once you get organized with your clinical schedule, you will become a more effective nurse and begin to have the time to perform the type of nursing care that you were taught. Often you will hear nurses complain about not having enough time in clinical to provide the type of bath or teaching they would like to do because of the lack of time. Check them out; often they are the most guilty of wasting time (e.g., taking time to gossip after report, wasting time complaining that they do not have enough time, not delegating effectively, allowing unnecessary interruptions, not organizing their patient care, or not delegating when appropriate). Wow, all the things that this chapter is all about!

BIBLIOGRAPHY

Branden N: *The power of self-esteem*. Deerfield, Fla, 1992, Health Communications.

Buscaglia L: *Born for love: reflections on loving*, Thorofare, NJ, 1992, Random House.

Covey S: *Seven habits of highly effective people*, New York, 1989; 2004, Simon & Schuster.

Goleman D: *Emotional intelligence*, New York, 1995, Bantam Books.

Gustafsson C, Fagerberg I: Reflection, the way to professional development? *J Clin Nurs* 13(3):271-280, 2004.

Johns C: *Becoming a reflective practitioner*, Malden, Mass, 2004, Blackwell Publishing.

Kernan WD, Wheat ME: Nursing students' perceptions of the academic impact of various health issues, *Nurse Educator* 33(5):215-219, 2008.

Keyes R: *Timelock: how life got so hectic and what you can do about it*. New York, 1991, HarperCollins.

Lerner R: *Daily affirmations*. Pompano Beach, Fla, 1985, Health Communications.

Patel CJ et al.: Work-family conflict, job satisfaction and spousal support: an exploratory study of nurses' experience, *Curationis* 31(1):38-44, 2008.

Peck MS: *The road less traveled*, New York, 1978, Simon & Schuster.

Stark MA, Maning-Walsh J, Vliem S: Caring for self while learning to care for others: a challenge for nursing students, *J Nurs Educ* 44(6):260-270, 2005.

Teekman B: Exploring reflective thinking in nursing practice, *J Adv Nurs* 31(5):1125-1135, 2000.

Additional resources are available online at *http://evolve.elsevier.com/Zerwekh/nsgtoday/.*

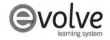

CHAPTER 3

Mentorship, Preceptorship, and Nurse Residency Programs

Ashley Zerwekh Garneau, PhD, RN

> *Mentoring is a brain to pick, an ear to listen, and a push in the right direction.*
> —JOHN CROSBY

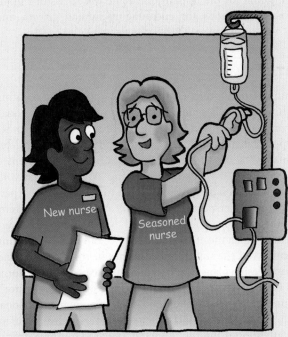

New nurse

Seasoned nurse

Mentoring is one of the broadest methods of encouraging human growth and potential.

After completing this chapter, you should be able to:

- Describe the difference between mentoring, coaching, and precepting.
- Identify characteristics of effective mentors, mentees, and preceptors.
- Implement strategies for finding a mentor.
- Discuss the types of mentoring relationships.
- Examine components of a nurse residency program.

■ ASHLEY

It was my first day as a nurse extern in a busy medical intensive care unit. As I walked into my new place of work, I observed nurses on the phones, talking with doctors, and running in and out of patients' rooms with stern looks on their faces. So many questions were going through my head. Which one of these nurses was my preceptor? What would my preceptor expect from me? Would he or she be receptive to helping me develop into my role as a nurse? I entered the room where the nurses receive report from the night staff. It was there that I had my first encounter with Julie, who would become my preceptor, nursing role model, and mentor in the months ahead.

HISTORICAL BACKGROUND

Did you ever wonder where the word *mentor* originated? It originated from Greek mythology. Mentor was the name of a wise and faithful advisor to Odysseus. When Odysseus (or Ulysses, as the Romans called him) left for his long voyage during the Trojan War, he entrusted the direction and teaching of his son, Telemachus, to Mentor. According to mythology, through Mentor's guidance, Telemachus became an effective and beloved ruler (Shea, 1999). Mentor's job was not merely to raise Telemachus, but to develop him for the responsibilities he was to assume in his lifetime. Mentoring is one of the broadest methods for encouraging human growth and potential.

WHAT MENTORING IS AND IS NOT

Mentoring is often confused with coaching or precepting. *Coaching* is an approach of assisting an individual's growth through partnership with a colleague or other individual who is an equal. In coaching, one person focuses on the unique and internal qualities observed within the other person that may not be recognized or appreciated. In the business world, executives often refer to themselves as coaches rather than managers, thus fostering a collaborative team-oriented approach. The International Coach Federation (2008) defines coaching as, "partnering with patients in a thought-provoking and creative process that inspires them to maximize their personal and professional potential." From a nursing perspective, Yoder (2007) asserts that coaching is geared to all nursing staff to promote their professional growth and development. She refers to coaching as an ongoing two-way process in which the nurse manager and staff nurse are willing to invest time and energy in the development of the staff nurse. Coaches help individuals find new ways to solve problems, reach goals, and design plans of action to motivate people to perform at the "top of their game." According to Guest, "The strength of mentoring lies in the mentor's specific knowledge and wisdom, in coaching it lies in the facilitation and development of personal qualities. The coach brings different skills and experience and offers a fresh perspective, a different viewpoint. In both cases one-to-one attention is the key" (1999, p 7). Based on these definitions, "A good coach will mentor; and, a good mentor will coach, according to the situation. In considering the best fit, therefore, the two approaches should be regarded as synergistic and complementary, rather than mutually exclusive" (Guest, 1999, p 4).

What about preceptors? The term *preceptor* simply means "tutor" and generally refers to a more formal arrangement that pairs a novice with an experienced person for a set period of time, with a focus on policies, procedures, and skill development. Preceptors serve as role

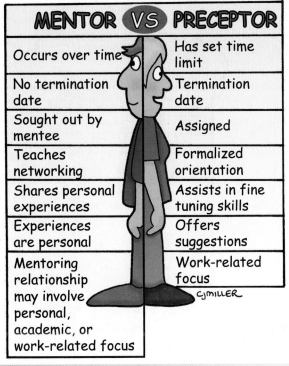

MENTOR VS PRECEPTOR	
Occurs over time	Has set time limit
No termination date	Termination date
Sought out by mentee	Assigned
Teaches networking	Formalized orientation
Shares personal experiences	Assists in fine tuning skills
Experiences are personal	Offers suggestions
Mentoring relationship may involve personal, academic, or work-related focus	Work-related focus

CJMILLER

FIGURE 3-1

Mentor versus preceptor.

models and precept during their regularly scheduled work hours, which is part of their work assignment, in contrast with mentors, who are chosen, not assigned, and focus on fostering the mentee's individual growth and development over an extended period of time. Mentors develop a professionally based, nurturing relationship, which generally occurs during personal time (Figure 3-1).

What Is a Preceptorship?

A preceptorship is a clinical teaching model in which a student is assigned to a preceptor, usually during the student's last semester of nursing school (Billings and Halstead, 2009). Nursing schools sometimes use the term **capstone course** synonymously with the term **preceptorship**. In a capstone course, the senior-level student works one-on-one with a preceptor who is a competent and experienced registered nurse (Figure 3-2). The preceptor guides, observes, and evaluates the student's ability to perform clinical skills with competency and begin applying critical thinking and organization skills in managing a group of patients in a specific setting. The preceptor and the nursing student identify goals and work in a collaborative fashion toward meeting the goals. Typically, the nursing student undertakes the preceptorship in an area of interest that he/she anticipates working in following nursing school as it provides an opportunity for the

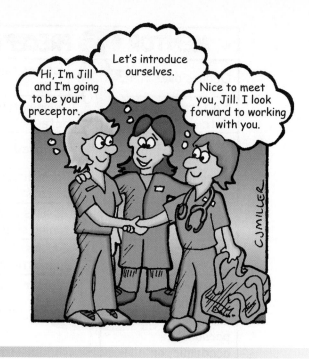

FIGURE 3-2

Capstone course.

student to acquire and master nursing skills common to the specialization area, and begin practicing clinical decision making and prioritization (Emerson, 2007). The preceptorship experience promotes role transition and socialization for the nursing student while fostering professional leadership skills in the preceptor. For example, a student may begin to role-model characteristics of prioritizing patient care based on observations of how the preceptor plans and prioritizes patient care activities. In turn, the preceptor gains leadership traits by communicating and role-modeling professional behaviors. Preceptors have also been referenced in the literature as clinical coaches where they foster critical thinking, safe practice, and socialization during the first year of practice for the new nurse (Bratt, 2009).

What Happens if I Experience a Challenge during My Preceptorship?

When the time arrives for you to complete your preceptorship at the end of your nursing education program, rest assured that those feelings of uncertainty and anxiety that you experienced on your first day of nursing school are normal and will subside with time. As you establish a professional relationship with your preceptor, it is important to understand your role and responsibilities as preceptee as well as the preceptor's role and responsibilities. But, what happens when you are placed with a preceptor who doesn't share the same excitement and interest as you do in participating in the preceptorship? Or, what happens when your personalities do not blend well? What do you do?

First, it is important to identify the issues you are having with your preceptor. It may be helpful to write down what is concerning you and share this information with your clinical site supervisor prior to communicating your concerns to the preceptor. *A word of advice: Never approach an issue with anyone (this includes your preceptor) when your emotions are running high. Give yourself a little time to cool off.*

After you have discussed your concerns with the clinical supervisor, arrange a time to meet with your preceptor to communicate your concerns in a professional tone, while also providing suggestions for a possible solution to the issues you are having with your preceptor. Oftentimes, expressing your concerns to your preceptor will help the preceptor recognize and see your perspective on an issue. Equally important, is for you to provide an opportunity for the preceptor to provide you feedback on any concerns or issues related to the preceptorship experience. If neither you nor the preceptor are able to resolve the issue(s), then reach out to your clinical site supervisor for guidance and support. For additional strategies for resolving conflict, refer to Chapter 13, Conflict Management.

A preceptorship has also been identified as a partnership between an experienced nurse and a new graduate nurse in which the graduate nurse receives training and orientation to the unit that he or she is working in for a specified amount of time. Considering this, a regulatory transition to practice model for new graduate nurses is being proposed by the National Council State Boards of Nursing (NCSBN) that would require newly licensed nurses to complete during the first 6 months after they begin working (see Figure 1-2). After 6 months, the nurse will show evidence supporting their completion of the transition program in order to remain licensed (NCSBN, 2008b). Nurse residency programs are now being implemented across many practice settings to assist new graduate nurses with their transition into the workplace setting.

What is a Nurse Residency Program?

The moment has finally arrived; you have passed the NCLEX-RN® and obtained your RN license. Now, the next step in your professional career path as a nurse begins as you land your first job position. Making this step (but, what might feel like a big leap!) in your nursing career is like a moment of passage. Gone are the days of nursing school; you are no longer a student, but a competent professional nurse. The expectations that your employer expects from you, are high – as they should be. To that end, it is no surprise that you might be feeling a little bit scared or anxious as you start your first day working on the unit at your new place of employment. Remember your first day of nursing school? Similar feelings are sure to surface again as you begin working as a new graduate nurse.

In an effort to ease the transition into the clinical practice setting and reduce job-turnover rates of new graduate nurses, nurse residency programs are now being employed by many healthcare organizations as a mandate for all newly hired new graduate nurses. You might be asking yourself, what exactly is a nurse residency program? A nurse residency program is a formalized orientation that varies in length (anywhere between 5 and 16 months, but usually for about one year), where a new graduate nurse works full-time on the unit he/she will be working on following completion of the residency program. Nurse residency programs vary at each institution, but essentially serve the same purposes, which are to assist the new graduate nurse with transitioning into their new role by providing orientation to the unit to which the new graduate nurse is hired, and working with a dedicated and experienced nurse throughout the residency that serves as both a mentor and coach. In addition, residency programs provide additional specialty training,

BOX 3-1   Relevant Websites and Online Resources

American Association of Colleges of Nursing (AACN) and University HealthSystem Consortium (UHC). (2012). Nurse Residency Program. Retrieved from http://www.aacn.nche.edu/education-resources/nurse-residency-program

American Association of Colleges of Nursing (AACN). (2010). Accredited Nurse Residency Programs. Retrieved from http://apps.aacn.nche.edu/CCNE/reports_residency/resaccprog.asp

Institute of Medicine of the National Academies (IOM). (2010). The Future of Nursing: Leading Change, Advancing Health (Consensus report). Retrieved from http://www.iom.edu/Reports/2010/The-Future-of-Nursing-Leading-Change-Advancing-Health.aspx

NHLBI (National Heart Lung and Blood Institute) (2012). eMentoring: An online mentoring initiative. Retrieved from http://www.nhlbi.nih.gov/ementoring/index.htm

Twibell, R.. St. Pierre, J., Johnson, D., Barton, D., Davis, C., Kidd, M., & Rook, G. (2012). Tripping over the welcome mat: Why new nurses don't stay and what the evidence says we can do about it. American Nurse Today, 7(6). Retrieved from http://www.americannursetoday.com/article.aspx?id=9168&fid=9138

U.S. Department of Health & Human Services. (2012). HHS Mentoring Program: Become a Mentor/Mentee. Retrieved from https://mentoring.hhs.gov/mentors.aspx

certification, and courses that may be a unit specific requirement for the newly hired graduate nurse. Twibell et al. (2012) added that nurse residency programs include a focus on curriculum and specific clinical experiences grounded in evidence-based practice as well as offer new graduate nurses an opportunity for professional growth and socialization as a member of the healthcare team (Box 3-1). Following completion of a nurse residency program, you will be working on the unit where you completed your residency. The American Association of Colleges of Nursing offers a listing of nationally accredited nurse residency programs (Box 3-1).

Further support for requiring all new graduate nurses to complete a nurse residency program following completion from a prelicensure degree program has been proposed by the Institute of Medicine (IOM). The IOM in collaboration with the Robert Wood Johnson Foundation conducted a two-year initiative examining how nursing practice and education will transform the delivery of healthcare. In the 2010 IOM report, *The Future of Nursing: Leading Change, Advancing Health,* the IOM recommended that state boards of nursing and health care organizations should implement and support nurse residency programs.

In 2008, The American Association of Colleges of Nursing (AACN) in collaboration with the University HealthSystem Consortium (UHC), developed a nurse residency program for post-baccalaureate nurses following completion of their educational program (AACN/UHC, 2012). The UHC/AACN nurse residency program is one year long and uses an evidence-based curricular framework for preparing new graduate nurses to transition their role from novice to competent practitioner. At the time of this publication, 89 practice sites in 29 states currently offer the UHC/AACN nurse residency program (Evidence-Based Practice Box 3-1).

As you begin your career as a professional nurse, here are a few questions you may want to ask your employing institution or agency:

- Is a formalized orientation program, preceptorship, internship, and/or nurse residency program available to graduate nurses? If so, what is the duration of the nurse residency program?
- Will I be paired with one or several preceptors?

BOX 3-1   EVIDENCE-BASED PRACTICE

Nurse Residency Program

PRACTICE ISSUE

The clinical environment presents an engaging and rewarding experience for nursing students to begin applying nursing concepts and skills learned in the classroom setting to the practice setting. However, changes impacting health-care, decreased clinical site availability, increased student enrollment and faculty shortages, has required key stakeholders in both academe and practice to develop alternative models of clinical education that will prepare tomorrow's professional nurse to practice competently and safely. Nurse residency programs are a move in that direction, where a graduate nurse participates in a one year program that fosters role transition and clinical decision-making skills grounded in evidence-based practice. Providing a smooth transition into practice has also contributed to increased retention of new graduate nurses and decreased job burnout following completion of the nurse residency program (AACN/UHC, 2012).

IMPLICATIONS FOR NURSING PRACTICE

- Healthcare organizations consider adopting a nurse residency program where new graduate nurses are required to participate in at the beginning of their employment.
- Implement an evidence-based curriculum under the nurse residency program that focuses on development of critical thinking behaviors and aligns to established core competencies implemented by the healthcare institution.
- Collaborate with academic institutions to align nurse residency program objectives with nursing educational program outcomes.
- New graduate nurses who have completed the one year nurse residency program reported an increase in confidence, competence, organization and prioritization, communication, leadership, and a reduction in stress levels (AACN/UHC, 2008, para 4).
- Since its inception, UHC facilities has a 94.3% retention rate for first-year employed nurses (AACN/UHC, 2008, para 4).

Considering This Information:

What are your thoughts on completing a nurse residency program as a requirement by your employer following graduation from nursing school?

References

American Association of Colleges of Nursing (AACN) and University HealthSystem Consortium (UHC): (2012). Nurse Residency Program. Retrieved from http://www.aacn.nche.edu/education-resources/nurse-residency-program

American Association of Colleges of Nursing (AACN) and University HealthSystem Consortium (UHC): (2008). Executive Summary. Retrieved from http://www.aacn.nche.edu/leading-initiatives/education-resources/NurseResidencyProgramExecSumm.pdf

- What is the structure of the nurse residency program? Face-to-face? Online? Hybrid Simulation?
- Is the nurse residency program nationally accredited?

■ ASHLEY

When I was in nursing school, I thought that *preceptor* was just a fancy term for mentor. However, I found out these two terms are very different from each other.

In nursing, the word *mentor* has become synonymous with trusted advisor, friend, teacher, guide, and wise person. There have been many attempts at deriving a single definition of mentoring. Gibbons (2004) provides a detailed listing of 16 (yes, 16!) different definitions for mentor. What makes mentoring so different, so "special," and more encompassing than precepting and coaching?

- Mentoring requires a primary focus on the needs of the mentee and an effort to fulfill the most critical of these needs.
- Mentoring requires going the extra mile for someone else. The rewards of mentoring are enormous: a sense of personal achievement, mentee appreciation, and a sense of building a better organization.
- Mentoring is a partnership created between two people; the mentor possesses the educational degree to which the mentee aspires (Shea, 1999).

As you read through this chapter, begin to develop your own definition of a mentor.

Storytelling is an important way that we have taught one another since the beginning of time. Following is a story about a starfish:

A beachcomber is walking along the beach one morning when he sees a young man running up and down by the water's edge throwing something into the water. Curious, he walks toward the runner and watches him picking up the starfish stranded by the tide and tossing them back into the ocean. "Young man," he says, "there are so many starfish on the beach. What difference does it make to save a few?" Without pausing, the young man picks up another starfish, and flinging it into the sea replies, "It made a difference for this one."

That is what mentors do. They make a difference for one person at a time.

According to Peddy, the process of mentoring can be described in eight words, "Lead, follow, and get out of the way" (2001, p 16). What does this mean?

Lead. Mentors are leaders. They encourage another's growth and development, professionally and personally. Mentors help and inspire mentees by acting as role models. The focus is on wisdom and judgment. The mentor plays a very active role: teaching, coaching, and explaining, while supporting and shaping critical thinking skills, providing invaluable advice when asked, and introducing the mentee to committees, advancements, and honors.

Follow. This is where mentees need to "get their feet wet." At this stage, the mentor and mentee walk the path together, but the advisor (mentor) assumes a more passive role. It is now up to the learner (mentee) to actively seek the advice or listening ear of the mentor.

Get Out of the Way. This means knowing when it is time to let go. If you have ever taught a child to swim or ride a bike, you know how hard it is to "let go" and let the child soar on his or her own. A helping relationship is a freeing relationship. This does not mean the relationship has to end; you share common values and beliefs in lifelong learning.

This process of mentoring is dynamic, not static. A mentor's task of self-development, learning, and mastery is never done. Each person in the mentoring process has a role. Mentors generally have more experience and are dedicated to helping mentees advance in their careers, especially in work and/or life skill issues. Mentoring is a two-way street, a partnership, with both parties freely contributing to the relationship as equals—working together in mutual respect.

■ JOANN

On a personal note, when I think about mentors that I have had, one person comes to mind: Satora. She was my first mentor when I started working in the ICU after graduating with my diploma in nursing. She personified all that a new graduate would want in a mentor. She was understanding, patient, and compassionate, and she possessed extensive experience. She made an important, long-lasting impact on my nursing career. She nurtured me and encouraged me to reach within myself to become the nurse that I am today. I will never forget her.

Approximately 25 years after I left the ICU, I had the opportunity to talk with Satora by phone. It was one of those coincidences or synchronistic moments in which I was able, via a mutual friend, to find out where she was working. I had lost contact with her over the years and in the several moves that I had made to different places. She was so surprised that I had called, and I shared with her how important our mentoring relationship had been to me. It made me feel good to pass along my gratitude for her willingness to mentor me.

How to Find a Mentor

The key to finding a mentor is having an open mind, being flexible, and remaining optimistic. As you finish nursing school and while you are in school, write down the goals you feel a mentor might help you achieve. Keep this list of goals with you while you are working, and try to get a feel for the different personality types that you will see as a nurse among your coworkers.

■ ASHLEY

During my orientation program as a newly licensed professional registered nurse, my mentor Julie shared with me a saying that I will share with you: "Always remember, the patient comes first." This stuck with me because it helped me gain greater awareness of the profound impact that we, as nurses, have in our patients' lives and in assisting them to an optimal level of wellness.

As you progress through your nursing program, consider establishing a mentoring relationship. Having the feeling of comfort and building trust with this person is crucial to the process of mentoring. Here are some ideas and strategies to think about:

- Look for common background in either nursing education or an area of expertise/practice or interest.
- Tell the person about yourself. When you disclose something about yourself, it is especially helpful if you can laugh about yourself in a given situation. This sets the tone of the interaction. It is helpful to keep it light, friendly, and positive.
- Find out the best mode for communicating (i.e., in person, by e-mail, phone) with your mentor.

- Ask broad, open-ended questions such as, "How are things going?" that stimulate open discussion rather than direct questions such as, "Do you like working here?" or "What kind of problems are you having?" that may make the other person feel vulnerable.
- By starting out with these basic questions, you can begin to determine a level of comfort about the person. Next, let us examine the characteristics of a successful mentor.

What Are the Characteristics of a Successful Mentor?

When I think about the desired characteristics or competencies of a successful mentor, the following qualities come to mind:

- A mentor communicates **high expectations.** Mentors push mentees and provide avenues and opportunities for them to grow. They allow the mentees to learn through many of their own failures. The mentee grows and develops through active listening, role modeling, and open communication with the mentor. When mentors act as sources of intellectual stimulation and encouragement, they encourage their mentees to trust their own abilities and skills. Mentors open doors and encourage their mentees to search out and seek professional avenues that mentees might not have known about or would have taken longer to discover on their own. Rather than being the "sage on the stage," the mentor is the "guide on the side."
- A mentor is also a **good listener.** Mentors provide a nonjudgmental, listening ear (without taking on the mentee's problems, giving advice, or joining the mentee in a game of "Ain't it awful?"). This can serve as a powerful aid to a mentee. Many mentors believe that respectful listening is the premier mentoring act. When two people really listen to each other, a wonderful sense of synergy is created.
- A mentor has **empathy.** A mentor possesses a degree of sensitivity and perception as to the needs of the mentee and has an ability to teach others in an unselfish, respectful way that does not blame, but stays neutral. Mentors know what it is like to be the "new kid on the block."
- A mentor offers **encouragement.** By providing subtle guidance and reassurance of decisions made by the mentee, the mentor values the mentee's experience, ideas, knowledge of how things work, and special insights into problems. Mentors strive to promote independence in their mentees by offering suggestions, but not pushing—mentors know that growth depends on the mentee solving his or her own problems.
- A mentor is **generous.** Mentors are willing to share their time and knowledge with others. Much of what the mentor offers is personal learning or insight (Shea, 1999) (Critical Thinking Box 3-1, Figure 3-3 and Box 3-1).

What Is a Mentoring Moment?

Have you ever experienced a flash of insight or a revelation? Peddy (2001) calls this a "mentoring moment." How do you know when that moment arrives? Someone once said, "When the student is ready, the teacher appears" (Peddy, 2001, p 52). According to Peddy, mentoring is often built on a just-in-time principle, whereby the mentor offers the right help at the right time. A potential

CRITICAL THINKING
BOX 3-1

- Which of these traits appeal to you the most?
- Which ones would be the most important for your mentor to have?

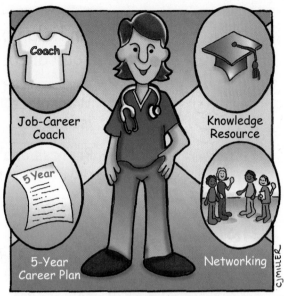

FIGURE 3-3

Expectations of a mentor.

mentor must recognize when the mentee feels free to expose a deep-felt need, thereby enabling the mentor to provide the right help at the right time to the best of the mentor's ability.

When Do We Need Mentors?

A mentor is an established professional (selected by you) who takes a long-term personal interest in your nursing career. The mentor not only serves as a role model or counselor for you but also actively advises, guides, and promotes you in your career. A mentor can be any successful, experienced nurse who is committed to a professional career and to being a key figure in your life for a number of years while you are going through school, as well as when you graduate. Mentors should have your best interest at heart and bolster your self-confidence. Mentors should be able to give feedback in a highly constructive, supportive atmosphere. As a result, trust and caring are hallmarks of the bonding that occurs between mentor and mentee. In short, a mentor is "a wise and trusted adviser" who can serve you well as you progress through school (Figure 3-4).

A mentoring relationship is an evolving, personal experience for both mentor and mentee. It involves a personal investment of the mentor in the direction of the mentee's professional development. The mentor also benefits from the association by gaining an awareness and perspective of the recent mentee's role in nursing. Take note of the characteristics of successful mentors listed in Box 3-2.

What Is the Role of the Mentee?

As a mentee, you will be learning and absorbing the useful information that the mentor provides. Before seeking a mentor, there are a few questions you may want to ask yourself that may help you get exactly what you need from the mentoring relationship (Critical Thinking Box 3-2) (Shea, 1999).

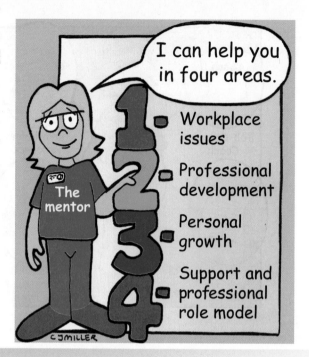

FIGURE 3-4
The mentor role.

BOX 3-2	Characteristics of Successful Mentors

- Make a personal commitment to be involved with mentee for an extended period of time
- Are trustworthy and sincere
- Show mutual respect
- Are not in a position of authority over the mentee
- Promote an easy, give-and-take relationship and are flexible and open
- Able to listen and accept different points of view
- Are experienced
- Have values and goals compatible with those of the mentee
- Are able to empathize with mentee's struggles
- Are nurturing
- Have a good sense of humor and enjoy nursing

CRITICAL THINKING
BOX 3-2

- What are my objectives for developing this mentoring relationship?
- What are my goals?
- How can a mentor help me achieve my goals?
- What is the best way for me to approach a possible mentor to gain his or her interest in developing a mentoring relationship?

TABLE 3-1 Mentee Checklist						
WHEN MEETING WITH YOUR MENTOR, DO YOU ...	ALWAYS	FREQUENTLY	USUALLY	SELDOM	NEVER	SCORE
Communicate clearly						
Welcome your mentor's input (express appreciation or tell him or her how it will benefit you)						
Accept constructive feedback						
Practice openness and sincerity						
Take initiative to maintain the relationship with your mentor						
Actively explore options with your mentor						
Share results with your mentor						
Listen for the whole message, including mentor's feelings						
Be alert for mentor's nonverbal communication, and use it as data						

Score yourself as follows: always = 10; frequently = 8; usually = 6; seldom = 4; never = 2. According to Shea, a score of 80 or better means you are among the limited group of individuals who have good mentee interaction skills (Shea, 1999, p 46).
Adapted From Shea GF: *Making the most of being mentored: how to grow from a mentoring relationship*, Lanham, Md: Crisp Publications, 1999.

What Are the Characteristics of a Mentee?

Just exactly what are important characteristics that you, as a mentee, should project in your interpersonal communications with your mentor? Use the checklist in Table 3-1 to answer the questions in the table.

How did you score? Are there areas that you need to improve in your interpersonal skills to make you a better mentee?

What Are the Types of Mentoring Relationships?

There are several types of mentoring relationships that you may experience when you develop an active relationship with your mentor (Table 3-2). Formal, informal, and situational mentoring relationships are three types that are commonly encountered (Shea, 1999).

TABLE 3-2 Types of Mentoring Relationships			
	FORMAL	INFORMAL	SITUATIONAL
Structure	Traditional/structured	Voluntary/very flexible	Brief contact/often casual
Characteristic	Driven by organizational needs	Mutual acceptance of roles	A one-time event
Effectiveness	Results measured by organization frequently	Periodic check-ups by supervisors	Results assessed later

Adapted from Shea GF: *Making the most of being mentored: how to grow from a mentoring partnership, Lanham,* Md: Crisp Publications, 1999, pp 73-75.

Mentoring Through Reality Shock

The hospital setting is the largest setting where nurses work. In this setting, formal preceptorship programs are usually established, and a mentoring environment is fostered for the new graduate to address the issues of reality shock. This type of mentoring setting appeals to many new graduates, because it provides support from other health care team members. Remember Kramer's phases of reality shock in Chapter 1? Let us see how an effective mentorship relationship could address each of the phases.

Honeymoon Phase. The mentor can be supportive by listening and understanding when the mentee shares the excitement of starting their new position and passing the NCLEX Exam. The mentor can act as an intermediary with other staff members and as a role model.

Shock or Rejection Phase. Mentors can encourage mentees to discuss their feelings of disillusionment and frustration, as well as share their own personal transition process through this phase. Asking mentees to write down their feelings (keep a reflection journal) or discuss ideas to make changes to the situation can be helpful in mitigating the feelings associated with this phase.

Recovery Phase. The mentor's role during this phase, as mentees begin to accept the reality of the situation and put issues in perspective, is to maintain an open channel of communication and encourage mentees to "step outside their comfort zone" and try new things.

Resolution Phase. Mentors are very instrumental during this phase to reinforce positive qualities that the mentee possesses and to encourage the mentee in problem-solving any issues relating to the desire to either change nursing positions or to stay put. *It is important to remember that any nurse may experience reality shock throughout her or his career when she or he enters a new work area* (Brunt, 2005).

What Does the Future Hold?

The future of mentoring programs is changing. Because of technological advancements that have made it possible to offer nursing programs online, a new wave of mentoring has evolved, known as E-mentoring. The term *E-mentoring* simply means any type of mentoring partnership that takes place in an online modality (National Heart Lung and Blood Institute, 2012). The National Heart Lung and Blood Institute (NHLBI) has launched an E-mentoring program for all college students and graduate students continuing their education in a science-related field (NHLBI,

2012, para 1.). An advantage of E-mentoring is that mentoring can occur at anytime; there are no time or physical constraints that may occur in a face-to-face mentoring partnership (Evidence-Based Practice Box 3-2).

Peer mentoring programs are developing in campuses throughout the United States. These programs allow senior-level nursing students to mentor entering freshman nursing students. Peer mentoring can be an effective collaborative clinical teaching model for use as a capstone course or preceptorship for senior-level nursing students (Evidence-Based Practice Box 3-3, and Box 3-1).

BOX 3-2   EVIDENCE-BASED PRACTICE

E-Mentoring

PRACTICE ISSUE

Formalized orientation programs traditionally are offered onsite at the new graduate nurses employing institution following their hire. Throughout the orientation, the new nurse is paired with a preceptor, and begins to acquire increased confidence and problem-solving abilities by working with the preceptor in delivering patient care, performing nursing skills, delegating, and communicating with other members of the health care team for a set period of time. A shortage of nursing staff coupled with an increase in the number of nurses retiring from the workforce and limited educational resources pose as a myriad of factors affecting the new graduate nurse's transition into practice.

IMPLICATIONS FOR NURSING PRACTICE

- Develop or adapt an e-mentoring model where a portion of the new graduate nurse's orientation program occurs in a blended learning environment consisting of both an online component and onsite at the institution.
- The online component would consist of the new graduate nurse and mentor. Seek mentors for the online course who possess leadership skills, are committed to communicating with the new nurse in an online environment, maintain professionalism, and are familiar with using the technology (e.g., e-mail, posting discussions in an online discussion thread).
- Miller and colleagues (2008) conducted a study on the effectiveness of e-mentoring in public health nursing by evaluating experiences gained of both students and mentors and concluded that the students (practicing nurses completing a public health nursing course) gained greater confidence in understanding population-based practice, and developed skills "in problem-solving, coordinating, and identifying best practices" (p 397) in public health nursing.

Considering This Information:

What are your thoughts on E-mentoring? What strategies would you use to maintain a consistent and open line of communication with your e-mentor? What do you feel you will benefit most from as a mentee in utilizing an e-mentoring approach?

Reference for the Evidence

Miller L, et al: E-mentoring in public health nursing practice, *J Contin Ed Nurs* 39(9):394-399, 2008. doi:10.3928/00220124-20080901-02.

BOX 3-3 EVIDENCE-BASED PRACTICE

Peer Mentoring

PRACTICE ISSUE

Peer mentoring involves a shared learning experience where a senior nursing student mentors a beginning or freshmen nursing student in fine-tuning nursing skills, assisting with test-taking strategies and study tips, and in sharing strategies for being successful in nursing school. According to Dennison (2010), peer mentoring has the potential to address the looming clinical site shortage and decreased number of faculty by having a component of the senior nursing student's clinical experience include a peer mentoring role in the nursing laboratory where he/she works with first and second-semester nursing students in learning how to operate medical equipment and perform nursing skills.

IMPLICATIONS FOR NURSING PRACTICE

- The mentors (senior nursing students) gain leadership skills and professional role development behaviors by mentoring other nursing students in the nursing program.
- The mentor maintains competency with nursing skills as he/she is continually teaching the skills to mentees in the nursing laboratory.
- The mentees (beginning or second-year nursing students) gain experience with learning nursing skills and may be more comfortable performing these skills in front of a student than a clinical instructor (Dennison, 2010).
- The mentee can take advantage of working one-on-one with a mentor in the nursing lab.
- Addresses decreased clinical site availability by including peer mentoring as a component of the student's capstone course.

Considering This Information:

What attributes would you look for in a peer mentor to assist you in performing various nursing functions in the skills lab? What do you feel might be a potential challenge(s) in working with a peer mentor? How will you plan to overcome these challenges?

Reference

Dennison S: Peer mentoring: Untapped potential, *Journal of Nursing Education* 49(6):340–342, 2010. doi:10.3928/01484834-20100217-04.

CONCLUSION

Here is one final note about mentorship: There is a short anecdotal story about "Everybody, Somebody, Anybody, and Nobody" that has become part of Internet lore. I think you will understand that Everybody has to realize the importance of advancing the field of nursing through mentorship; your task will be to find that Somebody willing to extend a hand to guide you through the process.

There was an important job to be done, and Everybody was sure that Somebody would do it. Anybody could have done it, but Nobody did it. Somebody got angry about that, because it was Everybody's job. Everybody thought Anybody could do it, but Nobody realized that Everybody wouldn't do it. It ended up that Everybody blamed Somebody, when Nobody did what Anybody could have.

Mentoring is a complex, interpersonal, emotional relationship. All parties involved in a mentoring relationship benefit from a mutual exchange of information, life experiences, and diversity. Mentoring is defined as a developmental, empowering, and nurturing relationship that extends over time (Vance and Olson, 1998). It involves mutual sharing, learning, and growth that occur in an atmosphere of respect and affirmation (Bower, 2000). A mentor has been described as a role model and guide who encourages and inspires. We leave you with this thought …

"There are two ways of spreading light: to be the candle or the mirror that receives it."
—EDITH WHARTON

BIBLIOGRAPHY

American Association of Colleges of Nursing (AACN) and University HealthSystem Consortium (UHC). (2012). Nurse Residency Program. Retrieved from http://www.aacn.nche.edu/education-resources/nurse-residency-program.

Billings D, Halstead J: *Teaching in nursing: a guide for faculty*, ed 3, St. Louis, 2009, Saunders.

Bower E: Mentoring others. In Bower EL, editors: *Nurses taking the lead*, Philadelphia, 2000, Saunders, pp 11–14.

Bratt M: Retaining the next generation of nurses: the Wisconsin Nurse Residency Program provides a continuum of support, *J Contin Ed Nurs* 40(9):416–425, 2009.

Brunt B: Beyond precepting: developing mentor skills. Retrieved from www.nursce.com/courses/1067/1067.htm.

Emerson, R. J. (2007). *Nursing education in the clinical setting*. St. Louis, MO: Elsevier.

Gibbons A (2004): Mentoring definitions. Retrieved from *www.coachingnetwork.org.uk/ResourceCentre/Articles/ViewArticle.asp?artId=54*.

Guest AB: A coach, a mentor … a what? *Success Now* 13, 1999.

Institute of Medicine of the National Academies (IOM). (2010). *The Future of Nursing: Leading Change, Advancing Health* (Consensus report). Retrieved from http://www.iom.edu/Reports/2010/The-Future-of-Nursing-Leading-Change-Advancing-Health.aspx

International Coach Federation (2008): What is coaching? Retrieved from *www.coachfederation.org*.

NCSBN (National Council of State Boards of Nursing) (2008b): NCSBN transition to practice report. Retrieved from *www.ncsbn.org/388.htm*.

NCSBN (National Council of State Boards of Nursing) (2008): NCSBN Transition to practice model. Retrieved from *www.ncsbn.org/TransitiontoPracticeRegulatoryModel_100209.pdf*.

NHLBI (National Heart Lung and Blood Institute) (2012). *eMentoring: An online mentoring initiative*. Retrieved from http://www.nhlbi.nih.gov/ementoring/index.htm

Peddy S: *The art of mentoring*, Houston, 2001, Bullion Books.

Shea G: *Making the most of being mentored: how to grow from a mentoring relationship*, Lanham, Md, 1999, Crisp Publications.

Vance, C, Olson RK: Discovering the riches in mentor connections, *Reflections on nursing leadership: Sigma Theta Tau International Honor Society of Nursing* 26(3):24–25, 1998.

Yoder LH: Coaching makes nurses' careers grow, *NurseWeek* 14(10):36–38, 2007.

Additional resources are available online at *http://evolve.elsevier.com/Zerwekh/nsgtoday/.*

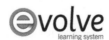

CHAPTER 4

Employment Considerations: Opportunities, Resumes, and Interviewing

JoAnn Zerwekh, MSN, EdD, RN

School is almost over and the dream of being paid as an RN (Real Nurse) will soon come true!

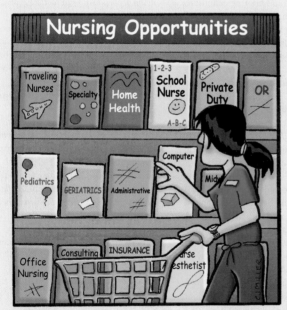

After completing this chapter, you should be able to:

- Assess trends in the job market.
- Identify the primary aspects of obtaining employment.
- Describe the key aspects of a resume.
- Describe the essential steps involved in the interviewing process.
- Discuss the typical questions asked by interviewers.
- Analyze your own priorities and needs in a job.
- Develop short-term career goals.

Nursing offers more job possibilities than any other aspect of health care. So if your first choice doesn't work out, select another specialty!

Thanks to the previous authors of this chapter, Alice B. Pappas, PhD, RN, and Jo Carol Claborn, MS, RN.

*W*ith graduation in sight, you are excited but probably a little anxious about moving into the workplace, looking for the perfect match to your hard-earned degree. As you consider possible employment opportunities, prepare for the upcoming job search as you would any graded class assignment: Do your homework! Careful preparation is the key to finding a job you really want. Very few worthwhile job offers come to someone who just happens to walk into the human resource department. The continued expansion of the health care field and the growing nursing shortage has created tremendous opportunities for recent graduates. You have developed marketable skills that are in demand, but to sell yourself successfully to prospective employers and get the job you really want, you must do some "homework."

> Take some time to brainstorm about a career—if you could go anywhere you wanted to in nursing, where would it be?

Give yourself plenty of time to consider what type of position you want and need, in addition to the possibilities and limitations of the job market under consideration. You can compare the process with the selection of a marriage partner, car, home, or any other major life choice. It is important for nurses to take the time to create a career plan. Your first professional position is a stepping stone in a long nursing career; it will help define who you are and influence your career path. Only *you* can determine the path you want to travel, so it is important that you become informed and selective in the process. Too often, new graduates accept their first job without sufficient awareness of their own needs or knowledge about the employer they select. Your work is a major factor in your life. If you simply go to work every day, put in your time, and go home, then your job will manage you. If your work enriches your life, is exciting, and you have a feeling of fulfillment, then you are in charge. As a graduate nurse, you have a choice—to do nothing or to take charge of the direction you want to go. However, as the Cheshire Cat was well aware, only Alice could make the choice as to the direction she should go (Figure 4-1). Although there is no guarantee that a job will be a perfect fit, career dissatisfaction and turnover can be decreased if careful consideration is given to possible job selection *before* you send out your resume and schedule an interview.

This chapter provides some guidelines to a thorough background preparation for your job search. Critical Thinking Box 4-1 will help you identify your clinical interests and the possible reasons for these preferences. Hint: This will also help you answer interview questions about your professional interests.

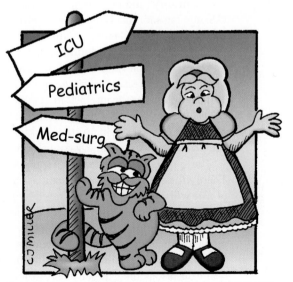

FIGURE 4-1

Choose carefully where you want to go.

CRITICAL THINKING BOX 4-1	ASSESS YOUR WANTS AND DESIRES, LIKES AND DISLIKES

Identify your interests and the possible reasons for them.

INTERESTS   **REASONS**

1. I prefer to work with patients whose age is
   _____.   _____

2. I prefer to work in a small hospital versus a large   _____
   medical center _____.   _____

3. I prefer rotating shifts versus straight shifts   _____
   _____.   _____

4. I prefer an internship versus general orientation   _____
   _____.   _____

5. I prefer to have a set routine or a constantly changing   _____
   environment _____.   _____

6. I prefer these areas (e.g., geriatrics, pediatrics,   _____
   community, health, medical)   _____

   _____.   _____

7. Which of my religious beliefs or values might have an   _____
   impact on where I work?   _____

   _____.

WHAT IS HAPPENING IN THE JOB MARKET?

For the last few years it has been impossible to read an article about the health field that does not mention the nursing shortage, the "looming nursing shortage," or the "worst nursing shortage in U.S. history" and despite the current easing of the nursing shortage due to the recession, the U.S. nursing shortage is projected to grow to 260,000 registered nurses by 2025 (Buerhaus et al., 2009). The "2008 Registered Nurse Population", a survey conducted every 4 years by Health Resources and Services Administration, noted that the average age of all licensed RNs increased to 47 years in 2008 from 46.8 in 2004, which represents a stabilization after many years of continuing large increases in average age. Nearly 45% of RNs were 50 years of age or older in 2008, a dramatic increase from 33% in 2000 and 25% in 1980 (HRSA, 2010). According to Carlson (2009), the recession has changed retirement plans for many older nurses. This means that experienced nurses are staying in the workforce; however, Buerhaus et al. (2009), point to a rapidly aging workforce as a primary contributor to the future projected shortage.

The graying of the American population will have a large impact on the health care industry. There will continue to be a substantial increase in the number of older patients, and their levels of care will vary widely from assisted living settings to high-technology environments.

What will happen with nursing employment, the job market, and health care when a large percentage of nurses become part of the older generation? What effort will hospitals make to retain older nurses as the economic recession recovers? Who will mentor the new nurses and help them develop critical decision-making skills at the bedside? How will the role of simulation help bridge the gap between textbook learning and clinical decision-making? The current and continuing shortage in nursing personnel will dramatically heighten the need for increased efficiencies in clinical education for new graduates and improved patient outcomes. How will

What changes have you observed as a result of the nursing shortage? What impact has the shortage had on salaries and staffing in your community? If the signs of a nursing shortage were beginning to surface in the late 1990s, why haven't we (education, health care employers, government) created effective solutions to this growing problem yet?

the job market continue to evolve for the graduate nurse during the next 5 years? Only one thing is certain—everything will continue to change at an increased pace (Critical Thinking Box 4-2).

SELF-ASSESSMENT

What Are My Clinical Interests?

Begin by jotting down possible settings where you could pursue your areas of clinical interest. Depending on your interests, there will be a number of possible paths to pursue. As you identify areas of clinical interest, try to prioritize them. This step may seem like a nonissue if you tend to "eat, sleep, and drink" one nursing specialty; however, many people have two or more strong interests, and this step helps to outline some possibilities. Believe it or not, some graduating students confess to liking *every* clinical rotation and feel pulled in multiple directions when they consider where to begin a job search. If that description fits you, hang in there—you are not alone! Keep in mind that all nursing experiences, both negative and positive, can contribute to your career in a productive way. The more areas you sample, the broader your knowledge base as you gradually build a career.

Recruiters like to see flexibility in new graduates, but let us try to narrow your professional interests just a bit before your actual job search. Perhaps you can identify what you liked about each clinical rotation through reflective journaling and then prioritize possible interests or identify common experiences.

What Are My Likes and Dislikes?

Another way to approach self-assessment involves identification of your likes and dislikes in the work setting. This is related to interests, but on a more personal level. The job you eventually select may have some drawbacks, but it should meet many more of your likes than dislikes in order to be a good "fit" (Figure 4-2).

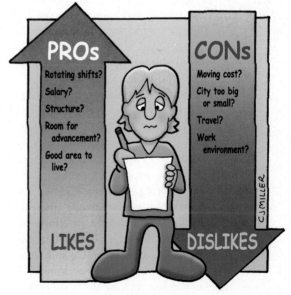

FIGURE 4-2

Assessing personal needs and interests. Is the job a good fit?

Write out your responses to the following questions:

1. Do you enjoy an environment that provides a great deal of patient interaction, or do you thrive in a technically oriented routine? Think back to your clinical rotations and see if you can find a pattern to what was most enjoyable or disagreeable.
   - I liked opportunities for using many technical skills.
   - I was bored with slower-paced routines (e.g., mother-infant care).
   - I liked to see the results of care as soon as possible (e.g., PACU).
   - I disliked the constant turnover of patients every day (e.g., ED).

2. Do you enjoy caring intensively for one or two patients at a time with a high acuity level and a potential rapid change in patient status, or do you prefer a patient assignment less acute with opportunities for family education and observing increased patient independence? Why did you like or dislike one type or the other? Discuss your responses with some friends who may have had other experiences and get their opinions. Consider how you will explain your preferences to a nurse recruiter on the phone, in an online cover letter, or in person.

3. Do you learn best in a highly structured environment or in more informal on-the-job training situations? Knowing your learning style can guide your interest and narrow your selection of an internship or orientation program. For example, internships range from formal classes with lengthy preceptorships to more informal orientations of fairly short duration. Remember, a program that meets your needs may not be the answer for your best friend. Write down what you would like from an orientation or internship program. Look over your list and prioritize what you need and want most.

4. Do you feel comfortable functioning with a significant degree of autonomy, or do you want and need more direction and supervision at this point in your professional development? Shortly, you will have completed nursing school, backed up by employment on a telemetry unit throughout your senior year. Are you ready to be a charge nurse on the 3 to 11 PM shift in a small rural hospital, or do you want a slower transition to such responsibility? If this situation was offered, would you be flattered, frightened, or flabbergasted? Write down your reaction and consider how you would respond to the recruiter who offers you such a position.

5. How much physical energy are you able and willing to expend at work? Running 8 to 12 hours a day may or may not act as a tonic. Think back to the pace of your clinical rotations, and consider how your body reacted (minus the anxiety associated with instructor supervision, if you can!). Would you prefer a unit that has some predictable periods of frenzy and pause, or do you thrive on the unpredictable for your entire work shift?

6. Are you a day, evening, or night person? Are there certain times of the day when you are at your peak of performance? How about your worst? Be honest and realistic with your answers. Very few people are equally efficient and effective 24 hours a day. If your body shuts down at 10 PM, or you resist all efforts to wake up before 9 AM, a certain shift may need to be eliminated. However, if the job market is tight in your area of interest, the available positions may be on a less-desirable shift and you may need to make adjustments in other areas of your life to temporarily acclimate better to a professional position.

7. Do you like rotating shifts, or, perhaps more realistically, can you work rotating shifts? One aspect of reality shock for many new graduates is the realization that working the day shift may have ended with the last clinical rotation in school. Hospital and long-term care staffing

is 24 hours a day, 7 days a week. It is a "24/7 profession"—a possibly unpleasant aspect of nursing, but a real one nonetheless. Assess your ability to work certain shifts and try to strike a flexible approach before you speak with nurse recruitment. Working 12-hour shifts (7 AM to 7 PM or 7 PM to 7 AM) can be very demanding on the days assigned, but this option is very popular with many nurses because of the increased days off.

8. Consider the impact of these choices on your family, your social life, and other needs. If there are certain shifts you must rule out, recognize that this may limit your job choices and plan accordingly. Giving some thought to your flexibility ahead of time will help you avoid committing to any and all shifts during an interview and will facilitate your job hunt. On the other hand, it is probably not realistic to request a Monday-through-Friday schedule in an acute care setting unless the organization has a separate weekend staff or a high level of personnel who request to work only weekends. Shift patterns may vary significantly within a city—and in different areas of the country as well—so do your homework online or through job fairs about available shifts before you go in for an actual interview.

9. Can you work long hours (e.g., 12-hour shifts) without too much tension and fatigue? The 12-hour staffing option offers flexibility (e.g., six 12-hour days of work in an 80-hour pay period) but leaves some people exhausted and irritable. Consider your personal needs outside of work when you respond to this item. Can you climb into bed or put your feet up after a nonstop 12-hour shift, or do you need to pick up family responsibilities as soon as you walk in the door? The 4 days off may well compensate for 3 days of fatigue, but map out your needs before you begin your job search.

10. Do you like making decisions quickly or generally favor a more relaxed approach to clinical problems? In general, ICU and step-down units require more immediate reactions than an adolescent psych unit or orthopedics. Does the ICU environment excite or overwhelm you? Would you prefer a slower pace? Do not criticize yourself for your likes or dislikes. Slower-paced units require different strengths, not less knowledge. You have nothing to gain by working in an ICU if you dislike the setting. Meet your own needs, not someone else's. You will spend a great deal of your time at work. Make the choice for you, not someone else's idea of the perfect job.

11. What do you need in a job to be happy? This question does not mean money or benefits, but rather the sense that the job is worth getting excited about. Think about past employment you have had, whether in health care or not. What did you like or dislike about the job? What made you stay? Possible answers include opportunities for growth, advancement, working with people you respect, or collegiality. Remember, your answers should include things that are important to you. These are the kind of issues that make you eager to go to work or to help you work through difficult clinical days. You may want to compare your answers with those of others whose opinions you value to gain a broader perspective.

What Are My Personal Needs and Interests?

A third aspect of self-assessment focuses on personal needs and interests. How much time and effort are you willing and able to give to your career at this point in time? Will work be a number-one priority in your life, or does family or continued education take precedence?

Is relocation a possibility? If you are considering relocation, decide how you will gather information on possible job opportunities in the area or areas under consideration. Include Internet websites, professional journals, and professional and family contacts as possible sources of information. In addition to reviewing online job possibilities, research the hospital's website for details about the organization's overall philosophy, its department of nursing, and a sense of "fit." Prospective employers want to know that applicants have taken the time to become knowledgeable about them and appreciate when applicants ask more informed questions about employment.

If this is a voluntary move, develop a list of pros and cons for each location under consideration. Include your personal interests in the decision (e.g., cost of living, commuting time, possible relocation allowance, access to recreational activities, opportunities for advanced education, and clinical opportunities).

What salary range are you willing to consider? Although starting salaries for new graduates are generally nonnegotiable, differentials for evenings, nights, and weekends create a range of salary possibilities. If you want an extended internship, a lower starting salary may be offered. Are you willing and able to trade this for the benefits of an extended internship? The quality of the internship may be worth a lower salary temporarily because of later advancement opportunities. Some areas of the country offer considerably higher salaries than others, but factor in the cost of living before you move out of town. You may be unpleasantly surprised by a monthly rent that swallows up a significant percentage of your salary.

What Are My Career Goals?

The final step of your self-assessment is the development of career goals. Yes, you really do need to have some goals! You are the architect of your professional future, so take pen to paper or fingers to the keyboard and start designing. Consider your answers to the following questions.

What do you want from your first nursing position? Possible answers might include developing confidence in decision making, more proficiency with technical skills, and increased organizational abilities.

What are your professional goals for the first year? Third year? Fifth year? If you cannot imagine your life, let alone your career, beyond 1 to 2 years, relax. Many people feel uneasy planning beyond their initial position and first paid vacation.

Develop a comfortable response to a question regarding your goals for the first year and consider what you might want to be doing after that time. Remember, it is far easier to gauge how your career is progressing if you have established some benchmark goals to which you can refer. This is also a favorite question posed during interviews, so spend some time thinking about it! Recruiters are interested in nurses with a plan.

RESEARCHING PROSPECTIVE EMPLOYERS

What Employment Opportunities Are Available?

You have a world of nursing to choose from; there are opportunities available to begin your practice as a graduate nurse. The largest employers are hospitals or acute care facilities. In hospitals, a wide variety of positions are available, although new graduates are almost always placed in staff nurse positions. If it is a general hospital, you need to choose what areas interest you most. Your first position may not be exactly what you want, but remember, it is the first step toward your career goal. As you build your competence and self-esteem, you may find just the position you want. In many hospitals, staff positions represent different levels of proficiency, especially if the hospital participates in clinical or career ladders (Figure 4-3).

The staff nurse position can be one of the most challenging. It can also be like an "incubator" from which to develop your nursing career.

Charge positions may involve responsibility for a particular staff or a particular day, or they may involve managing staff for an entire unit. New graduates should not be placed in charge positions until they have mastered a staff nurse role, but the marketplace may result in new graduates being offered the charge position, especially in more rural settings. If this is a situation that you will face soon after graduation, make sure that you identify your resources and consider whom you can contact for professional support and backup. Do not allow your ego to let you accept an unsafe position that could endanger patients and your hard-earned nursing license.

Entry-level positions in the hospital are usually staff nurse positions. Staff nurse positions in medical-surgical nursing are some of the most demanding—and rewarding—positions. Frequently, nurses begin their careers here with the intention of moving on to greener pastures; however, the rewards and challenges may more than fulfill their needs. It is important that your first position offers you an opportunity to further develop your nursing skills. Surely, you have heard at least one person in nursing school say to you, "You should get a year's experience in Med-Surg first." Is this a true statement? Yes and no. Yes, if you want to work in a medical-surgical field, and no, if you do not. Yes, the experience will help sharpen assessment skills and some technical skills, but every area of work has advantages and potential drawbacks. If you know in your heart that med-surg makes you miserable, turn around and go in a different direction. Life is too short to be miserable for 8 to 12 hours a day. Furthermore, chances are that you will not give your best to the patients if you are unhappy.

Whether it is working in the emergency department, day surgery, specialty units, or medical-surgical units, staff nurse positions give you a very valuable opportunity to polish your time management, patient care organization, and nursing skills. Once you are confident with skills, procedures, and the overall practice of nursing, you may be ready to move on to new challenges. This may take 6 months for some recent graduates. For others, it may take a year or more. Take the time to reinforce your nursing competencies; it will prepare you for your future practice in nursing. Other areas in which nurses may find employment include community health, home health care, and nursing agencies. Working in the community in such positions as occupational health, school health, and the

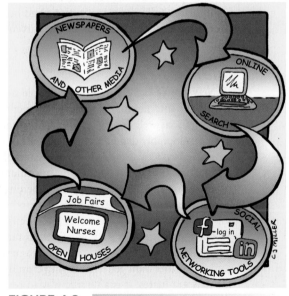

FIGURE 4-3

Ways to research prospective employers.

military may require a bachelor's degree in nursing and at least 1 year of hospital nursing. If you want to work in a community setting, concentrate initially on refining your assessment and critical thinking skills in the acute care setting, because the autonomy of the community setting means more decision making on your own without the immediate backup of experienced peers who are usually available in the acute care setting.

What About Advanced Degrees in Nursing?

There are many advantages to earning an advanced degree in nursing (review Chapter 7 for the different choices). One of the most important aspects of obtaining an advanced degree is using your experience as a nurse to help you determine in what direction you want to go. If you have an associate's degree, you might want to consider the basic requirements for your bachelor's degree, including what schools are available and what their requirements are. This is an area you can begin to work on immediately after graduation. As you interview for jobs, ask whether the prospective employer will work with your schedule if you decide to go back to school and if they provide tuition reimbursement for continuing education.

HOW DO I GO ABOUT RESEARCHING PROSPECTIVE EMPLOYERS?

Employment Considerations: How Do You Decide on an Employer?

In 1980, the American Academy of Nursing identified criteria for the designation of "magnet hospitals." This designation recognized certain hospitals for their lower turnover rates, their visionary leaders, the value they placed on education, and an ability to maintain open lines of communication. To identify magnet hospitals in your area, check the website *www.nursecredentialing.org/magnet/searchmagnet.cfm* (ANCC, 2010). In your search for a job, it is important to look for institutions and hospitals that create a work environment that supports professional nursing practice. In the current job market, locating magnet hospitals in your community is an important consideration in your job search.

Media Information

Newspapers. Although many people no longer look at the newspaper for information, preferring the Internet for data, the newspaper still remains a good place to access useful information about jobs, as well as articles about hospitals or other health care employment issues. This will vary considerably depending on the area of the country where you are hoping to work. Scan the advertisements to see whether any are targeted specifically to graduating seniors. Focus on these initially because they will include information on possible job fairs, internships, or specialized orientations, in addition to specific openings for graduate nurses.

Online Searches. Electronic job searches have replaced newspapers for many people as the top place to start looking for employment. This is an efficient way to search because you can access information for both local and distant nursing opportunities with the ease of a few clicks, assuming that sites are kept current. As a new graduate, consider the value of looking at employer websites rather than generic nursing employment sites because employer sites are better focused for new graduates. It is a terrific way to review the positions available within the entire institution. If you intend to use this method to follow up on a job posting, be prepared to submit your flawless resume electronically—and be sure to spell-check all of your correspondence before you click the "Send" button! Many institutions now require electronic applications, occasionally raising issues of software compatibility for applicants. Know and be prepared to comply with human resources requirements for submitting your resume and cover letter. Patience in the application process is essential for your professional success. With the availability of computer spell checking and editing support, there is no excuse for a poorly written resume or cover letter. Take the time to review your documents for errors. Recruiters pay attention to these details.

Social Networking. Social networking is the way the 21st century seems to communicate with each other in online websites that consist of a community of individuals with like-minded interests. According to the February 2010 PEW Internet report, approximately 72% of young adults use social network sites and some 40% of adults 30 and older use some type of social sites, such as Facebook, MySpace™, and Twitter™. The survey results also reported that among adults 18 and older, Facebook has taken over as the social network of choice; 73% of adult profile owners use Facebook, 48% have a profile on MySpace™, and 14% use LinkedIn® (Lenhart et al., 2010).

In a 2009 CareerBuilder Survey, it was reported that 45% of employers use social networking online websites to screen future employees. So, if you are trying to make a good impression, then your appearance on the social networking website will be what an employer first sees. Be sure to use a professional photo, perhaps just a headshot, and make your Facebook account private to prevent employers from searching for you, if you want to use the Facebook account for family and friends. Potential employers may dismiss you as a candidate after viewing inappropriate photographs or information. A recent study by ExecuNet found that 77% of recruiters run searches of candidates on the Web to screen applicants and 35% of these same recruiters say they have eliminated a candidate based on the information they uncovered. As the amount of personal information available online grows via sources such as MySpace™, Facebook, Twitter™, and the like, first impressions are being formed long before the interview process begins, warns David Opton, ExecuNet CEO and founder. "Given the implications and the shelf-life of Internet content, managing your online image is something everyone should address—regardless of whether or not you're in a job search," he says (Lorenz, 2009).

LinkedIn® is a site that is primarily for job networking. LinkedIn has become the place for reconnecting with colleagues and classmates, as well as powering your career with a vast network of contacts and employers looking for the right employee. As Copland (2007) says increasingly, if you're not LinkedIn®, you may be "left out" finding the right type of position, if you do not have a profile. LinkedIn® allows you to link to your professional Twitter™ or blog and upload your resume to your profile, which definitely comes in handy for interested employers.

Job Fairs/Open Houses. You may have the opportunity to attend a nursing job fair or hospital open house as a soon-to-be graduate nurse. Take advantage of this opportunity to collect information about specific employers and possibly make initial contacts for later interviews. Leave your jeans and tennis shoes at home on these occasions, however. Take some time with your appearance, because first impressions are important! (Figure 4-4)

Employee Contacts. If you have a friend or family member—or simply know someone—who works at an institution you are considering for employment, make an effort to speak with him or her about the job environment. As an insider, this person may be able to provide you with a perspective about the employer that the advertisement, recruiter, or interview cannot. Possible questions you may want to ask such an insider may include these: "Why do you enjoy working there? What was orientation like? How is employee morale? What is the turnover rate for nursing or for other employees?"

Recruitment Contacts

Letter-Writing Campaign. Plan to send your resume with a cover letter and triple-check both documents for grammatical errors. Your resume and cover letter are the first impression you will make with a prospective employer. Make it a positive one!

Telephone Contact. Before you pick up the telephone, get out your calendar and start planning likely dates for possible interviews, as well as the approximate date you want to begin working. Armed with this information, you can comfortably answer questions beyond the fact that you would like the employer to send you a brochure and an application. Depending on the institution you contact, the human resources or nurse recruitment department may want you to first submit a resume online or may ask you to set up an appointment for an interview. Do not commit to an interview if you are not ready.

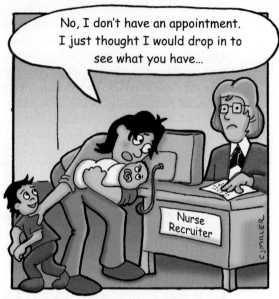

FIGURE 4-4

The first impression is a lasting one, so make it count for you, not against you.

Personal Contact. If you plan to just stop by human resources or nurse recruitment for a brochure and an application, make sure you give some thought to your appearance. Tee shirts, shorts, and jeans are not appropriate and have caused otherwise well-qualified applicants to be passed over for further consideration. Again, remember that first impression!

WHAT DO I NEED TO KNOW TO ASSESS THE ORGANIZATION?

Now that you have described yourself and have thought about the kind of setting in which you work best, continue these exercises on a consistent basis. This ongoing analysis will help you make decisions about the kind of organization that is best for you and put you in a position to determine what kind of organization fits you.

How Do You Go About Assessing an Organization to Find What You Want?

Talk to People in the Organization. One obvious answer is to ask the people who work in that organization. When you interview for a position, you can meet people who work in the specific setting in which you are interested. Ask questions that will help you learn about certain situations. Take some time to think about questions and situations you would like to present when you talk to people in various facilities. Keep in mind that the values of the organization will affect your work on a daily basis. If both patients and employees are valued, you will see this reflected in the quality of patient care and in the retention of nurses.

CRITICAL THINKING BOX 4-3	What are some observations that you could have during your interview process that would cause you to have second thoughts about accepting a position at the institution?

Read and Analyze the Recruitment Materials. Organizations also present themselves to you through their documents. Carefully analyze the materials presented to you—this is another way of determining the values the organization lives by and deems important. All of these materials are intended to make a statement to you about who they are.

Is There a Mission or Philosophy Statement? There are other written documents to examine. For example, a specific nursing unit may have a mission statement that tells you who they are and what they are about. The department of nursing will have a philosophy statement or possibly a nursing theory that should be the organizing framework around which the members structure themselves in delivering nursing care. In some organizations, the staff knows what this mission statement says and how it provides direction to them. In other organizations, the staff will be unfamiliar with the statement of philosophy and may react with confusion when you ask them. All of these written materials should send a message to you about the organization. Do your observations during the interview process support the organization mission/philosophy statements? (Critical Thinking Box 4-3)

Evaluate the Reputation of the Leadership. Organizations are guided by people at the top and take on the characteristics these people support. What do you know about the chief executive officer? This person sets the stage and the direction for the organization. You can gather information about the chief executive officer by checking the website and asking people during the interview what this person is like. People in the community will also be familiar with this person and can give you insight into the values and characteristics that this person represents.

The same can be said for the chief nursing officer (CNO). This person sets the direction for the nursing organization, either by active design or benign neglect, and sets into motion an organization that structures the beliefs about patients, staff, and nursing. It is important to talk with nurses who are working with the CNO to determine how they feel about the leadership in the organization. Has he or she had a successful track record? Is this person well respected? Can people point to a strategic direction and philosophy this person has given to the organization?

RESUME WRITING

How Do I Write an Effective Resume?

Design your resume by using the KISS principle: Keep It Simple, Sincerely! (That is, use concise wording and make it easy-to-read, informational, and simple.)

Your resume is the first introduction a prospective employer will have to you. It will give the employer a basic idea of who you are professionally and what your objectives are for your nursing career. While defining your strengths, it is important not to overstate your skills. Everything that

> **BOX 4-1   Resume Guidelines**
>
> - Catch all typos and grammatical errors. Have someone proofread your resume.
> - Present a clear objective that emphasizes your skills and strengths.
> - A good first impression is critical, so if written, your resume should be neat and printed on white or off-white paper.
> - Avoid using "I" or "me" in your resume.
> - Keep the information concise, preferably limited to one or two pages.
> - The rule of thumb on work experience is to show most current work experience. This generally means the last 10 to 15 years unless there is something in your more distant background that is critical to note.
>
> - Do not try to impress anyone with big words. Jargon specific to the profession is okay if everyone knows what it is.
> - Do not inquire about salary or benefits in your resume. It is not the right time or place for that.
> - Do not exaggerate about what you can and cannot do, because the potential employer will check it out.
> - Present yourself in a positive light.
> - Your resume should be neat and visually appealing.
> - Do not list all of your references. Be prepared to provide them on a separate list when asked. You may want to have different references for different types of positions.

you include on your resume should be true. Expect the employer to check all facts. Do not jeopardize a job possibility by intentional misstatements or careless attention to dates of prior employment or education.

Most employers are willing to train you on all or some of the components of the position you are applying for. A resume is a concise, factual presentation of your educational and professional history (Box 4-1). Do not be surprised if a recruiter suggests other areas to you in addition to what you have initially indicated on your resume or in your interview. Be open to suggestions; they may have some ideas or considerations you have not even thought about.

What Information Is Necessary for a Resume?

Here are the components of a resume. Be sure to proofread what you write for correct spelling and grammar. Do not forget that this is the first impression someone may have of you.

Demographic Data: Who Are You? Your name, address, telephone number, and e-mail address should be at the top of the page. Be sure to give correct, current information so that the employer can easily contact you. If you need to give an alternate telephone number or e-mail address, provide that person's name and advise the person that a prospective employer may be calling for you. Keep in mind that you never put personal information such as your social security number, marital status, number of children, or your picture on a resume. Your e-mail address conveys a message, so do not include anything that sends a "cutesy" or possibly offensive message to an employer. Consider the image you want to convey.

Professional Objective: What Position Are You Applying For? There is a wide variety of ways to address this element. However, it is very important that you describe the position you are applying for and specify what department or area of nursing you are interested in. With the widespread use of the Internet, it is easy to view job openings and be more educated and decisive about what you are looking for. You can identify several areas if you have more than one area of preference. This is your short-term goal. You may also state a long-term goal (e.g., transport, quality assurance, case management, transplant team).

Education: Where Did You Receive Your Education? List your education in chronological order, beginning with the most recent. List the month and year of graduation and what degree was received, if any. If you have degrees other than nursing, include these in the chronological order in which you received them. This section will contain any certifications and special training you have received, where you received them, and the date you completed them. If you are currently enrolled in school, be sure to include that as well.

Professional Experience: What Do You Know How to Do? "Easy to read" is the goal. It is very important to put this section in chronological order beginning with the present. You want the prospective employer to see what you have been doing most recently. List your current or previous employer, position held, dates from and to, and a brief description of your responsibilities. This is a good place to highlight special skills that you feel may be important to your prospective employer. This section will differ for an experienced nurse than for a recent graduate nurse. However, it is important to list your employment history through the past 7 years, including those areas of employment that may not be associated with nursing or the health care field. All the experiences you have had as an "employee" help to demonstrate your ability to work with people, handle stress, be flexible, and so forth. It is not necessary to list clinical rotations you have completed during nursing school, which are mostly standardized. If you have not had any work experience and this will be your first job, state that also. It is important for managers and staff educators to be aware of the levels of experience of recent graduates they consider. If you had an opportunity to take a clinical elective in a specialty area, include that information because it may enhance your application, especially if you apply for a position in that specialty.

Licensure: What Can You Do and Where Can You Do It? This is a very important area of information for nurses. With the implementation of the multistate Nurse Licensure Compact (see Chapters 5 and 20), you may only need to be licensed in one state. It is your responsibility to know which states will honor your license and which ones will require you to obtain a separate license. As a general rule, you will be required to be licensed in the state of your residence, then possibly in another state of practice, depending on the licensure compact of the states involved. List the state in which your license was issued and the expiration date. For security reasons, do not list your license number.

Professional Organizations: What Do You Belong To? You may list organizations in which you are a member or have held an office. You should list professional and community groups. Include any certifications that you have obtained (BLS, ACLS, PALS). This section is optional.

Honors and Awards: What Did You Receive Recognition For? If you have received recognition for special skills or volunteer work, you may want to include it here. You may also include any scholarships you have received. This is also an optional section.

References: Who Knows About You? Be prepared to provide a separate typed sheet that lists at least three references. Provide the names and telephone numbers of three professionals with whom you have worked. Always notify your references that you have listed them and that they may receive a telephone call about you. Look at the example of a resume in Figure 4-5 and adapt it to what works best for you. Make every effort as a new graduate to keep your resume

Linda Smith

123 Any Street

Dallas, TX 77777

972-555-5555

E-mail: lsmith@hotmail.com

Objective:

To obtain a staff nurse position in Hematology-Oncology.

Education:

Memorial High School, Dallas, Texas, graduated 5/2008.

El Centro College, Dallas, Texas

ADN, awarded June, 2011
Experience:

10/2008 to present–Baylor Hospital, Dallas, Texas–nurse tech, part-time

0/2005 to 5/2008–Kroger's Supermarkets, cashier

Licensure:

Eligible for NCLEX May 2008 (Texas)

Certifications: CPR expires 3/3012

Professional Organizations:

Texas Nursing Students Association

References: on Request

FIGURE 4-5
Resume.

on one page because recruiters generally scan the resume in less than 2 minutes. As you gain professional experience a longer resume may become necessary. If you need further examples of resumes or formats, check the Internet for samples *(www.resume.monster.com)*. Many word processing programs also have resume formats that you can access.

What Else Should I Submit with My Resume?

Along with your resume, you should enclose a cover letter that serves as a brief introduction (Box 4-2). Summarize your important strengths or give information regarding change of specialty, but remember that this letter should be brief—about three to five well-written paragraphs on one or two pages *(www.csuchico.edu/plc/cover-letters.html)*. If you have spoken with a recruiter and have a specific name, address the letter to him or her. However, you do not have to address it to a specific person; it will be distributed to the recruiter who handles the units in which you have indicated an interest. Simply addressing it to "Nurse Recruitment" will usually ensure that it gets to the right person. Large institutions may have several recruiters, so a general address to recruitment will often suffice.

What Are the Methods for Submitting Resumes?

There are a variety of ways to submit a resume: hand-carry it, submit it electronically by means of e-mail or the hospital website, or mail it through the post office. Your prospective employer will likely have a preferred method for submission. If their website states that electronic

BOX 4-2	Reminders for Cover Letters

- 8½- by 11-inch paper—white, off-white, or light blue
- Typed, with no mistakes (your first opportunity to wow them with professional style)
- No smudges
- 1½- to 2-inch margins on all sides
- Signed, usually in black ink
- No abbreviations
- Business letter format

submission is required, do not place a printed version in the mail. It is likely to be ignored. One of the most popular methods for nurses to send resumes is through the website of the medical institution where they are interested in obtaining an interview. This is an excellent way to submit your resume, but remember to follow up with a telephone call if you have not heard from a recruiter within 1 week. You can also directly e-mail your resume to a recruiter. E-mail addresses are readily available through business cards, websites, and word of mouth. But beware: Your e-mail first page will serve as the cover letter when you submit your resume by using e-mail. The same resume-writing principles apply to all electronically submitted resumes because your resume will be printed for review.

There are also many large job-search websites available on the Internet. You can post your resume on any of these by using their specific formats, but remember that businesses must pay a fee to search for applicants. It is important to remember that not all of the institutions belong to every job-search website. Use discretion regarding where you want to post your resume; if you are interested in a specific institution, it is best to review their website directly for positions available and guidelines for submitting resumes.

Now that you have your resume ready to submit, you will need to identify prospective employers. Remember, one of the first things you can do is network. Networking is contacting everyone you know and even some people you do not know to get information about specific organizations or institutions. Places where you can network are at your facility during clinical, at nursing student organization programs, at career days at colleges, and at career opportunity fairs. Attend local chapter meetings of nursing organizations. Read nursing journal employment sections. When you have identified the institutions where you would like to discuss possible employment, send them your resume. If you have not heard from them within 7 to 10 days, give them a call to make sure your resume was received and to schedule an interview. Keep a record of contacts and resumes sent so that you will have easy access to all of this information (Figure 4-6). It will be important to document your follow-up actions and results—do not forget to keep copies of correspondence and notes about any conversations with potential employers. Date all entries, briefly note any information received, and indicate all interviews requested and granted, resumes sent, and job offers received. Box 4-3 presents a summary of the steps to finding the job you want.

THE INTERVIEW PROCESS

How Do I Plan My Interview Campaign?

Set Up Your Schedule. Keep the following points in mind:
- Agencies usually have specific dates for orientations, internships, and preceptorships.
- Identify when you want to begin employment, and mark your calendar.

Employer Address and Phone Number	Interviewer and Title	Date Resume Sent	Date and Time of Interview	Inquiry of Application Letter	Application Submitted	"Thank You" Letter Sent After Interview	Job Offer Received	Confirmation of "No Thank You" Letter Sent	Comments or Notes

FIGURE 4-6

Record of employer contacts and resumes sent.

BOX 4-3   Your Checklist for Finding a Job

- Define your goals.
- Develop your resume.
- Identify potential employers.
- Send your resume and cover letter.
- Return a follow-up phone call.
- Schedule an interview.
- Send a follow-up letter.
- Keep a record of employer contacts (see Figure 4-6).
- Make an informed decision where to work.

- Work backward from this date to plan dates and times for interviews.
- Plan no more than two interviews in 1 day. If you do, beware of information overload and the risk of being late for at least one interview. Have two or three possible dates available on your calendar before calling the human resources or nurse recruitment office. Advance planning will keep you from fumbling on the telephone when they tell you that your first choice is unavailable!

While you are on the telephone, ask questions about the interview process. How much time should you plan for the interview? It may range from under 1 hour to a half day. If you have not already read the job description in the newspaper or online, ask about it when you call. Becoming familiar with both the job description and the prospective employer is critical to interview success.

What does the interview process involve? It may involve tours and multiple interviews including human resources, nurse recruitment, one or more clinical managers, and, possibly, staff nurses. If you are applying for an internship, it is not unusual to be interviewed by a panel of three or four people. Knowing this ahead of time may increase your anxiety, but it is less stressful than being surprised by this fact at the door.

Will more than one interview be required? Some institutions will use the first interview as a screening mechanism. You may be asked to come back for a follow-up interview.

How do you get to the human resources or nurse recruitment office? Ask for directions ahead of time if you are unfamiliar with the area. Have a good idea of the time involved for travel. Arriving late for an interview may create a very poor initial impression.

Will you be able to meet with clinical managers from different areas on the same day? Are there new graduates in the area with whom you can talk? This is important if you are interested in more than one clinical area.

Will a tour of the unit be included? If this is not a standard part of the interview process, express interest in having one so that you can get a more realistic idea of the setting and possibly meet some of the staff.

Prepare to Show Your Best Side. Develop your responses to probable interview questions. If you do not plan possible responses, you run the risk of looking wide-eyed as you fumble for an answer or ramble on around the subject. Despite the reality of a severe nursing shortage, organizations still give considerable weight to the interview, and an employment offer is far from automatic to anyone who walks in the door with a diploma or license in hand.

Critical Thinking Box 4-4 includes examples of interview questions with which you should be familiar. How would you answer these questions?

Rehearse the Interview. If you role-play a possible interview, it will probably increase your comfort level for the real thing. Following are some suggestions for a rehearsal:
- Dress for the part. It will add some authenticity to the situation.
- Choose a supportive friend or family member to role-play the interviewer.
- Practice your verbal responses to sample questions.
- Ask for constructive feedback regarding your appearance, body language, and responses.

Many applicants say they have no questions at the end of the interview. This may be true, or it may reflect the urge to end the interview and relax! Some words of advice: Prepare a few questions! This will be your opportunity to gather important details and possibly impress the interviewer with your interest. The following is a sampling of possible questions:
- What are your expectations for recent graduates?
- What is your evaluation process like?
- Who will evaluate me, and how will I get feedback about my performance?
- I would like some more information about your preceptorship program. How long will I have a preceptor, and what can I expect from the preceptor?
- What is the nurse-to-patient ratio on each of the shifts I may be working?
- What is your policy regarding weekend coverage?
- What opportunities are there for professional development?

Strategies for Interview Success

One of the most important strategies for successful interviewing is to dress for success (Box 4-4). Pay attention to your interviewing etiquette; your parents taught you to mind your manners, and this is an opportunity to put that education to good use. Also, make sure you know the name and title of the individual who is scheduled to meet with you.

CRITICAL THINKING

BOX 4-4

SAMPLE OF INTERVIEW QUESTIONS

The following is a sampling of interview questions you should be familiar with. Prepare your responses.

1. What area or areas of nursing are you interested in and why?
2. Tell me about your clinical experiences. Which rotations did you enjoy the most? Why?
3. What is the biggest mistake you ever made, and how was the problem resolved?
4. Tell me about yourself. What do you see as your strengths? Why?
5. How about your weaknesses? Why?
6. How would your most recent nursing instructor describe your performance in the clinical setting?
7. Tell me about your most challenging clinical assignment and what you learned from it.
8. What skills do you feel you have gained from your past work experiences that may help you in this position?
9. Tell me a little about yourself. How would others describe you?
10. What are your future career plans? Where do you expect to be in 2 or 3 years? In 5 years?
11. We do not have any openings at the present time in the areas in which you have indicated an interest. Would you be willing to accept a position in another area?
12. Tell me about a time when you had to establish priorities during one of your clinical experiences.
13. Tell me about a time when you went out of your way to assist a family or patient, even though you really did not have the time.

(Spend some time looking over your answers. Do they describe you accurately? Rework your answers until you feel comfortable with them, but do not try to memorize the words. They should serve as a guide for the upcoming interview.)

CRITICAL FIRST 5 MINUTES!

The decision to hire or not is usually made within the first 60 seconds. You will need to put your best foot forward from the start. Show up at least 10 to 15 minutes early. Smile at everyone you meet, and shake hands firmly (Restifo, 2002).

Arriving early may give you a chance to look over additional information about the institution or possibly give you more time for your interview. If you are delayed or cannot keep the appointment, call the interviewer as soon as possible to reschedule. Under no circumstances should you present yourself for an interview with your children or spouse in tow. They do not belong at a job interview and will create a negative impression with the interviewer. Human resources cannot provide babysitting services, and the presence of children in the waiting area is a safety concern without adult supervision. If you experience a childcare emergency, call and reschedule the interview.

BOX 4-4	The *Dos* and *Don'ts* of Dressing for Interviews

DO

- Look over your wardrobe and select a conservative outfit. Ladies, if you own a suit, consider wearing it, but do not blow your budget buying something you will never wear again. Other acceptable outfits include a business-type dress or skirt with coordinated top. The tried-and-true rule for job interview attire is this: Dress conservatively and professionally. Although a nursing shortage may loosen the rules a bit, the impression you convey by your appearance is likely to be remembered. Also, remember that you may be touring the facility, so wear comfortable shoes.
- Be conservative with your makeup and hairstyle.
- Wear minimal jewelry; you do not want to jingle and rattle with every move.
- Wear hose with a skirt or a dress; bare legs may be fashionable, but they are not appropriate for a professional interview.
- Men: consider a suit or jacket with coordinated slacks and shirt. A tie is optional.
- Take a few minutes to look yourself over in the mirror.

DON'T

- Wear casual clothes such as tee shirts, jeans, tennis shoes, or sandals. They may reflect the "real" you, but this is not the place to show that aspect of your personality.
- Be guilty of poor grooming or hygiene.
- Wear brand-new shoes, which may turn your day into a "painful" experience.
- Bring your children with you. You should leave them at home. Do not expect the staff to act as babysitters.
- Wear wrinkled or revealing clothing. This is not a date, and a bare midsection, though perhaps attractive in a casual setting, is inappropriate for a job interview.

Be aware of your body language; establish eye contact with the interviewer and maintain reasonable eye contact during the interview. Try to avoid or minimize distracting nervous mannerisms. Keep your hands poised in your lap or in some other comfortable position. If you tend to "talk with your hands," try not to do this continually. If you cross your legs, do not shake your foot. If offered coffee or another drink, decide whether this will relax you or complicate your body language. Show enthusiasm in your voice and body language. Do not chew gum or have anything in your mouth. Give a winning smile when you are introduced, and offer to shake hands. Women sometimes have a problem with shaking hands. Practice it at home to become more comfortable.

Demonstrate interest in what the interviewer has to say. Do not argue with or contradict the interviewer! Wait to ask about salary and benefits until all other aspects of the interview have been completed, including your other questions! Salary and benefits are important aspects, but they should not dominate your conversation. If the salary offer is lower than you expected, do not argue with the interviewer. You may point out that another institution is offering a higher starting salary, but do not try to use this information as a form of harassment or coercion. If you want to take some notes during the interview, ask the interviewer if he or she minds. This is generally quite acceptable. Bring along your list of questions, and if you cannot recall them when given the chance, ask to take out your list. Do not check off information during the interview as if you were grocery shopping!

PHASES OF THE INTERVIEW

The interview is generally divided into three areas, each of which serves a particular purpose. The first few minutes constitute the introduction. This is a "lightweight" section that is designed to help put you somewhat at ease. Some effort to "break the ice" will be made, and the communication may focus on the traffic, the weather, or the excitement you probably feel about your upcoming graduation. Take some slow, deep breaths and make a conscious effort to relax.

The second phase involves fact finding. Depending on the skill and style of the interviewer, you may be unaware of the subtle change in conversation, but questions about you will most likely now be asked. Your resume may be used as a source of questions, so make sure you can speak about its contents and that every item on the resume can be verified. Be prepared to offer your references and possibly explain why you have selected these particular individuals. If you have a tendency to give short responses or avoid answering questions, a skilled interviewer will reword the question or possibly note that you do not answer questions well. Interviewers strive to have the applicant talk about 90% of the time, so consider this your audition. They are really interested in getting to know you as a prospective "fit" with their institution, so you should be both enthusiastic and honest. Although many institutions offer a prolonged internship or preceptorship to increase both your confidence level and practical skill set, the interviewer is looking for prospective employees who are capable of being assertive team players—people who can be flexible but persistent. Critical Thinking Box 4-4 offers sample questions that you can practice with. Consider how you can best portray your background and experiences for the recruiter. Explaining how you have gone the extra mile for patients in a challenging situation is what a recruiter and nurse manager want to hear.

Some institutions are asking students or recent graduates to bring in a portfolio reflecting their school experiences. Included in this portfolio might be your skills check-off sheet, exemplar nursing care plans/concept maps, and any educational materials that showcase your best work. This is particularly beneficial if it is signed by the faculty with occasional positive comments. The closing is the last phase of the interview process. The interviewer may summarize what has been discussed and give you some ideas about the next step in the process (e.g., a tour, a meeting with clinical managers, or a follow-up interview). This is your time to ask questions. However, if you feel full of facts and unable to ask any questions at this time, leave the door open to future contacts by saying "I believe you answered all my questions at this time, but may I contact you if I have some questions later on?"

After the initial interview, you may have the opportunity to tour the area in which you will work. Show interest when this tour is offered, and use it as a chance to observe the surroundings for such things as professional behaviors as well as organizational and environmental factors. If you have the chance, interact with the staff, especially with recent graduates. Ask what they enjoy about their unit and job position. Before leaving, make sure you thank the interviewer for his or her time and interest.

HOW DO I HANDLE UNEXPECTED QUESTIONS OR SITUATIONS?

So, you did your homework and you are prepared for anything, but out of the blue you are asked a question you never expected. What should you do? Saying "No fair" is not a good answer! Take a deep breath, pause, and consider saying something like this: "That's an interesting question. I'd like to think about my answer for a minute if you don't mind. Can we come back to that subject later in the interview?" Given a temporary break, you will have time to develop your thoughts on the subject. Do not ignore the question, however, because a good interviewer will most likely bring it up again. Suppose you answer the question but feel your response was incomplete or off the mark. Look for an opportunity at the end of the interview to bring up the subject again, saying something like "I've had some time to think about an earlier question and want to add some additional information if you don't mind" (Box 4-5).

Now Can We Talk About Benefits?

At some point during the interview process, the interviewer will open the discussion on salary and the benefits the hospital has to offer. Salary, job responsibilities, and facility location are not the only major considerations in choosing an employer; do not forget to consider the total compensation package (that is, your benefits). Often, benefits are overlooked by new graduates because their value is less visible than an exciting new salary. Some organizations spend as much as 40% of their total employee payroll to provide this extra compensation. You should consider benefits as your "hidden paycheck" (Box 4-6).

Sign-On Bonuses. This has become a marketing tool for some institutions. Be cautious: carefully read and evaluate what is connected with the sign-on bonus. How long will you have to work for the institution to receive any or all of the bonus, and when will it be paid? Is the sign-on bonus in any way tied to the area in which you will be working? If you originally wanted to work in an intensive care unit but decided after 6 months that was not the area for you, can you transfer to another unit without losing your sign-on bonus?

BOX 4-5	Key Points to Remember About Your Responses During an Interview

- Answer honestly.
- Do not brag or gloat about your achievements, but do show yourself in a positive light.
- Remember that you are your best salesperson!
- Do not criticize past employers or instructors. It is more likely to reflect unfavorably on you than on them.

- Do not dwell on your shortcomings. Turn them into areas for future development: "I want to improve my organizational skills. Managing a group of patients will be a challenge, but I am looking forward to it."
- Demonstrate flexibility and a willingness to begin work in an area of second or third choice if the job market is limited in the area in which you are applying.

BOX 4-6	Benefit Package Options

Check with human resources regarding which benefits you are eligible to receive and when they are effective.

- Health and life insurance
- Accidental death and dismemberment coverage
- Sick or short-term disability pay
- Vacation pay
- Retirement plan
- Long-term disability leave

- Dental and/or vision care
- Parking
- Tuition reimbursement
- Loan programs
- Dependent care programs
- Health and wellness programs

When doing your job search, reviewing benefits is a major part of your decision. Therefore, as a new graduate, be sure to familiarize yourself with all the options that are available to you. The human resources department of the hospital or institution will be able to answer your questions. The decisions you make soon after graduation and in the early months of employment will have a far-reaching effect on your future.

JOB OFFERS AND POSSIBLE REJECTION

Let us consider a positive outcome first. If you are offered a position during or at the end of the interview, you are likely to have one of three possible reactions:

1. You are not ready to say yes or no. This is your first interview, and you have two more interviews scheduled.
2. You would like very much to work here. The job offer is just what you are looking for.
3. You do not want the position. It is not what you thought it would be, or something about the institution has created a negative impression.

Whichever decision you make about the job offer, the following are helpful tips for forming a response:

- Be honest. If you have other interviews to complete, say so. Be prepared to tell the interviewer when you will make your decision about the job offer.
- Avoid being pressured to say yes if you are not ready to commit to the job or feel that the position does not meet your needs.
- Be polite. Ask for some time to consider the offer if you are unsure of what you want to do at present.
- If you know the offer does not interest you, decline the offer graciously and express appreciation for the company's interest in you.
- Accept the offer and smile!

Suppose you receive a rejection or no job offer for the position, despite your interest and preparation. Before you leave in a state of dejection, find the courage to ask for a possible explanation if it has not been made clear at this point. If you do not find out about the rejection until later, consider calling the interviewer for this information. Check the following list for common reasons an institution may not offer you a job. Consider whether any of these factors might apply to you:

Lack of opening for your interests and skills. They liked you but could not find a spot right now, or a more qualified candidate was selected for the position.

Poor personal appearance, including inappropriate clothes. You stopped by for the interview on your way to the gym.

Lack of preparation for the interview. You were unable to answer questions intelligently or showed lack of knowledge of, or interest in, the employer. Your answers were superficial or filled with "I don't know."

Poor attitude. You conveyed an attitude of "What's in this for me?" instead of "How can I contribute to the organization?" Your first question focused on salary and perks.

Your answers and behavior reflected conceit, arrogance, poor self-confidence, or lack of manners or poise. They should hire you just because you showed up! Or you submitted a resume and responses that did not reflect initiative, achievements, or reliable work history.

You have no goals or future orientation. After all, you just want a job, and they should hire you because there is a nursing shortage.

Perceived lack of leadership potential. You like being a follower in all situations and do not want to make decisions. If this scenario sounds like you, rethink your approach. All nurses are expected to be leaders, whether in a formal or informal role. In your next interview, ask the interviewer how the organization supports the development of leadership in new graduates.

Poor academic record without a reasonable explanation. You worked as hard as you could in school, but the teachers did not like you; you lacked appropriate references; or your references were not available or did not reflect favorably on you. All experiences provide us with an opportunity for growth, especially the negative ones. Avoid blaming others for your shortcomings, and look for ways to grow from the experience.

Lack of flexibility. You were unwilling to begin work in an area that is not your first or second choice. Consider how rigid you can afford to be at this particular point in time or at this institution.

> If at first you don't succeed, try, try again.

Postinterview Process

Now that the interview is over, you may want to relax, celebrate, or jump in your car to make your next interview appointment. However, stop for a few minutes and jot down some notes about the interview. This is particularly important if you have another interview the same day. Critique the interview you just had. Consider the following questions:

1. What do you think were your strengths and weaknesses?
2. Is there anything you wish you had or had not said? Why?
3. Were there any surprises?
4. How do you feel you handled the situation?
5. What can you do differently the next time?

Write down details about the job, which will help you decide on its relative merits and drawbacks. If you do not do this, you may not be able to distinguish job A from job B by the time the interviews are finished. You may experience information overload after a number of interviews, but if you have taken notes about each, the sorting-out process will be easier.

After the interviews are over, rank your job offers against your personal list of priorities to make an informed choice. This may be an unnecessary step for you if you were sold on a particular interview. However, it is a good idea to consider interviewing with at least two institutions, if only to strengthen your decision about the first interview. It will help eliminate possible doubts about your choice later on. If there is a job you think you are really interested in, do a couple of other interviews first. This will give you some experience in interviewing. You may then be able to conduct a more positive interview for the position in which you are most interested. More interviews may also open your eyes to other possibilities.

Follow-Up Communication

Remember how nice it is to get a thank-you note in the mail or a telephone call of appreciation? Well, the same idea carries over to the work world: Write those letters!

Follow-Up Letter. Take a few minutes to write a note of thanks to the interviewer for the time and interest spent on your behalf. You may want to include additional information in the note: your continuing interest in the position if you hope an offer will be made, the date you will be making your job decision, additional thanks for any special efforts extended to you (lunch, individualized tour), and any change in telephone numbers and appropriate times when you can be reached. Use plain thank-you note cards, not frilly or cute ones. This is a situation where a handwritten note is certainly acceptable; just make sure it is legible and neat. Recruiters frequently comment on the positive aspect of a follow-up letter, and this attention to interpersonal communication may serve to keep your name at the top of the list. This step also helps to "separate you from the pack of applicants."

An electronic note of thanks is acceptable *(www.jobsearch.about.com/od/thankyouletters/a/ samplethankyou.htm)*. However, in the blur of daily e-mail, a personal handwritten note will particularly stand out.

Letters of Rejection. As soon as you make up your mind regarding job offers, notify other prospective employers of your decision. Decline their job offer graciously, and include an expression of appreciation for their interest in you. The format for this letter should follow the standard rules of business letters. Remember, you have accepted a position elsewhere, but your career could take a turn in the future that may bring you back to the institution you are now declining. Leave a positive impression with human resources and recruitment.

Telephone Follow-Up. On the basis of the interview, you should have a pretty clear idea of the "how" and "when" of further contact. A telephone call may be appropriate when you have not heard from a recruiter by an agreed-upon date. You can contact a recruiter or interviewer by telephone to decline a job offer, but a personal letter is preferable to leaving a telephone message. Remember to be unfailingly polite to everyone you speak to on the telephone. Administrative assistants and other support personnel will remember and pass on unfavorable impressions to their superiors. Recruiters do not want to hire staff members who are rude or impatient. They know that this behavior is likely to be shown toward patients and families as well. Assistants often act as gatekeepers for their boss and can be counted on to report both positive and negative perceptions of the job applicants with whom they have contact.

What If I Do Not Like My First Position?

It is not uncommon to experience frustrations during your first work experience. Return to Chapter 1 on transitions and reality shock, and review it for some suggestions on how to handle your situation. You also need to keep in touch with the nurse recruiter who hired you. Nurse recruiters can offer further support and assistance. Recruiters know where other recent graduates are working in the institution and may provide you with a network of individuals who can offer suggestions and support to improve your situation. In addition, recruiters know the staffing needs of other areas in the hospital and may suggest transferring. A good way to get an idea of other areas where you may be interested in working is to "shadow" a staff nurse in that area. This means you would spend a day observing this staff nurse performing his or her job. This provides you with a good insight as to what the job requires and the working conditions of that area. When you take your first position, plan on staying there for at least a year. You want to avoid "job hopping," or changing jobs whenever you do not like what is going on with your current position. Remember, other positions have their benefits and problems; the grass may not be greener on the other side of the fence.

November 1, 2010

Linda Smith
101 Anywhere Street
Dallas, TX 77777
214-555-8888

Ms. Joan Winter
Assistant Vice President
Children's Medical Center of Dallas
1935 Hospital Street
Dallas, TX 75235

Dear Ms. Winter:

It is with regret that I must submit my resignation. I have been offered a position with Hancock Hospital. My period of employment at Children's has been very positive. I feel I have gained much experience that will be of great benefit to me in my career. My last day of employment will be November 20, 2010.

Thank you for the opportunity to work at your facility and your kind consideration.

Sincerely,

Linda Smith
Linda Smith

FIGURE 4-7
Letter of resignation.

> Don't trade one set of problems for another set that may be even more difficult.

What If It Is Time for Me to Change Positions?

If you think it is time to change positions or explore other options, it is important to submit a letter of resignation (Figure 4-7). Give at least 2 weeks' notice. Check your contract to see whether you agreed to give more than that; if so, give 4 weeks' notice if possible. If you are leaving on less than amicable terms, do not express this in your resignation letter. You can always report grievances to the personnel or human resources department. As a means of improving retention, many institutions conduct an exit interview or call former employees sometime after resignation to explore reasons for leaving. If you are provided this opportunity, make every effort to provide objective feedback and avoid character assassination. Do not "burn any bridges" since you may want to work at the organization again later in your career. Maintain a professional attitude as you develop a network of contacts. Always "take the high road" and avoid petty comments.

CONCLUSION

Searching for and finding your niche in the workplace can sometimes be overwhelming. Take the plunge and start looking. Keep a positive outlook because the job you are looking for is out there. This is one of those situations in which a little preparation and investigation go a long way toward finding what you want. Get your resume together and start investigating what is out there for you. A basic understanding of the process of job hunting can minimize the frustrations and promote a positive first-job experience. Good luck with your job search.

> Success lies not in achieving what you aim at, but in aiming at what you want to achieve.

BIBLIOGRAPHY

American Association of Colleges of Nursing (2009): *Fact sheet: nursing shortage,* AACN. Retrieved from *www.aacn.nche.edu/media/FactSheets/NursingShortage.htm.*

American Nurses Association (2010): *Nursing Career Center.* Retrieved *www.nursingworld.org/careercenter.*

American Nurses Credentialing Center (2010): *Find a Magnet Organization.* Retrieved from *www.nursecredentialing.org/Magnet/FindaMagnetFacility.aspx.*

Borgatti J: Plan a career, not just a job, *Am Nurse Today* 47-48, 2007.

Buerhaus PI, Auerbach DI, Staiger DO: The recent surge in nurse employment: causes and implications, *Health Affairs* 28(4):657-668, 2009. Retrieved from *www.specialtystaffinc.com/news/headline/85.*

Carlson J: Nursing shortage eases …, *Modern Healthcare* 39(20):8-9, 2009.

Copland MV (2007): *The Missing Link.* Retrieved from *http://money.cnn.com/magazines/business2/business2_archive/2006/12/01/8394967/index.htm.*

Doyle A: *Thank you letter: job interview.* Retrieved from *http://Jobsearch.about.com/cs/thankyouletters/qt/thank.htm.*

Health Resources and Services Administration (2010): *The registered nurse population: initial findings from the 2008 national sample survey of registered nurses.* Retrieved from *http://bhpr.hrsa.gov/healthworkforce/rnsurvey/initialfindings2008.pdf.*

LaMaster MA, Larsen RA: Prepare for a behavioral interview, then ace it!, *AJN* 110(1):8, 10, 2010.

Larson SE: Create a good impression: professionalism in nursing, *Imprint* 53(5):50-52, 2006.

Lenhart A et al. (2010): *Social media and young adults. PEW Internet report.* Retrieved *www.pewinternet.org/Reports/2010/Social-Media-and-Young-Adults.aspx.*

Lorenz K (2009): *Warning: Social networking can be hazardous to your job search.* Retrieved from *www.careerbuilder.com.*

Restifo V: The successful interview how to market yourself for career advancement, *NSNA Imprint* 37-41, 2002. Retrieved from *www.nsna.org/Portals/0/Skins/NSNA/pdf/Career_successint.pdf.*

Thomas DO, Grossman VGA: Career compass, *RN* 70:18-24, 2007.

Additional resources are available online at *http://evolve.elsevier.com/Zerwekh/nsgtoday/.*

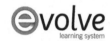

CHAPTER 5

NCLEX-RN® Examination and the New Graduate

JoAnn Zerwekh, EdD, RN

The way I see it, if you want the rainbow, you gotta put up with the rain.
—DOLLY PARTON

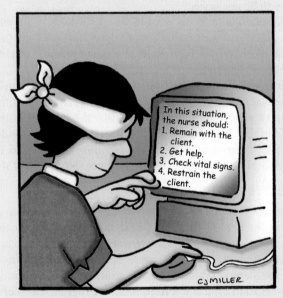

In this situation, the nurse should:
1. Remain with the client.
2. Get help.
3. Check vital signs.
4. Restrain the client.

CJ MILLER

Don't take any chances … understand the NCLEX Examination process.

After completing this chapter, you should be able to:

- Discuss the role of the National Council of State Boards of Nursing.

- Discuss the implications of computer adaptive testing.

- Identify the process and steps for preparing to take the National Council Licensure Examination for Registered Nurses (NCLEX-RN Examination).

- Identify criteria for selecting a NCLEX examination review book and review course.

- Identify the characteristics of the alternate item format questions on the NCLEX examination.

---

he National Council Licensure Examination for Registered Nurses (NCLEX-RN Examination)—this is the really big test you have been preparing for since you entered nursing school. Consider the opportunity to take the NCLEX-RN Examination a privilege; it took a lot of hard work to achieve this level, and there are a lot of people who never get there! Your passage through the "NCLEX Gate" will begin your transition into professional nursing. As with other aspects of transition, planning begins early, before you graduate. Planning ahead will help you develop a comprehensive plan on how you want to attack that mountain of material to review. When you plan ahead and know what is expected, your anxiety about the examination will be decreased. Being prepared and knowing what to expect will help you maintain a positive attitude.

THE NCLEX-RN EXAMINATION

Who Prepares It and Why Do We Have to Have It?

The National Council of State Boards of Nursing (NCSBN) is the governing body for the committee that prepares the licensure examination. Each member board or state determines the application and registration process as well as deadlines within the state. The NCLEX examination is used to regulate entry into nursing practice in the United States. It is a national examination with standardized scoring; all candidates in every state are presented with questions based on the same test plan. Every state requires the same passing level or standard. There is no discrepancy in passing scores from one state to another. In other words, you cannot go to another state and expect the NCLEX examination to be any easier.

According to the NCSBN, the NCLEX examination is designed to test "knowledge, skills and abilities essential to the safe and effective practice of nursing at the entry level" (NCSBN, 2010a). Upon successful completion of the examination, you will be granted a license to practice nursing in the state in which you applied for licensure. The status of state licensure continues to be in a transition process of its own. There are many nurses who maintain a current license in multiple states. The increase in nursing practice across state lines, the growth of managed care, and the advances in telehealth medicine prompted a research project conducted by the NCSBN in the late 1990s. Results of the research resulted in the development of the Mutual Recognition Model for Multistate Regulation. This is frequently referred to as the *Nurse Licensure Compact.* As of June 2010, the compact has been enacted through the legislatures of 24 states (NCSBN, 2013f).

How Will the Nurse Licensure Compact Affect Your License?

The nursing license in the participating compact states will function much like a driver's license. The individual holds one license issued in the state of residence but is also responsible for the laws of the state in which he or she is driving. The individual nurse will be licensed to practice in their state of residence, but may practice nursing in another state; however, the nurse must comply with the Nurse Practice Act of the state in which he or she practices. The transition process for the Nurse Licensure Compact began in 2002 and is continuing to progress. The Nurse Licensure Compact must be passed by the state legislature in each participating state. Watch your state nursing organization and Board of Nursing newsletters, or check the NCSBN website *(www.ncsbn.org)* to see where your state is in the process of implementing the Interstate Compact on Nurse Licensure (Critical Thinking Box 5-1).

CRITICAL THINKING BOX 5-1   What is the status of the Nurse Licensure Compact in your state?

Before the Nurse Licensure Compact is implemented, the respective states will continue to require the nurse to be licensed in the individual state of practice. Transfer of nursing licenses between states is a process called "licensure by endorsement." If you wish to practice in a state in which you are not currently licensed, you must contact the State Board of Nursing in the state in which you wish to practice. The State Board of Nursing will advise you of the process to become licensed in that state (see Appendix A, State Boards of Nursing, on the Evolve website). Transferring your license to practice from one state to another does not negate your successful completion of the NCLEX examination, nor do you have to take the examination again. All states recognize the successful completion of the NCLEX examination, regardless of the state in which you took the examination or where your initial license was issued. You can get the most recent list of State Boards of Nursing from the NCSBN website *(www.ncsbn.org).*

What Is the NCLEX-RN Examination Test Plan?

The content of the NCLEX examination is based on a test blueprint that is determined by the National Council. The blueprint reflects entry-level nursing practice as identified by research and the Practice Analysis Study of Newly Licensed Registered Nurses. This research study is conducted by the National Council every 3 years. The practice analysis research in 2011 indicated that the majority of new graduates were continuing to work in a hospitals with approximately 20% working in long-term care and community-based facilities. There was a trend noted of a decrease in newly licensed RNs working in hospitals with a subsequent increase seen in long-term care and community-based facilities since the previous practice analysis study. Most entry-level nurses indicated that they cared for acutely ill clients. The majority of entry-level nurses indicated they cared for adult and geriatric clients who were acutely ill, as well as adults and geriatric clients with stable and unstable chronic conditions. The majority of the new graduates surveyed responded receiving some form of formal orientation. Hospitals and long-term care facilities were the primary employers of new graduates. Respondents (50%) reported having a primary administrative position. Newly licensed RNs working in long-term care facilities were more likely to report having administrative responsibilities than those working in hospitals (61.2% in long-term care vs.6.5% in hospitals). The test plan in this chapter was implemented in April 2013 and will be used until April 2016. A new test plan is implemented every 3 years. This represents the time required to conduct the research, analyze the data, and implement the new test plan for the NCLEX examination.

The examination is constructed from questions that are designed to test the candidate's ability to apply the nursing process and to determine appropriate nursing responses and interventions to provide safe nursing care. The distribution of content is based on the areas of client needs.

Safe, Effective Care Environment	
Management of care	17%-23%
Safety and infection control	9%-15%
Health Promotion and Maintenance	6%-12%
Psychosocial Integrity	6%-12%
Physiological Integrity	
Basic care and comfort	6%-12%
Pharmacological and parenteral therapies	12%-18%
Reduction of risk potential	9%-15%
Physiological adaptation	11%-17% (NCSBN, 2013a)

The nursing process is integrated throughout the exam. There are four levels of client needs identified in the 2013 NCLEX-RN Detailed Test Plan (NCSBN 2013a). Each level of client need is assigned a percentage that reflects the weight of that category of client need on the NCLEX-RN examination. The approximate percentages of each area are as follows:

In April 1994, the NCSBN implemented computer-adaptive testing (CAT) for the NCLEX examination for both practical/vocational nurses (NCLEX-PN/VN) and registered nurses (NCLEX-RN). The information presented here is a brief introduction to the NCLEX-RN computer adaptive test (CAT). It is important that you download the NCLEX examination Candidate Bulletin for your testing year from *www.ncsbn.org* and carefully follow the instructions; you will receive additional information from your state board of nursing.

Pearson VUE is the company contracted by the NCSBN to schedule candidates, administer, and score the NCLEX examination. The NCSBN is responsible for the content and development of the test questions, the test plan, policies, and requirements for eligibility for the NCLEX examination. Pearson VUE will assist you in scheduling your examination and will provide a location and equipment for the administration of the examination.

What Does CAT Mean?

With CAT (computer adaptive test), each candidate receives a different set of questions via the computer. The questions are assembled interactively as the candidate progresses through the examination. The computer develops an examination based on the test plan and selects questions to be presented on the basis of the candidates' responses to the previous question. The number of questions each candidate receives and the testing time for each candidate will vary. As candidates answer questions correctly, the next question will be either a degree of difficulty equal to the previous question or a higher level of difficulty. All of the questions presented will reflect the categories of the NCLEX examination test plan (NCSBN, 2013a).

"Pretest" questions have been integrated into the examination in the past and will continue to be integrated into the current examination. The NCSBN Examination Committee evaluates the statistical information from each of these "pretest" questions to determine whether the question is valid and to identify the level of difficulty of the test item (NCSBN, 2013a). Do not be alarmed—these questions are not counted in the grading of your examination, and time has been allocated for you to answer these questions. It is impossible to determine which questions are "pretest" questions and which ones are "scored" test questions, so it is important that you answer every question to the very best of your ability. These pretest items ensure that each question that counts toward your score has been thoroughly evaluated for content as well as statistically validated.

What Is the Application Process for the NCLEX Examination CAT? In the beginning of the semester in which you will graduate, your school of nursing will have each student complete an application form and send it to the state board of nursing. Upon your completion of the nursing program, the school will verify your graduate status with the state board of nursing. After the forms have been processed, you will receive an Acknowledgement of Receipt of Registration. You will then receive your Authorization to Test (ATT) with instructions regarding how to schedule your examination with Pearson VUE. You cannot schedule your examination until you have received your ATT. Read your instruction packet and your *Candidate Bulletin* carefully (the Candidate Bulletin may be found at www.ncsbn.org, navigate to NCLEX Examination Candidates). Keep track of your ATT. It will be *required* for scheduling your testing date and for admission into the testing center. If you received your ATT letter via email, you must print the attachment and bring it with you on the day of your exam. Your ATT will contain your authorization number, candidate ID number, and an expiration date. The expiration date cannot be extended for any reason; *you must test within the dates on the ATT*. It is to your advantage to schedule your examination date shortly after receiving your ATT—even if you do not plan to take the test for several weeks. Testing centers tend to fill up early, if you wait too long you may not be able to get your desired testing date. Pearson VUE will send you a confirmation of your testing appointment (NCSBN, 2013b).

If you provide an e-mail address at the time you register for the NCLEX examination, all future correspondence from Pearson VUE will be via e-mail, regardless of whether you registered by telephone, mail, or via the Internet. If you do not provide an e-mail address, all correspondence will arrive via U.S. mail (NCSBN, 2013a).

Where Do I Take the Test? There are testing sites in every state. A candidate may take the test at any of the Pearson VUE testing sites listed in the *Candidate Bulletin*. However, the license to practice will be issued only in the state where the candidate's application was submitted. Information regarding the location of the centers can be found at the candidate area on the National Council website, as well as in the ATT. There will be multiple testing stations at each center.

When Do I Take the Test? After receiving the ATT, a candidate may contact the NCLEX examination Candidate Services at the phone number provided in the *Candidate Bulletin* or go to the NCLEX examination area of the Pearson VUE website *(www.pearsonvue.com/nclex)* to schedule the examination. The location and telephone numbers of the testing centers will be included in the information from the NCSBN. For most students, the ATT will be received approximately 2 to 3 weeks after graduation. Remember, you *must* test within the dates on your ATT. You may schedule your examination as soon as you receive the ATT. This means that you could receive the ATT on Wednesday, call or go online to the location of your choice, and if you wish, take the examination the next day, if there is space available. Or, you can call and/or go online and schedule your examination date within the next 2 to 3 weeks.

During the last 2 months of school, begin to make plans for when you would like to take the examination. The examination should be taken within approximately 4 to 6 weeks of graduation. Allow for some study time and consider whether you want to take a formal review course. It is important that you take the examination soon after graduation. If you wait too long, your level of comprehension of critical information will be decreased. Finish school, take a review course if you want to, get your ATT, and go take the examination. This is not a good time to plan a vacation, get married, or engage in other activities that could cause a crisis in your life (Critical Thinking Box 5-2).

How Much Time Do I Have and How Many Questions Are There? Each candidate is scheduled for a 6-hour time slot. You should plan to be at the site for 6 hours. Each candidate

CRITICAL THINKING BOX 5-2   When do you want to take your NCLEX examination? Refer to this book's Evolve website for information on selecting an NCLEX examination review course to help you get started on thinking about this process and assist you in deciding how to select a review book.

must answer at least 75 questions. Within those first 75 questions, there are 15 pretest items that are not scored on your examination. The number of questions you answer and the length of time that you test are not indications of whether you will receive a pass or fail score. The length of your examination depends on how you answered the questions. When the computer indicates that you are finished, regardless of how long you have been testing or how far past 75 questions you have gone, it just means you have "turned your test in," and your test is completed. The examination will end when the student:

- Measures at a level of competence above or below the established standard of competency and at least 75 questions have been answered
- Completes a maximum of 265 questions
- Has been testing for the maximum time of 6 hours (NCSBN, 2013d)

Do I Have to Be Computer-Literate? It is not necessary to study from a computer, nor is it necessary that you be "computer literate." Research has demonstrated that candidates who were not accustomed to working on a computer did as well as those who were very comfortable with the computer. So, previous computer experience is not a prerequisite to passing the NCLEX examination!

How Will I Keep the Computer Keys Straight and Deal with a Mouse? At the testing site, each candidate is given a tutorial orientation to the computer. This tutorial will introduce you to the computer; demonstrate how to use the keyboard and the calculator, as well as how to use the mouse to record your answers (Figure 5-1). It will also explain how to record the answers for the alternate item format items (more about this later). If you need assistance with the computer after the examination starts, a test administrator will be available. Every effort is made to ensure that you understand and are comfortable with the testing procedure and equipment.

There will be only one question on the screen at a time. You will read the question and select an answer. After the answer is selected, select "enter" from the lower right corner of the screen and the computer will present another question. Previously answered questions are not available

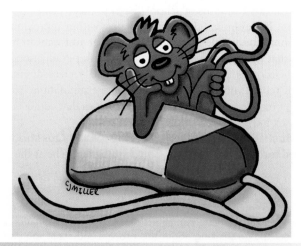

FIGURE 5-1

As of 2002, the use of the computer mouse makes navigating the CAT easier.

for review. There is an onscreen optional calculator built into the computer. The tutorial program will demonstrate the use of the calculator in calculating numeric answers.

What Is the Passing Score? Every state has the same passing criteria. Specific individual scores will not be available to you, your school, or your place of employment. You cannot obtain your results from the testing center. Your score will be reported directly to you as pass or fail. A composite of student results will be mailed to the respective schools of nursing. There is no specific published score or number that represents passing.

How Will I Know I Have Passed? The examination scores are compiled at the Pearson VUE center and transmitted directly to state boards of nursing. Most boards of nursing can advise the candidates in writing of their results within 3 to 4 weeks of taking the examination. Check your *Candidate Bulletin,* as well as online verification from your state board of nursing, regarding the availability of results online or from an automated telephone verification system. *Do not call* the state board of nursing, NCLEX examination Candidate Services, or the Pearson VUE Professional Centers to inquire about your pass or fail status; they cannot release information over the telephone.

What Kind of Questions Will Be on the NCLEX Examination?

Most of the questions are in multiple-choice format, with four options. Each question will stand alone and will not require information from previous questions to determine the correct answer. All of the information for the question will be available on the computer screen. You will be provided an erasable board for notes or calculations you would like to make. You may not take calculators into the examination; the "drop-down" calculator will be available on the screen for math calculations. Everyone will be tested according to the same test plan, but candidates will receive different questions. There is only one correct answer to each question; you do not get any partial credit for another answer—it is either right or wrong. All questions must be answered, even if you have to make a wild guess. The computer selects the next question based on your response to the previous question. (You do not get another question until the one on the screen is answered.) You will not be able to go back to a previous question once that question is removed from the screen. (This means you cannot go back and change your answer to the wrong one!) There will be an optional 10-minute break after 2 hours of testing. If you need to take a break before the 2 hours, notify one of the testing center administrators. A second optional break is offered after $3\frac{1}{2}$ hours of testing. The tutorial and all breaks are considered part of the 6 hours allowed for testing (NCSBN, 2010b).

There is not much storage space at the testing sites. There are some small lockers for your personal items. Therefore, do not take your textbooks, your notes from school, your lucky stuffed bear, or any other materials you have been carrying around in that pack for the past 2 years!

What Are Some of the Other Things I Really Need to Know About the NCLEX Examination?

What If I Need to Change the Time or Date I Have Already Scheduled? You can change your testing date and time if you advise NCLEX examination Candidate Services 24 hours or 1 full business day prior to your scheduled examination appointment. You may go to the NCLEX candidate website (www.Pearsonvue.com/nclex) to reschedule or your may speak with an agent at Pearson Vue and receive confirmation of the unscheduled/rescheduled appointment letter. The phone number will be listed in your *Candidate Bulletin*. You can then reschedule the test at no additional cost. If a candidate does not reschedule within this time frame or does not come at the scheduled testing time, the ATT is invalidated, and the candidate will be required to reregister and repay the $200 registration fee. There are *no exceptions* to this policy (NCSBN, 2013b).

What About Identification at the Testing Site? At the testing site, you will submit a digital signature and be digitally fingerprinted and photographed. An additional security screening recently implemented is the palm vein screening. It will be required for admission to the exam. You will also be required to provide one form of identification. All identification documents must be in the original form; no copies will be accepted. Be sure that the first and last name printed on your identification match exactly the first and last name printed on your ATT letter. The following are acceptable forms of identification (must be in English, valid and not expired, with a photograph and a signature):

- U.S. driver's license
- U.S. state-issued identification
- Passport
- U.S. military identification (NCLEX, 2012b)

What Are the Advantages of CAT for the Candidate? The environment is quiet and conducive to testing. The work surface is large enough to accommodate both right-handed and left-handed people, with adequate room for the computer. Each candidate can work at his or her own pace and is allowed to test up to 6 hours. Each candidate has his or her own testing station or cubicle. There should be a minimal amount of distraction, if any, by the other candidates who are testing at the same time. If a candidate has to retake the examination, the parameters for retesting are established by the respective state board of nursing. The National Council requires the candidate to wait at least 45 days prior to rescheduling the examination. Some individual boards of nursing require a waiting period of 90 days after the first examination before scheduling. Candidates who take the examination again will not be given the same questions (NCSBN, 2013d).

PREPARING FOR THE NCLEX-RN EXAMINATION

Where and When Should I Start?

Six Months Before the NCLEX Examination

Make Sure You Know the Dates and Deadlines in the State in Which You Are Applying for Licensure. Your school will advise you of the specific dates the forms are due to the state board of nursing. If you are registering individually, contact the state board of nursing in your state of residence (or in the state where you wish to file for licensure) and find out the filing deadlines. Make sure you follow the directions exactly. State boards of nursing do not respond favorably to applications that are not submitted on time or are submitted in an incorrect format. A listing of the state boards of nursing can be found on the Evolve website. If you plan to apply for licensure in a state other than the one in which you are graduating, it is your responsibility to contact the board of nursing in that state to obtain your papers for application. Plan early (at least 6 months ahead) to investigate the feasibility of taking the examination in another state.

Investigate Review Courses. Review courses can be an excellent resource in your preparation for the NCLEX examination. Review courses will assist you in organizing your study materials and identifying areas in which you need to focus your study time. These courses will help you to understand the NCLEX-RN Examination test plan. Understanding the test plan will help you to prioritize your studying.

Plan an Expense Account for the End of School and for the NCLEX Examination. Frequently, students face unexpected expenses at the end of school; one of these expenses may be the fees for the NCLEX examination. Start a small savings plan—maybe $10 a week—to help defray these expenses. For family and friends who want to give you something for graduation, you might tell them of your "wish list," including those expenses incurred at graduation (Box 5-1).

Two Months Before the NCLEX Examination: What Do I Need to Do Now?

If You Have a Job, Discuss Your Anticipated NCLEX-RN Examination Test Date with Your Supervisor. You can estimate your test date by checking your graduation date, determining from

---

BOX 5-1	Budget for the End of School and the NCLEX Examination: How Much Is It Going to Cost Me to Get Out of School?

REQUIRED EXPENSES

Graduation fees from college or university _____

Application fees for NCLEX-RN Examination _____

EXPENSES TO TAKE NCLEX-RN EXAMINATION

Travel (e.g., car, bus, airfare) _____

Hotel accommodations at NCLEX examination testing site _____

Miscellaneous (e.g., food, cab fare, parking) _____

OPTIONAL EXPENSES

School pin _____

Uniform or cap and gown for graduation _____

Graduation expenses passed on to graduate _____

Graduation pictures (class or individual) _____

Graduation invitations _____

Commercial exit testing _____

NCLEX-RN examination review course (need to plan this before school is out) _____

NCLEX-RN examination review books (get these early—they really help with the last year of nursing school!) _____

EXPENSES AFTER GRADUATION (IT'S NOT OVER YET!)

Professional organizations (most organizations will give a discount on new membership to the graduate nurse) _____

Professional journals _____

Uniform, scrub suits, and shoes to begin new job _____

Professional liability insurance (check with the school regarding transfer from school policy to individual policy) _____

previous students or nursing faculty the approximate time to receive the ATT in your state, and then considering review courses and study time and how these might affect when you want to schedule your examination. Remember, you can change your testing appointment, without penalty, as long as you do it within 24 hours (or one full business day) of your scheduled appointment and within the dates on the ATT. Submit your request for days off work in writing as soon as you have confirmed your examination date. This is something you want to make sure that your manager understands. Plan to take off the day or two before the examination and, if possible, the day after as well. This will allow you time to relax and, if necessary, travel to and from the testing site.

Decide How You Are Going to Get to the Test Site and Whether It Will Be Necessary for You to Stay Overnight. If the closest testing site is not easily accessible, is more than an hour's drive away, or involves driving through a heavily congested traffic area, you may want to consider staying overnight in a hotel room close to the site. For some graduates, this will prevent unnecessary hassle and may alleviate anxiety on the day of the examination.

Are You Going with a Group or By Yourself? How will you feel if the group is finished and you are still working on your examination? Will you feel rushed because everyone is waiting for you? Do not create a situation that will increase your anxiety at one of the most important times of your nursing career. If you are okay with the group waiting for you, and everyone understands the situation, then it may be a source of support for you. If a group of graduates is traveling together, and everyone is able to schedule the examination on the same day, consideration should be given to planning hotel accommodations, if they are necessary. Do not have a crowd in your room. Five people in a room designed for two or four will not be conducive to sleep the night before the examination. If you are rooming with another person, select someone you like and can tolerate in close quarters for a short period of time. Surround yourself with people who have a positive attitude; you do not need complainers and negative thinkers.

Develop a Plan for Studying. Do you need to study alone, or do you benefit from group study time? Set yourself a study schedule that you can realistically achieve. About 2 to 3 hours a day for 2 or 3 days a week is realistic; 8 hours a day on your days off does not work. If you take a formal review course, plan your study time to gain the most from the course. A review course is not meant to be your only study time. When you finish a review course, you should have a much better idea regarding what is going to be tested, how it will be tested, and where you need to focus some study time. Priority areas to study are those in which you are the weakest; focus on those first.

The Day Before the BIG DAY

Make Sure You Have All of the Papers Required for Admission. Read your information packet again. The ATT that you received from the testing service *will be required* at the testing site. The information packet that you receive should have all of the necessary information and directions needed for the test site. Check whether there is anything else you will need to take with you to the site.

Make a "Test Run" the Evening Before the Test. Go to the site and evaluate traffic patterns and driving time. Find the parking area. If your hotel is within four to six blocks of the test site, walk to the site; this is a terrific way to help reduce anxiety and get the blood circulating to your brain! Whether you drive or walk to the site, go the day before to make sure you know where you are going.

Go to Bed Early; Do Not Study, Cram, or Party! Plan to eat a light dinner, something that will not upset your stomach—you do not need to be up half of the night with heartburn and/or diarrhea!

The BIG DAY Is Here

Eat a Well-Balanced Breakfast, Not Sweet Rolls and Coffee. Protein and complex carbohydrates will help sustain you during the examination. Eat light, something that is nourishing, but not heavy. Do not drink a lot of coffee; you do not need to have the caffeine jitters or be distracted by frequent bathroom trips.

Dress Comfortably, but Look Nice. Anticipate that the temperature at the testing sites will be a little cool rather than too warm. Do not wear tight clothes that restrict your breathing when you sit down! Dress casually and comfortably; you may not wear hats, scarves, or jackets in the testing room. The National Council requests that you arrive at the testing site about 30 minutes early. This will allow you time to get checked in and prevent anxiety about being late. If you arrive more than 30 minutes after your scheduled appointment, you may be required to forfeit your examination appointment, as well as the examination fees (NCSBN, 2013b).

How Do I Select an NCLEX Examination Review Course?

There are many review courses available to assist the graduate nurse in preparing for the NCLEX examination. Before you sign up, evaluate which course will be most beneficial to you. In considering a review course, remember that the objective is review, not primary learning. (See Evolve website for Selecting an NCLEX Examination Review Course.)

What Types of Review Courses Are Available?

Live (Face-to-Face) Review Courses. Evaluate your geographic location. Which review courses are easily accessible? Are you considering traveling to another city to attend a review course? If you have a prospective employer, check with the nurse recruiter to determine whether the facility provides a review course. Collect data on all of the courses; then compare them to see which one best meets your needs and budget. Also, check with the nurse recruiter or the nursing manager regarding time off and scheduling. Plan ahead and make an intelligent decision regarding review courses. Do not feel that you must sign up with the first review company that contacts you!

NCLEX Examination Online Review Courses. How well do you study at the computer? If you find studying at the computer is very easy for you, then you may want to consider an online review course. When investigating online review courses, determine whether the course provides an online book, study questions, additional online study materials, as well as the availability of a review faculty. Most students need a resource person or faculty to answer questions (either about nursing content or the NCLEX examination) and to assist in developing a study plan. Consider the length of time the online course is available—is it over several weeks, or is it an indefinite time? With online courses, it is critical to set aside study time, plan how you are going to progress through the course, and evaluate how long you think you will need to complete the course. Online review courses can be beneficial if you plan your study time, take advantage of the course resources available, and follow the suggested activities within the online course.

Carefully evaluate your need for a review course. Are you the type of student who can plan study time, establish a study review schedule, and stick to it? Were you in the top 25% of your graduating class? Have you had experience working in a hospital with adult medical-surgical clients, other than while you were in school? As a new graduate, do you feel prepared for this examination? If you can answer "yes" to all of these questions, you may not need to consider a review course in your preparation for the NCLEX-RN Examination. Most graduates can say "yes" to one or two of these questions, but not to all of them.

What Are the Qualifications of the Review Course Instructors? To teach a review course effectively, the instructor needs to be familiar with the NCLEX examination. That ability is most often found in instructors who have teaching experience in a school of nursing. Some hospitals provide in-house review courses taught by excellent educators and clinical specialists. Determine whether these instructors are familiar with the NCLEX examination test plan. Information that is not a focus of the NCLEX examination test plan does not need to be included in a review course. It is also important to find out whether the review course instructor is from a school of nursing in your immediate area. It is possible that you will be paying for a review course to be taught by someone from your nursing school faculty. A review course may be more effective if it is taught by someone other than your school faculty. You need to hear information from a different perspective. This helps to anchor information and reinforce previous learning. Look for a course that brings faculty in from areas outside your school.

What Type of Instructional Materials Are Used in the Course? Are the materials required for the course an additional expense (or part of the registration fee)? Do you get to keep the materials after the course is over? Can you print copies of the materials if you are taking an online course? Are handouts, workbooks, CDs, audiotapes, books, and other materials used to enhance learning? Be concerned if there are no course outlines, workbooks, handouts, or books; you might spend all of your time writing and miss listening to the necessary information. Do the course materials include practice test questions that are similar in format to the NCLEX examination? Ask about the format used to organize the material (e.g., integrated, blocked, systems). How does the format compare with the NCLEX examination plan of client needs and nursing process that is described in your *Candidate Bulletin* from the National Council?

Does the Course Include Instruction in Test-Taking Skills and Practice? Test-taking skills and practice are a very important aspect of a review course. Graduates need to practice testing strategies and use them in answering questions written by someone other than their nursing school faculty. This is important to evaluate in the face-to-face review as well as in the online review.

How Much Does the Course Cost? Most review courses cost between $250 and $500. Frequently, there is a discount for early registration, and there may also be a discount for group registration. Make sure you understand the review company policy regarding deposit, registration fees, and the cancellation policy. Check out the possibility of organizing a group; some courses give a free review or a discount to the group organizer.

How Long Does It Last? Is the face-to-face course 3, 4, or 5 consecutive days? Is it given only in the evenings? Is it taught only on the weekend for 6 weeks? This is very important to determine early in your evaluation of review courses. Notify your employer as soon as possible if you need to fit the review course into your work schedule. Most hospitals will arrange the new graduate's schedule to allow attendance at a review course. It is important to provide adequate advance notice to your employer so that staffing schedules may be planned.

If you are considering an online course, how long will it take you to work through the course? Is the course set up in "real-time" similar to the face-to-face review or is it self-paced? How long does the provider recommend you spend in the course? Do you want to study for 2 to 3 hours every day for 4 weeks, or do you want to work faster and study 4 to 6 hours a day and complete it in 2 weeks? If you plan on studying 4 to 6 hours in 1 day, you should not plan on working that day.

Some hospitals even provide a review course or reimburse the review course registration fee as a benefit to the graduate nurse employee! Once you have determined which review course as well as what type of review course you wish to take, discuss it with your prospective employer or notify your current employer as soon as possible.

Where Is the Face-to-Face Course Held? Are you going to have to drive for an hour every day? Will you need to arrange for a hotel room? Ask about parking. What is the availability of inexpensive restaurants in the area? These are additional expenses you must consider if you plan on taking a live review course.

What Are the Statistics Regarding the Pass Rate for the Company? It is very appropriate to inquire about how the pass rate statistics are determined by the review company. Check the NCSBN website *(www.ncsbn.org/index.htm)* to determine the most current statistics for passing the NCLEX examination. The review company must obtain NCLEX examination results directly from course participants or from schools of nursing. The National Council will not provide this information to review companies. Find out whether the advertised pass rate is based on actual responses from participants or on projected figures from the company.

Does the Review Company Offer any Type of Guarantee? Some review companies will offer you a guaranteed "refund," a free review course, or further assistance if you are not successful on the examination. Find out what the guarantee means and who is eligible for it. Sometimes the "guaranteed refund" is not easily accessible. Make sure you get in writing what you must do to be eligible and to file for the benefit.

When Is the Course Offered? Some graduates prefer to take a review course just before the examination so that the information is still fresh in their minds. Most graduates prefer to take the review within 1 to 2 weeks before the examination. This time frame generally works very well; the review course may be scheduled during the time you are waiting for your Authorization to Test. When you receive your authorization, you have completed your review course, and you are ready to schedule the examination. This schedule allows time to organize and study those areas that are your weakest. If you have only one review course available, how does it fit with your plans for scheduling the examination? Another aspect to consider is your employment schedule. Arrange your review course time so that you can truly focus on the material. If you have to work nights or evenings during the course, you will not benefit as much from the review.

Call the review company to get your questions answered. Does the representative spend time on the telephone with you, or is he or she in a rush to get you off the telephone? Or do you get an automated response instead of a live conversation? Is the company representative friendly and knowledgeable, and does that person demonstrate concern for answering all of your questions?

The online review course eliminates the problem of scheduling a specific time you have to take a review course. However, you must still plan the time to spend working through the online course in order for the review to be beneficial. Ultimately, each graduate must decide whether to take a review course as well as what type of review course. The more informed you are regarding a review course, the more intelligent a decision you can make.

NCLEX-RN Examination Review Books: Which One Is Right for You?

It is important to select a review book that meets your study needs. The first step is to check out your choices. Nursing faculty, friends with review books, the school library, and the local nursing

| **BOX 5-2** | **Selecting an NCLEX Examination Review Course** |

Here are some questions to consider:

WHERE AM I GOING TO WORK?

Will the institution pay for the review? _____

Will the institution pay the initial fee, or do I need to plan for reimbursement? _____

DOES THE INSTITUTION PROVIDE AN ON-SITE REVIEW?

Who teaches it? _____

Is it organized and presented by an independent company or hospital employees? _____

REVIEW COURSE INSTRUCTORS

Who will teach the class? Your faculty from school? Or review course faculty trained by the review company? _____

WHAT TYPE OF INSTRUCTIONAL MATERIAL IS USED?

Does it cost extra beyond the registration fee? _____

If it is additional to the registration fee, where do I get it? _____

Can I keep all of the instructional materials (e.g., books, testing booklets, audiotapes, DVDs, CDs)? _____

Does the instructional material include practice test questions in the NCLEX examination format? _____

HOW ARE THE CLASSES CONDUCTED?

How many days? _____

Are days consecutive or spread over several weeks? _____

What are the hours each day? _____

What is the teaching style (e.g., group work, lecture, home study, group participation, testing practice)? _____

What is the average-size class for the area? _____

HOW MUCH DOES IT COST?

What is the total price? _____

Does this include all of the class materials? _____

Are there group rates? If yes, what are they? _____

Are there early registration discounts? _____

When does the money have to be in? _____

Are there any "extra incentives"? _____

HOW DO I PAY FOR IT?

Is there a payment plan? _____

Can I make an early deposit to hold my space? _____

When is the deposit due? When is the final amount due? _____

If I change my mind after I make the deposit, can I get the deposit back? _____

IS THERE A GUARANTEE?

What is the guarantee? _____

Can I take the review again? _____

Does it have to be in the same location as the first time? _____

What do I have to do to qualify for the guarantee? _____

WHAT IS THE PASS RATE, AND HOW IS IT DETERMINED?

How does the company determine the pass rate for the review course? (Remember—the review company does not have access to NCLEX examination results)_____

Is it a company survey of review participants after the NCLEX examination? _____

Is it based on all participants or only the first-time takers? _____

Is it based on the company projected success rate? _____

Did the review company answer all of my questions in a courteous manner and seem interested in my business? _____

Do you know anyone who has taken a review? What are their recommendations?

textbook stores are all sources of information regarding review books. There are two types of nursing review books: those with content review and those that consist totally of review test questions. Evaluate how you are going to use the book. Is it for study during school, or is it specifically for review for the NCLEX examination? For example, if you bought the review book to study pediatric nursing, you may be disappointed. The focus of the NCLEX examination is not on pediatrics; therefore, it is not often a strong component in review books. If you wish to use a review book to identify priority aspects of care in the medical-surgical client, a review book can be of great benefit. The following discussion of review book selection is directed primarily toward review books that contain content review. Take notes as you read the different selections; it is hard to remember all the positive and negative points of each book (Box 5-2) (see "Selecting a Review Book: Where Do I Start?" in Evolve resources). Frequently, students find the review books to be of great benefit during school in assisting them to organize and consolidate a large amount of information. Plan to purchase a review book while you are still in nursing school.

Scan the Table of Contents. Is the information presented in a logical sequence? How is the information organized? It is important that the information be organized in a manner that is logical to you. The NCLEX examination is based on an integrated format, with a focus on the nursing process and client needs. Read the introduction to see how these areas were considered in the organization of the text. Quickly scan the table of contents and check the number of pages in various areas of subject material. Where is the focus of the material?

Evaluate Chapter Layout. How well is the material organized within the chapter? Are there major headings and subheadings to assist you in finding information quickly? Some texts use boxes or color to highlight divisions of content or priority information. These characteristics help to decrease the monotony of constant reading and to increase interest in the material presented.

Evaluate Content. Select a topic or topics you would like to read about in each of the review books you are considering. Select the priority nursing concepts and interventions you want to identify (e.g., nursing care of a client with diabetes). Evaluate the information regarding the adult, pediatric, and obstetric client. How does the information compare in the review books you are considering? Is the material logically organized? Does it contain the major concepts of care for that particular example? The focus of the review book should be toward nursing concepts and delivery of safe nursing care. In evaluating the currency of content, keep in mind that you cannot expect information that came out last month to be reflected in any textbook. The purpose of the NCLEX examination is to determine whether a candidate can perform safely and effectively as an entry-level nurse. This is the content that should be included in the review book. Based on the detailed test plan and the areas where new graduates are employed, the NCLEX examination is more heavily weighted toward the medical-surgical adult client.

Evaluate the Index. Look up several common topics in the index. A good index is critical to finding information in a timely manner.

Test Questions. Are test questions included in the text? Questions may be found after each of the main chapters or grouped together at the end of the book. Check to see if a rationale for the correct answer is included for each question. Does a computer disk of questions or an online test bank come with the book? How many questions are available?

Test-Taking Strategies. Does the book include information on test-taking strategies for multiple-choice and alternate item format questions? Test-taking strategies help you to be more "test-wise." These strategies can be of great benefit while you are still in school, in addition to practicing them as a method to prepare for the NCLEX examination.

Test Anxiety: What Is the Disease? How Do You Get Rid of It?

Frequently, students and graduates focus on their "test anxiety" as the reason for not doing well on examinations. Test anxiety is something that only you can change. You are the one allowing the anxiety to affect you in a negative way. The only person responsible for your test anxiety is you, and the only one who can do anything about it is you. Address your test anxiety while you are still in school. Look at some simple steps to decrease your anxiety regarding testing.

- **Plan ahead.** Do not wait until the last minute to read 150 pages in your textbook, all your classroom notes, and the 10 articles assigned for the test. Plan study time, and stick to it!
- **Set aside study time for when you are at your best.** Frequently, study time is squeezed in only after everything else (laundry, meals, housecleaning, yard work, and so on) has been completed. You are defeating your purpose and increasing your anxiety when you try to study at a time when you are tired and not receptive to learning.
- **Study smart.** Plan for 45 minutes to an hour of review on the day after a 90-minute class lecture. This will greatly enhance your retention of the classroom information. Plan for an hour to review/scan assigned reading or information before class so that you will know where information is located and what you will need to take notes on in class.
- **Give yourself a break!** Plan your study time to include a break about every hour. Your retention of information begins to decrease after about 30 minutes and is significantly decreased after an hour.
- **Think positively!** If your friends are "negative thinkers," do not plan to study with them. Go to the movies or play sports with them, but do not study with them. Anxiety and negative thinking are contagious—do not expose yourself to the disease!
- **Do not cram.** Whether you are studying for a unit examination in school or for the NCLEX examination, cramming is not an effective study method and it will increase your anxiety. The NCLEX examination is not written to evaluate memory-based information. Test questions focus on the higher levels of cognitive ability. Application of principles and the analysis of information will be required to determine an appropriate nursing response or action. Do not jeopardize your critical thinking skills by staying up late and cramming.

Just thinking about an examination can cause some students an increase in anxiety. It seems as though during the last year of school, particularly the last semester, tests become a major source of anxiety. Everyone knows fellow students who become obsessed with the idea that they are going to fail an important examination. View an examination as a positive step—an opportunity to demonstrate your knowledge.

Put yourself in charge of your feelings.
Get rid of those negative thought "tapes"!
Replace negative thoughts and ideas with positive ones:
  I WILL pass this test!
  I will be so glad to get this test behind me.

Write down positive affirmations and put them on your bathroom mirror, on your refrigerator, anywhere you will see them often. Potential employers, state boards of nursing, your spiritual advisers, and your neighbors are not going to think less of you if you are not at the top of the class. Keep in mind that your employers and the state boards do not care what your grades were in school or on the NCLEX examination—they just want to know that you can pass the NCLEX examination and practice nursing safely. Give yourself permission to be in the middle— an average student on grades, but one who is concerned about professional, safe nursing practice.

What Kind of Questions Can I Expect on the NCLEX Examination?

On the NCLEX examination, it is anticipated that most of the questions will be in a multiple-choice format; they have a stem in which the question is presented and four options from which to choose an answer. Of these four options, three are meant to distract you from the correct answer. With the four-item, multiple-choice questions, there is only one correct answer. The multiple-choice NCLEX examination questions give you the choice of four answers, not a combination of the four options (Figure 5-2).

> The focus of the NCLEX examination is on nursing care. The questions will ask you to use nursing concepts and judgment in the situation presented.

What Are "Alternate Item Format" Questions and Why the Big Fuss About Them? In October 2003, different types of questions (other than four-option multiple-choice questions) were introduced as "scored" questions on the NCLEX examination. These questions

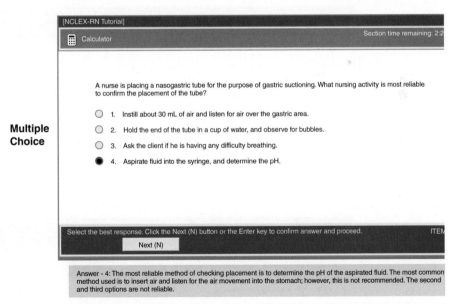

FIGURE 5-2
Sample of multiple-choice test question.

are frequently referred to as "alternate item format" questions and are included in the test bank of questions that will be used to select the test items for a candidate's examination. There is no preset number of alternate item format questions that will be presented to a candidate; the question or items will be randomly selected as the adaptive testing process selects questions that meet the parameters of the test plan.

There is no special or additional nursing knowledge needed to answer the alternate item format questions. There is no attempt to hide or camouflage the questions; they are randomly selected to be included in a candidate exam. The same nursing concepts are being tested, and the questions are based on the same test plan. The question is simply asked in a different format. You do not need to do anything differently with regard to the alternate item format questions; just be aware of types of format and implement good testing strategies to answer the question (NCSBN, 2013c).

What Are the Different Types of Alternate Item Format Questions?

Fill-in-the-Blank. These are questions in which a short answer is required. This may be a question that requires a drug calculation, or an intake and output calculation, or an assessment scoring. In these cases, only the numbers should be entered in the space provided. No units of measurement can be included with the answer, because the unit of measurement is already on the screen (Figure 5-3).

Multiple-Response Item. This is a different type of multiple-choice question. There will be more than four options presented, and the question will very clearly ask you to select all of the options that correctly answer the question. With the mouse, you will select each option you want to include in the answer and then click enter to confirm your answer and continue to the next question. There is only one correct combination of answers (Figure 5-4).

Fill in the Blank

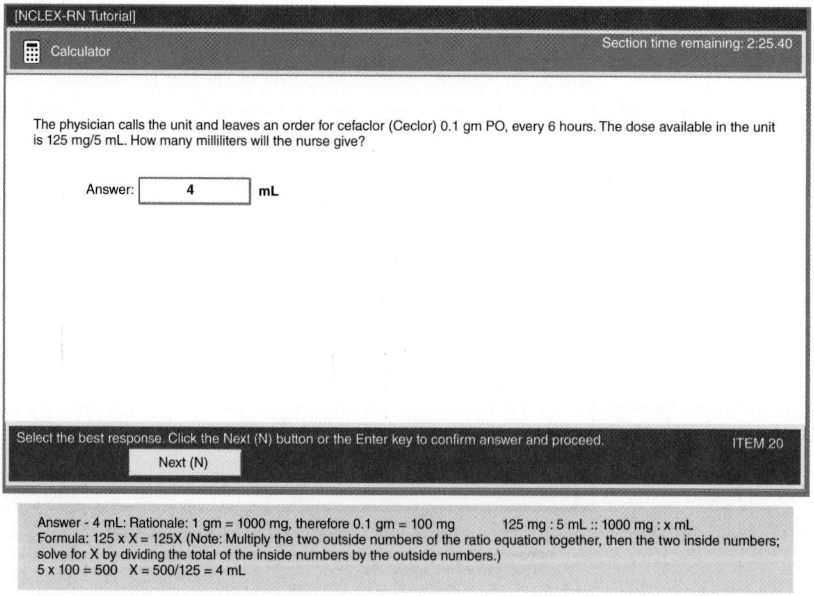

[NCLEX-RN Tutorial]

⊞ Calculator   Section time remaining: 2:25.40

The physician calls the unit and leaves an order for cefaclor (Ceclor) 0.1 gm PO, every 6 hours. The dose available in the unit is 125 mg/5 mL. How many milliliters will the nurse give?

Answer: [4]   mL

Select the best response. Click the Next (N) button or the Enter key to confirm answer and proceed.   ITEM 20

Next (N)

Answer - 4 mL: Rationale: 1 gm = 1000 mg, therefore 0.1 gm = 100 mg   125 mg : 5 mL :: 1000 mg : x mL
Formula: 125 x X = 125X (Note: Multiply the two outside numbers of the ratio equation together, then the two inside numbers; solve for X by dividing the total of the inside numbers by the outside numbers.)
5 x 100 = 500   X = 500/125 = 4 mL

FIGURE 5-3
Fill-in-the-blank.

[NCLEX-RN Tutorial]

Calculator   Section time remaining: 3:15.20

The nurse is caring for an 85-year old client who has a diagnosis of Vancomycin resistant enterococci (VRE). What precautions will the nurse implement in assisting the client with morning care?

Select all that apply:

1. ☑ Wear clean gloves.
2. ☐ Remove all extra suctioning supplies from the room.
3. ☐ Dispose of the gown and mask in container outside client's door.
4. ☑ Wear face mask when working within 3 feet of the client.
5. ☑ Put on a gown prior to entering the room.
6. ☐ Remove the stethoscope from the room if it did not come in contact with the client.

Select the best response. Click the Next (N) button or the Enter key to confirm answer and proceed.   ITEM 21

Next (N)

Answer: The answer is based on standard precautions, plus respiratory precautions for the pneumonia. Nothing should be removed from the room and the gown should be removed prior to leaving the room, not outside the room.

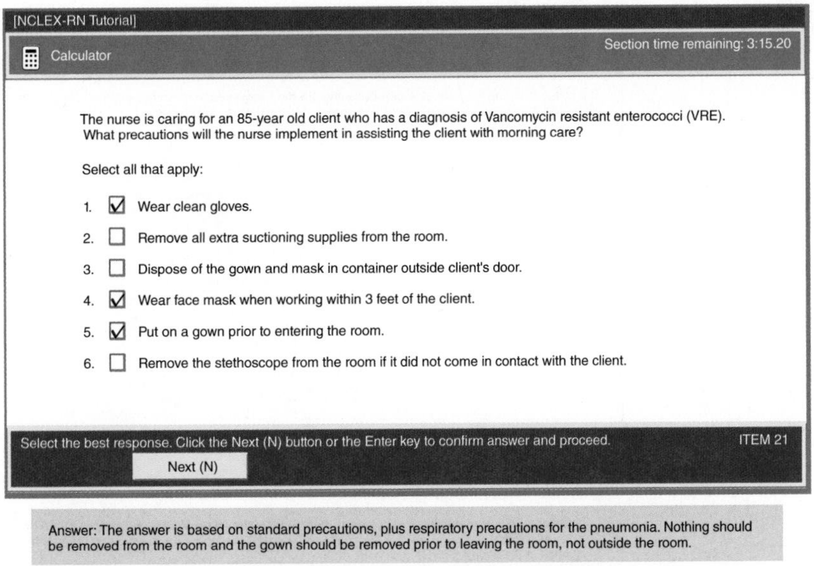

FIGURE 5-4

Multiple response.

Hot Spot. These items present a diagram or a graphic and require you to select an area on the diagram to answer the question. For example, let's assume that the diagram is an illustration of the anterior thorax. The question for this diagram might ask you to click on the area where you would place the stethoscope to listen for the apical heart rate or to click on the area where you would listen for the characteristic sounds of the mitral valve (Figure 5-5).

Ordered Response (Drag-and-Drop). For this type of question, you will be presented with a list of activities, clients, or steps in a procedure. The question will ask you to click on each item and "drag" it to another area of the screen, placing the items, for instance, in the order in which they would be performed or in order of priority of care. Pay close attention to how the question asks you to rank the options. After you have determined how your answer should be ranked, click on the option you want to place first, "drag" that option over, and place it in the box. You will then select the next option you want to place second, "drag" that option over, and place it in the box. You will continue this process until you have used all of the options present. You can change your answer any time before you click the Next button. This type of question is called an "ordered response" (Figure 5-6).

Chart/Exhibit Item. These questions will present a problem, then provide exhibit information stored in tabs. You will click on each tab to find information that will assist you in solving the problem that is presented. The tabs frequently contain information from a chart or data collection from the client. There will still be four options from which to select the correct answer, but you will need to evaluate the data in each of the tabs to determine the correct answer. Do not attempt to select the correct answer without evaluating all of the information provided on each of the tabs (Figure 5-7).

Audio Item. In this type of item, you will be presented with a question that has an audio component. You will put on the headset provided and click the "Play button" to listen to the

Hot Spot

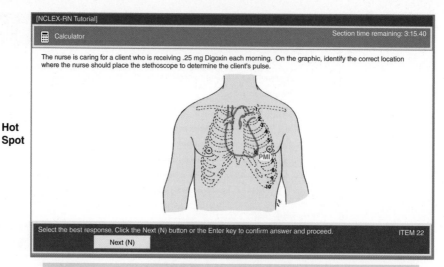

FIGURE 5-5

Hot spot.

Drag and Drop

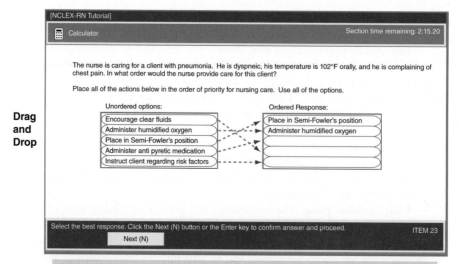

FIGURE 5-6

Drag and drop (ordered response).

audio for the information required to answer the question. The volume may be adjusted and you can click the Play button to repeat the audio information. Listen carefully to the audio clip and select the option that best answers the question (Figure 5-8).

Graphic Options. The graphic option type of alternate item format presents you with graphics instead of text for the answer options. You will be required to select the correct answer from the graphics presented at the end of the question (Figure 5-9).

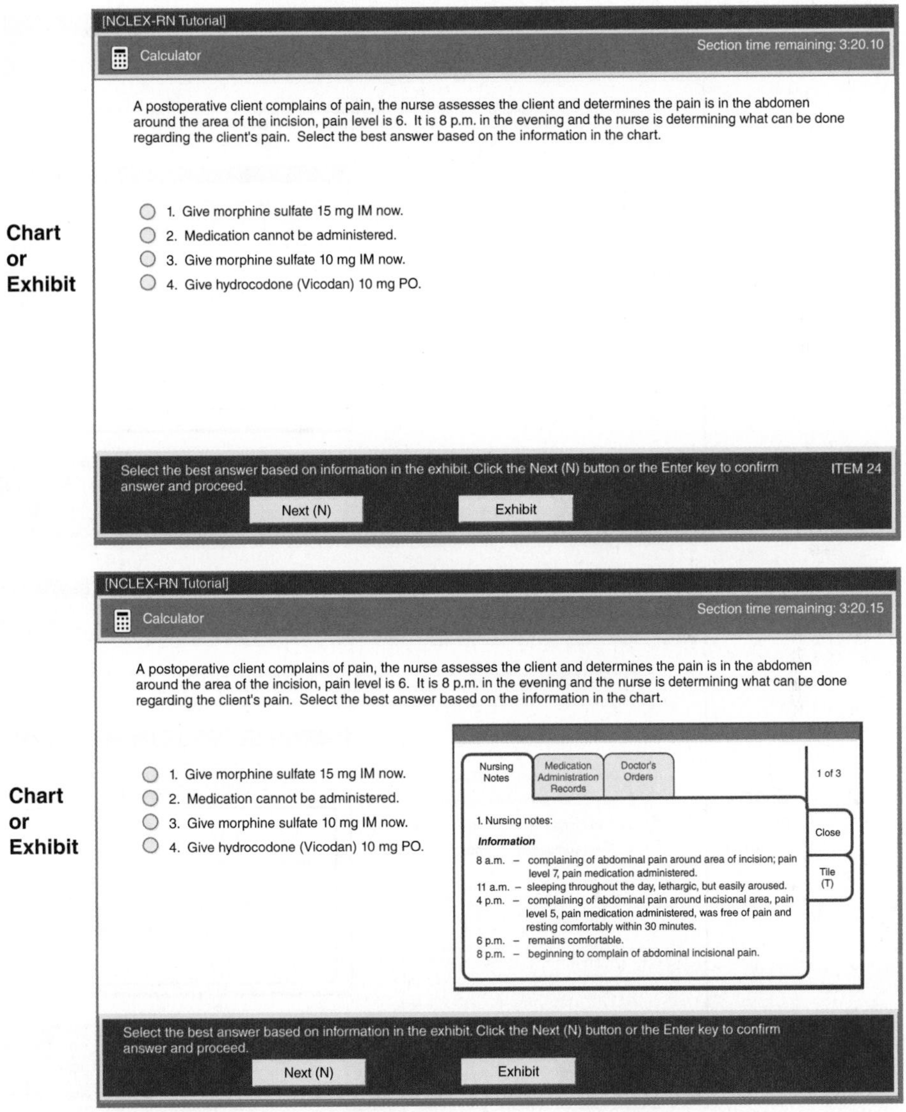

Chart or Exhibit

[NCLEX-RN Tutorial]

Section time remaining: 3:20.10

▦ Calculator

A postoperative client complains of pain, the nurse assesses the client and determines the pain is in the abdomen around the area of the incision, pain level is 6. It is 8 p.m. in the evening and the nurse is determining what can be done regarding the client's pain. Select the best answer based on the information in the chart.

○ 1. Give morphine sulfate 15 mg IM now.
○ 2. Medication cannot be administered.
○ 3. Give morphine sulfate 10 mg IM now.
○ 4. Give hydrocodone (Vicodan) 10 mg PO.

Select the best answer based on information in the exhibit. Click the Next (N) button or the Enter key to confirm answer and proceed.   ITEM 24

Next (N)   Exhibit

Chart or Exhibit

[NCLEX-RN Tutorial]

Section time remaining: 3:20.15

▦ Calculator

A postoperative client complains of pain, the nurse assesses the client and determines the pain is in the abdomen around the area of the incision, pain level is 6. It is 8 p.m. in the evening and the nurse is determining what can be done regarding the client's pain. Select the best answer based on the information in the chart.

○ 1. Give morphine sulfate 15 mg IM now.
○ 2. Medication cannot be administered.
○ 3. Give morphine sulfate 10 mg IM now.
○ 4. Give hydrocodone (Vicodan) 10 mg PO.

Nursing Notes	Medication Administration Records	Doctor's Orders

1 of 3

1. Nursing notes:

Information

8 a.m. – complaining of abdominal pain around area of incision; pain level 7, pain medication administered.
11 a.m. – sleeping throughout the day, lethargic, but easily aroused.
4 p.m. – complaining of abdominal pain around incisional area, pain level 5, pain medication administered, was free of pain and resting comfortably within 30 minutes.
6 p.m. – remains comfortable.
8 p.m. – beginning to complain of abdominal incisional pain.

Close

Tile (T)

Select the best answer based on information in the exhibit. Click the Next (N) button or the Enter key to confirm answer and proceed.

Next (N)   Exhibit

FIGURE 5-7

Exhibit.

As the NCSBN continues to research the development of test items that evaluate the reasoning and nursing judgment of nursing graduates, other types of alternate item format questions will be developed. Don't be alarmed if you should encounter one of these alternate item format questions—focus on what the question is asking, follow the directions, and select the option that reflects the best client care.

Chart or Exhibit

[NCLEX-RN Tutorial]

Calculator — Section time remaining: 3:20.15

A postoperative client complains of pain, the nurse assesses the client and determines the pain is in the abdomen around the area of the incision, pain level is 6. It is 8 p.m. in the evening and the nurse is determining what can be done regarding the client's pain. Select the best answer based on the information in the chart.

1. Give morphine sulfate 15 mg IM now.
2. Medication cannot be administered.
3. Give morphine sulfate 10 mg IM now.
4. Give hydrocodone (Vicodan) 10 mg PO.

Nursing Notes | Medication Administration Records | Doctor's Orders — 2 of 3

Close / Tile (T)

2. Medication administration record (MAR):

Morphine sulfate 10 mg IM administered at 8 a.m.

Hydrocodone 10 mg, PO administered at 4 p.m.

Select the best answer based on information in the exhibit. Click the Next (N) button or the Enter key to confirm answer and proceed. ITEM 24

Next (N)   Exhibit

Chart or Exhibit

[NCLEX-RN Tutorial]

Calculator — Section time remaining: 3:20.30

A postoperative client complains of pain, the nurse assesses the client and determines the pain is in the abdomen around the area of the incision, pain level is 6. It is 8 p.m. in the evening and the nurse is determining what can be done regarding the client's pain. Select the best answer based on the information in the chart.

1. Give morphine sulfate 15 mg IM now.
2. Medication cannot be administered.
3. Give morphine sulfate 10 mg IM now.
4. Give hydrocodone (Vicodan) 10 mg PO.

Nursing Notes | Medication Administration Records | Doctor's Orders — 3 of 3

Close / Tile (T)

3. Doctor's orders:

Orders for the last 24 hours include:

Morphine sulfate 10-15 mg q 3-4h PRN severe pain.

Hydrocodone (Vicodan) 10 mg PO, every 3-4 hours moderate pain.

Select the best answer based on information in the exhibit. Click the Next (N) button or the Enter key to confirm answer and proceed. ITEM 24

Next (N)   Exhibit

FIGURE 5-7, cont'd
Exhibit.

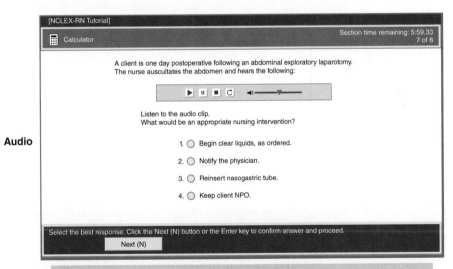

[NCLEX-RN Tutorial]

Calculator   Section time remaining: 3:20.40

A postoperative client complains of pain, the nurse assesses the client and determines the pain is in the abdomen around the area of the incision, pain level is 6. It is 8 p.m. in the evening and the nurse is determining what can be done regarding the client's pain. Select the best answer based on the information in the chart.

Chart or Exhibit

○ 1. Give morphine sulfate 15 mg IM now.
○ 2. Medication cannot be administered.
○ 3. Give morphine sulfate 10 mg IM now.
● 4. Give hydrocodone (Vicodan) 10 mg PO.

Select the best answer based on information in the exhibit. Click the Next (N) button or the Enter key to confirm answer and proceed.   ITEM 24

[Next (N)]   [Exhibit]

Need to know: Analysis of information.
Client received Demerol 50 mg IM at 11 a.m. and he was lethargic and sleeping for the next 5 hours. He received hydrocodone PO at 4 p.m. and he was comfortable for the next 4 hours. The doctor's orders are current for both the IM and the PO medication for pain. Give the hydrocodone, PO for pain at this time. It held him for 4 hours the last time, and the doctor's order is current.

FIGURE 5-7, cont'd
Exhibit.

[NCLEX-RN Tutorial]

Calculator   Section time remaining: 5:59.33
                                                                                                    7 of 8

A client is one day postoperative following an abdominal exploratory laparotomy. The nurse auscultates the abdomen and hears the following:

[▶ II ■ C   ◀━━━●━━]

Listen to the audio clip.
What would be an appropriate nursing intervention?

Audio

1. ○ Begin clear liquids, as ordered.

2. ○ Notify the physician.

3. ○ Reinsert nasogastric tube.

4. ○ Keep client NPO.

Select the best response. Click the Next (N) button or the Enter key to confirm answer and proceed.

[Next (N)]

Answer 1: Bowels sounds are noted on the audio clip, which means that peristalsis has returned to the gastrointestinal tract and the client can begin a clear liquid diet. If bowel sounds are present, there is no need to notify the physician; keep the client NPO or reinsert the nasogastric tube. Laparoscopic procedures are associated with lower rates of postoperative complications, earlier diet progression, and shorter hospital stays.

FIGURE 5-8
Audio.

What Difference Do Test-Taking Strategies Make?

Knowing how to take an examination is a skill that is developed through practice. Look back at the beginning of nursing school and your first nursing examination; you have come a long way from there! How many times during school have you reviewed a test and discovered you knew the right answer but marked the wrong one? Nursing faculty and those responsible for the NCLEX examination are not sympathetic to your claim that you "really meant this answer and not the one I marked." How many times did you go back and change an answer from the correct response to the wrong one? If these are common errors you experience during nursing school, you need to incorporate test-taking strategies into your testing skills. Some of the testing practices you have developed over the years may be positive, whereas others may be negative. Information on test-taking strategies can be of benefit to you now and later. Start using testing strategies while you are still in school. This will help you with your current examinations, and the testing strategies will be second-nature by the time you take the NCLEX examination. Take the time to implement good testing practices—get the question right the first time! Analyze where you are with testing skills, get rid of the negative, and retain the positive.

What Are Strategies for Answering Multiple-Choice Questions?

Read the Question (Stem) Carefully. Do not read extra meaning into the question. Avoid asking yourself, "What if the client should … ?" Or, "What if the client does … ?" Make sure you read the "stem" correctly and understand exactly what information is being requested. (Do you tend to make the client sicker than he really is by the time you finish the question?)

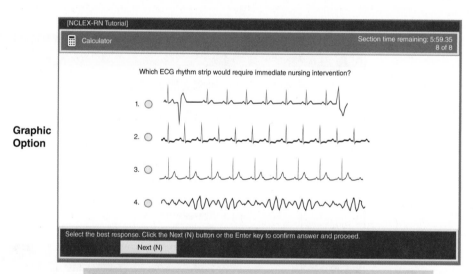

Graphic Option

FIGURE 5-9

Graphic option. *(Figures 1, 2, 3, and 4 from Lewis et al:* Medical-Surgical Nursing, *7e. St. Louis, Elsevier, 2007, pp 846, 851, 853, and 854, respectively.)*

Create a Pool of Information. What are the concepts of care regarding a client with the condition or problem presented? Get a general idea of the condition and type of care required before you read the options. Do not try to predict a correct answer.

Look for Critical Words. Evaluate the question for critical words that make a difference in what the question is asking. Watch for *priority, initial, first action, side effect,* and/or *toxic effect.*

Evaluate All the Options in a Systematic Manner. Focus on what information is being requested, and then carefully go through each option. Do not stop with the first correct answer; the last option may be more correct or more inclusive of information.

Eliminate Options You Know Are Not Correct. And leave them alone! Once you have eliminated an option, do not go back to it unless you have gained more insight into the question. Frequently, your initial response in evaluating an option is correct. Go through all of the options and eliminate incorrect ones. What is left is frequently the correct answer, even if it is not what you were looking for.

Identify Similarities in the Options. Look for an option that is unique from the rest. For example, in a question dealing with a low-residue diet, three of the options might contain a vegetable with a peeling, but one might not—that one is probably the correct answer. Evaluate options that contain several suggested client activities. Are three of the activities similar and one different from the rest? The option that is different may be the correct answer.

Evaluate Priority Questions Very Carefully. Keep in mind the nursing process and Maslow's hierarchy of needs. You must have adequate assessment information before proceeding with the nursing process. If assessment information is presented in the stem of the question, then the answer may require a nursing intervention. If a client is presented in the question as experiencing severe chest pain, it would not be appropriate to conduct a cardiac assessment prior to putting the client to bed and starting the oxygen! (*If in distress, don't assess!*—If a client is presented in a distressed condition, then adequate assessment data have already been provided in the stem of the question, so you will need to look for an immediate nursing intervention to address the problem). According to Maslow, physical needs must be met before psychosocial needs—the physical needs of your mental health client must be met before you can focus on the mental health needs. When considering the physical needs, respiratory needs are a priority. (You've got to breathe first!) But a word of caution here—do not give a client a respiratory problem if he does not have one!

Select Answers That Focus on the Client. Choices that focus on hospital rules and policies are most often not correct. Consider that you have enough time and adequate staff to perform whatever action necessary for safe client care.

Analyze your testing skills so that you will know where to start to improve them. Once you have identified your testing weaknesses, organize a plan to correct the problem areas. One of the most difficult things to do is to change the way you are used to doing something, even when the change makes life easier. Get an early start on evaluating testing skills; it can make a significant difference in the remaining examinations in nursing school.

NCLEX Examination Testing Tips

NCLEX Hospital. For the NCLEX examination to be appropriate to all candidates nationwide, it is important that there be a base for the vast knowledge that is to be tested. Therefore, when you are taking the NCLEX examination, consider yourself working in the "NCLEX Hospital." It is a great place to work; everything you need is provided—great equipment that works the way it is supposed to, plenty of staff, and enough time to provide the best and safest nursing care possible. The clients (*patients* are most frequently referred to as *clients* on the NCLEX examination) all have conditions that respond just as the book says they are supposed to respond. Study according to your textbooks. Your clinical experience is complementary with your academic study. Do not focus on the unusual, unexpected, or strange things that happened to you during clinical rotations.

NCLEX Clients. Focus on the client in the question you are working on. As far as the NCLEX Hospital is concerned, that is the only client you are to be concerned about. Do not worry about the five or six other clients you may have assigned to your care. In the NCLEX Hospital, you are taking care of one client at a time, unless it is stated otherwise. Your priority concern is the client in the current question you are trying to answer.

Medication Administration. Know the Six Rights and the common nursing implications of medications. The generic name will be in the question and the trade name in parenthesis (NCSBN, 2013e). A good strategy is to study the medications according to the classification. For example, study the nursing implications regarding administration of corticosteroid medications and be able to identify common corticosteroid medications and their nursing implications.

Calling for Assistance. Be careful with questions for which the right answer appears to be to call someone else to take care of the problem. This is a nursing examination; therefore, identify the best nursing management. This includes questions that include calling the doctor, respiratory therapist, housekeeping, chaplain, or social worker. Be sure there is not something you need to do for the client before notifying someone else regarding the problem. If the client is experiencing difficulty, his condition is changing, and there is nothing you can do, call the doctor. This is particularly true in situations in which the client is experiencing a problem with circulatory compromise. However, if the client is having difficulty breathing, the priority focus may be to position the client to maintain an open airway, and/or to begin oxygen as well as quickly assess the status of the client before calling the doctor.

Positioning. Watch for questions that have particular positions in the stem of the question or those that include positions in the options. Is the client's position necessary to prevent complications or treat a current problem, or is it primarily for comfort? As you are reviewing, be aware of questions that include conditions that require a specific position in the care of that client.

Delegation and Supervision. The NCLEX examination includes questions in these areas. Check out the delegation decision tree developed by the Ohio Board of Nursing (*www.ncsbn.org/delegationtree.pdf*). Some common considerations to make when evaluating these questions:

- Delegate to someone else the care of the most stable client with the most predictable response to care.
- Delegate tasks to the most qualified person to perform the task.
- Delegate to nursing assistants those tasks that have the most specific guidelines (e.g., collecting a urine sample, feeding, providing hygiene, ambulating).

Setting Priorities with a Group of Clients. A question may present a group of clients and ask you to determine which client you would take care of first or to rank the clients according to when you would take care of them. Determine the most unstable client who requires nursing care to prevent immediate problems—take care of this client first. Keep in mind Maslow's hierarchy of needs.

Doctor's Orders. For most of the questions, you can consider that you have a doctor's order to perform any of the options presented in the question. However, you should watch for questions that may be specifically asking for a "dependent nursing action" where you will have to consider whether you need a doctor's order to perform the nursing action. It would be difficult to present questions and continue to repeat that a physician's or health care provider's order was present. Standing orders and state nurse practice acts all have implications on orders. This is a standardized test that is administered nationally and therefore, there has to be consistency; consequently, unique aspects of nurse practice acts and standing orders are not tested.

> Be aware that the answer you are looking for frequently will not be included in the options! This is not uncommon on NCLEX examination questions. Consider the principles and concepts of care for a client with the problem presented. Eliminate the wrong answers and evaluate what is left.

CONCLUSION

Wow! NCLEX examination deadlines, review courses, testing skills, review books, money, license—and you thought all you needed to do was graduate from nursing school! A lot happens between graduating from nursing school and being successful on the NCLEX examination. The key to surviving it all with a smile is careful planning and implementing those plans during your role transition. (That sounds a lot like the nursing process, doesn't it?) The NCLEX-RN Examination is one of the most incredible opportunities of your life. Box 5-3 provides a listing of relevant websites and online resources. This examination will open the doors for you as you begin one of the most fantastic experiences of a lifetime: a career in nursing.

> Just say to yourself, "I can do it. I can pass the NCLEX examination!"

BOX 5-3	Relevant Websites and Online Resources

National Council of State Boards of Nursing http://www.ncsbn.org
- Candidate bulletin https://www.ncsbn.org/2013_NCLEX_Candidate_Bulletin.pdf
- Detailed Test Plan https://www.ncsbn.org/2013_NCLEX_RN_Detailed_Test_Plan_Candidate.pdf
    Pearson Vue Testing http://www.pearsonvue.com/nclex/ Also location for Online Tutorial for the NCLEX Exam

BIBLIOGRAPHY

National Council of State Boards of Nursing: *2011 Practice Analysis: Linking the NCLEX-RN Examination to Practice*, 2012. Retrieved from https://www.ncsbn.org/12_RN_Practice_Analysis_Vol53.pdf

National Council of State Boards of Nursing: 2013 NCLEX-RN detailed test plan. National Council of State Boards of Nursing, 2013a, Retrieved from https://www.ncsbn.org/2013_NCLEX_RN_Detailed_Test_Plan_Candidate.pdf

National Council of State Boards of Nursing: 2013 NCLEX examination candidate bulletin, National Council of State Boards of Nursing, 2013b. Retrieved from https://www.ncsbn.org/2013_NCLEX_Candidate_Bulletin.pdf

National Council of State Boards of Nursing: Alternate Item Formats Frequently Asked Questions, 2013c, National Council of State Boards of Nursing. Retrieved from https://www.ncsbn.org/2334.htm

National Council of State Boards of Nursing: NCLEX Candidate Frequently Asked Questions, 2013d, National Council State Boards of Nursing. Retrieved from https://www.ncsbn.org/2321.htm

National Council of State Boards of Nursing: NCLEX Exam Development Frequently Asked Questions, 2013e, National Council of State Boards of Nursing. Retrieved from https://www.ncsbn.org/2324.htm

National Council of State Boards of Nursing: Nurse licensure compact, 2013f, National Council of State Boards of Nursing. Retrieved from https://www.ncsbn.org/nlc.htm

National Council of State Boards of Nursing: Practice Analysis Frequently Asked Questions, 2013g, National Council State Boards of Nursing. Retrieved from https://www.ncsbn.org/2322.htm

National Council of State Boards of Nursing: The eight steps of the NCLEX examination process, 2013h, Retrieved from https://www.ncsbn.org/2013_Eight_Steps_of_NCLEX.pdf

Pearson VUE (2009): State of the art identification: Palm vein pattern recognition for the NCLEX examination. Retrieved from www.pearsonvue.com/nclex/NCLEX_PalmVeinFAQ.pdf.

Pearson VUE (2013). The NCLEX Examination. Retrieved from http://www.pearsonvue.com/nclex/

Additional resources are available online at http://evolve.elsevier.com/Zerwekh/nsgtoday/.

Additional resources are available online at *http://evolve.elsevier.com/Zerwekh/nsgtoday/.*

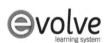

CHAPTER 6

Historical Perspectives: Influences on the Present

JoAnn Zerwekh, MSN, EdD, RN

> *History repeats itself because each generation refuses to read the minutes of the last meeting.*
> —ANONYMOUS

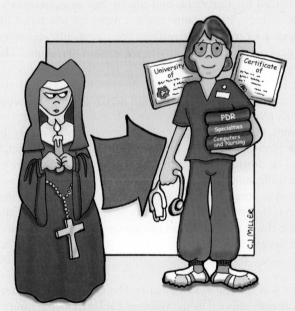

After completing this chapter, you should be able to:

- Explain the early European contributions to nursing.

- Explain the forces that have affected the roles of American nurses.

Nursing has come a long way; it is not what it used to be.

o, you have to study the history of nursing. Generally, the topic is considered boring. Well, be prepared for a different approach to the topic. Knowing the history of our profession guides our understanding of why we do what we do today. This understanding can be useful to us as we set our professional goals. Threads of nursing history can be found throughout the book. Understanding the history can often help in deciding what changes are needed, what changes are helpful, and what changes may be unnecessary. Let us begin with a look at where nursing began.

NURSING HISTORY: PEOPLE AND PLACES

Where Did It All Begin?

Most nursing historians agree that nursing, or the care of the ill and injured, has been done since the beginning of human life and has generally been a woman's role. A mother caring for a child in a cave and someone caring for another ill adult by boiling willow bark to relieve fever are both examples of nursing. The word *nurse* is derived from the Latin word *nutricius,* meaning "nourishing."

Roman mythological figures included the goddess Fortuna, who was usually recognized as being responsible for one's fate and who also served as Jupiter's nurse (Dolan, 1969). Even before Greek and Roman times, ancient Egyptian physicians and nurses assembled voluminous pharmacopoeia with more than 700 remedies for numerous health problems. Great emphasis was placed on the use of animal parts in concoctions that were generally drunk or applied to the body. The physician prescribed and provided the treatments and usually had an assistant who provided the nursing care (Kalisch and Kalisch, 1986). Some ancient medicine was based on driving out the evil spirit rather than curing or treating the malady. The treatments were often very foul and frequently included fecal material. By now you may be thinking of the saying, "The treatment was successful, but the patient died."

Advancement of medical knowledge halted abruptly after the Roman Empire was conquered and the Dark Ages began. Any medical and health care knowledge that survived these dark times did so only through the efforts of Jewish physicians who were able to translate the Greek and Roman works (Kalisch and Kalisch, 1986). One bright spot was in Salerno, where a school of medicine and health was established for physicians and women to assist in childbirth. In fact, a midwife named Trotula wrote what may be considered the first nursing textbook on the cure of diseases of women (Dalton, 1900). Generally, nursing was performed by designated priestesses and was associated with some type of temple worship. Little information has survived about this early period. Historians have assumed that Hippocrates was assisted by women, but there is little information to support that. From these roots, nursing began to develop as a recognized and valued service to society (Jamieson and Sewall, 1949).

Why Deacons, Widows, and Virgins?

Paralleling the fall of the Roman Empire was the rise of Christianity. The early organization of the young Christian church, which was directly affected by the vision of Paul, included a governing bishop and seven appointed deacons. These individuals assisted the apostles in the work of the Church (the word *deacon* means "servant"). The deacon was directly responsible for distributing all the goods and property that apostles relinquished to the Church before they "took up the cross and followed." The apostles were required to give up all material resources to achieve full status in the Church.

Women sympathetic to the Christian cause of aiding the poor were encouraged in this work by the bishops and deacons. Eventually, the deacons relinquished this work to women and established the position of deaconess for that purpose. To maintain a pure heart, these women were required by the Church to be either virgins or widows. The stipulation for widows, however, was that they had to have been married only once (Jamieson and Sewall, 1949). The deaconesses carried nursing forward as they ministered to the sick and injured in their homes. Phoebe, a friend of Paul's and the very first deaconess in the young Christian church, has been called the first visiting nurse (Dana, 1936).

Treatments continued to be a mixture of scientific fact, home remedies, and magic. Eventually, an order of widows evolved that was composed of women who were free from home responsibilities and thus able to commit fully to working among the poor. The widows, although not ordained, continued to do the same work as the deaconesses. This was soon followed by the creation of the Order of Virgins as the Church began placing greater value on purity of body. Although deaconess orders were abolished in the Mediterranean countries, they thrived in other European countries. The traditional commitment to care for the poor and sick became invaluable in a society that generally had neither the time nor the inclination to aid them. Eventually, these women became known as *nuns* (from *non nuptae*, meaning "not married").

This was a time of tremendous upheaval in the world. Wars, invasions, and battles were constant, and as a result of these encounters, the number of widows was significant. Society during this time did not have the sophistication or the means to deal with the dependents of the soldiers killed in battle. As a means of survival, women joined the nuns as a form of protection from starvation and poverty. This was a dark and dreary time in which superstition, witchcraft, and folklore were predominant influences. Because of the need for physical protection, convents were built to shelter these women (Jamieson and Sewall, 1949). The convents became havens to which women could withdraw from ignorance and evil and be nurtured in traditional Christian beliefs (Donahue, 1985). The deaconesses, widows, and virgins continued to minister to and nurse the ill within the safety of the convent.

How Did Knighthood Contribute to Nursing?

The Holy Wars furthered the development of nursing in a rather interesting way. Because many Christian crusaders became ill while in Jerusalem, a hospital known as the Hospital of St. John was built to accommodate them. Those who fought in these Holy Wars had taken oaths of chivalry, justice, and piety and were known as knights. Often the knights were accompanied into battle by men trained in the healing arts. These male nurses cared for wounded or otherwise stricken knights. They usually wore a red cross emblazoned on their tunics so that in the heat of battle they could be easily identified and avoid injury or death (Bullough and Bullough, 1978).

The Hospital of St. John gave excellent nursing care. Many of the nurses who survived stayed to work with the hospital organizers. As the battles in the Holy Land continued, the nurses and knights organized a fighting force with a code of rules and a uniform consisting of a black robe with a white Maltese cross, the symbol of poverty, humility, and chastity. They ventured out to rescue the sick and wounded and transport them to the hospital for care; thus they became known as the Hospitalers (Kalisch and Kalisch, 1986). Male nurses dominated these orders. Other orders that emulated the Hospitalers developed in Europe, and more hospitals were opened based on the Hospital of St. John model (Donahue, 1985).

The altruistic spirit of nursing was also seen in the craftsmen's guilds. Although their primary purpose was to provide training and jobs through the practice of apprenticeship, the guilds provided care and aid for their members when they became old and could no longer work at their trade. The guilds also assisted members and their families in times of illness and injury. The apprenticeship system—in which experience is gained on the job but no formal education is provided—once served as a model for the training of nurses (Donahue, 1985). This system is no longer used and is now considered to have been detrimental to the evolution of nursing.

What nursing gained during this period of history was status. The altruistic ideal of providing care as a service performed out of humility and love became the foundation for nursing. The recognition of the value of hospitals grew; all across Europe, cities were building their own hospitals. A general resurgence in the demand for trained doctors and nurses contributed to the building of medical schools and the development of university programs in the art and science of healing.

What About Revolts and Nursing?

Revolts—not the kind that led to battles, but revolts of a social nature—were common. There were battles too; however, the social revolts had a more direct impact on nursing. The revolution of the spirit, more commonly known as the Renaissance, ushered in new concepts of the world: the discovery of the laws of nature by Newton, the exploration of unknown lands, and the growth of secular interests (humanism) over spiritual ones. In this era emerged several outstanding humanists who were to become saints (Donahue, 1985). Interestingly, in depictions of these saints, they are shown as needing nursing care or as giving care to a wounded or injured person.

In Europe, the Protestant Reformation began primarily as a religious reform movement, but ended with revolt within the Church. Many hospitals in Protestant countries were forced to close, and those loyal to the Church that operated them were driven out of the country, resulting in a significant shortage of nurses (mostly nuns) to care for the ill and injured. The poor and ill were considered a burden to society, and those hospitals that remained operational in the Protestant countries became known as "pest houses." To fill the need for nurses, women (many of whom were alcoholics and former prostitutes) were recruited. Generally, during this period, a nurse was a woman serving time in a hospital rather than a prison (Donahue, 1985; Jamieson and Sewall, 1949).

The industrial and intellectual revolutions that followed the Reformation all had significant impacts on nursing. During the Industrial Revolution, as production of much-needed goods was streamlined through industrial innovation, craftsmen left the rural life to work in factories. The intellectual contributions of scientists, many of whom were physicians, combined with the inventions of the microscope, thermometer, and pendulum clock, advanced our knowledge and understanding of the world. The invention of the printing press allowed for easier sharing of information, which further contributed to experimentation. Finally, a disease that was feared worldwide was conquered when Edward Jenner (1749-1823) proved the effectiveness of the smallpox vaccination.

Throughout these revolutions, however, the maternal and infant death rates continued to be high. In fact, before his pioneering work in antisepsis in obstetrics, Ignaz Phillipp Semmelweis (1818-1865) observed that patients giving birth in hospitals under the care of educated physicians had significantly higher death rates than women giving birth at home or in clinics with the assistance of midwives.

Despite all the knowledge gained during this time of revolution, society was generally callous toward the plight of children. Children were abandoned without apparent remorse, and infanticide was practiced by poor families desperate to reduce the number of mouths to feed. These families had no reliable form of birth control except abstinence. Because it was common practice for the woman hired as a wet nurse to sleep with the infant, many infants were inadvertently suffocated. Donahue (1985) reported that, during this period, 75% of all children baptized were dead before they reached the age of 5 years. Because of the persistence of these sad conditions, children's and foundlings' hospitals were established. Eventually, laws were enacted to aid these unfortunate victims (Donahue, 1985).

Existing health care conditions for the ill and injured continued to contribute to high mortality rates. Some sources reported hospital mortality rates as high as 90%. Conditions in the armies were no better. In any military action, mortality rates were high. Reports from the battlefront during the Crimean War suggested that battles were postponed because there were too few able-bodied soldiers to fight. Dysentery and typhoid were the military's nemeses. If a soldier was wounded, infection invariably resulted. Hospitals generally offered no guarantee of survival. In any event, these occurrences had a serious effect on military strategies. If men are ill or injured, battles cannot be won.

Upon this scene entered Florence Nightingale.

Florence Nightingale: The Legend and the Lady

First, let us discuss the legend. Published works about Florence Nightingale before the 1960s generally presented the legend. Most authors agreed that she was beautiful, intelligent, wealthy, socially successful, and educated. She certainly had an ability to influence people and used every Victorian secret to accomplish her desires. Although Nightingale believed it improper to accept payment for her services, she did demand financial support for materials, goods, and staff to accomplish her programs and goals. Some historians believe that it was through Nightingale's influence that Jean Henri Dunant, a Swiss gentleman, provided the aid to the wounded that lay the foundation for the organization of the International Red Cross (Bullough et al, 1990; Dodge, 1989; Dossey, 2000).

Regardless of what actually happened between Dunant and her, Nightingale's interest and ambition lay in becoming a nurse. Her family was in an uproar over this decision. As described by Dossey (2000), Florence (or "Flo" as her family and friends called her) began her journey as a mystic when she was 16 years old. Her experience of a sudden, inner "knowing" took place under two majestic cedars at Lebanon in Embley (England), one of her sacred spots for contemplation. She claimed to receive the following in her awakening moment: "That a quest there is, and an end, is the single secret spoken." Energized by her contact with the Divine Reality or Consciousness, Florence "worked very hard among the poor people" with "a strong feeling of religion" for the next 3 months (Dossey, 2000, p 33) (Critical Thinking Box 6-1, Figure 6-1, and Box 6-1).

Nightingale's parents felt that hospitals were terrible places to go and that nurses were, in most cases, the dregs of society. Hospitals were certainly not places for women of proper social

CRITICAL THINKING BOX 6-1   Consider all that you have heard about Florence Nightingale. Now, think about the idea that she was a mystic. What does that mean?

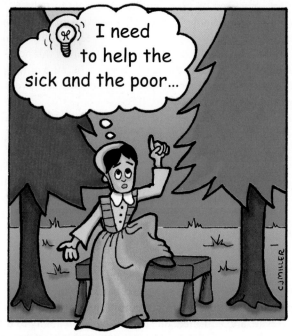

FIGURE 6-1
Florence Nightingale: The legend (mystic, visionary, healer) and the lady.

| BOX 6-1 | Nightingale and Mysticism |

What is mysticism? It is considered to be a universal experience of enlightenment obtained via meditation or prayer that focuses on the direct experience of union with divinity, God, or Ultimate Reality, and the belief that such experience is a genuine and important source of knowledge. It is characterized by a call to personal action, because the person is uncomfortable with the world as it is. Underhill (1961) describes five (nonlinear or nonsequential) phases in the spiritual development of a mystic: awakening, purgation, illumination, surrender, and union.

Awakening: At age 16, Nightingale experienced her first call from God, and again on three other occasions later in life when she heard the voice of God again.

Purgation: Nightingale spent her later teen years and young adulthood (approximately 17 years) separating herself from the affluent lifestyle and worldly possessions that characterized her early life.

Illumination: For Nightingale, this period began when she accepted her first superintendent position at Harley Hospital in London, which propelled her to battle for better conditions during the Crimean War invasion and later, when she returned to England, to fight for reform of the army medical department.

Surrender: This "dark night of the soul" period for Nightingale is thought to have begun approximately 6 years after the Crimean War when she was in her late 30s and continued to her late 60s, a time characterized by her chronic ill health and episodes of stress, overexertion, and depression.

Union: The last 20 years of Nightingale's life (ages 70 to 90) were engendered with an appreciation of the blessings in her life and feelings of peace, joy, and power. The driving force in her life was no longer spurred by social action and issues.

From Dossey B (2005): *Nursing as a spiritual practice: the mystical legacy of Florence Nightingale.* Retrieved from *www.altjn.com/perspectives/spiritual_practice.htm*; Underhill E: *Mysticism.* New York: Dutton, 1961.

upbringing. Although she was forbidden to do so, Nightingale studied nursing (in secret). After a fortuitous meeting, a relationship developed between Nightingale and Sidney and Elizabeth Herbert, an influential couple who were interested in hospital reform. Impressed with Nightingale's analytical mind and her ability to apply nursing knowledge to the critical situation in the hospitals (Bullough and Bullough, 1978; Bullough et al, 1990), they encouraged her to study nursing at Kaiserswerth School, run by Lutheran deaconesses (Dolan, 1969). Her family, of course, was very unhappy. In fact, Dodge (1989) reported that the event precipitated a family crisis because they threatened to withdraw financial support.

Nightingale accepted a position as administrator of a nursing home for women, the Institution for the Care of Sick Gentlewomen in Distressed Circumstances. She hired her own chaperone and went to work at reforming the way things were done. Nightingale's interest in hospital reform was insatiable. She visited hospitals and took copious notes on nursing care, treatments, and procedures. She sent reports on hospital conditions to Sidney Herbert, the British Secretary of War. Secretary Herbert then assigned her other hospitals to review. The reviews always included recommendations for improving nursing care. From this early background of experiences, Nightingale was now ready for her greatest mission—the Crimean War. The legend was on the way (Bullough et al, 1990).

In 1854, soldiers were dying, more from common diseases than from bullets. Bullough and colleagues (1990) reported that the Crimean War was a series of mistakes. No plan was made for supplying the troops, no plan was in place to maintain the environment in camps, and no provisions were available to care for the injured after the battle. When Herbert appointed Nightingale as head of a group of nurses to go to Crimea, she had already developed a plan of action. In fact, some historians believe that she was already planning to go in an unofficial capacity. The announcement caused a sensation, and when Nightingale began a rigorous selection process for accepting nurses, many volunteered, but few were chosen. She cleaned up the kitchens, the wards, the patients, and the mess. From there, the legend grew.

She was clever; after demonstrating the effectiveness of her methods, she withdrew her services. Naturally, all that she had accomplished was done under the scrutiny, skepticism, suspicion, and anger of the physicians. Without the services of the nurses, the abominable conditions quickly returned, and finally the physicians begged her to do whatever she wished—just help! Nightingale responded to the pleading. The actual number of soldiers who benefited from the care of her nurses was immeasurable.

> The nurses made rounds day and night, and the legend of the lady with the lamp was born.

Nightingale's great success prompted her to begin developing schools of nursing based on her knowledge of what was effective nursing. Eventually, many schools in Europe and America used the Nightingale model for nursing education. The program was generally 1 year in length, and classes were small. Many women wanted to become nurses; however, only 15 to 20 applicants were accepted for each class. The goals of her programs included training hospital nurses, training nurses to train others, and training nurses to work in the district with the sick poor (Dolan, 1969). Nightingale had changed society's view of the nurse to one of dignity and value and worthy of respect. As a tribute to Nightingale, Lystra Gretter, an instructor of nursing at the old Harper Hospital in Detroit, Michigan, composed "The Nightingale Pledge," which was first used by its

BOX 6-2   Nightingale Pledge
I solemnly pledge myself before God and in the presence of this assembly, to pass my life in purity and to practice my profession faithfully. I will abstain from whatever is deleterious and mischievous, and will not take or knowingly administer any harmful drug. I will do all in my power to maintain and elevate the standard of my profession, and will hold in confidence all personal matters committed to my keeping and all family affairs coming to my knowledge in the practice of my calling. With loyalty will I endeavor to aid the physician, in his work, and devote myself to the welfare of those committed to my care.

graduating class in the spring of 1893. It is an adaptation of the Hippocratic Oath taken by physicians (Box 6-2).

In any legend, the truth is often mixed with myth. The stories surrounding Florence Nightingale are many. What is interesting is that, before the 1970s, authors tended to deify Nightingale or establish her as a saintly person. These myths make for interesting reading. Early nurse historians also contributed to these myths by their interpretations of Nightingale's work. But myths have a purpose. They can be used to explain world views of groups of people or professions at a given time, and they provide explanations for practice beliefs or natural phenomena. Myths tend to maintain a degree of accuracy when the truth is lost. The trick is to separate myth from fact and story from legend and to draw conclusions regarding the occurrences. This is no easy task when one studies Florence Nightingale. Therefore, it is important to read a variety of studies across several time periods before drawing conclusions about the legend and the lady.

In summary, Florence Nightingale had certain characteristics that assisted her in becoming successful during the strict Victorian times in which she lived. She was extremely well educated for her time. She had traveled throughout the world and had the advantage of personal wealth and a gift for establishing relationships with persons of influence and philanthropic spirit. Most portraits depict her as an attractive woman with pleasant features. Contemporary historians agree she had tremendous compassion for all who suffered. She was very strong-willed, a characteristic that carried her through the period of the Crimean War. She had the ability to analyze data and draw relevant conclusions, on which she based her recommendations. Her students of nursing received better preparation than most physicians. She was 36 at the end of the war, and when she returned home, she became a virtual recluse until she died at age 90. She did have some physical ailments: Crimean fever, sciatica, rheumatism, and dilation of the heart, each of which could have crippling side effects and contributed to her becoming bedridden (Bullough et al, 1990). According to Dossey (2000), "In 1995, D.A.B. Young, a former scientist at the Wellcome Foundation in London, proposed that the Crimean fever was actually Mediterranean fever, otherwise known as Malta fever; this disease is included under the generic name brucellosis" (p 426). Because of the widespread Crimean fever that the soldiers encountered, it is thought that Nightingale was most likely exposed to this disease through ingesting contaminated food, such as meat or raw milk, cheese, or butter. It seems a logical assumption that Nightingale's 32-year history of debilitating, chronic symptoms is compatible with a diagnosis of chronic brucellosis. In any event, the legend and the lady had a significant effect on American nursing as we know it today (Bullough and Bullough, 1978; Bullough et al, 1990; Dodge, 1989; Dolan, 1969; Dossey, 2000).

AMERICAN NURSING: CRITICAL FACTORS

What Was It Like in Colonial Times?

In colonial times, nursing responsibilities were shared by all able-bodied persons; however, when there was a choice, women were preferred as nurses. Early colonial historians described care for the ill and house chores as the responsibilities of nurses. Although most women of this era were considered dainty (Bradford, 1898), nurses were usually depicted as willing to do hard work. Some colonies organized nursing services that sought out the sick and provided comfort to those who were ill with smallpox and other diseases (Bullough and Bullough, 1978). There were few trained nurses, however, and most of the individuals who delivered nursing care in the five largest hospitals were men (Dolan, 1969). Eventually, women were hired at the command of George Washington to serve meals and care for the wounded and ill. The era ended with the enactment of the first legislation to improve health and medical treatment and to provide for formal education for society as a whole (Dolan, 1969).

What Happened to Nursing During the U.S. Civil War?

The period of the U.S. Civil War witnessed an improvement in patient care through control of the environment in which the patient recovered. The greatest problems for the Army stemmed from the poor sanitary conditions in the camps, which bred diseases such as smallpox and dysentery. The results were many deaths from inadequate nutrition, impure water, and a general lack of cleanliness.

Nurses who had some formal training were recognized as being major contributors to the relative success of hospital treatments. It was in this era that the value of primary prevention, or the prevention of the occurrence of disease by measures such as immunization and the provision of a pure water supply, became understood. Volunteer nurses, mostly women, served in hospitals caring for those wounded soldiers fortunate enough to have survived the trip from the battlefield. Their patients were nursed in a clean environment and were provided with adequate nutrition. The likelihood of their recovering was significantly improved. Astute physicians observed that patients cared for by nurses generally recovered well enough to return to the battlefield. Families, too, saw that when nurses had control over the environment, their ill or injured loved one was more likely to recover—and return home.

As the United States moved into the industrial age of the early 1900s, Victorian values began to permeate the middle and upper-middle classes. Social concerns focused on protecting families from the diseases of the crowded urban areas, and the demand for improved health care increased.

How Did the Roles of Nurses and Wives Compare During the Victorian Era?

The Victorian era had a significant effect on nurses, primarily because they were women. The parallelism between the idealized view of the Victorian woman and the traditional nurse is stunning. The effect of many of the values and beliefs of this era, some historians report, is still felt by women today.

The typical upper-class Victorian household consisted of a husband, who earned a living outside of the home and maintained total control of the family finances, and his wife, who maintained harmony within the home and raised their children. Women's work was generally restricted to philanthropic and voluntary work; women attended teas and other social functions to raise money for organizations and people in need.

Most women were considered fragile and dainty. They were often ill. It has been suggested that some women used illnesses and frailty as a form of birth control to prevent the numerous pregnancies that most women experienced. Some historians concluded that it was through their weaknesses that women gained control and attention. If the wife was ill or frail, maids or servants were hired, but if the wife were healthy, the husband would expect more from her. The Victorian wife was expected to "be good." She was esteemed by her husband but had limited power within the confines of the home and society. She was expected to be hard-working and able to maintain harmony while at the same time being submissive to the demands of her husband. Generally, this fostered dependence on the dominant male figure—the Victorian husband (Rybczynski, 1986).

Let us examine nursing during this same time, especially within the hospital organization. Nurses generally were women who wanted to avoid the drudgery of a Victorian marriage. They were required to be single to make a complete commitment to their vocation. Schooled in submission, women were expected to be equally accommodating within the hospital organization. A good nurse worked for harmony within the hospital. She was expected to be hard-working and submissive. The doctor and the hospital administrator were frequently the same person, usually a man who expected position and power to go hand in hand. Patients were admitted only if they had income and could afford to pay for the services. It was the physician who generated income, and good nurses were expected to help him continue to maintain power. Because the system rewarded people for being ill, there was little incentive to be healthy. Social values contributed to dependence on the health care system. From this milieu came the reformers (Bullough and Bullough, 1978; Davis, 1961; Kalisch and Kalisch, 1986; Stewart, 1950).

Who Were the Reformers of the Victorian Era?

The Victorian era, although a time of repression for women, was also a time of reform. A list of important names in nursing reform includes M. Adelaide Nutting, Minnie Goodnow, Lavinia L. Dock, Annie W. Goodrich, Isabel Hampton Robb, Lilian D. Wald, Isabel M. Stewart, and Sophia Palmer, among others (Jamieson and Sewall, 1949; Kalisch and Kalisch, 1986). These women, who had in common a comfortable upper middle-class background, intelligence, and education, also had in common a desire to reach beyond the constraints that society imposed on them. As society began to realize the important role that nurses played in treating the ill and injured, it also began to understand the need for training programs that would educate better nurses. Reformers focused on establishing standards for nursing education and practice. Among their accomplishments were the organization of the American Nurses Association and the creation of its journal, the *American Journal of Nursing*, and the enactment of legislation to require the licensure of prepared nurses. This protected the public from inadequate care given by people who were not trained to nurse (Christy, 1971; Dock, 1900).

How Did the Symbols (Lamp, Cap, and Pin) of the Profession Evolve?

As mentioned previously, Florence Nightingale acquired the nickname "Lady with the Lamp" while caring for soldiers during the Crimean War. Throughout the night, she would carry her lamp while checking on each soldier. For many historical scholars, this image of Nightingale more accurately represents Longfellow's poetic imagination in his 1857 Santa Filomena than the historical record (Grypma, 2010). Here is a link to this famous poem: *www.theatlantic.com/past/docs/unbound/poetry/nov1857/filomena.htm*.

The nurse's cap design evolved from the traditional garb of the early deaconesses or nuns who were some of the earliest nurses to care for the sick. More recently, the cap's original use was to keep a female nurse's hair neatly in place and present a professional appearance. There were two types of cap styles: one was a long nurse's cap, which covered most of the nurse's head; the other was a short nurse's cap, which sat on top of the head. The design of the cap identified the nurse's alma mater, which differentiated graduates from their respective nursing programs. Typically, a black band sewn on the cap signified a senior level student or graduate status, and sometimes identified the head nurse on a clinical unit. The origin of the black or navy band is unknown; some historical scholars believed the black band was a sign of mourning for Florence Nightingale. By the late 1970s, the hat had disappeared almost completely, as have "capping" ceremonies when the new student passed a probationary period of the program to receive their nursing cap. Also, the rapid growth of the number of men in nursing also necessitated a unisex uniform.

The nursing pin is a 1000-year-old symbol of service to others (Rode, 1989). The Maltese cross worn by the knights and nurses during the Crusades is considered the origin of the nursing pin. The most recent ancestor of the pin is the hospital badge that has been worn to identify the nurse since its inception more than 100 years ago. The nursing pin was given by the hospital school of nursing to the graduating students to identify them as nurses who were educated to serve the health needs of society. As schools of nursing flourished, each designed their own unique pin to represent their unique philosophy and beliefs. The pin is still worn as part of the nurse's uniforms today.

HISTORY OF NURSING EDUCATION

What Is the History of Diploma Nursing?

The oldest form of educational preparation leading to licensure as an RN in the United States is the diploma program. Education in diploma schools emphasized the skills needed to care for the acutely ill patient. Graduates received a diploma in nursing, not an academic degree. From 1872 until the mid-1960s, the hospital diploma program was the dominant nursing program. Currently, there are approximately 59 diploma programs accredited by the National League for Nursing (NLN); this represents the smallest percentage of all basic RN programs (NLNAC, 2007). Perhaps one of the reasons for this decline was that the courses offered by hospitals frequently did not earn college credit. Although most diploma programs are associated with institutions of higher learning, where the graduates receive some college credit, they still may not receive college credit for the nursing courses.

What Is the History of Associate Degree Nursing?

The associate degree nursing program has the distinction of being the first and, to date, only educational program for nursing that was developed from planned research and controlled experimentation. Since its beginning in 1951, the associate degree nursing program has grown to more than 880 programs, producing more graduates annually than either diploma or baccalaureate programs.

In 1951, Mildred Montag published her doctoral dissertation, *The Education of Nursing Technicians,* which proposed education for the RN in the community college. Dr. Montag suggested that the associate degree program be a terminal degree to prepare nurses for immediate employment. According to Dr. Montag, there was a need for a new type of nurse, the "nurse technician," whose role would be broader than that of a practical nurse but narrower than that of the professional nurse. The technical nurse was to function at the "bedside." The duties of the technical nurse, according to Dr. Montag, would include (1) giving general nursing care with supervision, (2) assisting in the planning of nursing care for patients, and (3) assisting in the evaluation of the nursing care given (Montag, 1951).

In 1952, an advisory committee was established by the American Association of Junior Colleges. Along with the National League for Nursing (NLN), this committee was to conduct cooperative research on nursing education in the community college. The goals of this Cooperative Research Project were threefold: (1) to describe the development of the associate degree nursing program, (2) to evaluate the associate degree graduates, and (3) to determine the future implications of the associate degree on nursing. The original project was directed by Dr. Montag at Teachers College of Columbia University and included seven junior colleges and one hospital from each of the six regions of the United States.

In the proposed technical nursing curriculum, there was to be a balance between general education and nursing courses. Unlike the diploma programs, the emphasis was to be on education, not service. At the end of 2 years, the student was to be awarded an associate's degree in nursing and would be eligible to take the state board examinations for RN licensure.

What Is the History of Baccalaureate Nursing?

The early baccalaureate nursing programs were usually 5 years in length and consisted of the basic 3-year diploma program with an additional 2 years of liberal arts. In 1919, there were eight baccalaureate programs. In a 2006-2007 survey conducted by the American Association of Colleges of Nursing (AACN) found that total enrollment in all nursing programs leading to the baccalaureate degree, both entry-level and RN degree completion programs, was 180,127—up from 163,706 in 2005 (AACN, 2008).

What Is the History of Graduate Nursing Education?

Graduate nursing programs in the United States originated during the late 1800s. As more nursing schools sought to strengthen their own programs, there was increased pressure on nursing instructors to obtain advanced preparation in education and clinical nursing specialties.

The Catholic University of America, in Washington, DC, offered one of the early graduate programs for nurses. It began offering courses in nursing education in 1932 and conferring a master's degree in nursing education in 1935.

The NLN's Subcommittee on Graduate Education first published guidelines for organization, administration, curriculum, and testing in 1957. These guidelines have been revised throughout the years and reflect the focus in master's education on research and clinical specialization.

Until the 1960s, the master's degree in nursing was viewed as a terminal degree. The goal of graduate education was to prepare nurses for teaching, administration, and supervisory positions. In the early 1970s, the emphasis shifted to developing clinical skills, and the roles of clinical specialists and nurse practitioners emerged. By the late 1970s, the focus again shifted back to teaching, administration, and supervisory positions (McCloskey and Grace, 2001).

In response to health care reform, the number of master's programs has increased. Enrollments in master's degree programs rose 18.1% (8337 students) bringing the total student population to 56,028. In research-focused doctoral programs, enrollments increased by 6.3% (231 students) with the total student population at 3927 (AACN, 2008).

THE NURSE'S ROLE: THE STRUGGLE FOR DEFINITIONS

What Do Nurses Do?

As a student, you study nursing texts that explain theories, skills, principles, and the care of patients. Every text has at least one introductory chapter that describes nursing and its significance. By examining many of these introductory chapters of nursing texts, you can generate a rather extensive list of roles (Anglin, 1991). From this list of roles, six major categories can be determined (Table 6-1). The most traditional role for nurses is that of caregiver. The nurse as teacher is often referred to when discussing patient care or nursing education. The role of advocate has been very controversial since 1900. Nurses were also expected to be managers ever since the first formal education or training program was instituted. Another interesting role for the nurse is that of colleague. The final role is that of expert.

What Is the Traditional Role of a Nurse?

The role of the nurse as caregiver has engendered the least amount of controversy. This role has been thoroughly documented, not only in writing but also through art, since early times. Nurses and nursing leaders agree that this is their primary role. As students, your caregiving skills will be measured constantly through skill laboratories, clinical evaluation proficiency, and eventually, through licensure testing and staff evaluations. All of these mechanisms are used to evaluate your ability to be a caregiver.

> Caregiving is probably the only role about which there is agreement as to what it means and how we do it.

TABLE 6-1 What Nurses Do

CAREGIVER	TEACHER	ADVOCATE	MANAGER	COLLEAGUE	EXPERT
Care provider	Patient	Interpreter	Administrator	Collaborator	Academician
Comforter	educator	Learner	Coordinator	Communicator	Historian
Handmaiden	Counselor	Protector	Decision maker	Facilitator	Nursing instructor
Healer	Patient	Risk-taker	Evaluator	Peer reviewer	Professional
Helper	teacher	Change	Initiator	Professional	educator
Nurturer		agent	Leader	Specialist	Researcher
Practitioner			Planner		Research consumer
Rehabilitator					Teacher
Support agent					Theorist
					Practitioner
					Leader

Imagine a nurse giving care. Generally, the picture that most often comes to mind is someone, usually female, in a white uniform caring for a patient who is ill. This picture is the romanticized version of caregiving continually portrayed in movies, television, and novels. We know that caregiving takes place in many settings: clinics, homes, hospitals, offices, businesses, and schools, among others. We can probably agree that caregiving is an important role for nurses and that it is why most of us chose nursing. Studies examining the role of caregiver continue, and our understanding of the role is expanding (Benner, 1984; Leininger, 1984; Watson, 1985). Without a doubt, this is an important role, one that is essential to nursing.

Did You Know You Would Be a Teacher?

Teaching patients about their therapy, condition, or choices is critical to the successful outcome of some prescribed treatments. For example, nurses have learned through research that knowledge can reduce anxiety before and after surgery. Teaching becomes especially important when patients have to make treatment choices and decisions about their care. With the volumes of information available regarding health care, it is even more important that nurses help patients understand what they need to know to make wise decisions. Discharge plans also provide for patient education. Home care includes teaching as a reimbursable activity. Agency charting procedures all require documentation of patient education. All nursing textbooks include sections on what the nurse needs to emphasize regarding patient education. With all this evidence, there is little doubt that the teacher role is an important one for the nurse (Figure 6-2).

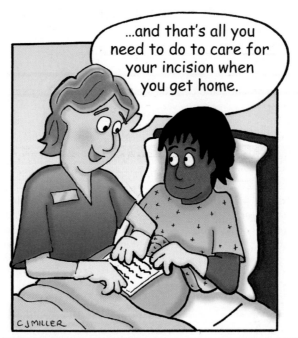

FIGURE 6-2
Did you know you would be a teacher?

Teaching is planned to strengthen a patient's knowledge of making decisions about treatment options and is an essential nursing intervention (Alfaro-LeFevre, 1998). In many ways, the nurse as teacher is also an interpreter of information, and this leads us to the next role for discussion.

When Did the Nurse Become An Advocate?

A useful definition of the term *advocate* is "one who pleads a cause before another." The first advocacy issue, arising early in the 1900s, concerned nursing practice. Public health and visiting nurses were the majority (approximately 70%), and hospital nurses were the minority (approximately 30%) of working nurses. Working as a private duty nurse or visiting nurse was a source of income for women who had no other means of support. Because there was no way to determine the credentials of the visiting nurse, many impostors worked in that capacity. Lavinia L. Dock, Sophia Palmer, and Annie W. Goodrich, three nursing leaders, deplored this situation and endeavored to protect the public from unscrupulous "nurses" (Dolan, 1969; Goodnow, 1936). Dock was an excellent nurse who believed in fairness to qualified nurses and to the public. She advocated that all practicing nurses be measured by a "fair-general-average standard," as determined by written examination, and rewarded with licensure upon attainment of the standard (Christy, 1971).

Palmer's proposed solutions were similar. Many hospitals were sending out inexperienced undergraduates to do private duty nursing while keeping the income. She advocated a training school in which students of nursing would learn to give care under a qualified nurse and supported the implementation of a registration process for all qualified nurses to protect the public from incompetent, unqualified nurses.

Goodrich advocated compulsory legislation that would ensure that graduates or trained nurses would be the only ones who could work as nurses. She pleaded for the registration of qualified nurses, not only for the protection of the nurse, but for the protection of the community. Goodrich also fought against correspondence or home-study programs for nurses, which were a greater menace to the public's safety than people realized. Such legislation, she believed, would encourage talented young women who were intellectually prepared for scientific education to select nursing as a career. The role of the advocate, as understood by these three early nursing leaders, was to protect the public from unqualified nurses (Christy, 1969; Dock, 1900; Palmer, 1900).

From this beginning, the role of advocate grew. Public health nurses served as advocates in factories and communities during the Industrial Revolution. Many municipal boards of health hired visiting nurses to work as inspectors in the factories to protect the workers from health hazards and to help prevent accidents. Communities were finding that the nurse as advocate for the factory worker had inestimable value. Visiting nurses were also proving very effective in preventing the spread of communicable diseases. Hospital nurses also worked as advocates for the patients while giving care. Nurses were crucial in protecting patients from harm when they were too ill to protect themselves. Nurses were also responsible for providing measures to relieve pain, and they strove to make their patients happy and comfortable, even if it meant breaking the rules sometimes (Hill, 1900). During the 1970s and 1980s, the responsibility of the nurse as advocate was expanded to include speaking for their patients when they could not speak for themselves (Sovie, 1978). Nurses returned to work in churches in the primary role of advocate under the Granger Westberg model for parish nursing. The members of the congregation where a parish nurse practiced found affirmation and support as they reached to improve their physical, emotional, and spiritual health (Striepe, 1987).

However, consumers, administrators, and courts do not share the perception of the nurse as advocate. The findings of a study done in 1983 indicated that consumers did not recognize the nurse as an initiator of health care (Miller et al, 1983). Consumers also believed that physicians would protect the rights of the patient. Miller and colleagues (1983) concluded that although nurses were serving as mediators between patients and institutions, changes rarely occurred within the institutions as a result of this role. Patient advocacy was directly related to the power and authority allowed the nurse by the particular system. Nurses generally became advocates whenever the issue was care; however, they had little power to be truly effective as an advocate when the concerns involved the medical regimen or health care services (Miller et al, 1983). Examples of advocacy included questioning doctors' orders, promoting patient comfort, and supporting patient decisions regarding health care choices.

> Advocacy is a critical role for nurses today. Nurses are in a vital position to be effective in this role.

With the need for informed consent, advance directives, and treatment choices, patients more than ever need an advocate to interpret information, identify the risks and benefits of the various treatment options, and support the decision they make. Being an advocate does involve taking personal and professional risks. When the issue is care, nurses are willing advocates, but when the issue is the profession, nurses seem reluctant (Anglin, 1991).

Why Are Nurses Managers?

Even Florence Nightingale recognized the need for nurses to be managers. She insisted that nurses needed to organize the care of the patient so that other nurses could carry on when they were not present. There were four major eras in the development of the nurse as manager. During the first period, lasting until about 1920, a nurse manager was known as the *charge nurse*. Charge nurses were responsible for teaching the nursing students what they needed to know and for directing the care that the students gave. The charge nurse was autocratic. This nurse had absolute authority over the student.

During the second era, lasting until 1949, the term *supervisor* was used to describe the role of nurse manager. The supervisor continued to be responsible for the students; however, the role had expanded to include enforcing agency policies, developing improvements in the care of the ill, and being responsible for the effective use of the ward's resources. Nurses were more involved in the patient care process. Hospital administrators were relying on nursing expertise to establish policies for patient care and hospital administration. This era ended with the publication of Esther Lucille Brown's report (1948) recommending that nursing education be separated from hospital administration.

During the third period, lasting until 1970, the nurse was referred to as a *coordinator*. The nurse coordinator no longer had responsibility for the nursing education of the students but was expected to motivate staff, be innovative, and solve problems. Coordinators were active in improving patient care and were expected to maintain harmony within the institution. Many nurse coordinators had few skills in and little knowledge of middle management. They basically learned by trial and error how to be effective.

The last period, from 1970 to the present, is a series of waves. Nurses gained recognition as managers and were able to function in that role. Hospital nurses gained middle-management positions and proved their abilities. The period before diagnostic-related groups (DRGs) saw escalating hospital costs and growth in the numbers of employees and services. From this growth came significant efforts to control the costs of health care. The term *manager* is used most often now in the nursing literature, but you may find it used to describe any of the four periods.

> No matter what era in history you study, the expectation is that the nurse-manager will coordinate patient care and supervise nurses in the delivery of quality care.

Can Nurses Be Colleagues?

The role of colleague is a vital one in any profession. The status of colleague within health care generates pictures of nurses, doctors, and pharmacists discussing, on an equal basis, problems and concerns related to health care. In nursing, however, a review of our history reveals that we have not quite achieved the status of colleague. Interdisciplinary collegial relationships currently are tenuous. More surprising is that, even among nurses, intradisciplinary collegial relationships are strained.

Between 1960 and the present, the term *collaborator* has been adopted for this role. The root of this word means, "to exchange information with the enemy." This may be the most fitting description of the role. Nurses were interested in developing collaborative relationships with doctors, pharmacists, and other health professionals. The literature is abundant with discussions of these relationships and consistently describes these relationships as collaborative (Hahm and Miller, 1961; Kelly, 1975; Quint, 1967; Seward, 1969; Tourtillott, 1986; Wisener, 1978).

Where Does This Leave the Role of Colleague?

Nursing education has promoted the term *collaborator* over *colleague*. The dilemma is that employers neither recognize nor reward the role. Students in their educational experiences are seldom offered the opportunity to practice the role of colleague and therefore have only a vague understanding of the role. However, public health nurses throughout American history have not only understood the role, but probably have attained a greater degree of collegiality than any other practice area of nursing. Public health nurses are not the majority within the profession. Nevertheless, they continue to enjoy and maintain the essence of the role (Anglin, 1991). As a colleague, one recognizes nurses with expertise and relies on those nurses for their expertise in the interest of improving patient care and advancing the profession. The essence of the role is mutual respect and equality among professionals, both intradisciplinary and interdisciplinary (Anglin, 1991). Until nurses can respond to each other with respect, it will be difficult to move from collaborator to true colleague.

What About Experts?

There is one other role in which nurses are often found. For lack of a better name, this role is called *expert*. It is a conglomerate of advanced formal or informal education, certification, and acquired or recognized expertise. The role includes academicians, historians, nursing educators, clinicians, professional educators, researchers, research consumers, theorists, nurse technologists, and the leaders within the profession. The American Academy of Nursing recognizes some of these individuals and votes to bestow on them the honor of Fellow. There are many nurses who are experts in an area of practice, whether it be in clinics, at the bedside, in nursing homes, or in other settings. As nurses with special expertise, they are called on to provide testimony in courts and at government hearings or to share information and knowledge with other nurses, which is their obligation to the profession. This sharing can be done through mentoring, guest-speaking, performing in-services, offering continuing-education programs, contributing to publications, and writing technical articles. These experts are usually the nurses who create the momentum that moves the profession forward. This is a role that should be recognized, encouraged, and rewarded.

CONCLUSION

The history of nursing provides a wealth of knowledge about where we have been and illustrates for us the lessons that have been learned. Few of us know the specifics of how nursing evolved into the discipline that it is today; however, the study and review of our rich history provides the context of where we will be tomorrow.

What do nurses do? There is no simple answer. We agree that nurses care for patients—hence nurses are caregivers. We agree that nurses teach patients what they need to know to make informed choices—and therefore nurses are teachers. We also agree that the role of manager exists in some form, and so we manage our practice and patients' care. We can even define the role of advocate; yet, based on the history of the role, nurses are reluctant to take risks to fully carry the role into the future. The role of colleague is less clear. We are consistent in using the term *collaborator;* however, the term *colleague* is deemed more fitting for professionals, and that is the role to which we should aspire.

Finally, we have experts whom we may or may not recognize—and upon whom the profession depends to provide the leadership for the whole. These roles merely provide a beginning for you to understand the profession you have chosen—nursing. May you become proficient in these roles and develop into an expert who will then provide the leadership for nursing in the future.

> The future is not the result of choices among
> Alternative paths offered;
> It is a place that is created,
> Created first in the mind and will,
> Created next in activity.
> The future is not some place we are going to,
> But one we are creating.
> The paths to it are not found, but made.
> And the activity of making them
> Changes both the maker and the destiny.
> —Anonymous, 1987

BIBLIOGRAPHY

Aikens CA: *Studies in nursing ethics*, Philadelphia, 1935, Saunders.

Alfaro-LeFevre R: *Applying nursing process: a step-by-step guide*, New York, 1998, Lippincott Williams & Wilkins.

American Association of Colleges of Nursing: *2006-2007 Enrollment and graduations in baccalaureate and graduate programs in nursing*. Washington, DC, 2008, Author.

Anderson NE: The historical development of American nursing education, *J Nurs Educ* 20(1):18-36, 1981.

Anglin LT: *The roles of nurses: a history, 1900 to 1988*, Ann Arbor, Mich, 1991, University of Michigan.

Benner P: *From novice to expert: excellence and power in clinical nursing practice*, Menlo Park, Calif, 1984, Addison-Wesley.

Bradford W: *History of Plymouth Plantation: book II (1620)*, Plymouth, Mass, 1898, Wright & Potter.

Brown EL: *Nursing for the future*, New York, 1948, Russell Sage Foundation.

Bullough V, Bullough B: *The care of the sick: the emergence of modern nursing*, New York, 1978, Prodist.

Bullough V, Bullough B, Stanton MP: *Florence Nightingale and her era: a collection of new scholarship*, New York, 1990, Garland.

Christy TE: Portrait of a leader: Isabel Hampton Robb, *Nurs Outlook* 17(3):26-29, 1969.

Christy TE: First fifty years, *Am J Nurs* 71(9):1778-1784, 1971.

Dalton R: Hospitals: their origins and history, *Dublin J Med Sci* 109(3):17-19, 1900.

Dana CL: *The peaks of medical history*. New York, 1936, Paul B Hoeber.

Davis MD: I was a student over 50 years ago, *Nurs Outlook* 61:62, 1961.

Dock L: What may we expect from the law? *Am J Nurs* 1:9, 1900.

Dodge BS: *The story of nursing*, ed 2, Boston, 1989, Little, Brown.

Dolan JA: *History of nursing*, Philadelphia, 1969, Saunders.

Donahue MP: *Nursing: the finest art*, St. Louis, 1985, Mosby.

Dossey B: *Florence Nightingale: mystic, visionary, healer*, Springhouse, Penn, 2000, Springhouse.

Goodnow M: *Outlines in the history of nursing*, Philadelphia, 1936, Saunders.

Grypma S: Revis(it)ing nursing history, *J of Christian Nurs* 27(2):67, 2010.

Hahm H, Miller D: Relationships between medical and nursing education, *J Nurs Educ* 39:849-851, 1961.

Hamilton JA: Success or failure in nursing administration, *Am J Nurs* 49:496, 1949.

Hill J: Private duty nursing from a nurse's point of view, *Am J Nurs* 1(2):129, 1900.

Hodson J: *How to become a trained nurse*, New York, 1905. William Abbott.

Jamieson EM, Sewall MF: *Trends in nursing history*, Philadelphia, 1949, Saunders.

Kalisch PA, Kalisch BJ: *The advance of American nursing*, Boston, 1986, Little, Brown.

Kelly LY: *Dimensions of professional nursing*, ed 3, New York, 1975, Macmillan.

Lawman JH: The evolution and development of the nurse, *Am J Nurs* 8:8, 1907.

Leininger M: *Care: the essence of nursing and health*, Thorofare, NJ, 1984, Charles B Slack.

McCloskey J, Grace HK: *Current issues in nursing*, ed 6, St. Louis, 2001, Mosby.

Miller BK, Mansen TJ, Lee H: Patient advocacy: do nurses have the power and authority to act as patient advocate? *Nurs Leadersh* 6(2):56-60, 1983.

Montag ML: *The education of nursing technicians*, New York, 1951, GP Putnam's Sons.

National League for Nursing Accrediting Commission (NLNAC) (2007): *Online directory of accredited programs*. Retrieved from *www.nlnac.org/Forms/directory_search.htm*.

Palmer S: The editor, *Am J Nurs* 1(4):166-169, 1900.

Quint GC: Role models and the professional nurse identity, *J Nurs Educ* 6:1, 1967.

Rode MW: The nursing pin: symbol of 1,000 years of service, *Nurs Forum* 24(1):15-17, 1989.

Rybczynski W: *Home: a short history of an idea*, Middlesex, England, 1986, Penguin.

Seward JM: Role of the nurse: perceptions of nursing students and auxiliary nursing personnel, *Nurs Res* 18(2):164-169, 1969.

Sovie L: Nursing. In: Chaska N, editor: *The nursing profession*, New York, 1978, GP Putnam's Sons.

Stewart IM: A half-century of nursing education, *Am J Nurs* 50:617, 1950.

Striepe J: *Nurses in churches: a manual for developing parish nurse services and networks*, Spencer, IA, 1987, Iowa Lake Area Agency on Aging.

Tourtillott EA: *Commitment—a lost characteristic*, New York, 1986, JB Lippincott.

Watson J: *Nursing: human science and human care—a theory of nursing*, East Norwalk, Conn, 1985, Appleton-Century-Crofts.

Wisener S: *The reality of primary nursing care: risks, roles and research. Role changes in primary nursing*, New York, 1978, National League of Nursing.

Zander K: Nursing case management: a classic, *Definition* 2(2):1-3, 1987.

Zander K: Managed care within acute care settings: design and implementation via nursing case management, *Health Care Supervisor* 6(2):24-43, 1988.

Additional resources are available online at *http://evolve.elsevier.com/Zerwekh/nsgtoday/*.

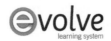

CHAPTER 7

Nursing Education

Gayle P. Varnell, PhD, APRN, CPNP-PC

Education should not be a destination—but a path we travel all the days of our lives.
—ANONYMOUS

Education is the ability to listen to almost anything without losing your temper or your self-confidence.
—ROBERT FROST

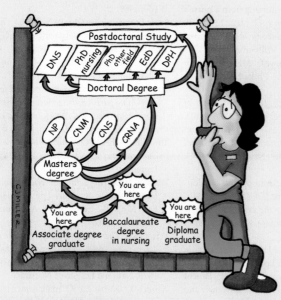

Pathway to career goals.

After completing this chapter, you should be able to:

- Compare the various types of educational preparation for nursing.

- Describe the educational preparation for a graduate degree.

- Compare the alternative options provided by career ladder or bridge programs, external degree programs, Bachelor of Science in Nursing programs, accelerated programs, and online universities.

- Describe the purpose of nursing program accreditation.

 fter struggling to complete your basic educational preparation for nursing, you are probably looking forward to that first paycheck as a registered nurse. The last thing on your mind is returning to school for more education! The purpose of this chapter is not to discuss the issue of entry into practice or to debate which educational program is best. Instead, the goal of this chapter is to help you look at where you are educationally and to offer direction regarding educational opportunities to enhance your career goals. Before looking down the path at the variety of educational offerings available to help you meet those goals, let us look at the variety of pathways that lead to the basic educational preparation for an RN.

Which path did you travel? There are three primary paths (diploma, associate's degree, and bachelor's degree) that lead to one licensing examination: the National Council Licensure Examination for Registered Nurses (NCLEX-RN Examination). These programs usually require a high school diploma or the equivalent for admission. Some of the other paths include master's and doctoral nursing degree programs, both of which accept college graduates with liberal arts majors. Other paths are becoming more popular, including career ladder programs (from practical nurse to associate degree nurse), two-plus-two programs (from associate's degree to bachelor's degree), and the increasingly popular accelerated baccalaureate program for nonnursing college graduates. Still another source for nursing education is the online option. Online programs are particularly popular for people who are place-bound and unable to travel to distant sites to obtain or continue their education. Some of these programs require brief visits to a campus, whereas others are completely online.

The distribution of the RN population according to basic nursing education is illustrated in Figure 7-1. In 1980, the diploma education track was the highest level of education for most nursing graduates. Since 1996, there has been a continued increase in the number of RNs receiving their initial preparation in either an associate's degree or a baccalaureate program. The most recent 2008 survey indicates that initial preparation in a diploma program accounted for 20.4%, the associate's degree accounted for 45.4%, and the baccalaureate degree program accounted for

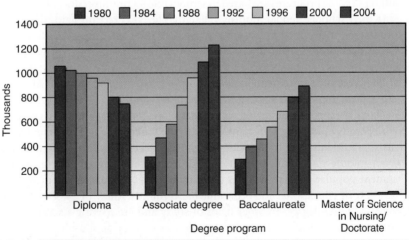

FIGURE 7-1

Distribution of RNs according to basic nursing education, 1980-2004. (*Source: Health Resources and Services Administration. [2010]: The registered nurse population: Findings from the March 2008 National Sample Survey of Registered Nurses. Washington, DC: U.S. Department of Health and Human Services. Retrieved from* www.bhpr.hrsa.gov/healthworkforce/rnsurvey/initialfindings2008.pdf.)

34.2% of the registered nurses. Furthermore, it is estimated that 0.5% of RNs received their initial nursing education at either a master's or doctoral level.

PATH OF DIPLOMA EDUCATION

What Is the Educational Preparation of the Diploma Graduate?

The current preparation of a diploma nurse varies in length from 2 to 3 years and takes place in a hospital school of nursing. This type of program may be under the direction of the hospital or incorporated independently. The diploma program may include general education subjects such as biology and physical and social sciences, in addition to nursing theory and practice. Graduates of diploma programs are prepared to function as beginning practitioners in acute, intermediate, long-term, and ambulatory health care facilities. Because there is a close relationship between the nursing school and the hospital, graduates are well prepared to function in that institution. On graduation, many diploma graduates are employed by that same hospital and therefore may experience an easier role transition.

Standards and competencies for diploma programs are developed and maintained by the National League for Nursing (NLN) Council of Diploma Programs. Graduates of diploma programs are awarded a certificate and are eligible to take the NCLEX-RN examination for licensure.

PATH OF ASSOCIATE DEGREE EDUCATION

What Is the Educational Preparation of the Associate Degree Graduate?

The current preparation of an associate degree nurse usually begins in a community college, although some programs are based in senior colleges or universities. The associate degree program is 18 to 21 school calendar months in length. The NLN recommends that associate degree nursing programs consist of 60 to 72 semester credits (90 to 108 quarter credits) and that there be a balanced distribution of no more than 60% of the total number of credits allocated to nursing courses (NLN, 2001). In some programs, the student must complete the general education and science course requirements before beginning the nursing courses. At the end of the program, the student receives an associate's degree in nursing.

Associate degree nursing education has helped to bring about a change in the type of student who enrolls in nursing programs. Prior to the emergence of associate degree nursing programs, nursing students were traditionally single, white females younger than 19 years of age who came from middle-class families (Kaiser, 1975). Associate degree programs attract a more diverse student population that includes older individuals, minorities, men, and married women from a variety of educational and economic backgrounds. Many of these individuals have baccalaureate and higher degrees in other fields of study and are seeking a second career. Along with their maturity, these students bring life experiences that are applicable to nursing. The students tend to be more goal-oriented and have a more realistic perspective of the work setting. The community college curriculum is conducive to students who want to attend school on a part-time basis.

Standards and competencies for associate degree programs are developed and maintained by the NLN Council of Associate Degree Programs. At the NLN 1998 Education Summit, the associate's degree in nursing (ADN) competencies were revised to include multiculturalism, long-term care, systems management, and interdisciplinary collaboration. Graduates of associate degree programs are eligible to take the NCLEX-RN examination for licensure.

Dr. Montag's original proposal for the associate degree program to be a terminal degree is no longer applicable. In 1978, the American Nurses Association proposed a resolution regarding associate degree programs that recommended they be viewed as part of the career upward-mobility plan rather than as terminal programs. The associate degree program has provided students with the motivation to further their education and the opportunity for career mobility. Although many nursing students end their education with an associate's degree, many others enter the associate degree program with every intention of continuing their nursing education to the baccalaureate level or even further.

PATH OF BACCALAUREATE EDUCATION

In this discussion, only the "generic" baccalaureate programs are addressed. A "generic student" is one who enters a baccalaureate nursing program with no training or education in nursing. A traditional generic baccalaureate program includes lower-division (freshman and sophomore) liberal arts and science courses with upper-division (junior and senior) nursing courses. RNs entering baccalaureate programs are discussed later in this chapter.

What Is the Educational Preparation of the Baccalaureate Graduate?

The current preparation of a baccalaureate nurse is 4 to 5 years in length (120 to 140 credits) and emphasizes courses in the liberal arts, sciences, and humanities. Approximately one-half to two-thirds of the curriculum consists of nonnursing courses. To qualify for a baccalaureate program, the student must first meet all of the college's or the university's entrance requirements. Usual entrance requirements include college preparation courses in high school (e.g., foreign language, advanced science, and math courses) and a specified cumulative grade-point average (GPA). Most colleges also require a college entrance examination such as the Scholastic Aptitude Test (SAT) or the American College Test (ACT).

During the first 2 years of a traditional baccalaureate nursing program, the student is usually enrolled in liberal arts and science courses with other nonnursing students. It is usually not until late in a student's sophomore or early junior year that nursing courses are introduced. However, some baccalaureate programs incorporate nursing courses throughout the 4-year nursing curriculum. The emphasis in the baccalaureate nursing program is on developing critical decision-making skills, exercising independent nursing judgment, and acquiring research skills.

The graduate of a baccalaureate program must fulfill both the degree requirements of the nursing program and those of the college. On completion of the program, the usual degree awarded is a Bachelor of Science in Nursing (BSN).

The graduate of a baccalaureate program is prepared to provide health promotion and health restoration care for individuals, families, and groups in a variety of institutional and community settings. Graduates of baccalaureate nursing programs are eligible to take the NCLEX-RN examination for licensure. BSN graduates are also prepared to continue their education by moving directly into graduate education. An increasing number of BSN graduates are continuing their nursing education by going directly into graduate programs.

OTHER TYPES OF NURSING EDUCATION

What Are the Other Available Educational Options?

In the 1960s, baccalaureate programs made it very difficult for the RN to return to school to earn a baccalaureate in nursing. Most of the time, these nurses found themselves receiving no credit for their past education or experience. A resolution was passed in 1978 by the American Nurses Association (ANA) that helped to change this philosophy. This resolution urged the creation of quality career-mobility programs with flexibility to assist individuals desiring academic degrees in nursing. Several basic patterns are available for achieving upward mobility in nursing; within these basic patterns are many variations. Career ladder programs or bridge programs, BSN-completion programs, external degree programs, accelerated programs, and online universities are the basic patterns that will be addressed in this section. In assessing the available educational options, one source of information is the All Nursing Schools website *(www.allnursingschools. com/find/)*. Potential students should also contact individual schools for information regarding their particular programs.

The career ladder or bridge concept focuses on the articulation of educational programs to permit advanced placement without loss of credit or repetition. There are many variations on this type of program. Multiple-exit programs provide opportunities for students to exit and reenter the educational system at various designated times, having gained specific education and skills. An example is a program that ranges from practical nurse to RN at the associate's, baccalaureate, master's, and doctoral levels. A student in such a program may decide to leave the educational system at the completion of a specific level and be eligible to take the licensure examination applicable to that educational level. On termination, the student may choose to work for a while and later return for more education at the next level without having to repeat courses on previously acquired knowledge or skills.

A growing number of basic nursing education programs within the community college setting are beginning to offer career ladder programs, affiliating themselves with upper-division colleges in the area. A student can enter the community college to spend 1 year studying to become a practical or vocational nurse. After a year, the student can decide to stop and take the practical nurse licensure examination or continue and complete the associate's degree in nursing. At the end of the second year, the student is eligible to take the RN licensure examination and may choose either to exit with an associate's degree or to attend an affiliated upper-division college to obtain a bachelor's degree (Figure 7-2).

What Is a BSN/MSN Completion Program?

A BSN-completion program is a baccalaureate program designed for students who already possess either a diploma or an associate's degree in nursing and hold a current license to practice as an RN. Depending on the part of the country, these programs may also be known as RN baccalaureate (RNB) programs, RN/BSN programs, baccalaureate RN (BRN) programs, two-plus-two programs, or capstone programs. There are more than 620 BSN-completion programs In addition to the BSN-completion programs, 161 RN-to-master's degree program options are available and there are 27 additional nursing schools planning to implement a BSN/MSN completion program in the near future (AACN, March 2010b). In most of these programs, nurses receive transfer credit in basic education courses taken at other institutions plus either some

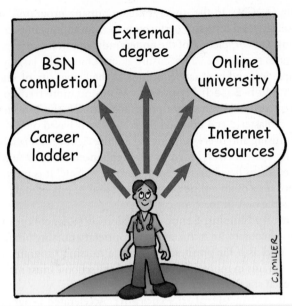

FIGURE 7-2
What are other available education programs?

transfer credit for their previous nursing courses or the opportunity to receive nursing credit by passing a nursing challenge examination.

The usual length of such programs is 1 to 2 years, depending on the number of course requirements completed at the time of admission to the program. To meet the needs of the returning student, many BSN-completion programs offer flexible class scheduling, which allows the student to continue working while going to school. Another innovation being implemented to address the needs of individuals seeking baccalaureate degrees in outlying geographic areas is telecommunication-assisted studies and Internet courses. More than 400 programs have part of their curriculum online while there are an increasing number of programs available completely online (AACN, March 2010b).

What Is an External Degree Program? In the early 1970s, the external degree program was a nontraditional program that allowed a student to gain credit, meet external degree requirements, and obtain a degree from a degree-granting institution without attending face-to-face classes. One of the earliest external degree (or distance education) programs was offered through the New York Board of Regents external degree programs (REX), which is now Excelsior College. External degree programs may offer an ADN as well as a BSN and a master of science in nursing (MSN). These programs are designed to allow individuals to obtain a degree in nursing without leaving their jobs or their communities.

Nursing education online is a rapidly expanding part of the Internet. These external degree, or distance education, programs are accredited either by the National League for Nursing Accrediting Commission (NLNAC) or by the Commission on Collegiate Nursing Education (CCNE), which is an autonomous accrediting agency associated with the American Association of Colleges of Nursing (AACN). In the undergraduate nursing programs, all students are required to pass specific college-level tests and performance examinations in two components: general education and nursing. On completion of the undergraduate external degree programs, students are eligible in most states to take the RN licensure exam. One of the largest CCNE-approved programs for BSN completion and graduate education is the University of Phoenix online campus.

Online (Web-Based) Programs. More and more traditional colleges and universities are offering courses and even entire programs through the Internet. In fact, it is possible to earn ADN, BSN, master's, and doctoral degrees in Web-based or Web-enhanced formats. At times, it can be confusing and overwhelming to find the right programs. Several sites are available to help users locate specific Web-based or Web-enhanced courses (and course descriptions). See the Internet resources listed on this book's Evolve website. It is important to take into consideration the cost not only of an online program, but also of out-of-state tuition when considering which program is the best fit for your career goals.

Proprietary Nursing Schools. In addition to the colleges and universities that are offering these types of courses, an influx of new proprietary nursing programs has emerged. A proprietary nursing school is a for-profit school with a nursing program. Many proprietary schools have nursing programs in more than one state; these schools must meet the different program requirements of each state's nursing board.

What Is an Accelerated Program? Accelerated programs are offered at both the baccalaureate and master's degree levels; they are designed to build on previous learning to help a person with an undergraduate degree in another discipline make the transition into nursing. In 2009, there were 230 accelerated baccalaureate programs and 65 accelerated master's programs available at nursing schools nationwide. In addition, 33 new accelerated baccalaureate programs are in the planning stages, and 6 new accelerated master's programs are also taking shape (AACN, 2010a).

NONTRADITIONAL PATHS FOR NURSING EDUCATION

What About a Master's Degree as a Path to Becoming an RN?

MSN programs are particularly attractive to the growing number of college graduates who decide later in their lives to enter nursing. Generally, the program is 24 to 36 months in length. On graduation these students are expected to demonstrate the same entry-level competencies in nursing as baccalaureate graduates. MSN graduates from these programs are then eligible to take the NCLEX-RN. Currently, there are 65entry-level master's programs in the United States (AACN, 2010c).

What About a Doctoral Path to Becoming an RN?

The last, and the least common, path leading to the RN licensure examination is the doctoral degree, where the graduate has a nonnursing baccalaureate degree. This program began in 1979 at Case Western Reserve University in Cleveland, Ohio. Rush University in Chicago initiated a similar program in 1988, and the University of Colorado began one in 1990 (Forni, 1989). These programs, such as the one at the University of Texas at Austin, provide basic nursing courses, along with advanced nursing courses. On completion, the graduate is eligible to take the NCLEX-RN examination.

GRADUATE EDUCATION

What About Graduate School?

Whatever path you chose to become an RN, there is one thing for certain: It was not easy. After putting life, liberty, and the pursuit of happiness on hold while you worked toward becoming an RN, it may seem like pure insanity to subject yourself to more education!

Graduate nursing education, like other graduate programs, is responding to changes in social values, priorities in the public sector, and student demographics, in addition to technological advances, knowledge development, and maturity of the profession (McCloskey & Grace, 2001). According to the National Sample Survey of Registered Nurses (2008), 32% of RNs with a baccalaureate or higher degree listed their initial RN education as diploma or associate's degree, indicating that RNs in the workforce are recognizing the need to further their education and are returning to college to further their education either in nursing or nursing-related fields such as public health and health care administration.

Graduate education programs are available on either a part-time or a full-time basis. Graduate programs require a good grade-point average at the undergraduate level. Prerequisites for most graduate programs are satisfactory scores on the Graduate Record Examination (GRE) or the Miller Analogies Test (MAT). Although an increasing number of graduate programs are waiving the entrance examination requirements, it is strongly recommended that all students, whether they plan to pursue graduate studies or not, take the GRE after completing their undergraduate studies. Taking another test may be the last thing you want to do, but it is much easier to do it now, while the information is current in your mind, than later, when you decide that you want to continue your education.

Why Would I Want a Master's Degree?

You've got to be kidding! More school?

Sure, an advanced degree may not be in your career plans right now, but later on, after you have been practicing nursing, you may change your mind. Policy statements from the nursing profession reflect the need for more education in preparation for the changing role of nursing, a result of health care reform. As care delivery moves increasingly from the acute care center to the community setting, there will be an increased need for advanced clinical practice nurses. Nursing programs are already responding to this changing need.

Master's nursing programs vary from institution to institution, as do the admission and course requirements and costs. The master of science (MS) and the MSN are the most common degrees. The usual requirements for admission include a baccalaureate degree from an NLN-accredited program in nursing, licensure as a registered nurse, completion of the GRE or MAT, and a minimum undergraduate GPA of 3.0.

The majority of programs are at least 18 to 24 months of full-time study. Unlike undergraduate students, master's students usually choose an area of role preparation, such as education or administration, as well as an area of clinical specialization, such as pediatrics or adult health. Some of the more common areas of role preparation include education, administration, case management, health policy/health care systems, informatics, and the increasingly popular advanced clinical practice roles. Still another evolving area of role preparation is that of the clinical nurse leader (CNL). According to the AACN White Paper on the Education and Role of the Clinical Nurse Leader (AACN, 2007), the CNL role is different from the role of manager or administrator. The CNL is prepared as a generalist managing the health care delivery system across all settings.

Areas of specialty within the master's nurse practitioner programs include family, acute care, pediatric, psychiatric, geriatric, school health, and adult nursing practice. There are more family nurse practitioner programs than any other program.

According to the 2008 National Sample Survey of Registered Nurses prepared for advanced practice, there are an estimated 158,348 nurse practitioners, 59,242 clinical nurse specialists, 18,492 nurse-midwives, 34,821 nurse anesthetists, and 14,689 nurse practitioner/clinical nurse specialists (Figure 7-3). To take advantage of these trends and better position yourself in the job market, you might find that the benefits of returning to school far outweigh the sacrifices. See Table 7-1 for typical educational preparation and responsibilities of various advanced practice nurses.

The National Council of State Boards of Nursing APRN Advisory Committee and leading professional nursing organizations formed an APRN Consensus Work Group to work toward establishing clear expectations for licensure, accreditation, certification, and education (LACE) for APRNs. This work group has been meeting for several years and in July 2008 the landmark document, *Consensus Model for APRN Regulation: Licensure, Accreditation, Certification, & Education* was finalized. This document will be used to shape the future of APRN practice across the nation and allow APRNS to practice to the full extent of their education. APRNS will be educated in one of the four roles, certified registered nurse anesthetist (CRNA), certified nurse-midwife (CNM), clinical nurse specialist (CNS), or certified nurse practitioner (CNP) and in at least one

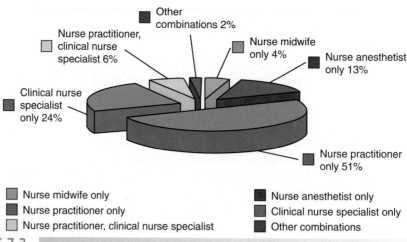

FIGURE 7-3

Registered Nurse Population National Sample Survey, March 2008. *(Source: Health Resources and Services Administration. [2010]: The registered nurse population: Findings from the March 2008 National Sample Survey of Registered Nurses. Washington, DC: U.S. Department of Health and Human Services. Retrieved from www.bhpr.hrsa.gov/healthworkforce/rnsurvey/initialfindings2008.pdf.)*

TABLE 7-1   Advanced Practice Nursing

	EDUCATION	WHAT THEY DO
Nurse practitioner (NP)	Most of the approximately 150 NP education programs in the United States today confer a master's degree. The majority of states require NPs to be nationally certified by ANCC, ACNP, or a specialty nursing organization. In 2008, 158,348 of advanced practice nurses were NPs.	Working in clinics, nursing homes, hospitals, HMOs, private industry or their own offices, NPs are qualified to handle a wide range of basic health problems. Most have a specialty—for example, an adult, family, or pediatric health care degree. At minimum, NPs conduct physical examinations, take medical histories, diagnose and treat common acute minor illnesses or injuries, order and interpret laboratory tests and radiographs, and counsel and educate patients. In all states they may prescribe medication according to state law. Some work as independent practitioners and can be reimbursed by Medicare or Medicaid for services rendered.
Certified nurse-midwife (CNM)	An average 1.5 years of specialized education beyond nursing school, either in an accredited certificate program or at the master's level. In 2008, there were an estimated 18,492 nurses prepared as CNMs in the United States.	CNMs provide well-woman gynecological and low-risk obstetrical care, including prenatal, labor and delivery, and postpartum care. In 2004, there were 13,684 formally prepared CNMs in the United States (a 48.2% increase from 2000), and 93.7% had national certification. The number of CNM-attended births has increased every year since 1975. An ANA meta-analysis of CNM care found that nurse-midwives performed fewer fetal monitors, episiotomies, and forceps deliveries; administered fewer intravenous solutions; delivered fewer low-birth-weight and premature infants; and had shorter patient hospital stays. CNMs have prescriptive authority in all 50 states.

Continued

TABLE 7-1 Advanced Practice Nursing—cont'd		
	EDUCATION	WHAT THEY DO
Clinical nurse specialist (CNS)	CNSs are registered nurses with advanced nursing degrees—master's or doctoral—who are experts in a specialized area of clinical practice such as mental health, gerontology, cardiac or cancer care, or community or neonatal health. There was a decrease in the number of CNSs from the 2004 to 2008 survey. In 2008, there were an estimated 59,242 CNSs in the United States.	CNSs work in hospitals, clinics, nursing homes, their own offices, and other community-based settings, such as industry, home care, and HMOs. Qualified to handle a wide range of physical and mental health problems, CNSs provide primary care and psychotherapy. They conduct health assessments, make diagnoses, deliver treatment, and develop quality-control methods. In addition to delivering direct patient care, CNSs work in consultation, research, education, and administration. Some work independently or in private practice and receive reimbursement.
Certified registered nurse anesthetist (CRNA)	CRNAs are registered nurses who complete a graduate program and meet national certification and recertification requirements. There are an estimated 34,821 CRNAs in the United States.	In this oldest of the advanced nursing specialties, CRNAs safely administer approximately approximately 32 million anesthetics to patients each year in the United States. CRNAs are the sole anesthesia providers in more than two thirds of all U.S. rural hospitals (AANA, 2009). This enables health care facilities to provide obstetric, surgical, and trauma stabilization services. CRNAs provide anesthetics to patients in collaboration with surgeons, anesthesiologists, dentists, podiatrists, and other qualified health care professionals.

of six population foci: family/individual across the lifespan, neonatal, pediatrics, adult-gerontology, women's health/gender-related or psych/mental health. All four of these roles will be given the title of advanced practice registered nurse (APRN). It is important for all potential APRNs to read this document because it will change how APRNs are educated in the future *(www.aacn.nche.edu/education/apn.htm).*

In the more traditional master's degree programs, the student takes the courses required for the degree and then, depending on institutional requirements, may also be required to take a written or oral comprehensive examination or write a thesis, or both. There are also nontraditional models that include outreach programs, summers-only programs, and programs for RNs who have bachelor's degrees in other fields.

Advances in technology have also made it possible for graduate programs to become more creative in the way courses are being offered. It is now possible for students to obtain all or part of their course offerings by means of the Internet, distance learning, computer-based programs, and teleconferencing. This flexibility makes it easier for students in rural communities and part-time students to obtain advanced degrees.

How Do I Know Which Master's Degree Program Is Right for Me?

Your career goals and interests will help you to determine which choice is best for you. Do some reading on your area of special interest and find out how advanced education would help you to obtain your career goals. As an example, in most nursing programs, a nurse with a nonnursing master's degree would need to complete a master's in nursing to become an advanced practice nurse. If you think that you might want to become a nurse practitioner at some point in your life, be sure that you obtain your master's in nursing. You can always go back and obtain a post-master's certificate as a nurse practitioner. If your master's degree is in another field, this would not be possible.

Once you have decided on a master's degree, there are several resources available online, such as the *Peterson's Guide (www.petersons.com)*, to help you find the right school. Consider all the options and do your homework. If you are considering an advanced practice degree, be sure to check with the Board of Nurse Examiners for the state in which you reside to see what the requirements are to be recognized as an advanced practice RN in your state. Believe it or not, the requirements are NOT the same for every state. After all, if you are going to expend the time, energy, and finances to obtain a graduate degree, you want to get the most from it.

Why Would I Want a Doctoral Degree?

Power, authority, and professional status are usually associated with a doctoral degree. Nurses with doctoral degrees provide leadership in the improvement of nursing practice and in the development of research and nursing education programs. It is no secret that the role of the nurse is changing and will continue to change as health care reform continues to be implemented. There is a growing need for administrators, policy analysts, clinical researchers, and clinical practitioners in the community and in governmental agencies. Nurses need to position themselves to take on these new leadership roles, and the way to do this is through advanced education, particularly at the doctoral level.

Until recently, there were two basic models of doctoral education in nursing: the academic degree, or Doctor of Philosophy (PhD), and the professional degree, or Doctor of Nursing Science (DNS, DSN, or DNSc). For either of these degrees, you must first have a master's in nursing. Nurses have other doctoral degree options available to them, such as the Doctor of Education (EdD), the Doctor of Public Health (DrPH), the Doctor of Philosophy (PhD) in a discipline besides nursing, the nontraditional external degree doctorate, and the practiced-focused Nurse Doctorate (ND), which was initiated as an entry-level degree.

In October 2004, the AACN published a position statement on the practice doctorate in nursing (DNP). The term *practice doctorate* would be used instead of *clinical doctorate,* and the ND degree would be phased out. The DNP would become the educational preparation for all advanced practice nurses. This move toward a DNP is to take place over a 15-year period (AACN, 2009). There are currently 92 DNP programs with more than 102 additional nursing schools considering starting a DNP program (AACN, 2009).

How Do I Know Which Doctoral Program Is Right for Me?

As with the master's degree, it is important to look at your career goals before deciding which doctoral program is best for you. To help you with that task, look at the NLN publications specific to doctoral education. Ask yourself how much time you can devote to obtaining a doctorate degree. Can you be a full-time student, or must you continue to work? What do you plan to do with the degree once you get it?

Is there an institution available to you that offers a doctorate in nursing, or would you have to consider moving? What are your career and professional goals? Do you want to teach? The PhD is considered the research-focused degree. It prepares an individual for a lifetime of intellectual inquiry and has an increased emphasis on postdoctoral study. In contrast, the DNP is viewed as the practice-focused degree. The goal of this program is to prepare an advanced practitioner for the application of knowledge with an emphasis on research. The original intent of the DNS was to prepare nurses to do clinical research.

CREDENTIALING: LICENSURE AND CERTIFICATION

What Is Credentialing?

In the early days of nursing before the Nightingale era, anyone could claim to be a nurse and practice the "trade" as he or she wished. It was only during the past century that nursing became a credentialed profession. A credential can be as simple as a written document of an individual's qualifications. A high school diploma is a credential that indicates a certain level of education has been attained. A credential can also signify a person's performance. The attainment of a title—such as Fellow of the American Academy of Nursing (FAAN)—signifies excellence in performance; a postgraduate degree from an institution of higher learning (PhD or EdD) indicates success in terms of academic achievement and advanced nursing knowledge.

In nursing, the educational credentials that an individual holds indicate not only academic achievement, but also the attainment of a minimum level of competency in nursing skills. Academic achievement is represented by an ADN, a diploma in nursing, or a baccalaureate degree in nursing (BSN or BS). After academic preparation and successful completion of NCLEX, you will have a legal credential—your nursing license—that permits you to practice as an RN. Additional nursing credentials may reflect practice in special areas, such as Critical Care Registered Nurse (CCRN) and Certified Addictions Registered Nurse (CARN). Figure 7-4 summarizes how professional and legal regulations affect the individual, the institution, and the public.

What Are Registration and Licensure?

Licensure affords protection to the public by requiring an individual to demonstrate minimum competency by examination before practicing certain trades. By 1923, all 48 states had some form of nursing licensure in place. Nursing licensure is a process by which a governmental agency grants "legal" permission to an individual to practice nursing. This accountability is maintained through state boards of nursing, which are responsible for the licensing and registration process. Boards of nursing vary in structure and are based on the design of the nurse practice act within each state. State boards of nursing also exercise legal control over schools of nursing within their respective states. In 1978, all boards of nursing formed a national council, the National Council

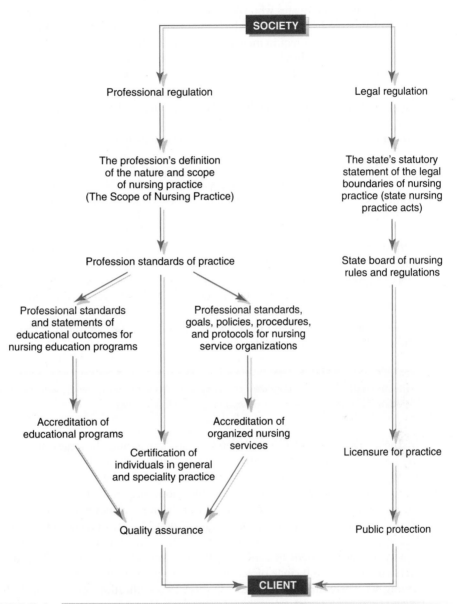

FIGURE 7-4

Flow chart on professional and legal regulation of practice. *(From American Nurses Association:* The scope of nursing, *Kansas City, Mo: ANA, 1987.)*

of State Boards of Nursing (NCSBN), to present a more collective front on nursing education and licensure.

Foreign nurse graduates who want to practice nursing in the United States must contact the board of nursing in the state in which they want to practice to obtain licensure, because each state controls its own requirements for licensure. The state's board of nursing will review the candidate's nursing education and determine requirements needed to obtain a license in that respective state. Most states require that foreign nurses take the Committee on Graduates of Foreign Nursing Schools (CGFNS) examination before the NCLEX-RN examination. This examination determines proficiency both in nursing and the English language, thus assisting in the prediction of success on the NCLEX-RN examination. All foreign graduates, regardless of licensure in their home countries, must successfully complete the NCLEX-RN examination.

What Is Certification?

In the classic article on credentialing published by the ANA in the late 1970s, certification is defined as a "voluntary process by which a nongovernmental agency or association certifies that an individual licensed to practice a profession has certain predetermined standards specified by that profession for specialty practice" (ANA, 1978-1979). Certification is a different credential from licensure and has a variety of interpretations—both for the nursing profession and the public.

The movement toward certification in nursing practice areas has grown significantly within the past 40 years. It was in 1946 that credentialing was first required for entry into practice as a nurse anesthetist (i.e., Certified Registered Nurse Anesthetist [CRNA]). Twenty-five years later, nurse-midwives followed suit by requiring certification through the American College of Nurse Midwives as an entry-level credential.

> The nursing license is recognized as indicating minimum competency, whereas the certification credential indicates preparation beyond the minimum level.

In August 2000, the ANCC issued a press release concerning the largest study ever conducted in the United States and Canada with credentialed nurses. The study indicated that nurses who have professional certification made fewer health care errors (ANCC, 2003).

Since the establishment of the first certification program by the ANA in 1973, certification is the credential that provides recognition of professional achievement in a defined functional or clinical area of nursing practice. More than 75,000 advanced practice nurses are currently certified by ANCC (ANCC, 2006). Credentials, such as professional certification, are the stamps of quality and achievement to communicate professional competence. The process of becoming certified engages a full circle of accountability to patients and families, along with professional colleagues. There are over 40 areas of specialty certification areas available from the ANCC (2006).

What Is Accreditation?

The term *accreditation* is often confused with certification. The term is defined as "a process by which a voluntary, nongovernmental agency or organization approves and grants status to institutions or programs (not individuals) that meet predetermined standards or outcomes." The accreditation of nursing programs by either the NLNAC or the Commission on Collegiate Nursing Education (CCNE) is an activity that you, the recent graduate, may have been involved with during your nursing education.

Accreditation is a peer review and voluntary process. The use of standards and criteria are supported by member schools for the evaluation peer review process. The process of accreditation is similar for both accrediting organizations—the CCNE and the NLNAC. The NLNAC is the only organization that accredits all levels of nursing program education from the practical nurse to the graduate-level nurse.

Why should you be concerned whether the nursing program you are attending, or thinking about attending, is accredited? Accreditation assures you, the student, and the public that the program has achieved educational standards over and above the legal requirements of the state. It guarantees the student the opportunity to obtain a quality education. Accreditation is strictly a voluntary process. The U.S. Department of Education approves the professional association that is allowed to accredit nursing schools. Until 1997, the NLN was the only accrediting body for nursing programs. In 1997 the NLNAC was established, and responsibility for all accrediting activities was transferred to this new independent subsidiary. Around the same time, the AACN sought recognition from the U.S. Department of Education to accredit baccalaureate and graduate degree nursing programs, because membership in AACN is restricted to deans and directors of baccalaureate and graduate programs. The CCNE was established by AACN as their autonomous accrediting agency.

Some graduate nursing programs require completion of an NLNAC- or CCNE-approved undergraduate program as a prerequisite for admission to their master's or doctoral program. The NLNAC and CCNE both publish an official complete list of accredited programs annually. Accreditation becomes a major concern as more and more courses and programs are offered by means of distance learning.

With two organizations offering accreditation to schools of nursing, it was difficult for schools of nursing to develop competency statements that were consistent. Rather than listing competency statements for three levels of nursing, the competency statement accepted by the 1996 annual meeting of the NCSBN is presented. According to the NCSBN, "Competence is defined as the application of knowledge and the interpersonal, decision-making and psychomotor skills expected for the practice role, within the context of public health, safety and welfare" (NCSBN, 1996, p 47). The NCSBN continues work on the concept of continued competence exploring its regulatory role.

"Boards of nursing cannot go it alone. This has to be a collaborative effort. Nurses, employers, educators, nursing organizations, CE providers, consumers and boards of nursing are all stakeholders and have perspectives to share and expertise to offer. Stakeholder buy-in to any regulatory model is important. But the bottom line is that only governmental licensing boards have the authority to enforce change" (NCSBN, 2005).

The promotion of competency requires a collaborative approach; it involves the individual nurse, employers of nurses, nursing educators, and the regulating board of nursing. The roles of each of these in competence accountability are described in Figure 7-5.

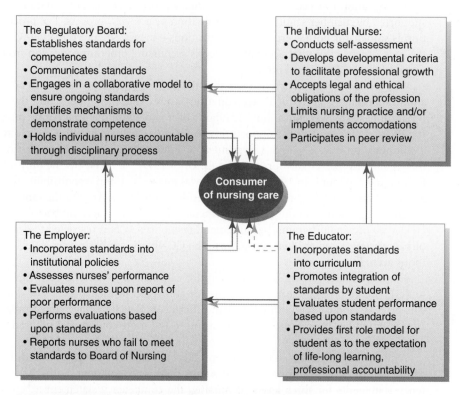

The Regulatory Board:
- Establishes standards for competence
- Communicates standards
- Engages in a collaborative model to ensure ongoing standards
- Identifies mechanisms to demonstrate competence
- Holds individual nurses accountable through disciplinary process

The Individual Nurse:
- Conducts self-assessment
- Develops developmental criteria to facilitate professional growth
- Accepts legal and ethical obligations of the profession
- Limits nursing practice and/or implements accomodations
- Participates in peer review

Consumer of nursing care

The Employer:
- Incorporates standards into institutional policies
- Assesses nurses' performance
- Evaluates nurses upon report of poor performance
- Performs evaluations based upon standards
- Reports nurses who fail to meet standards to Board of Nursing

The Educator:
- Incorporates standards into curriculum
- Promotes integration of standards by student
- Evaluates student performance based upon standards
- Provides first role model for student as to the expectation of life-long learning, professional accountability

Actions of boards of nursing that ensure competence to the public:
1. Establish competence requirements for safe and effective practice.
2. Communicate standards to the consumers, nurses, nursing educators, employers, and other regulators.
3. Hold individual nurses accountable for continued competence.
4. Engage in collaborative activities with nurses, educators, employers, and consumers to ensure nurses practice safely and effectively.
5. Identify a variety of techniques nurses may use to demonstrate competence.
6. Discipline nurses who fail to meet standards for safe and effective practice.
7. Inform the public of disciplinary actions taken against nurses.
8. Establish nondisciplinary model to monitor and/or limit the practice of nurses who demonstrate an inability to carry out essential nursing role functions.

FIGURE 7-5

Competence accountability. *(From National Council of State Boards of Nursing: Annual meeting. In:* Book of reports, *Chicago: National Council of State Boards of Nursing, 1996, p 51.)*

NURSING EDUCATION: FUTURE TRENDS

Education is a lifelong process and an empowering force that enables an individual to achieve higher goals. Student access to educational opportunities is paramount to nursing education. A chapter on nursing education would not be complete without taking a look at the future.

The Changing Student Profile

Future nursing programs will need to be flexible to meet the learning needs of a changing student population. It has previously been stated that there is a growing population of nontraditional students—individuals who are making midlife career changes in part because of job displacement or job dissatisfaction. The student population tends to be older, married, and with families. Minority individuals, foreign students, and the poor are looking toward nursing education for career opportunities. There are a growing number of students choosing to attend school part-time.

These changes mean that nurse educators will have to further address the needs of the adult learner. More programs will be needed that permit part-time study and allow students to work while attending school. One option may be for more night or weekend course offerings. There will continue to be a need for emphasis on remedial education such as developmental courses in math, English, and English as a second language. The diversity in the student population means diversity in learning rates, which may be addressed with more self-paced learning modules (Figure 7-6).

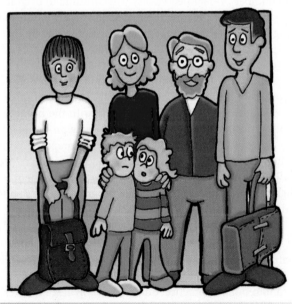

FIGURE 7-6

The changing student profile.

Educational Mobility

Educational mobility will also need to be addressed further. A growing number of individuals in health care are seeking more education. The issue is not one of entry into practice, but rather of how to best facilitate the return of these individuals to nursing school for educational advancement. The growth of Web-based (online) courses may facilitate educational mobility.

A Shortage of Registered Nurses

According to the AACN (2010d) *AACN Fact Sheet on the Nursing Shortage,* despite the economic downturn leading to more nurses remaining employed and new graduate nurses having a difficult time finding employment, the shortage is going to continue to intensify. The U.S. Bureau of Labor Statistics predicts that registered nursing will have more than 587,000 new RN jobs created through 2016. The creation of new jobs coupled with a rapidly aging nursing workforce make the prediction of a nursing shortage reaching 800,000 by the year 2020 not unlikely. These predictions place nursing at the top of the list in terms of projected job growth in the United States.

A Shortage of Qualified Nursing Faculty

Data on faculty reported by the AACN (2010e) indicate that the "average ages of doctorally prepared faculty holding the ranks of professor, associate professor, and assistant professor were 60.1, 56.9, and 52.1 years, respectively. For master's degree-prepared nurse faculty, the average ages for professors, associate professors, and assistant professors were 56.9, 55.7 and 50.6 years, respectively" (para. 3). There are fewer nurses entering the profession that are choosing a teaching role. Because of decreased numbers of new teachers, along with the number of current faculty retiring, the number of qualified faculty will continue to decline. An NLN Survey conducted in 2002 found three trends affecting the future of nursing education over the next decade:

1. The aging of the nurse faculty population. Approximately 75% of the current faculty population is expected to retire by 2019. Approximately 1800 full-time faculty members leave their positions each year.
2. The increasing number of part-time faculty. The percentage of full-time faculty teaching in nursing programs dropped from 71% to 61%, and the number of part-time faculty grew from 29% to 39% during a 10-year period, along with the number of budgeted unfilled full-time faculty positions in all types of RN and graduate programs rose from 860 to 1106.
3. The large number of nursing faculty who are not prepared at the doctoral level. Approximately 50% of full-time faculty in baccalaureate and higher degree programs hold a doctoral degree. Doctorally prepared faculty account for only 6.6% of the nursing faculty in ADN programs with slightly more than 5% in diploma programs. Only 350 to 400 nursing students receive doctoral degrees each year (NLN, 2002).

Technology and Education

Educational learning will continue to change with advances in telecommunication and technology. Nurses and nurse educators will need education to implement these advances into the curriculum and into nursing practice. Cable television and the Internet have significantly extended the boundaries of the classroom; these technologies will facilitate the offering of courses to meet the lifestyle of the changing student population.

Changing Health Care Settings

There has been a major shift from inpatient to outpatient nursing services as health care and nursing focus on maintaining health rather than dealing with illness. However, with an increase in the age of the population, more inpatients have multiple chronic health problems. Society is now developing a variety of new health care settings. Are nurses educated for these new roles? What will be the role of the advanced nurse practitioner? Will there be enough nurses educationally prepared to meet these new challenges?

The Aging Population

There is a growing aging population. According to the Administration on Aging (2007), by 2030 there will be approximately 71.5 million people over the age of 65 years, representing 20% of the population. This is more than twice the number in 2000. Naisbitt and Aburdene stated in their book *Megatrends 2000,* published in 1991, "If business and society can master the challenge of daycare, we will be one step closer to confronting the next great care giving task of the 1990s—eldercare" (p 83). This is still a critical issue in the 21st century. Already, the United States has well over 2000 adult daycare centers. Nursing educators need to address the provision of health care to the elderly and include it in the curricula.

> What great opportunities in nursing!

CONCLUSION

The future of nursing looks bright and exciting. With technological advances, changes in health care settings, increased demand for the services of the RN, and the shift back to the acute care setting, nurses now have increased opportunities to chart their own destinies.

Nurses who have career plans and career goals will see the future trends in health care as a challenge and an opportunity for growth in roles such as case manager, independent consultant, nurse practitioner, nursing education, policy maker, and entrepreneur. In contrast, nurses without career goals may find themselves displaced or obsolete. There has never been a more exciting time to be entering the profession of nursing than right now. Opportunities in nursing are wide open to those with the sensitivity and the creativity to embrace the future.

BIBLIOGRAPHY

Administration on Aging (2007): Retrieved from *www.aoa.gov.*

APRN Consensus Work Group and the National Council of State Boards of Nursing APRN Advisory Committee. Consensus Model for APRN Regulation (2008): *Licensure, accreditation, certification, and education.* Retrieved from *www.aacn.nche.edu/education/apn.htm.*

American Academy of Nurse Practitioners Fact Sheet (2010): *Nurse practitioner facts.* Retrieved from *www.aanp.org/NR/rdonlyres/32B74504-2C8E-4603-8949-710A287E0B32/0/NPFacts2010.pdf.*

American Association of Colleges of Nursing Fact Sheet (2010a): *Accelerated Baccalaureate and Master's Degrees in Nursing.* Retrieved from *www.aacn.nche.edu/media/factsheets/acceleratedprog.htm.*

American Association of Colleges of Nursing Fact Sheet (2010b): *Degree completion programs for registered nurses: RN to master's degree and RN to baccalaureate programs.* Retrieved from *www.aacn.nche.edu/media/factsheets/DegreeCompletionProg.htm.*

American Association of Colleges of Nursing (2010c): *Research and data fact sheet.* Retrieved from *www.aacn.nche.edu/Education/pdf/APLIST.PDF.*

American Association of Colleges of Nursing (2010d): *Nursing shortage fact sheet.* Retrieved from *www.aacn.nche.edu/media/factsheets/nursingshortage.htm.*

American Association of Colleges of Nursing (2010e): *Nursing faculty shortage fact sheet.* Retrieved from *www.aacn.nche.edu/media/factsheets/nursingshortage.htm.*

American Association of Colleges of Nursing fact sheet (2009): *The Doctor of Nursing Practice (DNP).* Retrieved from *www.aacn.nche.edu/Media/FactSheets/dnp.htm.*

American Association of Colleges of Nursing fact sheet (2009): *Nursing shortage.* Retrieved from *www.aacn.nche.edu/Media/FactSheets/NursingShortage.htm.*

American Association of Colleges of Nursing: *2007-2008 Enrollment and Graduations in Baccalaureate and Graduate Programs in Nursing.* Washington, DC, 2008, AACN.

American Association of Colleges of Nursing: White Paper on the Education and Role of the Clinical Nurse Leader February 2007 (revised and approved by AACN Board of Directors July 2007). Retrieved from *www.aacn.nche.edu/cnl/index.htm.*

American Association of Nurse Anesthetists (AANA) (2009): *2009 practice profile survey.* Retrieved from *www.aana.com/ataglance.aspx.*

American Nurses Credentialing Center (2006): *ANCC certification statistics.* Retrieved from *www.nursecredentialing.org/faculty/PDFs/2006CertificationStatistics.pdf.*

Forni PR: Models for doctoral programs: first professional degree or terminal degree? *Nurs Health Care* 10(8):429-434, 1989.

Kaiser JE: *A comparison of students in practical nursing programs and in associate degree nursing programs,* National League for Nursing Publication No. 23-1592, New York, 1975, National League for Nursing.

McCloskey J, Grace HK: *Current issues in nursing,* ed 6, St. Louis, 2001, Mosby.

Montag ML: *The education of nursing technicians,* New York, 1951, GP Putnam's Sons.

Montag ML: *Community college education for nursing,* New York, 1959, McGraw-Hill.

Naisbitt J, Aburdene P: *Megatrends 2000: new directions for tomorrow,* New York, 1991, William Morrow.

National Council of State Boards of Nursing: Definition of competence and standards for competence, National Council of State Boards of Nursing annual meeting, *Book of reports,* Chicago, 1996, National Council of State Boards of Nursing.

National Council of State Boards of Nursing (2005): *Meeting the ongoing challenge of continued competence.* Retrieved from *www.ncsbn.org/Continued_Comp_Paper_Testing Services.pdf.*

National League of Nursing (2002): *Nurse faculty shortage fact sheet–2002 survey.* Retrieved from *www.nln.org/governmentaffairs/pdf/NurseFacultyShortage.pdf.*

National League for Nursing, Council of Associate Degree Nursing Competencies Task Force: *Educational competencies for graduates of associate degree nursing programs,* book code 1404-6, New York, 2001, National League for Nursing.

National Sample Survey of Registered Nurses (2008): *Initial findings.* Retrieved from *www.bhpr.hrsa.gov/healthworkforce/rnsurvey/initialfindings2008.pdf.*

Raines C, Taglairene M: Career pathways in nursing: entry points and academic progression, *Online Journal of Issues in Nursing* 13(3), 2008 Sep. Retrieved from *www.nursingworld.org.MainMenuCategories/ANAMarketplace/ANAPeriodicals/OJIN/TableofContents/vol132008/No3Sept08/CareerEntryPoints.aspx.*

Rowland HS, Rowland B: *The nurse's almanac,* ed 2, Rockville, MD, 1984, Aspen.

U.S. Bureau of Labor Statistics (2007): *Occupational employment and wages for 2006.* Retrieved from *www.bis.bov/news.release/pdf/ocw.age.pdf.*

Additional resources are available online at *http://evolve.elsevier.com/Zerwekh/nsgtoday/.*

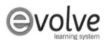

CHAPTER 8

Nursing Theory

Ashley Zerwekh Garneau, MS, RN

> *The only good is knowledge and the only evil is ignorance.*
> —SOCRATES (469 BC-399 BC)

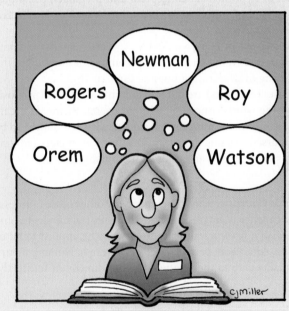

There are many nursing theories available to help guide my practice.

After completing this chapter, you should be able to:

- Identify the purposes for nursing theory.

- Describe the origins of nursing theory.

- Describe some of the key words associated with nursing theory.

- Identify some of the more well-known and well-developed nursing theories.

- Discuss some of the main points of each of these theories.

ust mentioning the word theory, let alone nursing theory, can make many nurses' yawn reflexes start to work overtime. What is theory? Who are nursing theorists? What are the different nursing theories? Most nurses are not aware of theory, nor can they name a nursing theorist. Nursing theories are a way to organize and think about nursing, and the people who wrote theories are part of our nursing history. Theory provides an overall "theme" to what nurses do. In this chapter, the key words related to theory are defined, and the main elements of eight nursing theories are summarized.

> Buckle your seatbelts—we might be in for a bumpy ride. And no yawning!

NURSING THEORY

What Is Theory?

Quite simply, theories are words or phrases (concepts) joined together in sentences, with an overall theme, to explain, describe, or predict something. A more complex definition of a theory is "a set of interrelated concepts, definitions, and propositions that present a systematic way of viewing facts/events by specifying relations among the variables, with the purpose of explaining and predicting the fact event" (Kerlinger, cited in Hickman, 2003).

Theories help us understand and find meaning in our nursing experience and also provide a foundation to direct questions that provide insights into best practices and safe patient care. Ellis (1997) stated, "A theory is a coherent set of hypothetical, conceptual and pragmatic principles forming a general frame of reference for a field of study" (p 373). You might see theory referred to as a conceptual model or a conceptual framework.

Nursing theory is, according to Meleis (cited in Hickman, 2003), "an articulated and communicated conceptualization of invented or discovered reality in or pertaining to nursing for the purpose of describing, explaining, predicting or prescribing nursing care" (p 16).

The bottom line is that words and phrases (concepts) are put together into sentences (propositions that show the relationships among the words/concepts), with an overall theme, to create theories. Theories also have some basic assumptions (jumping-off points; what is assumed to be true), such as the idea that patients need nurses. Nursing theories also define four metaparadigms (metaparadigms refer to big, comprehensive concepts) and address the nursing process.

What Nursing Theory Is Not

Nursing theory is *not* managed care, primary nursing, team nursing, or any other more business-related method of delivering care. Nursing theory is *not* obstetric nursing, surgical nursing, home health nursing, or any other nursing specialty; however, nursing theory can be applied to all of areas of nursing, including administration, education, patient care, and research. Nursing theory is by nurses and for nurses, providing quality care to their patients, either directly or indirectly.

Why Theory?

Consider all that you do as a nurse. What you do is based on principles from many different professions, such as biology, sociology, medicine, ethics, business, theology, psychology, and philosophy. What is specifically based on nursing? Also, if nursing is a science (and it is), there must be some scientific basis for it. Furthermore, theory helps define nursing as a profession (Figure 8-1).

Theory is a means to gather information, to more clearly and specifically identify ideas, to guide research, to show how ideas are connected to each other, to make sense of what we observe or experience, to predict what might happen, and to provide answers. A nurse is not a "junior physician," although for years nursing care has been based on the medical model. Because nursing is a science (as well as an art) and a unique profession in its own right, nurses need nursing theory on which to base their principles of care (Critical Thinking Box 8-1; Evidence-Based Practice Box 8-1).

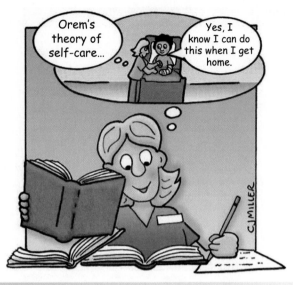

FIGURE 8-1
Theory guides both research and nursing practice.

 CRITICAL THINKING BOX 8-1 What are some advantages and disadvantages that you can see to using nursing theory?

What Is the History of Nursing Theory?

In studying nursing theories and the people who created them, it is important to look at the background of the theorist, as well as how life experiences, beliefs, and education influenced the resulting theory. What are the overall theme and main ideas of the theory, and how does the theorist define the four nursing metaparadigms (Box 8-1)?

The four metaparadigms for nursing are nursing, person, health, and environment.

Florence Nightingale is considered to be the first nursing theorist. She saw nursing as "A profession, a trade, a necessary occupation, something to fill and employ all my faculties, I have always felt essential to me, I have always longed for; consciously or not … The first thought I can remember, and the last was nursing work …" (cited in Dunphy, 2002). Now, you might not feel that dedicated, but Nightingale also stated, "Nursing is an art … It is one of the Fine Arts; I had almost said, the finest of the Fine Arts" (cited in Dunphy, 2002).

Nightingale had various influences, including her education (which was fairly comprehensive for a 19th century English woman), her religion (Unitarianism), the history of the time (the Crimean War and invention of the telegraph), and her social status. The Unitarian belief involved

BOX 8-1   **EVIDENCE-BASED PRACTICE**

Nursing Theory

PRACTICE ISSUE

While the focus of health care institutions in improving patient outcomes is based on evidenced-based practice, little research has been done on utilization of a theoretical framework guided by nursing theory in examining patient perceptions in living with a physical life-altering injury.

Desanto-Madeya (2006) examined perceptions of family members in individuals who had sustained a spinal cord injury about the "meaning of living" (p 240) using Roy's Adaptation Model. In her qualitative ethnographic study, seven themes emerged from the data analysis in addressing the following research question of what the meaning of living means to the family of an individual with a spinal cord injury.

"The seven themes were (a) looking for understanding to a life that is unknown, (b) stumbling along an unlit path, (c) viewing self through a stained glass window, (d) challenging the bonds of love, (e) being chained to the injury, (f) moving forward in a new way of life, and (g) reaching normalcy" (Desanto-Madeya, 2006, p 241). Using Roy's adaptation model, each theme was categorized into one or more modes of adaptation.

IMPLICATIONS FOR NURSING PRACTICE

Implementation of a nursing theory to examine patient and family experiences when faced with an unexpected illness or injury that causes both physical and emotional life-altering changes can serve as a framework for nurses in guiding their practice.

Nurses can assist patients and their families in adapting to the physiological and psychosocial factors affected by a life-altering injury and/or illness.

Nursing theories can assist nurses in providing holistic nursing care.

Reference for the Evidence

DeSanto-Madeya S: A secondary analysis of the meaning of living with spinal cord injury using Roy's adaptation model, *Nursing Science Quarterly* 19(3):240-246, 2006.

salvation through health and wholeness, or our modern-day "holism." Nightingale believed that there was no conflict between science and spirituality. Science was necessary for the development of a mature concept of God. She also studied many other religions throughout her lifetime and considered starting a Protestant religious order of nuns (Dunphy, 2002).

Nightingale came from a very wealthy family and enjoyed traveling throughout Europe, one of the destinations being Kaiserwerth in Germany, where she observed and was moved by nuns caring for the ill. Nightingale felt a "calling" to care for others and began training with various groups, usually nuns who cared for the sick. When the Crimean War broke out, Nightingale was asked and volunteered to go to care for the wounded English soldiers. The Crimean War was the first war since the invention of the telegraph, so news of the war was more immediate than had been previously experienced (Dunphy, 2002).

The overall theme of Nightingale's theory was that the person is influenced by the environment. When she went to help soldiers during the Crimean War, her initial intent was to feed the soldiers healthy food and to clean the place (Figure 8-2). When soldier mortality rates fell, a legend was born (Dunphy, 2002)!

Nightingale believed that nursing was separate from medicine and that nurses should be trained (although we prefer the word *educated*). She also believed that the environment was

---

BOX 8-1   Definition of Metaparadigms

PERSON

Individuals, families, communities, and other groups who are participants in nursing.

ENVIRONMENT

A person's significant others and physical surroundings, as well as the setting in which nursing occurs, which ranges from the person's home to clinical agencies to society as a whole. All local, regional, national, and worldwide cultural, social, political, and economic conditions that are associated with the person's health.

HEALTH

A person's state of well-being at the time that nursing occurs, which can range from high-level wellness to terminal illness.

NURSE

The actions taken by nurses on behalf of or in conjunction with the person and the goals or outcomes of nursing actions. Nursing actions typically are viewed as a systematic process of assessment, labeling, planning, intervention, and evaluation.

From Fawcett J: *Analysis and evaluation of contemporary nursing knowledge: nursing models and theories,* Philadelphia, 2005, FA Davis.

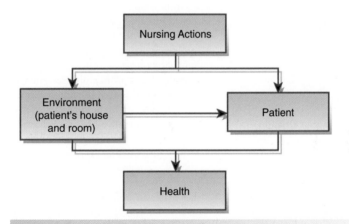

FIGURE 8-2

Nightingale's conceptual model of nursing. *(From Fitzpatrick J, Whall A:* Conceptual models of nursing: analysis and application, *ed 3, Stamford, Conn, 1996, Appleton & Lange, p 38.)*

important to the health of the person and that the nurse should support the environment to assist the patient in healing (Dunphy, 2002).

To define the metaparadigms, Nightingale noted that the person is the center of the model and incorporated a holistic view of the person, someone with psychological, intellectual, and spiritual components. The nurse was a woman (because only women were nurses in Nightingale's day) who had charge of the health of a person, whether in providing wellness care, such as with a newborn, or in providing care to the sick. Health was the result of environmental, physical, and psychological factors, not just the absence of disease (Dunphy, 2002).

No other theories were identified or published until the 1950s when Peplau published her theory based on the interpersonal process. Other nurses were working on theories during that time and into the 1960s. In the 1970s, nursing was beginning to see itself as a scientific profession based on theoretical ideas (Table 8-1). In 1972, the National League for Nursing (NLN) required that nursing curricula be based on conceptual frameworks (McEwen, 2011).

TABLE 8-1	Nursing Theories	
YEAR	THEORIST	THEORY DESCRIPTION
1860	Florence Nightingale	Although her model did not have a specific name, the basic underpinnings revolve around how a person is influenced by the environment. Nursing was a "calling" to help the patient in a reparative process by directly working with the patient or indirectly by affecting the environment to facilitate health and recovery from illness.
1952	Hildegard Peplau	Interpersonal Relations Model—describes the four phases of the dynamic relationship between nurse and patient: orientation, identification, exploitation, and resolution.
1960	Faye Abdellah	Patient-Centered Approach—develops a list of 21 unique nursing problems related to human needs; promoted the use of a problem-solving approach to practice rather than merely following physician orders. Responsible for changing the focus of nursing theory from a disease-centered to a patient-centered approach and moved nursing practice beyond the patient to include care of families and the elderly.
1961	Ida Jean Orlando	Theory of Deliberative Nursing Process—focuses on the interpersonal process between nurse and patient through a deliberative nursing process; most concerned with what was uniquely nursing.
1966	Virginia Henderson	One of her main topics is the "unique functions of nurses." All of her materials provide a focus for patient care via 14 basic needs.
1969	Myra Estrin Levine	Conservation Model—focuses attention on the wholeness of the person, adaptation, and conservation, which is guided by four principles (conservation of energy, structure, personal integrity, and social integrity).
1970	Martha Rogers	Science of Unitary Human Beings—an abstract model addressing the complexity of the "unitary human being," which allows for the examination of phenomena (energy fields, paranormal) that other theories do not describe, as nurses promote synchronicity between human beings and their environment/universe.
1971	Dorothea Orem	Self-Care Nursing Theory—three interwoven theories of self-care, self-care deficit, and nursing system help the nurse to identify strategies to meet the patient's self-care needs.

TABLE 8-1   Nursing Theories—cont'd

Year	Theorist	Theory Description
1971	Imogene King	Theory of Goal Attainment—patient goals are met through the transaction between nurse and patient involving three systems (personal, interpersonal, and social).
1972	Betty Neuman	Neuman Systems Model—focuses on wellness and mitigating stress within three levels of prevention: primary, secondary, and tertiary.
1974	Sister Callista Roy	Roy's Adaptation Model—individual seeking equilibrium through the process of adaptation; identified six physiological needs (exercise and rest; nutrition; elimination; fluid and electrolytes; oxygenation and circulation; and regulation of temperature, senses, and endocrine system).
1976	Josephine Paterson and Loretta Zderad	Humanistic Nursing Theory—focuses on the nurse and the patient; dignity, interests, and values are of greatest importance; belief that there is more to nursing that is not explainable by scientific principles.
1978; 1991	Madeline Leininger	Theory of Culture Care Diversity and Universality—a grand theory that considers the impact of culture on the person's health and caring practices.
1979	Margaret Newman	Theory of Health as Expanding Consciousness—every person in every situation is ever-changing in a unidirectional, unpredictable, all-at-once pattern involving movement, time, space, and consciousness; emphasizes the importance of viewing patients in the context of their holistic patterns.
1979	Jean Watson	Theory of Human Caring—identifies 10 "carative" factors focusing on the interactions between the one who is caring and the one who is being cared for.
1980	Dorothy Johnson	Behavioral Systems Model—focuses on human behavior rather than the person's state of health; this theory helped clarify the differences between medicine and nursing.
1981	Rosemarie Rizzo Parse	Theory of Human Becoming—focuses on the human-health-universe; views nursing as a participation effort with the patient that focuses on health.
1983	H. Erickson, E. Tomlin, and M. Swain	Modeling and Role Modeling Theory—uses the understanding of the patient's world to plan interventions that meet the patient's perceived needs and that will assist the patient to achieve holistic health; focus is on the person receiving the care, not the nurse, not the care, and not the disease.
1984	Pat Benner	Professional-Advancement-Model—applies the Dreyfus model of skill acquisition to nursing; area of concern is not how to do nursing but rather, "How do nurses learn to do nursing?"; identifies seven domains: practice-helping, teaching/coaching, diagnosing and monitoring, managing changes, administering and monitoring therapeutic interventions, monitoring quality care, and organizing to enact the work role.

From Fawcett J: *Analysis and evaluation of contemporary nursing knowledge: nursing models and theories,* Philadelphia, FA Davis, 2005; Alligood MR, Marriner Tomey A: *Nursing theorists and their work,* ed 7, St. Louis, 2010, Mosby.

Among the most well-known and well-formulated theories or models are those by Dorothea Orem, Martha Rogers, Sr. Callista Roy, Dorothy Johnson, Betty Neuman, Imogene King, Jean Watson, and Madeleine Leininger (see the *Definitions of the Metapardigms* by these theorists in the Evolve website). Each theory has been around for at least 20 years, and each theorist has practiced nursing at the bedside, in the community, and in administration or education.

WHO ARE THE NURSING THEORISTS?

Selected Nursing Theorists

Dorothea Orem—Self-Care Nursing Theory. Orem's theory includes the overall theme of self-care. She sees the person as composed of physical, psychological, interpersonal, and social aspects. Nursing consisted of those actions to overcome or prevent self-care limitations (self-care deficits) or to provide self-care for someone who is unable to do so. A nurse may need to do everything for the patient (wholly compensatory, such as for a patient who is under general anesthesia or is critically ill), to do some things for the patient (partly compensatory, such as with a patient who is 2 days post-op and may be able to do some things, but not everything, independently), or to educate the patient (supportive educative, such as with postpartum parents). Health, to Orem, is the internal and external conditions that permit self-care needs to be met. The environment is anything outside of or external to the person. Thus, in assessing a patient, a nurse using Orem's theory would ask, "What can the patient do for himself or herself? And what do I, as the nurse, need to do for the patient? What are the patient's self-care deficits (or things that he or she cannot do)?" (Hood, 2009).

Orem's nursing process includes assessing the patient, deciding whether nursing care is needed, and if so, determining which self-care deficits are present. Does the patient need wholly or partly compensatory or supportive-educative nursing care? The nurse needs to identify interventions and decide which interventions the patient can do (if any) and which interventions the nurse will do. The nurse describes which helping methods are used for the interventions (acting for or doing for another, guiding and directing, providing physical or psychological support, providing a therapeutic environment, or teaching) (Foster et al, 2003). And all interventions fall under one of those five helping methods (Figures 8-3 and 8-4).

Martha Rogers—Science of Unitary Human Beings. Martha Rogers is one of the most original thinkers of the nursing theorists. Her overall theme is that the person and environment are one thing and cannot be separated. Rogers takes holism to a new level. The person, for Rogers, is an energy field that exhibits patterns (think of electrocardiogram [ECG] patterns, fetal heart rate patterns, biorhythms, auras). Health is an "indication of the complexity and innovativeness of patterning of the energy field that is the person" (Hood, 2009). Rogers, however, did not like to define the word *health,* because she believed it was a value judgment (e.g., what your patient thinks is healthy about himself may not be what you think is healthy about the patient). The environment for Rogers was also an energy field that was interacting constantly with the energy field of the person (similar to what Nightingale thought). The role of nursing was to repattern the person and environment to achieve maximum health potential for the person. While this may all sound a little far-fetched, many nurses, when first entering a patient's room in a hospital, will assess the patient and rearrange or clean up the room to make it more convenient or therapeutic for caring for the patient. That is, the patient and environment are "repatterned" to achieve maximum health for the patient (Hood, 2009).

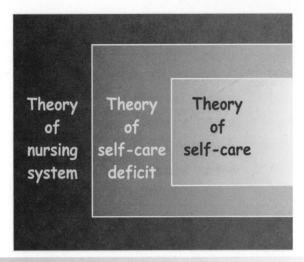

FIGURE 8-3

Orem's self-care deficit model. *(From Orem DE:* Nursing concepts of practice, *ed 6, St. Louis, 2001, Mosby, p 141.)*

Rogers' theory is grounded in the science of physics and the ideas of matter and energy. Rogers was very interested in space travel and envision nurses as providing care for people on earth or in space. She felt that some pathologies were due to our being earthbound, (e.g., osteoporosis and arthritis), but that these diseases would not be an issue in outer space because of the changes in gravity. Rogers also believed in the value of nurses using creative therapies, such as touch, color, sound, motion, and humor. The use of alternative therapies fit very well with Rogers' ideas. The nursing care plan that Rogers developed, but was not sold on, included Pattern Manifestation Knowing-Assessment (our idea of *assessment*), Voluntary Mutual Patterning (whereby the nurse and patient pattern the environmental energy to promote health—or interventions), and Pattern Manifestation Knowing-Evaluation (our idea of *evaluation*) (Muth Quillen, 2003).

Rogers' theory entitled, "Principles of Homeodynamics" examines the wholeness of humans and their interactions with the environment. Under homeodynamics, three principles exist further defining the environmental conditions humans experience and they are resonancy, integrality, and helicy. Resonancy is the "continuous change from lower to higher frequency wave patterns in human and environmental fields" from Rogers' in *Nursing Science and the Space Age* (as cited in Alligood & Marriner Tomey, 2010).

Integrality looks at how human beings and environment are continuously and simultaneously interacting. This interaction influences the changing life process that humans experience in their everyday activities. Helicy looks at the continuous, unpredictable change "between the human-environmental field" (Alligood & Marriner Tomey, 2010, p 246) (Figure 8-5).

Sister Callista Roy—Adaptation Model. Sister Callista Roy saw the person as a bio-psychosocial being (yes, it does seem like these theorists make up their own words), seeking equilibrium. Her overall theme was adaptation. The four adaptation modes represent the behavior responses exhibited by the individual and include, "*physiological-physical, self-concept-group identity, role function,* and *interdependence*" (Tiedeman as cited in Fitzpatrick and Whall, 2005, p 152). As nurses, we are to assess how well the person is coping and adapting to stimuli. The

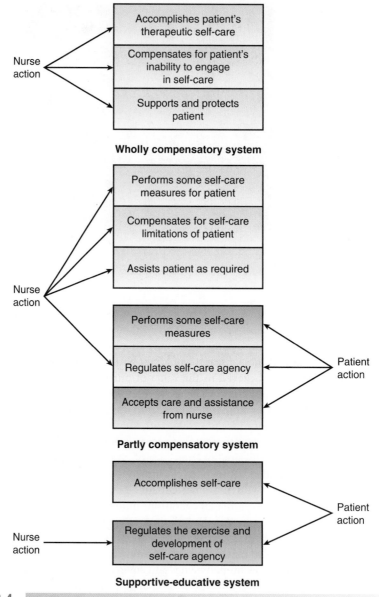

FIGURE 8-4

Orem's basic nursing systems. *(From Orem DE: Nursing concepts of practice, ed 6, St. Louis, 2001, Mosby, p 351.)*

stimuli could be any stressors that are making a person ill, or causing the person to not adapt. The stimulus could be focal (the stimulus that is the greatest concern at the moment—e.g., labor pain), contextual (all other stimuli in the area that contribute to the effect of the focal stimulus, such as noise in the background), or residual (a stimulus that is unknown to the nurse but is bothering the patient—e.g., memories of past labors and births).

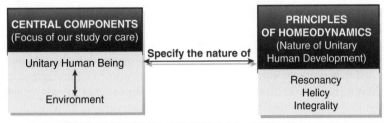

FIGURE 8-5

Roger's science of unitary human beings. *(From Fitzpatrick J, Whall A:* Conceptual models of nursing: analysis and application, *ed 3, Stamford, Conn, 1996, Appleton & Lange.)*

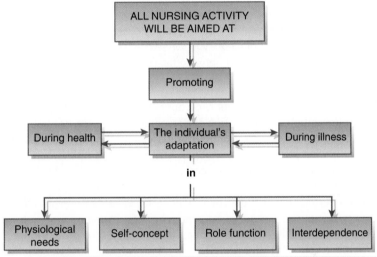

FIGURE 8-6

Roy's adaptation model. *(From Pearson A, Vaughan B, Fitzgerald M:* Nursing models for practice, *ed 3, Edinburgh, 2005, Butterworth & Heineman, p 129.)*

Health is defined as successful coping with stressors, and the environment is defined as the influences that affect the development of a person. Illness is unsuccessful coping. The nursing process is a problem-solving approach that encompasses steps to gather data, identify capacities and needs of the human adaptive system, select and implement approaches for nursing care, and evaluate the outcome of the care provided. In Roy's nursing process, she adds two assessment parts: (1) What is the stimulus? and (2) What is the person's response to the stimulus? The nurse's role is to influence stimuli to improve successful coping (Alligood & Marriner Tomey, 2010) (Figure 8-6).

Dorothy Johnson—Behavioral Systems Model. Dorothy Johnson was one of Roy's teachers at UCLA. Johnson's theme was balance; her theory is that the person is a behavior system and a biological system seeking balance. The environment is anything outside the person or behavior system. Health is balance or stability. The nurse's role is to restore or maintain the balance in the person or behavior system. A visual example would be learning to use crutches after a leg fracture. The person needs to learn to balance (literally) on crutches, but also needs to learn to "balance" the other aspects of his or her life that are affected by the broken leg (Hood, 2009).

Johnson views the nursing process as assessment, diagnosis, intervention, and evaluation. The person's seven subsystems are assessed. These subsystems are the achievement subsystem, which includes mastery or control of the self or environment; the aggressive/protective subsystem, which includes protecting oneself or others; the dependency subsystem, which includes obtaining attention or assistance from others; the eliminative subsystem, which includes not only physical elimination from the body, but also being able to express one's feelings or ideas; the ingestive subsystem, which includes eating, as well as "taking in" other things such as pain medication or information; the attachment/affiliation subsystem, which includes relating to others or achieving intimacy; and the sexual subsystem, which includes activities related to sexuality, such as procreating and sexual identity (Holaday, 2002) (Figure 8-7).

Consider how patients for whom you care would fall into each of these seven subsystems, or which subsystems would most apply to the patients for whom you provide care.

Betty Neuman—Systems Model. Betty Neuman's conceptual model focuses on prevention, or prevention as intervention as a response to stressors. Primary prevention is what a person does to prevent illness—for example, exercise, sleep 8 hours, eat a balanced diet. Secondary prevention is what is done when an illness strikes. For example, when a person with a myocardial infarction comes into the emergency department, what is done by the staff to prevent this person from dying or from having further heart damage? Tertiary prevention is what is done to rehabilitate a person after an illness or accident, such as cardiac rehabilitation or stroke rehabilitation. Tertiary prevention can move the person back to primary prevention again. The nurse's role is helping to reduce the stressors through the three levels of prevention.

Neuman also talks about the flexible lines of defense, the normal lines of defense, and lines of resistance. The flexible lines of defense are the outermost boundary and serve as the initial response to stressors. Neuman describes these lines as accordion-like, in that they can expand and contract depending on our health practices (e.g., lack of sleep, lack of eating well). Our normal lines of defense are what usually protect us from stressors—for example, our age, physical health, genetic make-up, spiritual beliefs, and gender. When the flexible lines of defense and the normal lines of defense can no longer protect us from stressors, our equilibrium is affected, and a reaction occurs. The lines of resistance come into play to help restore balance, similar to how the body's immune system works. The person, for Neuman, has physiological, psychological, sociocultural, developmental, and spiritual variables (Alligood & Marriner Tomey, 2010).

Think of how Neuman's ideas accurately portray the life of a student. The student struggles to keep up with coursework, work, and family life, but may find himself or herself sleeping less, eating less or eating poorly, and then getting sick or having less energy. Neuman's nursing process has just three steps: diagnosis, nursing goals (interventions are included with this step), and nursing outcomes. Neuman also has a unique way of looking at the environment, which she identifies as internal, external, and the created environment. The created environment is developed by the patient and serves as his or her protective device (Alligood & Marriner Tomey, 2010). The created environment can be a healthy adaptation (e.g., someone relaxing through

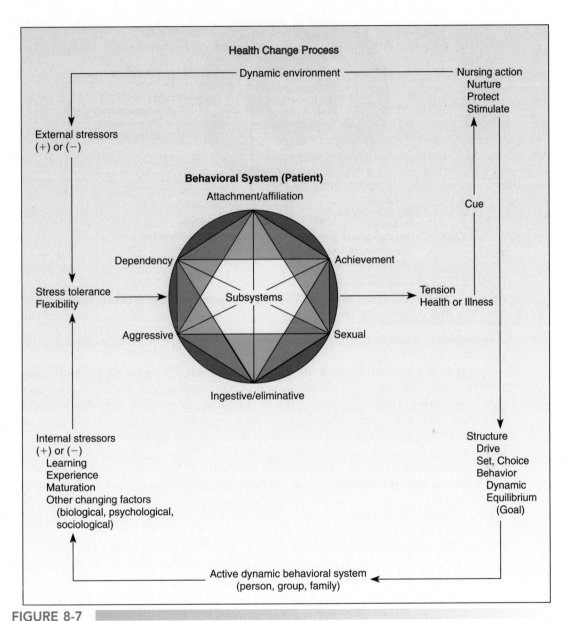

FIGURE 8-7

Johnson's behavioral systems model. *(From Alligood MR & Marriner Tomey A:* Nursing theorists and their work, *ed 7, St. Louis, 2010, Mosby, p 374.)*

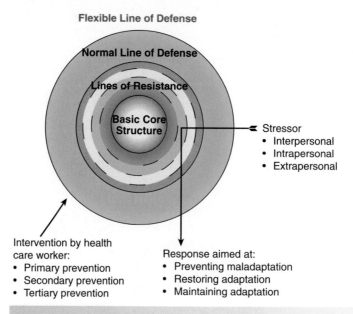

Flexible Line of Defense

Normal Line of Defense

Lines of Resistance

Basic Core Structure

≽ Stressor
- Interpersonal
- Intrapersonal
- Extrapersonal

Intervention by health care worker:
- Primary prevention
- Secondary prevention
- Tertiary prevention

Response aimed at:
- Preventing maladaptation
- Restoring adaptation
- Maintaining adaptation

FIGURE 8-8

Neuman systems model. *(From Pearson A, Vaughan B, Fitzgerald M:* Nursing models for practice, *ed 3, Edinburgh, 2005, Butterworth & Heineman, p 145.)*

visualization, or it can be maladaptive (e.g., someone with a type of psychosis, such as schizophrenia) (Figure 8-8).

Imogene King—Goal Attainment Model. The theme of Imogene King's theory is interaction and goal attainment. The person interacts with the environment, and health is a dynamic state of well-being. The nurse interacts with the patient to set mutually agreed-upon goals for the patient's health. The nurse and the patient are recognized as each bringing his or her own set of knowledge, values, and skills to the interaction. King also emphasizes that the nurse and patient usually first come together as strangers and through the interactions, both verbal and nonverbal, develop a relationship, based on their perceptions (Alligood & Marriner Tomey, 2010). King's nursing process looks very similar to what nurses are already familiar with: assessment, diagnosis, plan, intervention, and evaluation. King would like her model to be used as the basis of the U.S. health care system and would like the entry of a person into the health care system to be via nursing assessment! (King, 2002) (Figure 8-9)

Jean Watson—Theory of Human Caring. Jean Watson's theory is all about caring—finally, a theory about caring. Watson sees the person as a mind-body-soul connection. Health is unity and harmony within the mind, body, and soul. The nurse comes in contact with the person in a "caring occasion" or "caring moment" and promotes restoration of a sense of inner harmony through Watson's 10 "carative" factors. Caring to Watson is a moral idea, rather than an interpersonal technique (Alligood & Marriner Tomey, 2010).

Here are Watson's 10 carative factors (see what nursing interventions you can identify with each one):

1. The formation of a humanistic-altruistic system of values
2. The instillation of faith-hope

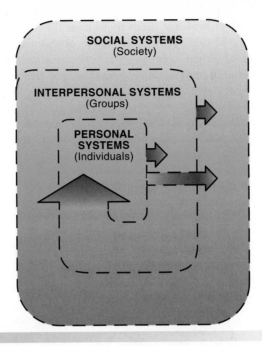

FIGURE 8-9

King's goal attainment model for nursing. *(From Pearson A, Vaughan B, Fitzgerald M:* Nursing models for practice, *ed 3, Edinburgh, 2005, Butterworth & Heineman, p 162.)*

3. The cultivation of sensitivity to one's self and to others
4. The development of a helping-trust relationship
5. The promotion and acceptance of the expression of positive and negative feelings
6. The systematic use of the scientific problem solving methods for decision making
7. The promotion of interpersonal teaching-learning
8. The provision for a supportive, protective, and corrective mental, physical, sociocultural, and spiritual environment
9. Assistance with the gratification of human needs
10. The allowance for existential-phenomenological forces (Alligood, 2010; Wills, 2011)

Madeleine Leininger—Culture Care Theory. Madeleine Leininger's overall theme is culture. Leininger is the "Margaret Mead of the health field" and has traveled widely and studied many cultures. She sees the person as caring and capable of being concerned with the welfare of others. Nursing is a transcultural caring discipline and profession. Nurses need to be mindful of folk practices or generic health care practices. (Think of health care practices that were practiced when you were a child that would be considered folk or generic health care practices—e.g., Vick's VapoRub applied to your chest for a cold; not drinking hot or cold beverages, depending on the illness; not sitting too close to the TV set because it was "bad" for your eyes.) The nurse needs to be aware of and use culture care data that are influenced by religion, kinship, language, technology, economics, education (both formal and informal), cultural values and beliefs, and the physical (or ecological) environment. Leininger believes that there can be no curing without caring. Health is culturally defined (Alligood & Marriner Tomey, 2010).

The health care professional needs to examine the prescribed health care requirements and decide if there can be culture care preservation or maintenance (where the relevant care values can be retained), or if there needs to be culture care accommodation or negotiation (where the cultural practices need to be adapted or negotiated to return the patient to health), or if culture care repatterning or restructuring is required (where the patient needs to change or significantly alter culturally based health practices to promote good health). Leininger's theory can be summarized in her Sunrise Model. The upper half of the model is for collecting data, and the lower half is for decision-making (Alligood & Tomey, 2010, p. 466) (Figure 8-10).

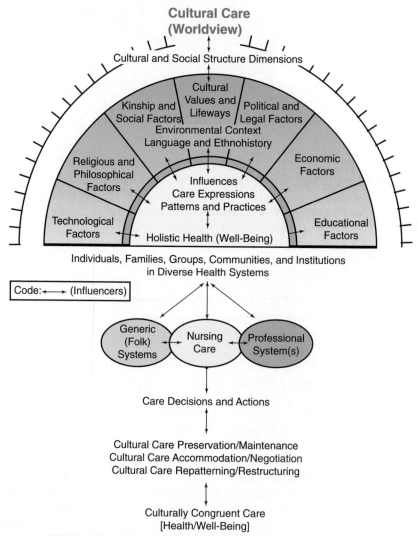

FIGURE 8-10

Leininger's sunrise model. *(From Alligood MR & Marriner-Tomey A: Nursing theory: utilization and application, ed 4, St. Louis, 2010, Mosby, p 415.)*

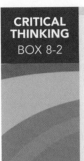

In reviewing the theories, which one would best fit in your clinical practice?
  Which theory most appeals to you and why?
  Which theory/theories would fit best with the following patient settings and why?
- Preop patient
- Labor patient
- Psychiatric patient
- Nursing curriculum
- Managing a nursing unit
- Organizing an internal medicine clinic
- Organizing a computer generated acuity form
- Pediatric patients
- Home health
- Hospice care
- Long-term care facility
- Rehabilitative therapy

CONCLUSION

In reviewing these nursing theories, you may find that some especially appeal to you and others do not. That is okay. What is important is to understand that nursing theories are a rich part of our nursing history and that they are a way to organize, deliver, evaluate, and ultimately improve the care we provide (Critical Thinking Box 8-2).

BIBLIOGRAPHY

Alligood MR, Marriner Tomey A: *Nursing theorists and their work*, ed 7, St. Louis, 2010, Mosby.

Alligood MR: *Nursing theory: utilization and application*, ed 4, St. Louis, 2010, Mosby.

Dunphy LH: Florence Nightingale caring actualized: a legacy for nursing. In Parker ME, editor: *Nursing theories and nursing practice*, Philadelphia, 2002, FA Davis, pp 31-53.

Ellis R: Characteristics of significant theories. In Nicoll LH, editor: *Perspectives on nursing theory*, Philadelphia, 1997, Lippincott, pp 373-381.

Foster PC, Bennett AM, Dorothea E. Orem. In University of Phoenix College of Health Sciences and Nursing, editor: *Theoretical foundations of nursing practice*, Boston, 2003, Pearson Custom Publishing, pp 137-168.

George JB: *Nursing theories: the base for professional nursing practice*, ed 4, Norwalk, Conn, 1995, Appleton & Lange.

George J: Betty Neuman. In University of Phoenix College of Health Sciences and Nursing, editor: *Theoretical foundations of nursing practice*, Boston, 2003a, Pearson Custom Publishing, pp 243-267.

George J, Madeleine M: Leininger. In University of Phoenix College of Health Sciences and Nursing, editor: *Theoretical foundations of nursing practice*, Boston, 2003b, Pearson Custom Publishing, pp 289-303.

Hickman JS: An introduction to nursing theory. In University of Phoenix College of Health Sciences and Nursing, editor: *Theoretical foundations of nursing practice*, Boston, 2003, Pearson Custom Publishing, pp 15-28.

Holaday B: Dorothy Johnson: behavioral system models of nursing. In Parker ME, editor: *Nursing theories and nursing practice*, Philadelphia, 2002, FA Davis, pp 83-101.

Hood L: *Leddy and Pepper's Conceptual bases of professional nursing*, ed 7, Philadelphia, 2009, Lippincott.

King I, Imogene M: King: theory of goal attainment. In Parker ME, editor: *Nursing theories and nursing practice*, Philadelphia, 2002, FA Davis, pp 273-286.

McEwen M: Overview of theory in nursing. In McEwen M, Wills EM, editors: *Theoretical basis for nursing*, ed 3, Philadelphia, 2011, Lippincott, pp 21–45.

Muth Quillen S: Rogers' model: science of unitary persons. In University of Phoenix College of Health Sciences and Nursing, editor: *Theoretical foundations of nursing practice*, Boston, 2003, Pearson Custom Publishing, pp 309-323.

Tiedeman ME: Roy's adaptation model. In Fitzpatrick JJ, Whall AL, editors: *Conceptual models of nursing: analysis and application*, Upper Saddle River, NJ, 2005, Prentice Hall, pp 146-176.

Wills E: Grand nursing theories based on interactive process. In McEwen M, Wills EM, editors: *Theoretical basis for nursing*, Philadelphia, 2011, Lippincott, pp 148-182.

Additional resources are available online at *http://evolve.elsevier.com/Zerwekh/nsgtoday/*.

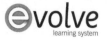

CHAPTER 9

Image of Nursing: Influences of the Present

Margi Schultz, PhD, RN, CNE, PLNC

> *The past is not simply the past, but a prism through which the subject filters his own changing self-image.*
> —DORIS KEARNS GOODWIN

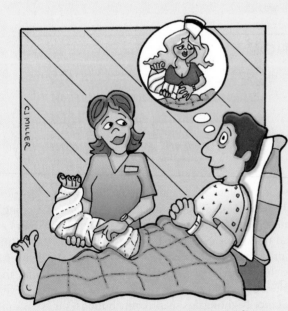

Nursing image—how is nursing perceived?

After completing this chapter, you should be able to:

- Discuss the effect of image on the public perception of nursing

- Describe different sociological models that characterize "professionalism."

- Apply Pavalko's characteristics as a framework to describe modern-day nursing practice.

- Identify the role that nursing organizations have in professional practice.

- Describe the role of credentialing and certification in professional practice.

Thanks to the previous author of the chapter—Linda Stevenson, PhD, RN, FNP.

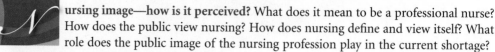

ursing image—how is it perceived? What does it mean to be a professional nurse? How does the public view nursing? How does nursing define and view itself? What role does the public image of the nursing profession play in the current shortage? Historically, nurses have struggled to define the image of nursing and the professional role of the nurse. There are many different views and opinions, but nurses are definitely gaining ground when it comes to defining the profession of nursing. The annual Gallup survey for professions noted that for honesty and ethical standards nursing has been rated at the top of the list for the past several years. Eighty three percent of the American public rate the standards held by nurses as either high or very high (Saad, 2008). The image of nursing is evolving and changing with nursing being promoted as an intellectual, autonomous profession that demands a high level of commitment, focus, and a dedication to continued education and scholarly activity.

Modern-day nursing has many dimensions, one of which includes the debate surrounding its identification as a profession. One ongoing challenge in nursing is to diligently foster and enhance the public image and the self-image of the nurse. In this chapter, the development of nursing into a profession is discussed, and the present and future dimensions of nursing's "image" are explored. Historical knowledge about our "rites of passage" gives us an appreciation of where nursing is today as a profession and what the future of nursing may hold for the recent graduate in this complex and evolving health care world.

PROFESSIONAL IMAGE OF NURSING

What Do We Mean by the "Image" of Nursing?

> *Santa Filomena*
> *Lo! in that hour of misery*
> *A lady with a lamp I see*
> *Pass through the glimmering gloom,*
> *And flit from room to room.*
> —Longfellow, 1857

Nursing has been identified as an "emerging profession" for at least 150 years. The historical context of nursing's image is often traced back to Florence Nightingale, the "founder of nursing." Florence Nightingale is recognized as a nurse, statistician, and writer who became known for her groundbreaking work during the Crimean War. Nurse Nightingale was also called the "Lady with the Lamp," as she was reported to have made rounds on her patients at night by the light of a lantern. International Nurse's Day is celebrated each year on her birthday, May 12, and the Nightingale Pledge is still solemnly repeated by new nursing graduates around the world. Even though much has been written about Florence Nightingale's many contributions, she is undeniably remembered as the pioneer of nursing education (Bostridge, 2008).

Who are today's role models for nursing? What qualities should a nursing role model exemplify? Are these qualities different from 10 years ago? 25 years ago?

The image of professional nursing continues to evolve and is significantly affected by the media, women's issues and roles, and a high-technology health care environment. How nursing views itself in the evolution of the profession and how actively nurses are involved in the definition process will continue to determine the image and role of nursing in the future.

Nurses are professionals who are science driven, technically skilled, and caring (Dukes, 2003). Dombeck (2003) noted that "the portrayal of nurses generally parallels the portrayal of women in the media" (p 351). That image of nursing has continued to demonstrate a general lack of knowledge regarding the role of professional nurses (Ward et al, 2003). As more men enter the profession and there is a push to increase minorities in nursing, will the image of nursing change (Critical Thinking Box 9-1)?

Nurses should be thought of as autonomous and competent decision makers within their nursing practice areas. Throughout the 1990s, a nationwide advertising campaign supported by the National Commission on Nursing Implementation Project produced radio and television ads that said, "If caring were enough, anyone could be a nurse." Nurses of America, an advocate organization sponsored by the National League for Nursing (NLN), implemented a very successful program directed toward improving the image of nursing as depicted on television, on radio, in print, and on lecture circuits. Consultants were contracted to work with executives, politicians, and celebrities on presenting nursing in a positive manner. This approach reinforced the image of the modern-day professional nurse as having critical thinking, decision-making, and problem-solving skills.

In a 2002 study, Turow and Gans found that on U.S. television programs, it was common for only physicians to be heard when health care policy was discussed; nurses and other health care team members were noticeably absent. The American Academy of Nursing (*www.aannet.org*, 2008) through the *Raise the Voice campaign* has brought nursing policy innovators to the forefront of health care policy debates. A concentrated effort by individuals and organizations is raising awareness of what nurses do and heightening the image and voice of nursing as a profession. As noted by Groves (2007), accurate portrayals of nurses as professional members of the healthcare team are rare, but it takes time to change perceptions. The continued trend of building

---

CRITICAL THINKING BOX 9-1

THINK QUICK!

Picture in your mind your image of a nurse—did you just think of a female, tidy hair, professional looking scrubs, serviceable white shoes, stethoscope around the neck, determined look in the eyes, energetic walk, clipboard in hand? Or … did you just envision a male nurse with many of those same attributes? The image of nursing is changing and many media depictions now include men as nurses. There have always been men in nursing, but with the increasing respect for the profession, and the high-touch, high-technicality in the field of nursing, more men than ever are looking to become nurses. Indeed, many men who enter nursing are interested in fighting the same stereotypes that woman have battled over the years. The term "male nurse" is considered an unnecessary distinction, much like saying a "female physician"—the gender bias is simply not a critical element (Wilson, 2009). The first step in turning the tide of thought about gender in nursing is for members of the profession to alter their own perceptions.

a positive, intelligent, competent, and professional image of nursing must continue. Nurses who are new to the profession need to be aware of the extraordinary challenges and opportunities that they will face. It is equally important for nurses to improve the self-image of the professional nurse. The behaviors and ethics displayed by nurses on a day-to-day basis can do much to elevate the present and shape the future image of nursing (Cohen & Bartholomew, 2008).

Nursing associations are working together to promote a positive image and deal with nursing shortage issues. Nurses for a Healthier Tomorrow, an alliance of 37 nursing organizations, has launched a national media campaign that demonstrates, through print and broadcast media, the many opportunities for the career of nursing. One tangible example of this effort is the website *www.nursesource.org.* Sigma Theta Tau International, the International honor society for nursing, is the coordinator of Nurses for a Healthier Tomorrow. Check out their website at *www.nursingsociety.org.* The American Nurses Association published a flyer titled *Every Patient Deserves a Nurse*, along with other promotional materials for the lay public. The promotional message of these materials reinforces the positive image of nurses as patient advocates and critical resources both to patients and families, while also emphasizing the right of people to a safe health care environment.

In 2002, the Johnson and Johnson Company developed a nationwide campaign to support the nursing profession. This program, titled "The Campaign for Nursing's Future," was developed along with health care leaders and nursing organizations such as the National Student Nurse's Association (NSNA), the American Nurse's Association (ANA), the American Organization for Nurse Executives (AONE), the National League for Nursing, and Sigma Theta Tau. The goal of this program is to increase the number of young adults entering nursing through raising the visibility of nurses of varied races, gender, and roles. The website for the campaign can be found at *www.discovernursing.com.*

The negative images of nursing, those of the "naughty nurse" or the "Nurse Ratchet" that are depicted in the media are still prevalent, but these erroneous portrayals do offer professional nurses the opportunity to educate the public in what nurses truly do. Nursing is not the only profession that struggles with a skewed media image. Some of these erroneous depictions may be related to the largely female population who seek these professions; consider the sexual media images that are often illustrated by flight attendants, massage therapists, or secretaries (*www.truthaboutnursing.org*, 2009). Other occupations that suffer from poor media portrayals include the "mad scientist" role (chemist or researcher), construction worker (often a sexual male image), or consider the negative images that both female and male lawyers are often faced with! Devaluation of the nursing profession by demeaning or comical images only extend the nursing shortage and further discourage talented people from entering the nursing profession. It is up to each individual to continue to display professional role modeling and provide public education on what nurses really do to empower the professional image of nursing (Cohen & Bartholomew, 2008).

How can nurses change the image of nursing? How can the image of nursing become more congruent with the actual role the nurse plays in today's health care? Nurses outnumber all other professions in health care. Mee (2006) suggests that nurses can promote the professional image of nursing by the following:

Patient Interactions. One by One. During the first 60 seconds that a patient sees the nurse, a lasting impression may be formed. Take a moment before meeting a new patient and portray confidence in your role and a respect for the patient from the beginning. Many health care institutions require nurses to wear nursing uniforms in a distinct color that separates them from nurse assistants and respiratory therapists.

Personal Interaction with the Public. Have a quick response ready in case someone asks about nursing. Present nursing in a positive image and relate what an important role nurses have in society as health care providers.

Public Speaking and Community Activities. Consider speaking at or visiting schools on Career Day. You don't have to be an expert at public speaking to discuss the role of the nurse with local community groups. A brief, interactive presentation at an elementary or high school can stimulate interest in nursing early—for both male and female students!

Participation in Political Activities. Increase the positive visibility of nurses through politics by becoming actively involved as a nurse lobbyist. Be aware of the current health care issues on the community, state, and national level. Get to know the elected officials and talk to them about the role of the nurse. This may be a valuable opportunity to present nursing in a very positive manner. Remember that most elected officials do not understand the role nurses play in health care (Mee, 2006).

Creating a professional image incorporates effective communication skills, positive attitude, and professional appearance. When you first meet patients, family members, or potential employers, your professional appearance has an impact on how they perceive you as a nurse. Dress appropriately and be prepared to ask and answer questions that reflect a confident, positive image (Larson, 2006).

The image of nursing continues to evolve as the many roles of nurses are portrayed through the media in the restructuring of health care environments and in a variety of settings, from emergency rooms to war zones. Studies continue to verify that competent nursing care affects mortality rates in critical care patients, and the future for many nursing jobs lies in the expanding role of nursing into emergency and disaster preparedness and integration of technology and informatics into practice settings (Health Resources and Services Administration [HRSA], 2009). The role and image of the nurse will continue to change as the many facets of health care delivery evolve during this century. The current nursing shortage will play a significant role in the creation of the future image and role of the nurse. How will nurses respond to these changes? How will you present yourself as a professional?

What Constitutes a Profession?

There are many ways to describe a "professional." What meaning does the word have for you as a graduate professional nurse? Controversy over the definition of the term *professional* as it relates to nursing is not a new issue. Strauss (1966), a noted sociologist, found the word *professional* used in reference to nursing in a magazine article published in 1892 titled "Nursing, a New Profession for Women." The nurses of the 20th and 21st centuries owe a great deal to Isabel Adams Hampton (later Isabel Hampton Robb) for her visionary focus in the late 1800s. She was an outstanding advocate for the professionalization of nursing. In the textbook *Nursing Ethics* (1901), she wrote:

> The trained nurse, then, is no longer to be regarded as a better trained, more useful, higher class servant, but as one who has knowledge and is worthy of respect, consideration, and due recompense ... She is also essentially an instructor; part of her duties have to do with the prevention of disease and sickness, as well as the relief of suffering humanity ... These are some of the essentials in nursing by which it has

become to be regarded as a profession, but there still remains much to be desired, much to work for, in order to add to its dignity and usefulness.

In Caplow's classic work from the early 1950s, *The Sociology of Work,* several steps in the process of "becoming professional" were defined further, and the value of forming an association that defined a special membership was addressed. Caplow suggested that making a name change to clarify an area of work or practice would subsequently produce a new role. With the creation of this new role, the group would then establish a code of ethics and legal components for licensure to practice and educational control of the profession (Caplow, 1954). This process of becoming professional was taking place in nursing in 1897 with the establishment of the ANA. Other aspects of professionalization were also beginning to develop. For example, the *Code for Nurses* was suggested as early as 1926, although it was not written or published by the ANA until the early 1950s. Revisions were made in 1956, 1960, and 1976, with changes made in 1985 that included interpretative statements. In the summer of 2001 at the ANA convention, delegates again updated the code and changed the name to the *Code of Ethics for Nurses with Interpretive Statements (www.ana.org/ethics/ecode.htm).*

Almost 20 years after Caplow's work, Pavalko (1971) described eight dimensions of a profession. Pavalko's dimensions of a profession and their specific application to nursing are examined in more detail later in this chapter. Nursing continues to apply these dimensions to support nursing's move away from the occupational focus to a professional focus. Is nursing a profession or semiprofession?

By responding to the questions in Critical Thinking Box 9-2 (which presents Levenstein's model, a fourth model of professionalism), you will identify common themes in describing a profession. What are your thoughts about the nursing profession in light of these criteria?

Others have written about professions and their development, but these sociological models present some logical characteristics for you to use to examine professionalism. According to Henshaw, a noted nursing leader and researcher, a profession includes "self-regulation and autonomy with ultimate loyalty and accountability to the professional group" (cited in Talotta, 1990). Nursing is a dynamic profession and continues to strive to enhance a professional image—which leads us to the next question.

Is Nursing a Profession?

Eunice Cole, a past president of the ANA, described nursing as a dynamic profession that has established a code of ethics and standards of practice, education, service, and research components. The standards for both the professional and practical dimensions of nursing are continually reviewed and updated. Nurses, strong in numbers but splintered professionally in many ways, represent the largest group of health care providers in the United States. There are more than 3 million registered nurses in the workforce with an average age of all licensed RNs increased to 47 years in 2008 from 46.8 years in 2004, which demonstrates a stabilizing of age. Although the number of RNs younger than 40 dropped steadily between 1980 and 2004, there was an increase in 2008 and they now comprise 29.5% of all RNs. Most RNs are actively practicing nursing (84.8%—highest in the history of the survey) and most are working full time (63.2% vs. 58.4% in 2004—the first increase since 1996). The majority of nurses (45.4%) complete their initial education preparation at the associate degree level. A little more than one-third (33.7%) have a

LEVENSTEIN'S CHARACTERISTICS OF A PROFESSION

What do you think about ...
- The element of altruism
  How do you define caring in your clinical practice?
- Code of ethics
  Are you familiar with the ANA Code of Ethics?
- Collaboration with groups and individuals for the benefit of the patient
  What other groups do you work with in your clinical setting that affect the health needs of the patient and family?
- Colleagueship demonstrated by:
  An organization for licensing
  - What is the role of the State Board of Nursing in your state?
  A group that helps ensure quality
  - Are you aware of the role of national nursing organizations that accredit nursing programs?
  - There are two national nursing organizations that accredit nursing programs; do you know what they are?
  Peer evaluations of practitioners
  - What is the role of job evaluations in terms of professional growth?
- Accountability for conduct and responsibility for practice decisions
  Who monitors professional conduct issues from a legal and ethical point of view? Does shared governance reflect more control of one's nursing practice?
- Strong research program
  Are you aware that a national center for nursing research is now operating in Washington, DC?

bachelor's degree, up from 31% in 2004, noting a trend of increasing education. There was significant growth (46.9% increase since 2000) in the numbers of RNs with a master's or doctoral degree in nursing or a related field (HRSA, 2010).

Examine the issues that challenge nursing as a profession by using Pavalko's eight dimensions to describe a profession.

1. **A Profession Has Relevance to Social Values.** Does nursing exist to serve self or others? Nursing historically had its roots in true altruism with lifelong service to others. As nurses, we focus not only on the treatment component of patient care, but also on wellness and health promotion issues, as a part of our nursing practice. The goal is to shift the focus of health care so that primary prevention becomes more valued. As this shift occurs, nurses will become increasingly important because of their ability to be teachers of health promotion activities and managers of wellness, activities that have an impact on social values.

2. **A Profession Has a Training or Educational Period.** According to Florence Nightingale, a nurse's education should involve not only a theory component, but also a practice component. An educational process for any professional is critical because it transmits the knowledge base of the profession and, through research and other scholarly endeavors, advances the practice of the profession. The diversity of educational programs for nurses has stimulated

debate regarding the entry practice level for registered nurses. Some questions surrounding the issues include the following:

- What is the future of associate degree nursing programs? Diploma or hospital-based nursing programs?
- How critical is it to complete a 4-year bachelor of science in nursing (BSN) program to handle the challenges of the health care environment, complex patient-family needs, and the expanding community-based settings for clinical work?
- Will the doctor of nursing degree that was pioneered at Case Western University become the minimum background for entry into the profession? Will the practice doctorate in nursing (DNP) degree clarify or confuse advanced-practice roles in nursing?

These questions have been debated since the publication in 1965 of an ANA position paper that charged the profession with the goal of establishing nursing education at the baccalaureate level within 25 years. Almost 40 years have passed since then, and the issue continues to challenge the profession. The inability of nursing organizations and educational systems at all levels to come to agreement on this issue has affected the solidarity of the profession.

In the mid-1990s, some states (e.g., Maine and Idaho) engaged in debate over regulatory issues concerning the BSN as the entry credential. Beyond this generic-degree controversy are the issues associated with specialization: What degree should serve as the entry level into advanced nursing practice—the master of science (MSN) degree, a doctorate (PhD) degree, or the DNP? This issue was not resolved in the 20th century. Will the 21st century bring a resolution?

3. Elements of Self-Motivation Address the Way in Which the Profession Serves the Patient or Family and Larger Social System. In 1990, the Tri-Council of Nursing, along with the American Association of Colleges of Nursing, designed a "Nursing Agenda for Health Care Reform" to collectively express the views of nurses concerning health care. Endorsed by 39 major specialty nursing organizations, along with the ANA and the NLN, the Tri-Council emphasized a restructured health care system that would provide universal access to health care, direct health care expenditures toward primary care, and reduce costs.

Political activity is a way of translating social values into action. Nursing faces special challenges when, for example, nurses must go on strike for better pay and benefits or demonstrate a united front to gain federal funding rather than continuing a passive role in such issues. It is time for the nursing profession to define a new narrative that reflects how much the profession has changed, how critical nursing skills are to today's patient care, how the profession has stayed abreast of medical and technological innovation, and what nursing is going to look like in the future (Kaplan, 2005).

4. A Profession Has a Code of Ethics. Nursing, like other professions, has ethical dimensions. As noted earlier in the chapter, the nursing *Code of Ethics* published by the ANA dates to the 1950s. Key points of the code are provided in Box 9-1. The *Code of Ethics* is discussed in more detail in Chapter 19.

5. A Professional Has a Commitment to Lifelong Work. By this statement, Pavalko means that a professional sees his or her career as more than just a stepping-stone to another area of work or as an intermittent job. Government data show that 83% of the nearly 2.9 million registered nurses work in health care (HRSA, 2004). Nursing constitutes the largest health care occupation, and more jobs are expected for registered nurses than for any other occupation. This faster-than-average growth is being driven by technological advances. Thus, nursing as a career

BOX 9-1	Code of Ethics for Nurses

The ANA House of Delegates approved these nine provisions of the new Code of Ethics for Nurses at its June 30, 2001, meeting in Washington, DC. In July 2001 the Congress of Nursing Practice and Economics voted to accept the new language of the interpretive statements, resulting in a fully approved revised Code of Ethics for Nurses with Interpretive Statements, as follows:

1. The nurse, in all professional relationships, practices with compassion and respect for the inherent dignity, worth, and uniqueness of every individual, unrestricted by considerations of social or economic status, personal attributes, or the nature of health problems.
2. The nurse's primary commitment is to the patient, whether an individual, family, group, or community.
3. The nurse promotes, advocates for, and strives to protect the health, safety, and rights of the patient.
4. The nurse is responsible and accountable for individual nursing practice and determines the appropriate delegation of tasks consistent with the obligation to provide optimum patient care.
5. The nurse owes the same duties to self as to others, including the responsibility to preserve integrity and safety, to maintain competence, and to continue personal and professional growth.
6. The nurse participates in establishing, maintaining, and improving health care environments and conditions of employment conducive to the provision of quality health care and consistent with the values of the profession through individual and collective action.
7. The nurse participates in the advancement of the profession through contributions to practice, education, administration, and knowledge development.
8. The nurse collaborates with other health professionals and the public in promoting community, national, and international efforts to meet health needs.
9. The profession of nursing, as represented by associations and their members, is responsible for articulating nursing values, for maintaining the integrity of the profession and its practice, and for shaping social policy.

Reprinted with permission from American Nurses Association: *Code of ethics for nurses with interpretive statements.* Copyright 2001, *nursebooks.org*, Silver Spring, Md.

has great potential for financial rewards, involvement in a variety of professional endeavors, several different areas of practice, and a commitment to lifelong work.

6. Members Control Their Profession. Nurses are not entirely autonomous. Although nurses have the challenge to ensure that members of the profession honor the trust given by society, they also work under professional and legislative control. Among these controls, are the 50 state boards of nursing, which regulate the scope of nursing practice within each state and professional practice standards that are supported both at local and national levels. In 1973, the ANA wrote the first *Standards of Nursing Practice* and since then has had a leadership role in the development of general and many specialty nursing practice standards. Moreover, specialty organizations maintain standards for certification.

Another publication by the ANA, the *Standards of Clinical Nursing Practice* (2003), discusses the use of nursing process and professional practice standards. The development of professional practice standards indicates to the larger social system that nursing can define and control its quality of practice. These national standards are incorporated into institutional standards to help guide nursing practice. Most recent publications by the ANA can be found on their website (*www.nursingworld.org*). The issue at hand, however, is that these professional practice standards authorize nurses to practice nursing. Nurses are expected to take responsibility for their own actions and not just follow orders without thinking critically.

Nurses practice in varied settings, and the advanced practice nurse functions in a more autonomous professional role, such as the nurse-midwife, psychiatric clinical specialist, nurse practitioner, or certified nurse educator. In 1992, there were 100,000 advanced practice nurses in the United States. Fifty percent of RNs have achieved a baccalaureate or higher degree in nursing or a nursing-related field in 2008, compared to 27.5% in 1980 (HRSA, 2010). These changes represent the largest-growing segment of specialty nursing practice. Advancing one's education level is often paired with increased autonomy.

Most nurses in the United States work within a structured setting; three out of five jobs are in hospital, inpatient, or outpatient settings. Trends in those settings are slowly changing to give nurses a stronger voice. For example, nursing care delivery systems that have case management and shared governance reflect more progressive and autonomous environments (see Chapter 15). Nursing can control its scope of practice through professional organizations and published documents, along with an active voice in regulatory bodies, such as state boards of nursing.

7. A Profession Has a Theoretical Framework on Which Professional Practice Is Based. Nursing continues to be based in the sciences and humanities, but nursing theory is evolving. It was not until the 1950s that nursing theory was "born." In 1952, Dr. Hildegard Peplau published a nursing model that described the importance of the "therapeutic relationship" in health and wellness. Since then, other nursing theorists such as Martha Rogers, Sister Callista Roy, Dorothea Orem, and Betty Neuman have contributed to our evolving theory-based nursing science.

8. Members of a Profession Have a Common Identity and a Distinctive Sub-culture. The outward image of nursing has changed remarkably within the past 50 years. Nurses were once identified by how they looked rather than by what they did. The nursing cap and pin reflected the nurse's school and educational background. The modern-day trend emphasizes that it is not what is worn but what is done that reflects one's role in the nursing profession. The struggle to shift out of rigid dress codes was a major issue in the 1960s. Clothing and other symbols identify a subculture, and changes in that identification process occur slowly. What kind of an image do you want to project as a professional nurse (Critical Thinking Box 9-3)?

CRITICAL THINKING BOX 9-3

WHAT DO YOU THINK?

WHAT KIND OF IMAGE DO YOU WANT TO PROJECT AS A "PROFESSIONAL?"

- Should nurses wear visible body jewelry or tattoos?
- What do professionals call each other in the clinical setting?
- Do you wear your name badge with proper credentials? Are the doctors on your unit called by their first or last names? How are you addressed in a professional setting?
- Are your credentials visible to indicate additional degrees or certifications?
- Are the nurses on your unit certified in their specialty area? Is this recognized by your facility?
- What do your peers wear?
- Do you think scrubs look professional?
- Can a nurse wearing cartoon character scrubs be taken seriously? Why? Why not?
- Should nurses leave the hospital in their scrubs and go run errands?
- What other professions are associated with a "uniform?"

Nursing colleagues reflect attitudes and values about the profession. Many schools of nursing have alumni associations, student nurse associations, and nursing honor societies or clubs on campus. These groups provide social interaction during the nursing education years and are great ways to network later in one's career. Sigma Theta Tau International sponsors the Chiron Mentoring program to assist individual nurses to achieve their professional goals related to leadership, scholarship, and evidenced-based nursing *(www.nursingsociety.org/programs/ chiron.html)*. Belonging to a professional organization (such as the ANA) or a specialty organization helps professional nurses maintain certifications and network with peers, and it enhances collegiality.

> "Nurses should choose optimism, making positive strides each day to celebrate who they are and the differences they make. Just a nurse—no, never."—Melissa Fitzpatrick, 2001

When will the conflicts in educational preparation be resolved? How will we use further refinement and application of nursing theories in our clinical practice? What can nurses do to have more control of nursing practice regardless of the clinical setting? Will there be an increase in the percentage of people who are choosing nursing as a career? What are the forces that will help nursing "come together" and become not only a true profession but the largest and most powerful of all the health care professional groups? (Remember, there is always strength in numbers.)

NURSING ORGANIZATIONS

What Should I Know About Professional Organizations?

Nursing organizations have significant roles in empowering nurses in their emerging professionalism (Figure 9-1). Yet many nurses do not belong to a national organization such as the ANA or to their state affiliate organization, or even to specialty-focused groups such as the American Association of Critical-Care Nurses (AACN) or the National Black Nurses Association (NBNA). Of the 3.1 million registered nurses, membership in the constituent associations in ANA represents less than half of the nurses (ANA, 2007; HRSA, 2010). During the past few years, researchers have examined the issue of belonging to a professional organization, with no conclusive findings regarding why or how nurses choose nursing organizations. Some have suggested that organizations representing nursing as a whole, such as the ANA and the NLN, do not meet the needs of the individual nurse practicing in today's changing health care environment.

Affiliation with a nursing organization to facilitate networking with colleagues is valuable and meaningful. As a recent graduate, you will need to examine your options for joining a professional group and then demonstrate your professional commitment by active involvement. The question should be "Which ones should I join?" rather than "Should I even join an organization?" (Box 9-2). In the next section, various organizations are reviewed, with some historical notes to assist you in making the best choice as you begin your nursing career. A more complete directory of nursing organizations can be found on the Evolve Resource website (also see Critical Thinking Box 9-4).

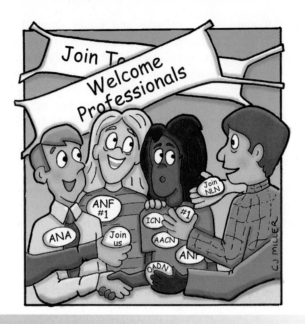

FIGURE 9-1

There is a nursing organization to fit your needs.

BOX 9-2	The Benefits of Belonging to Your Professional Organization

- Representation and influence in the legislature
- Continuing education
- Develop leadership skills
- Resources
- Personal benefits
- Networking
- Having a voice in the future of nursing

CRITICAL THINKING
BOX 9-4

WHAT DO YOU THINK?

- How are nurses in your organization socialized?
- Is there an informal initiation process?
- Is there a formal orientation process?
- How can new nurses be mentored?

What Organizations Are Available to the Recent Graduate?

A few of these key professional organizations for individual and organizational membership are described in the next section in alphabetical order. Many of these organizations publish a newsletter or professional journal, and most have websites. Individual membership in your professional nursing organization and a specialty organization is a great way to maintain current knowledge about changes in your career field (see Box 9-2).

American Nurses Association. The ANA is identified as the professional association for registered nurses. It was through the early efforts of Isabel Hampton Robb and others that the Nurses Associated Alumnae of the United States and Canada was formed. At the World's Fair in 1890, a group of 15 nursing leaders began discussions about forming a professional association. Six years later, alumnae from the training schools organized the professional association now known as the ANA. Canadian members split from the original group in 1911 and formed their own professional association. The organizational structure of the ANA has undergone many changes over the years.

Currently, when an individual joins the ANA, he or she joins the national organization along with the constituent associations at the state and local level. This method geographically groups smaller clusters of members together according to their practice interests. According to the ANA website, the current membership is almost 180,000 individual registered nurses (ANA, FAQ—Membership, 2010).

In 1974, an amendment to the Taft-Hartley Act allowed professional nursing organizations to be considered labor unions. United American Nurses is the collective bargaining organization representing the ANA. After this significant event, some nursing administrators and managers withdrew their memberships in ANA because of the potential conflict of interest between professional affiliation and the workplace. However, this change generated the development of other major nursing organizations: the Center for the American Nurse (CAN) and the American Association of Nurse Executives (AONE).

The ANA has been at the forefront of policy issues and represents nursing in legislative activities. The cabinets and councils of the ANA have provided standards of practice for both the generalist and the specialist. The 1988 *Social Policy Statement* document defined nursing practice at both the generalist and specialist levels; this is echoed in the current 2010 *Social Policy Statement*. The certifying organization of the ANA is the American Nurses Credentialing Center (ANCC), which has certified more than 250,000 RNs in different practice areas at both the generalist and specialist levels, along with over 75,000 advanced practice nurses (ANCC, 2007). The ANCC, a subsidiary of the ANA since 1991, identifies its mission as improving nursing practice and promoting quality health care service through several types of credentialing programs. The ANCC has created a modular approach to certification that enables the nurse to be recognized for multiple areas of expertise, not simply for competency in a core clinical specialty. There are 26 generalist care clinical specialties or advanced practice care areas. As a result of their "open door 2000" program, all qualified registered nurses, regardless of their educational preparation, can become certified as generalists in any of the following specialty areas: gerontology, medical-surgical, pediatrics, perinatal, and psychiatric-mental health nursing.

In addition to certifying individual nurses, the organization also accredits educational providers (i.e., organizations that issue continuing education credits for professional programs), recognizes excellence in Magnet nursing services through the ANCC Magnet Recognition Program®, and educates the public about credentialing and professional nursing. This organization is electronically linked on the home page of the ANA *(www.nursingworld.org)*.

American Nurses Foundation and the American Academy of Nursing. Two other organizations associated with the ANA are the American Nurses Foundation, founded in 1955, and the American Academy of Nursing (AAN), founded in 1973. Briefly described, these organizations serve special purposes in support of research and recognition of nursing colleagues. The American Nurses Foundation was established as a tax-exempt corporation to receive money for nursing research. With the establishment of the National Nursing Research Institute, the focus has changed to one of support in the areas of policy making and research or educational activities. The AAN has a membership of more than 1,500 nursing leaders and was established as an honorary association for nurses who have made significant contributions to the nursing profession. When a nurse is elected to the AAN, she or he is called a Fellow, and the credential following the nurse's name is FAAN. You may have had instructors who were faculty in the American Academy of Nursing, or you may be working with a nurse who is an FAAN. These nurses can provide valuable mentorship for the new graduate. The official publication of this organization is *Nursing Outlook*.

International Council of Nurses. The International Council of Nurses (ICN), established in 1899, is the international organization representing professional nurses. The focus of this nursing organization is on worldwide health care and nursing issues; it meets every 4 years and is headquartered in Geneva, Switzerland. The ICN has been involved in the development of ethical guidelines for the recruitment of nurses from low-income nations. Many European nations have adopted an ethical code and restrict their recruiting from 150 low-income nations (Anderson and Isaacs, 2007).

National League for Nursing. The NLN was established in 1952, however the beginning of NLN can be traced back to the 1893 organization of the American Society of Superintendents of Training Schools for Nurses of the United States and Canada. Between the late 1800s and the early 1900s, seven nursing organizations formed and joined under the collective name and function of the NLN. One of the unique features of the NLN is that both individuals and agencies are members. The NLN adopted a strategic plan in 1995 to place community-based health care education and health care delivery at the center of its focus and activities (NLN, 1995). The NLN continues to foster improvement in nursing services and nursing education and offers annual educational summits for nursing faculty and leaders in all types of nursing education programs to come together. Non-nurses can also join the NLN, fulfilling its purpose of promoting the consumer's voice in some nursing policies. The NLN has a biennial convention and publishes *N&HC: Perspectives on Community* (called *Nursing & Health Care* before 1995), NLN Update, and numerous other publications that can be obtained by calling 800-669-1656 or by visiting their website at *www.nln.org*.

Before 1997, the NLN functioned as an accrediting body in all levels of nursing education. In 1997, the NLN created an independent organization called the National League for Nursing Accrediting Commission Inc. (NLNAC) to accredit educational and professional nursing programs. This organizational change was in response to new standards established by the U.S. Department of Education. This step was taken to separate accrediting activities from membership activities and to respond to the Higher Education Act Amendment of 1992. Is your school an NLNAC-accredited institution? To find out, visit their website at *www.nlnac.org*.

National Student Nurses' Association. The National Student Nurses' Association is a fully independent organization with a membership of approximately 50,000 nursing students nationwide. NSNA mentors the professional development of future nurses and facilitates their entrance into the profession by providing educational resources, leadership opportunities, and career guidance.

The organization was formed in 1952. Becoming a member of the NSNA may be viewed as a way to begin the "professional" socialization process. There are local school chapters as well as state and national level membership. Often, members of the NSNA serve on selected committees of the ANA and speak to the ANA House of Delegates regarding student-related issues. The quarterly journal, *Imprint*, is published by the NSNA. Visit their website at *www.nsna.org*.

National Organization for Associate Degree Nursing. This group was organized in 1986 as an outgrowth of several state organizations. Texas was the first state to have a chapter, which was started in 1984. Membership in the National Organization for Associate Degree Nursing (NOADN) is open to associate degree nursing graduates, educators, and students. Individuals, states, agencies, and other organizations may also join. There are state and national chapters. The mission of this organization is to be the advocate for associate degree nursing education and practice. NOADN strives to maintain eligibility for RN licensure for graduates of associate degree (AD) programs, to promote AD nursing programs in the community, to provide a forum for discussion of issues affecting AD nursing, to develop partnerships and increase communication with other health care professionals, to increase public understanding of the AD nurse, to participate in state and national levels in the formation of health care policies, and to facilitate legislative action supporting the activities of NOADN. Visit their website at *www.noadn.org*.

American Association of Colleges of Nursing. This organization is the national voice for university and 4-year college educational programs in nursing and has a membership of more than 500 colleges. The mission of the organization is to serve the public interest by assisting deans and directors in improving and advancing nursing education, research, and practice. This organization publishes a newsletter and a bimonthly nursing journal called the *Journal of Professional Nursing*. In the past few years, it has formed a subsidiary for credentialing purposes. That organization is the Commission on Collegiate Nursing Education (CCNE). This autonomous accreditation agency serves only baccalaureate and higher degree programs in the accreditation process. Additional information on either organization can be found at *www.aacn.nche.edu*.

American Board of Nursing Specialties. The past 15 years have demonstrated significant growth in specialty practice in nursing. Throughout the 1980s and 1990s, specialty organizations met annually as the National Federation of Specialty Nursing Certifying Organization to discuss issues in certification and nursing practice. This organization dissolved, and many of the specialty organizations joined the American Board of Nursing Specialties (ABNS) in 1991. The ABNS was established to create uniformity in nursing certification; it now represents more than 25 specialty nursing organizations that promote specialty practice and address certification issues associated with specialty practice. The ABNS functions as a consumer advocate in promoting nursing certification.

As a recent graduate, are you interested in a particular specialty nursing practice area? How and when do you anticipate obtaining specialty certification? How will you include membership in a professional organization in your 5-year career-educational plan? Do you know the benefits of being a certified nurse? Do you work with nurses who are certified in their specialty?

The American Red Cross. This is an international organization of approximately 120 Red Cross organizations around the world. Nurses of the American Red Cross pioneered public health nursing in the early 1900s. The American Red Cross is a voluntary agency that is supported by contributions and plays an important role in providing disaster relief and education in first aid and home health and in organizing volunteers to assist in hospitals and nursing homes. Nurse volunteers with the Red Cross play a significant role in assisting those who have been affected by natural disasters.

In summary, professional organizations play a significant role in enhancing the image of nursing. Their impact is seen in both educational and practice issues for generalist and specialist nurse roles. Organizations provide a voice for nursing in policy issues and serve to unite nurses as a group of professionals. Ultimately, it may be nursing organizations that will serve as the catalyst for change in the health care system, and their impact will be felt in the next century.

CONCLUSION

Over the past century, the image of nursing has undergone many changes. The portrayal of nurses in the media has impacted the public perception of both male and female professional nurses. How will nurses continue to refine, intensify, and manage the image of nursing for the future? Will the self-image of nursing change public perception? Nursing will continue to define itself as a profession. Participation in the political side of health care, active involvement in professional organizations, and a commitment to the improvement of nursing's self-image are all ways to meet the upcoming challenges both in the nursing profession and in the rapidly changing health care environment.

The questions will go on and on, and the answers will come from nurses in clinical practice, education, and research. These issues, which have a significant impact on nursing's professional image, must be resolved so that nursing can move forward as a profession. As a recent graduate, you are the future of this exciting transition. The question to ask yourself is, what can I do to improve and maintain the image of nursing and the integrity of the profession? Change can and does begin with one person who is willing to step forward and make a difference. Is that you?

BIBLIOGRAPHY

American Nurses Association: *Code of ethics for nurses with interpretive statements*, Silver Spring, Md, 2001, ANA. Retrieved from *nursebooks.org.*

American Nurses Association: *Standards of clinical nursing practice*, Kansas City, Mo, 2003, ANA.

American Nurses Association (2010): Frequently asked questions, *NursingWorld.* Retrieved from *www.nursingworld.org/FunctionalMenuCategories/FAQs.aspx#about.*

American Nurses Association: *Social policy statement*, Kansas City, Mo, 2010, ANA.

American Nurses Association (n.d.): *The importance of belonging to your professional nursing organization.* *PowerPoint presentation.* Retrieved from *www.nursingworld.org/EspeciallyForYou/Educators/TheImportanceofBelonging.aspx#276.*

American Nurses Credentialing Center (2007): *Why ANCC Certification?* Retrieved from *www.nursecredentialing.org/cert/index.htm.*

Anderson B, Isaacs A: Simply not there: the impact of international migration of nurses and midwives—perspectives from Guyana, *J Midwifery Womens Health* 28(6):392-397, 2007. Retrieved from *http://web.ebscohost.com.ezproxy. baylor.edu/ehost/detail?vid=11&hid=10 2&sid=04252468-7087-4df4-84a1-f2f55dc652ec%40sessionmgr104.*

Bostridge M: *Florence Nightingale: the woman and her legend*, London, 2008, Viking Press.

Caplow T: *The sociology of work*, Minneapolis, 1954, University of Minnesota.

Cohen S, Bartholomew K: *Our image, our choice: perspectives on shaping, empowering, and elevating the nursing profession*, Marblehead, Mass, 2008, HCPro.

Dombeck M: Work narratives: gender and race in professional personhood, *Res Nurs Health* 26:351-365, 2003.

Dukes ME (2003): Writer hopes to change nurses' image, *Stripe*. Retrieved from *www.dcmilitary.com/dcmilitary_ archives/stories/050803/23071-1.shtml.*

Groves B (2007:) An image problem: from TV to silver screen, *The Record*. Retrieved from *www.nursingadvocacy. org/news/2007/may/06_record.html.*

Health Resources and Services Administration: National sample survey of registered nurses, Bureau of Health Professions, Division of Nursing, Washington, DC, 2004, HRSA. Retrieved from *http://bhpr.hrsa.gov/ healthworkforce/reports/ rnsurvey04/3.htm.*

Health Resources and Services Administration (HRSA): National advisory council on nurse education and practice: Seventh Report to the Secretary of Health and Human Services and the Congress, Washington, DC, 2009, HRSA. Retrieved from *http://bhpr.hrsa. gov/nursing/nacnep.htm.*

Health Resources and Services Administration (HRSA): HRSA Study Finds Nursing Workforce is Growing and More Diverse, Washington, DC, 2010, HRSA. Retrieved from *www.hrsa.gov/ about/news/pressreleases/100317_hrsa_ study_100317_finds_nursing_ workforce_is_growing_and_more_ diverse.html.*

Kaplan M (2005): Speech: why isn't nursing more newsworthy? *Medscape Nursing.* Retrieved from *www.medscape.com.*

Larson SE: Create a good impression: professionalism in nursing? *Imprint* 53(5): 50-52, 2006.

Mee C: Painting a portrait: how you can shape nursing's image, *Imprint* 53(5): 44-49, 2006.

National League for Nursing: The in/visibility of nurses in cyberculture, *NLN updates*, New York, 1995, NLN. Retrieved from *www.nursing-informatics.com/visiblenurse7.html.*

Pavalko R: *Sociology of occupations and professions*, Itasca, Ill, 1971, Peacock.

Peplau H: *Interpersonal relationships in nursing*, New York, 1952, Putnam Press.

Saad L (2008): *Nurses shine while bankers slump in ethics rating.* Retrieved from *www.gallup.com/poll.*

Strauss A: *The structure and ideology of American nursing: an interpretation in the nursing profession*, New York, 1966, Wiley.

Talotta D: Role conceptions and professional role discrepancy among baccalaureate nursing students, *Image J Nurs Sch* 22(2):111-115, 1990.

Turow J, Gans R (2002): *As seen on TV: health policy issues in TV's medical dramas. A report to The Kaiser Family Foundation.* Retrieved from *www.kff. org/entmedia/3231-index.cfm.*

Ward C, Styles I, Bosco A: Perceived states of nurses compared to other health care professionals, *Contemporary Nurse* 15(1/2):20-24, 2003. Retrieved from *www.contemporarynurse.com/15-1p20. htm.*

What's the big deal about naughty nurse images in the media? (2010): Retrieved from *www.truthaboutnursing.org/faq/ naughty_nurse.html.*

Wilson D: Meet the men who dare to care, *Johns Hopkins Nursing* VII(2), 2009. Retrieved from *http://web.jhu.edu/ jhnmagazine.*

Additional resources are available online at *http://evolve.elsevier.com/Zerwekh/nsgtoday/*.

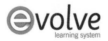

CHAPTER **10**

Challenges of Nursing Management and Leadership

Joann Wilcox, RN, MSN, LNC

> *Leaders don't force people to follow—they invite them on a journey.*
> —CHARLES S. LAUER

> *Outstanding leaders go out of their way to boost the self-esteem of their personnel. If people believe in themselves, it's amazing what they can accomplish.*
> —SAM WALTON

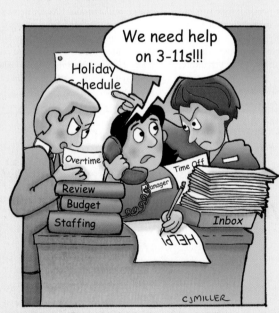

"I need help on the night shift!"

After completing this chapter, you should be able to:

- Differentiate between management and leadership.

- Describe theories of management and leadership.

- List characteristics of an effective manager and an influential leader.

- Identify distinguishing generational characteristics of today's workforce.

- Differentiate the concepts of power and authority.

- Apply problem-solving strategies to clinical management situations.

- Identify the characteristics of effective work groups.

- Discuss the change process.

- Discuss the value of using evidence-based management actions.

s you get closer to meeting your goal of becoming a graduate nurse, consideration should be given to understanding the role of the nurse as a manager and as a leader. You might be thinking:

I do not want to be a manager, I am just a recent graduate!
OR
I want to take care of patients, not be a paper pusher!
OR
Am I ready to be followed by others?

Consider this: Nursing, in any role, is a *people business. Management* is the process of effectively working with people. When you accept your first position as a graduate nurse, it is important to realize that you are becoming a part of a work group where members spend at least a third of their day interacting with each other. Therefore, nurses must be prepared to use interpersonal, leadership, and management skills to be effective in their role as a provider of patient care.

There are multiple levels of management that a nurse can practice. The specific level depends on the experience, competency, and defined role of the individual nurse. For instance, as a recent graduate, you will have primary *management* responsibility for the patients for whom you will be providing care. This will include planning and coordinating the care with other nursing personnel, health care staff, and with the patient and family members. This level of management is expected to be provided by all registered nurses who practice in the acute care environment. As you gain experience, you may assume the role of team leader with the addition of responsibility for managing a team of staff members who are managing and providing the care for a group of patients or you may be appointed to the role of charge nurse where you will assume management responsibility for an entire shift or unit.

MANAGEMENT VERSUS LEADERSHIP

What Is the Difference Between Management and Leadership?

Although the terms *management* and *leadership* are frequently interchanged, they do not have the same meaning. A leader selects and assumes the role; a manager is assigned or appointed to the role. Managers have responsibility for organizational goals and the performance of organizational tasks such as budget preparation and scheduling. Managers, as providers of care, supervise a team of people who are working to help patients achieve their defined outcomes.. Leaders are effective at influencing others. Although it is desirable for managers to be good leaders, there are leaders who are not managers and, more frequently, managers who are not leaders! So, let us discuss the actual differences in more detail.

The Functions of Management. *Management* is a problem-oriented process with similarities to the nursing process. Management is needed whenever two or more individuals work together toward a common goal. The manager coordinates the activities of the group to maintain balance and direction. There are generally four functions the manager performs: *planning* (what is to be done), *organizing* (how it is to be done), *directing* (who is to do it), and *controlling* (when and how it is done). All of these activities occur continuously and simultaneously, with the percentage of time spent on each activity varying with the level of the manager, the characteristics of the group being managed, and the nature of the problem and goal.

According to Rothbauer-Wanish (2009), planning is generally considered the most basic management function and one on which managers should spend a significant part of their time. The foundation for all planning begins with the development of goals that reflect the mission and vision of the organization and defining strategies that will be implemented to meet and maintain that mission and vision. The next level of planning is used on a daily basis as a part of determining the requirements for accomplishing the work to be done and how one ensures that what is needed is available. This planning must be congruent with the strategies for meeting the mission and vision of the organization. Along with this approach, a manager must also be able to plan for contingencies which, if not addressed, will interfere with accomplishing what needs to be done. When managing a patient-care unit, which needs specific resources 24 hours a day, one can be certain that the unexpected will happen. Being prepared for the unexpected is a key function of a nurse manager.

Staff nurses practice the elements of planning as the plans of care for each patient are developed. For this process, the patient's current status and goals are assessed determining what needs to occur during the time you will be assigned to provide care to him/her. The interventions needed to get the patient to the point of meeting his/her defined goals are selected. This process of management of patient care uses the same planning skills as those used by someone in the position of managing staff.

Organizing occurs as the manager aligns the work to be done with the resources available to do that work (Rothbauer-Wanish, 2009). This requires knowledge of all parts of the work, as well as a clear understanding of the competencies required of those who will be performing the assigned work. The manager must consider not only the licensing regulations but also the facility's policies when organizing the work to be assigned. For example, licensing regulations may allow a licensed practical nurse to administer defined intravenous medications, but the facility policy may not allow that level of employee to perform that procedure. Another example would be that the licensing regulations for registered nurses do not specify that a newly licensed nurse cannot be assigned to work in a critical care unit. However, facility policy may state that registered nurses who wish to work in a critical care unit need to complete one year of other experience before being assigned to that service. Knowing this information prevents the manager from making decisions that may be unacceptable.

The next phase of management is providing direction or supervision. The manager retains accountability for ensuring the work is completed in a timely and competent manner. Additionally, staff members need to complete assigned work according to standards, policies, and procedures with the understanding that the manager will provide sufficient observation and assessment of care being delivered to ensure that the care provided is safe and complete. When patient care falls below minimum standards, the manager has two actions to take. The first is to make certain the care/safety of the patient is addressed by ensuring the proper care is provided and secondly, actions need to be taken to address the performance of the staff who did not provide the care as assigned. Managers need to be able to make decisions regarding the level of supervision needed by each member of the staff. Managers must also be able to motivate staff toward reaching their full competence to perform the assigned work with minimal observation and direction.

Controlling is the last aspect of the planning function of the nurse manager. Most of the controls in health care facilities exist because health care is a highly regulated system and much of what must be done is dictated by governments, insurers, evaluating agencies, health policy, and institutional policy. The effective manager needs to be cognizant of the regulations that affect his or her area of practice and be able to clearly communicate the essence of these regulations to the staff. Staff members also need to have a thorough understanding of regulations and implications of noncompliance. An example of external controls imposed because of regulations is the elimination of the use of certain dangerous abbreviations when a physician writes a medication order (see Chapter 11 for a list of abbreviations). This regulation is a part of The Joint Commission (TJC) standards, as well as standards from the Centers for Medicare & Medicaid Services (CMS). Although the focus of this regulation is the physician; registered nurses may not implement an order that includes these eliminated abbreviations.

Control by the manager may also be demonstrated through data collected when reviewing quality of care to determine the level of compliance with standards and other quality monitors. These data give the manager the power of validation of observations since they can represent the outcomes of the care that has been provided. For instance, if the rate of hospital-acquired infections continues to be above the expected level, the manager has the information needed to implement and mandate interventions to reduce the number of infections.

Clancy (2008) adds a new dimension to the functions of management and that is directing. This is the "act of telling [staff] what to do" (p 61). Choosing the appropriate type of communication for these directives is dependent on the situation and the level of participation that can be allowed in the implementation. The level of communication ranges from making a decision without input by just announcing what will be done to allowing staff to function within limits defined by organizational policy. It is always best to allow input when possible. Then, when the situation calls for announcement only, staff will know that following the announcement is important and directly related to a situation requiring some direct action.

Florence Nightingale was an early nursing leader. What characteristics of a manager did she also demonstrate?

What Are the Characteristics and Theories of Management?

Active interest in management as a separate entity was first noted as part of the industrial revolution. The *traditional* theory developed at that time was based on the premise that there was a need to have the highest productivity level possible from each worker (Wertheim, n.d.). This theory is the basis for the hierarchy that has dominated much of management theory for almost two centuries.

The manager who functions under the traditional theory follows rules closely and understands the concept of the division of labor and the chain-of-command structure. Historically, this kind of functioning was thought to be efficient and clear and was considered necessary to achieve getting the most work from each employee. Throughout nursing history, this has been and continues to be, the theory on which the work of nurse managers is based. In the last two decades, movement from this traditional theory has been introduced and considered but not achieved in

90% of health care organizations today (Deming, 2000). Most facilities continue to expect management to function using the traditional theory since this is what fits with the prevailing hierarchical structures in place in these organizations. While many organizations have attempted to move from the hierarchy of management, multiple issues impacting the health care industry in the last 20 years has kept implementing other structures from occurring. There have been multiple management theories developed since the traditional theory was introduced. Each of these has attempted to build upon the others as additional issues are identified. For example, *behavioral theory* (also called human-interaction theory) evolved as it became more evident that the humanistic side of management needed to be addressed (Hellriegel et al, 1999). Employees seeking recourse from some of the rules of hierarchy looked for assistance outside of their place of work, for instance, in the growing labor unions. Employers recognized the need to consider the human side of productivity in order to maintain a stable, satisfied work force. This was followed by the introduction of *systems theory,* which considers inputs, transformation of the material, outputs, and feedback (Hellriegel et al, 1999). Systems theory is implemented when consideration is given to the impact of decisions made by one manager on other managers or parts of the system as a whole. This is important in health care because it helped management move from making decisions in the traditional manner, in which departments functioned as though they were independent. Recognizing that patients cannot be treated as though they are a number of separate and distinct parts has promoted the understanding and importance of systems theory. While behavioral theory as it relates to management considers the attitudes and needs of the employee, systems theory examines the possible outcomes of all individuals affected by a decision.

The last theory of management to be considered is the *contingency theory*, which is also referred to as the *motivational theory* (Hellriegel et al, 1999). This theory focuses on the manager being able to blend the elements of the earlier theories using those elements to determine what motivates people to make choices leading to the most effective methods to complete the work that needs to be done. All of these theories are directed toward ways to ensure that employees are as productive as possible—working in as timely a manner as possible—in order to meet the organizational goals or targets.

What Is Meant by Management Style?

You will experience a variety of management styles in your nursing practice. These styles follow a continuum from *autocratic* to *laissez-faire* styles (Figure 10-1).

The *autocratic manager* uses an authoritarian approach to direct the activities of others. This individual makes most of the decisions alone without input from other staff members. Under this style of management, the emphasis is on the tasks to be done, with less focus on the individual staff members who perform the tasks. The autocratic manager may be most effective in crisis situations when structure and control are critical to success, such as during a cardiac arrest or code situation. In general, however, the autocratic manager will have a difficult time in motivating staff to become a part of a satisfactory work environment because there is minimal recognition of the contributions of staff to the work that needs to be done. There is also minimal focus on the necessary relationships between the multiple disciplines that make up the successful health care team. Many individuals, particularly those from generations after the Baby Boomers, will not stay in a position in which autocracy is the major style of management.

On the other end of the continuum is the *laissez-faire manager,* who maintains a permissive climate with little direction or control exerted. This manager allows staff members to make and

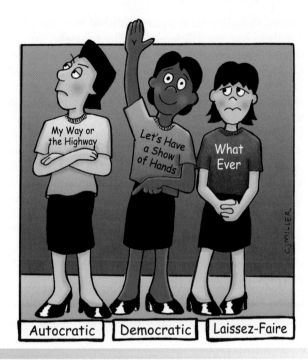

FIGURE 10-1

Management styles.

implement decisions independently and relinquishes most of his or her power and responsibility to them. Although this style of management may be effective in highly motivated groups, it may not be effective in a bureaucratic health care setting that requires many different individuals and groups to interact.

In the middle of the continuum is the *democratic manager*. This manager is people-oriented and emphasizes effective group functioning. The goals of the group are identified, and the manager is perceived as a group member who is also its organizer and who keeps the group moving in the defined direction. The environment is open, and communication flows both ways. The democratic manager encourages participation in decision making; he or she recognizes, however, that there are situations in which such participation may not be appropriate and is willing to assume responsibility for a decision when it is necessary. The democratic style is the blend of autocracy and laissez-faire with assurances that the extreme ends of the continuum are rarely, if ever, needed to be used.

One example of a democratic manager following either the behavioral or contingency theory would be a manager who creates a Nurse Practice Committee on his or her unit. This committee would have some defined authority and responsibility to address specific items in the practice environment such as schedules and practices on the unit. This type of committee supports the idea that staff and management are interdependent in governing the successful practice environment (Tonges et al, 2004).

To be a successful manager in today's hierarchical organizations, the nurse manager will need to adopt a democratic style of management, one that is flexible enough to adapt to the changing roles of nursing staff. The nurse manager should be willing and able to share power with the same people that he or she will supervise. The successful manager will also need to acquire an element of laissez-faire style for those components of governance that will be under the auspices of the staff. It will be important for staff nurses to develop a balanced combination of autocracy and laissez-faire as they implement shared governance (stakeholder participation in decision making) that will include quality of care and peer review. Both of these elements are necessary in order to create a safe environment for nurses (Institute of Medicine, 2004).

As you can see, the continuum of management styles includes approaches ranging from what might be considered total control to complete freedom for subordinates. In choosing a management style, the manager must decide on levels of control and freedom and then determine which trade-offs are acceptable in each particular situation. Behaviors vary from telling others what to do, to relinquishing authority for portions of the work to be done by another group within the organization. As a new staff nurse, your initial involvement in management occurs when you manage the care of a group of patients. The next involvement may be as a part of the shared governance model that may be developing in your facility. As you gain experience and knowledge, it is important for you to develop an understanding of which style you should use, depending on what you hope to be able to achieve.

> Look at managers on your clinical units. How do they fit into these categories?

Leadership, in contrast, is a way of behaving; it is the ability to cause others to respond, not because they have to but because they want to respond. Leadership is needed as much as management for effective group functioning but each role has its place. The manager determines the agenda, sets time limits, and facilitates group functioning. The leader focuses a group's efforts on indentifying goals and carrying out the activities needed to reach those goals.

What Are the Characteristics and Theories of Leadership?

The many attempts to define what makes a good leader have resulted in a variety of studies and proposals. Researchers have tried to identify the characteristics or traits necessary to be a good leader. Several of these studies have defined the concept of a *born leader,* implying that the desired traits are inherited. This is often referred to as the "Great Man" theory since it was first identified when leadership was generally thought to be a male quality, particularly as it related to military leadership (Van Wagner, 2007). With later research, it became clear that desired leadership traits could be learned through education and experience. It also became clear that the most effective leadership style for one situation was not necessarily the most effective for another, and that the effectiveness of the leader is influenced by the situation itself. As leadership theories continue to develop, emphasis is more on what the leader does rather than on the traits the leader possesses.

Several other theories of leadership are worth discussing. The first is *contingency leadership,* which says leadership should be flexible enough to address varying situations. Although this may sound complicated, it can be compared with your approach to patient care. As a nurse, you individualize a patient care plan on the basis of the needs of that individual. Then the plan is implemented, using available resources. The effective leader, using contingency leadership, brings the same flexible approach to each individual situation where leadership is required.

Situational leadership theory resulted from the study of the contingency theory and attempts to define functioning more closely to the situation being addressed. Blanchard and Hersey (1964) define the situational leader as one who analyzes the needs of the current situation and then selects the most appropriate leadership style to address that particular situation. The selected style depends on the competencies of each employee who will be helping address the current situation. The authors state that a good situational leader may use different styles of leadership for different employees who are all involved in addressing the same situation. This is not unlike what you, as a team leader, will be doing when assigning work to members of your work team. The assignments will need to be individualized based on the competencies of each member of the team to help ensure the patient care goals can be met.

Interactional leadership is the next theory to consider. With this theory, the focus is on the development of trust in the relationship (Marquis & Huston, 2003). Interactional leadership includes concepts of behavioral theories, which begin to address the fact that leaders are *made* and not *born*, since the needed behaviors can be taught and learned. Interactional leadership also includes the concepts of participative theories. Encouraging input and contributions from the group being led is the basis for interaction and the development of trust in the leader. Individuals who function based on the theory of interactional leadership use democratic concepts of management and view the tasks to be accomplished from the standpoint of a team member.

Leadership theory can also be described as *transactional* noting that the transactional leader is one who has a greater focus on vision, defined as the ability to envision some future state and describe it to others so they can begin to share that vision. The transactional leader holds power and control over followers by providing incentives when the followers respond in a positive way to the leader's vision and the actions needed to reach that vision. The basis for the relationship between leader and follower is that punishment and reward motivates people. Transactional leaders seek equilibrium so the vision can be reached and only intervenes when it appears that goals will not be attained (Sullivan & Decker, 2009).

This leadership theory does not sound like one that many would be encouraged to embrace or follow since the rewards are ultimately one-sided. However, the transactional approach to leadership still exists in most organizations, generally at the management level as incentives are provided to gain a defined level of productivity.

Transformational leadership occurs when the leader has a strong, clear vision that has developed through listening, observing, analyzing and finally by truly buying into the vision to dramatically change the way in which things are currently being done (Bass, 1990). Even though this theory was introduced as early as the 1970s, it is still in its infancy of use by particular industries such as health care. Transformational leadership will be implemented when it is clear to the strong, visionary leaders that the current situation(s) cannot be "fixed" using the traditional methods that have worked in the past.

If transactional leadership involves the use of leadership power over rewards and punishments to "lead," transformational leadership can be characterized as a process where leader and followers work together, in a way that changes, or transforms the organization, the employees/followers and the leader. It recognizes that real leadership involves transformation and learning on the part of follower *and* leader. As such, it is more of a partnership, even though there are power imbalances involved.

While transactional leadership involves telling, commanding, or ordering (and using contingent rewards), transformational leadership is based on inspiring, getting followers to buy-in voluntarily, creating common vision. Transformational leadership is what most of us refer to when we talk about great leaders in our lives and in society.

The nurse shortage is a good example of a problem in which the solution will most likely be found by transformational leaders. It is evident that the old ways of fixing the nursing shortage have not been effective. Managers, lawmakers, and organizations have tried increasing wages, paying bonuses, recruiting foreign nurses, mandating staff-to-patient ratios, adding nurse-extenders, and implementing flexible shifts. None of these methods has had any long-lasting effects because they do not address the conflicts that have occurred as newer generations of nurses have reached the level where they want control of their practice as granted by education and licensure. A transformational leader understands the basis for these conflicts and develops a vision, which will address the needs of the people involved in the conflict.

One might anticipate that the Chief Executive Officer and the Chief Nursing Officer of a hospital would both be transformational leaders. These leaders have a responsibility to see the bigger picture and to be able to describe that vision or picture to others. Porter O'Grady (2003b) describes this type of leader as one who can "stand on the balcony" (p 175). From this position, the leader can monitor the ebb and flow of the organization and determine which direction the organization is moving. To be effective, the transformational leader must have a vision that can be put into words for others to understand.

Although most leaders tend to lean toward one of the styles discussed above, fluctuations from one to another can occur, depending on the particular situation. In the health care setting, good leaders carefully balance job-centered and employee-centered behaviors to meet both staff and patient needs effectively (Critical Thinking Box 10-1).

A good leader works toward established goals and has a sense of purpose and direction. A good leader must also be aware of how her/his behavior impacts the workplace. Emotions, moods, and patterns of behavior displayed by the leader will create a lasting impression on the behavior of the team involved. It is critical for the leader to be aware of this impact if she or he is going to be effective in managing and leading a team (Porter-O'Grady, 2003a). Rather than push staff members in many directions, this leader uses personal attributes to organize the activities and *pull* the staff toward the goals.

The most current theory addressing the changing environment in which we work is the *complexity theory* of leadership. The complexity theory addresses the "unpredictable, disorderly, nonlinear and uncontrollable ways that living systems behave" (Burns, 2001, p 474). This theory indicates that we need to look at systems, such as those in health care organizations, as patterns of relationships and the interactions that occur among those in the system.

Complexity theory is complex! However, the basis of the thinking can most easily be understood by comparing traditional ways of analyzing an organization to the ways in which this analysis would be accomplished using the complexity theory. The traditional method used to understand an organization is to "break a system into smaller bits and when we believe we

CRITICAL THINKING BOX 10-1 Consider your educational and clinical experiences. What leadership theories and styles have you observed? What management styles have you observed? Are there specific personality traits that enhance a person's performance of these two roles?

understand the bits we put them all back together again and draw some conclusions about the whole" (IOM, 2004). Complexity theory examines the whole rather than the sum of its parts because the breaking a system apart removes all the impact of the human relationships that impact the whole.

Following complexity theory, one understands that organizations are "organic, living systems" (Anderson et al, 2005) in which people act quickly using knowledge sharing and patterns of relationships rather than the rules of a hierarchy. When leading according to the principles of complexity, an understanding is that change is successful when accomplished by individuals as they adapt to variations in the environment and not as the linear managers dictate. This is changing leadership from behaviors that are considered mechanical to behaviors that are dynamic and based on the current environment and the relationships operating within that environment.

As we complete the discussion on the theories and characteristics of leaders and managers, it becomes evident that there are more differences than those briefly identified in the opening paragraph of this discussion. According to Mannion (1998), the major differences are:

- Leaders focus on effectiveness, and Managers focus on efficiency.
- Leaders ask what and why, and Managers ask how.
- Leaders deal with people and relationships, and Managers deal with systems, controls, and policies.
- Leaders initiate innovation, and Managers maintain the status quo.
- Leaders look to the horizon, and Managers look to the bottom line (pp 3-7).

THE TWENTY-FIRST CENTURY: A DIFFERENT AGE FOR MANAGEMENT AND FOR LEADERSHIP

The face of leadership is changing, and this is very evident in nursing and health care. A major problem is that nursing continues to perform the same activities when there is clearly a demand for different processes. Changes in health care are altering some of the foundations of nursing practice. Shorter hospital stays and emerging therapeutics require less, but perhaps more intense, clinical time and challenge the need for certain nursing interventions that have become routine over time. Nurses are becoming increasingly frustrated with the reality that the nursing care they were taught to provide—and they feel they need to provide—is not possible given the decreased time spent with their patients (Porter-O'Grady, 2003b). This dissatisfaction may be compounded by the conflict between established nurses and upcoming generations of nurses. In general, younger generations of nurses have accepted the newer foundations of practice, whereas these changes are often resisted by tenured staff. Thus the task of learning how to bridge the gaps in a multigenerational staff must be added to the nurse manager's other responsibilities.

"For the first time in decades, there are four separate and distinct generations potentially working together in a stressful and competitive nursing work-place" (Boychuk-Duchscher & Cowin, 2004, p 493).

The leadership of health care in the 21st century has been and will continue to be significantly affected by the diverse generations in today's workplace. These generational groups have major differences in communication styles, in what motivates them, in what turns them off, and in their

BOX 10-1	Characteristics of Generations

- Silent or Veteran Generation: Born between 1925 and 1942—account for 10% of the current workforce
- Baby Boomers: Born between 1943 and 1960—account for 45% of the current workforce
- Generation X: Born between 1961 and 1979—account for 30% of the current workforce
- Generation Y: Born between 1980 and 2000—account for 10% of the workforce
- Generation Now: Born between 1995 and now—the newest group to the job market

workplace ideals (Boychuk-Duchscher & Cowin, 2004; Martin, 2004). Generational diversity has been recognized as one of the major factors precipitating conflict in the workplace. Great diversity exists in the beliefs, attitudes, and life experiences of the various generations (Scott, 2007). Box 10-1 lists general characteristics of the different generations in the current workforce.

"I honestly think there has always been a general tension among different generations, but it has never had a 'voice' like it has now" (Wieck, cited in Trossman, 2007, p 8).

The Silent or Veteran Generation

This oldest generation of nurses, which is also the group that is retiring or retired, was taught to rely on tried, true, and tested ways of doing things. Because of early experiences of these nurses with economic hardship and the Great Depression of the 1920s and 1930s, they place high value on loyalty, discipline, teamwork, and respect for authority (Boychuk-Duchscher & Cowin, 2004). This group also witnessed the destruction and genocide of World War II, the eradication of polio, and the control of many other diseases (tuberculosis, whooping cough) through the development of antibiotics and immunizations. Nurses from this generation have always worked within the hierarchy of management and leadership and are use to the autocratic style of leaders and managers.

The Baby Boomers

The Baby Boomers make up the largest group of nurses working today. Also, the majority of nurse management positions are filled by Baby Boomers. Members of this group have a multitude of family responsibilities, frequently spanning three generations. In fact, this group is frequently referred to as the "sandwich generation" because they are caught between caring for their children while also caring for their own aging parents. Nurses in this group are very ambitious. They put in long hours and have a strong sense of idealism, both at home and at work. Baby Boomers value what others think, and it is important that their achievements be recognized. They have set and maintained a grueling pace between their family and employment responsibilities. This group has embraced technology as a method of being more productive and to have more free time (Cordeniz, 2003).

The individuals of the Baby Boomer generation are still products of the hierarchical theory of leadership and management but are beginning to recognize and ask for some of the elements of the behavioral theory. They are also frequently challenged by nurses of younger generations, who see little value in hierarchical leadership in a system such as health care, which includes multiple groups and professions, some of whom have autonomy by licensure that is not recognized in a leadership hierarchy. By contrast, Baby Boomers are focused on building careers and are invested in organizational loyalty (Scott, 2007).

Generation X

Members of Generation X grew up in the information age; they are energetic and innovative. They are also hard workers, but unlike Baby Boomers, Gen X employees have little loyalty to, or confidence in, leaders and institutions. They value portability of their career and tend to change jobs frequently; they will stay in a position as long as it is good for them. This generation saw the downsizing of the 1990s, when organizational loyalty did not protect workers from loss of jobs or retirement. Thus they tend to have little aspiration for retirement. The use of technology has initiated an expectation of instant response and satisfaction. Their learning style has been shaped by technology; they want immediate answers from a variety of sources (Scott, 2007). They want different employment standards, such as opportunities for self-building and responsibility for work outcomes. They want extensive learning and precepting, and they want their questions answered immediately.

Gen X nurses value their free time; therefore, flexible scheduling and benefits (daycare centers, liberal vacations, working from home) are important. They claim to be motivated by work that agrees with their values and demands (Cordeniz, 2003). This group wants to work under motivational leadership with a democratic manager. If they do not find that kind of environment, they will have little reason to maintain employment in that institution.

Since most of the leaders and managers in health care are from the Baby Boomer generation, the conflict between these generations is certainly a significant contributor to the high turnover rate among younger nurses and the high rate of nurses finding employment outside of the hospital setting.

Generation Y

Members of Generation Y (also known as Generation Net, Nexters, or the Millennium Generation) were born between 1980 and 2000. This is the largest group, perhaps three times the size of Generation X; as such, this generation is having a formidable impact on the employment market. Those in their 30s are beginning to have an influence on how organizations are managed. This generation represents a large number of the children of the Baby Boomers. While the Baby Boomers were trying to master Windows, these kids were playing with computers in kindergarten!

The impact of this generation is still being defined, but with the speed of generational changes, the impact of Generation Y may soon be integrated with the newest generation, currently labeled Generation Now. The Y Generation is smart and believes education is the key to success. For this group, diversity is a given, technology is as transparent as air, and social responsibility is a business imperative (Martin, 2004). Members of Gen Y are optimistic and interactive; yet they value individuality and uniqueness. They can multitask, think fast, and are extremely creative.

Managing this group will require a vastly different set of skills than what exists in the market today. Generation Y nurses are not team players. They are in the driver's seat—they know that work is there for them if they want it. Focusing on understanding their capabilities, treating them as colleagues, and putting them in roles that push their limits will help managers recognize the potential of this group to become the highest-producing workforce in history (Martin, 2004). This is the most educated generation ever. Gen Y employees believe that they can either "start at the top or be climbing the corporate ladder by their sixth month on the job" (NAS, 2006, p 6). They learn quickly and adapt quickly. The hierarchy of health care leadership and management is generally not what they are seeking as a part of their employment.

Generation Now

The newest generation is being called the Generation Now or the I Generation——since they have never lived without the Internet and other forms of rapid communication. This means they have never known a world without immediacy (IMedia, 2006). The impact of this generation is already being felt in all aspects of our society and world. The way those in the I generation or Gen Now think, act, find information, negotiate, and make decisions may make our present theories of leadership and management obsolete and just a part of our long history.

The challenge to nursing will be to develop a workplace, as well as a profession, that will be attractive to all these generations, particularly those who represent the mainstream of the workforce. According to Lynn Wieck, who has been studying the different generations and the impact they have on nursing, "The younger nurses also want to know who, what, and why a policy was decided, and they want input into the process" (cited in Trossman, 2007, p 8). Wieck's research has validated the generational differences and the impact these differences are having on nursing (Trossman, 2007). The key is to learn the art of compromise as these generations continue to learn to work together calling on the wisdom of the more experienced generation and the enthusiasm of the youngest of us to demonstrate that excellent care can be provided while making the work "more ergonomic, economical and eco friendly" (Malleo, 2010, para 9). These Gen Now staff can show a new way to accomplish the work that is different from the task orientation of the older generations—both of which were/are appropriate for the system at the time.

Initially, there must be a focus on recruiting the younger generations into the health care fields, specifically into nursing. Emphasis must also be placed on retention of experienced nurses. These nurses are necessary to mentor the younger generations, and their experience is invaluable. Eric Chester works with young people and has outlined strategies for managing and motivating the younger generations (Boxes 10-2 and 10-3).

Review these strategies—they are not new, nor are they exclusive to young employees. These strategies make sense for every generation and every organization at any time (Verret, 2000) (Critical Thinking Box 10-2).

The changes in the way the younger generations relate to leadership and management may well be part of the reason more hospitals are becoming Magnet-certified. Magnet is a comprehensive program relating to many aspects of nursing and nursing practice, but the basis for most of the success of the program is the acceptance of a change in the way practice is governed and

CRITICAL THINKING BOX 10-2

What generation do you belong to? How do your work values and personal characteristics fit that generation?

BOX 10-2	Motivational Strategies for Generations X and Y

1. Let them know that what they do matters.
   - When was the last time a letter from a patient who was very pleased with the care on a unit was shared with the staff? When was the last time management sat down with all of the unit personnel to tell them what a good job they are doing? When was the last time the Chief Executive Office complimented the staff on a job well done?
2. Tell them the truth.
   - When did the managers on a unit acknowledge to the staff exactly what was going on? For example, the surgery schedule is going to be heavy this next week, there are going to be a lot of new admissions, as well as a lot of patients who will be going home. Acknowledge that the work level is going to increase, and ask whether any of the staff have suggestions for improving the coordination and workload assignments.
3. Explain why you are asking them to do it.
   - When a difficult time is anticipated, explain to the staff what is happening and why. Maybe a particular area of the hospital is overloaded and additional staff are being pulled from their regular units to help out. These patients must be accommodated and cared for—this is why the hospital is there, and maintaining patient census is what pays the bills.
4. Learn their language.
   - When was the last time the unit manager, head nurse, or other manager actually sat down with the staff (all levels) to find out who they are and what they like to do? What are their priorities? Their family situations? What do they do on their days off?
5. Be on the lookout for rewarding opportunities.
   - When did a staff member handle a particular difficult patient situation very well and the staff member was acknowledged at that time? Give positive feedback when opportunities arise. Do not wait for a performance evaluation to do so.
6. Praise them in front of their peers and other staff.
   - Acknowledge a job well done at a staff meeting or in the presence of people who are important to that person.
7. Make the workplace fun.
   - Making the hospital work environment fun can sometimes be a little difficult, but there are opportunities for humor if we just look for them. Patients share a lot of humor with the staff. Is the staff encouraged to share that with the rest of the unit personnel? When something funny happens to staff, are they encouraged to laugh and share with others?
8. Model behavior.
   - Does the behavior of the unit manager or head nurse model the behavior the manager is expecting others to exhibit? What about confidentiality? Is it expected of the personnel? Does the manager practice it as well?
9. Give them the tools to do the job.
   - What about effective communication skills, or perhaps good customer service skills. The health care industry is in the business of providing a service for the customer—the patient. Training is offered for the technical skills—new equipment, procedures, policies—but what about training for the skills necessary in dealing with people? How about skills to deal effectively with the angry patient, the difficult doctor, the outraged family? (Verret, 2000)

These strategies are from Eric Chester, as presented by Carol Verret in her article, "Generation Y: Motivating and Training a New Generation of Employees." Data taken from Verret C (2000): Generation Y: motivating and training a new generation of employees. *Hotel Online: Ideas and Trends.* Retrieved from *www.hotel-online.com/Trends/CarolVerret/GenerationY_Nov2000.html.*

BOX 10-3	Motivational Strategies for Generation Now

In addition to Box 10-2, consider these strategies specific to Generation Now:
1. Look at where they are going for information.
   - They are always on the lookout for something new. It is the job of the leader or manager to stay current to keep up with them.
2. Make your message relevant.
   - They know when they are being "talked to." They consider their time precious, and they want you to use their time wisely.

controlled. Magnet facilities demonstrate a true implementation of shared governance in which the nursing staff has control of the clinical practice of nursing and practice aspects of the work environment (HCPro, 2006).

Up to this point, leadership has been considered primarily as a part of management. In 2004, the American Association of Colleges of Nursing (AACN) brought a group together to develop a position of clinical nurse leader (CNL) (Stanley et al, 2008). The rationale for this position was that with the changing health care needs of this society, the system does not seem to be "making the best use of its resources leading to a need to educate future practitioners differently" (Stanley et al, 2008, p 615). It was thought that this was critical to successfully addressing the many significant clinical issues facing the system during a time when resources are becoming limited. Having a highly prepared individual in the clinical setting is meant to positively impact the current patient safety issues by identifying and managing risk while meeting standards of quality clinical care.

As stated by Tornabeni and Miller (2008), "Improved patient care requires more nurses, better educated nurses and revised systems and environments for delivering patient care" (pp 608-609). Many factors support this need since it is known that with shorter lengths of stay as well as care and treatment becoming more complex, stability in the delivery of nursing care is essential for reaching the defined outcomes of that care. This also has to be accomplished in a manner that maximizes the use of available resources while minimizing patient hand-offs and risks as these outcomes are reached. The clinical nurse leader is a master's degree-prepared registered nurse who is expected to:
- Improve the quality of patient care through evidence-based practices
- Improve communication among all team members
- Provide guidance for less experienced nurses
- Assure the patient has a smooth flow through the health system (Stanley et al, 2008, p 618).

This role is a combination of a bedside nurse, case manager, clinical educator, and team leader. The introduction of the clinical nurse leader role also addresses a long-standing complaint about acute care nursing practice. Within the clinical setting, the two major opportunities for advancement were to assume a management position or to become a clinical educator. Both essentially remove individuals from the bedside, which is the heart of our practice. With this new clinical role, nurses who wish to advance to a different role while providing direct patient care now have the opportunity to do so.

POWER AND AUTHORITY IN NURSING MANAGEMENT

Do You Know the Difference Between Power and Authority?

To have power means having the ability to effect change and influence others to meet identified goals. Authority relates to a specific position and the responsibility associated with that position. The individual with authority has the right to act in situations for which one is held responsible within the institutional hierarchy. This is a role most often assumed as a part of management.

> Power and responsibility always go hand in hand!

What Are the Different Types of Power?

There are many different types of power, so let us discuss those that are most common. *Legitimate power* is power connected to a position of authority. The individual has power as a result of the position. The head nurse has legitimate power and authority as a result of the position.

Reward power is closely linked with legitimate power in that it comes about because the individual has the power to provide or withhold rewards. If supervisors have the power to authorize salary increases or scheduling changes, then they have reward power. *Coercive power* is power derived from fear of consequences. It is easy to see how parents would have coercive power over children on the basis of the threat of punishment. This type of power can also be used against staff members when, for example, there is the threat of receiving unfavorable assignments. However, in considering the characteristics of the upcoming generations, this may not be effective with them.

Expert power is based on specialized knowledge, skills, or abilities that are recognized and respected by others. The individual is perceived as an expert in an area and has power in that area because of this expertise. For instance, the enterostomal therapist has expertise in the care of individuals who have had ostomies. Therefore, staff nurses seek out the therapist as a resource and use the expert's knowledge to guide the care of these patients.

Referent power is power that a person has because others closely identify with that person's personal characteristics; they are liked and admired by others. Individuals who have knowledge that is needed by others to function effectively in their roles possess *information power*. This type of power is perhaps the most abused! An individual may, for example, withhold information from subordinates to maintain control. The leader who gives directions without providing needed information on rationale or constraints is abusing information power.

Leadership power is the "capacity to create order from conflict, contradictions, and chaos" (Sullivan & Decker, 2009, p 42). This is possible when the staff or people involved in the conflicts have a trust for that leader who is able to influence people to respond because they want to respond!

Leaders and managers need to understand the concept of power and how it can be used and abused in working with others. Nurses, on the whole, need to identify ways to increase their power within the health team. Graduate nurses need to be aware of and willing to implement methods and resources to increase their personal power. As they gain experience in the staff nurse role, they can develop expert power by increasing competency in their roles and clinical skills.

> "If you really want to see the best use of power, see a nurse who is actually providing the care that a patient needs and how many times he or she has to manage the system, massage the system, and find ways through the system just to get good care for patients. That's power."
> —Beverly Malone, PhD, RN, FAAN (cited in Mendez, 2006, p 55)

Refining interpersonal skills that enhance the ability to work with others can expand many types of power, such as information, referent and leadership power. These skills include communicating what people need to know clearly and completely while gaining support for work to be done either through delegating or by encouraging staff to step forward to do what needs to be done to accomplish the stated goals. Demonstrating a willingness to give and receive feedback while providing positive communication is also important when working to develop and enhance power in working with others.

It is also important to recognize what detracts from power. Impressing others as disorganized, either in personal appearance or in work habits, engaging in petty criticism or gossip, and being unable to say *no* without qualification are some of the behaviors that can detract from power.

Today there is much discussion in nursing about the importance of power and the concept of *empowerment*. To *empower* nurses is to provide them with greater influence and decision making in their roles. The realization of greater power in the profession depends on the willingness of administrators to allocate this power and of nurses to accept it, along with the accompanying responsibility.

The basis for practice in Magnet-credentialed facilities is the empowerment of staff to make decisions that directly affect the practice of registered nurses who are providing direct care. This is accomplished through the development of a culture supporting the decentralization of management, power, and authority in all places in which registered nurses are providing care. A clearly delineated structure for accomplishing the appropriate decision making and clearly communicating these decisions must be in place and accessible to all registered nurses in the organization. Additionally, the responsibility for monitoring compliance and outcomes is also shared by the registered nurse staff rather than leaving this important function solely to management.

MANAGEMENT PROBLEM SOLVING

How Are Problem-Solving Strategies Used in Management?

Management is a *problem-oriented* process. The effective manager analyzes problems and makes decisions throughout all the planning, organizing, directing, and controlling functions of management. Problem solving can be readily compared with the nursing process (Table 10-1). This is because the nursing process is based on the scientific method of problem solving. The two are essentially the same, as can be seen by comparing the steps of one to the other.

As with the nursing process, problem solving does not always flow in an orderly manner from one step to the next. Throughout the process, feedback is sought, which may indicate a need for altering the plan to reach the desired objective. The most critical step in either process is identifying the problem (identified as the *nursing diagnosis* in the nursing process). Frequently what was originally identified as *the problem* may be too broad or unclear. Only the symptoms of the

TABLE 10-1 Nursing Process vs. Problem Solving	
NURSING PROCESS	PROBLEM SOLVING
Assessment	Data gathering
Analysis/nursing diagnosis	Definition of the problem
Development of plan	Identification of alternative solutions
Implementation of plan	Implementation of plan
Evaluation/assessment	Evaluation of solution

problem may be seen initially, or there may be several problems overlapping. If an approach is used to relieve only the symptoms, the problem will still exist. The good manager will guide the process of identifying the problem by asking questions such as "What is happening?" "What is being done about it?" "Who is doing what?" and "Why?" It is important to differentiate among facts and opinions and to attempt to break down the information to its simplest terms. Think of it as being a detective looking for every clue!

Once the problem is clearly identified, the group should *brainstorm* all possible solutions. Often the first few alternatives are not the best or most practical. Identifying a number of viable alternatives usually provides more flexibility and creativity. All possible solutions must fall within existing constraints, such as staff abilities, available resources, and institutional policies. The more complex the problem, the more judgment is required. In some cases the problem may extend beyond the manager's scope of responsibility and authority; therefore, it may be necessary to seek outside help.

After identifying all the alternatives, each must be evaluated in relation to changes that would be required in existing policies, procedures, staffing, and so forth, as well as what effect these changes would have. Ask "What would happen if …" questions to clarify the short- and long-term implications of each alternative. Keep in mind that the perfect solution is not possible in most situations.

Problem solving represents a choice made between possible alternatives that are thought to be the best solutions for a particular situation. At its best, problem solving should involve ample discussion of the possible solutions by those who are affected by the situation and who possess the knowledge and power to support the possible solution. Once an alternative has been selected, it should be implemented unless new data or perspectives warrant a change. Feedback should be sought continuously to provide ongoing evaluation of the effectiveness of the solution. Remember that simply choosing the best alternative does not automatically ensure its acceptance by those who work with it!

Evidence-Based Management Protocols and Interventions

Just as nurses are expected to practice using evidence-based protocols and interventions for clinical decision making, managers are expected to use those management practices that are not simply based on conventional wisdom but on demonstrated outcomes. This may be difficult to accomplish as management practices are often deeply imbedded in the culture of an organization. Changing these practices to what is known to work from those that may have worked in the past may be considered as challenging the core philosophy of that organization.

Pfeffer and Sutton (2006) state:

If a manager is guided by the best logic and evidence and if they relentlessly seek new knowledge and insight, from both inside and outside their organizations, to keep updating their assumptions, knowledge and skills, they can be more effective.

To accomplish this, the manager needs to be able to develop a commitment to searching for, and using, processes and solutions that are factually based leading to the ability to make what will be decisions that lead to the intended outcomes (Pfeffer & Sutton, 2006). It is believed that there is much peer-reviewed information regarding managing organizations that is not used because of the desire to do things as they have always been done—knowing that they do work some of the time.

The example given in an article in the *Harvard Business Review* relates to the use of stand-up meetings versus the traditional sit-down meetings. Evidence indicates that stand-up meetings took 34% less time to make decisions (Pfeffer & Sutton, 2006). Using this model could save an organization many hours a year that can be put to another productive use or could be eliminated from the payroll. However, very few organizations use this model for meetings even in the face of the clear evidence of the impact it would have on the organization.

Nurses who have been prepared to practice using evidence-based clinical information may find using these same skills and approaches to management as the norm. This will require a collaborative working relationship with the tenured management staff who may see that this may result in a shift of power to the staff who do use evidence-based management practices as a regular part of decision-making.

A model program for preparing novice nurses for management and leadership has been developed in Florida when the need for evidence-based leadership was noted. This resulted in the creation of the Novice Nurse Leadership Institute program whose purpose is to "create a pool of future nurse leaders to serve the community by developing a leadership mindset" (Dyess & Sherman, 2010, p 30). The program content includes a defined list of 42 evidence-based projects related to managerial decision making that need to be completed. Programs such as this are certain to become more widespread and will ultimately change the way in which effective management decisions are made and implemented.

Frequently, implementing the solution to a problem causes several other problems to arise. This can be avoided if the selected solutions are evidence-based and if they are tested before implementation to identify any areas that may be negatively affected by the new solution. This testing should be a formal process following the steps of a Failure-Mode-Effects-Analysis, which is meant to identify and address those risk points that may not have been evident when the solution was selected. Many of you will be given the opportunity to work with others to complete an analysis of new procedures, for example, before that new procedure is fully implemented. If problems arise after the analysis, testing, and implementation, the new problems should not be allowed to impede the implementation process. Instead, pause and consider each problem individually, solve it, and then return to the plan that was tested. The old adage "If at first you don't succeed, try, try again" is most appropriate when applying the problem-solving process but using evidence-based solutions should keep this to a minimum of repeat trials. Remain positive, confident, and flexible! Let us apply the process to an actual problem.

John is the head nurse on a busy medical-surgical unit with 32 patients. Staff members have complained to him that too much time is being spent during morning change-of-shift report. After asking questions

and seeking out additional information, John determines that a more clear definition of the problem is that the night charge nurse does not give a clear, concise report. Researching the peer-reviewed literature for solutions addressing end-of-shift communication and involving the night charge nurse in the problem-solving process helps to define the problem. Is it because the nurse does not have adequate knowledge of how to give a change-of-shift report. Or, is it a flaw in the report system that does not allow for adequate communication to occur?

Can you see how, once the problem has been clarified, it becomes more amenable to an acceptable, and perhaps even easy, solution?

How Do We Relate Problem Solving and Decision Making?

By definition, problem solving and decision making are almost the same process, with one very notable difference. Decision making requires the definition of a clear objective to guide the process. A comparison of the steps of each illustrates this difference (Table 10-2). Although both problem solving and decision making are usually initiated in the presence of a problem, the objective in decision making may not be to solve the problem, but only to deal with its results. It is also important to distinguish between a good decision and a good outcome. A *good outcome* is the objective that is desired, and a *good decision* is one made systematically to reach this objective. A good decision may or may not result in a good outcome. Although it is desirable to have both good decisions and good outcomes, the good decision maker is willing to act, even at the risk of a negative outcome.

Susan is the evening charge nurse on a medical unit that has a total of 24 patients. One of the patients is terminally ill and seems to be having a particularly difficult evening. The patient requires basic comfort measures but little complex care. Susan has a choice of assigning the patient to another RN or delegating care to a nursing assistant. If she assigns the RN, the workload for the other staff will be heavier and she herself will be assigned to the terminally ill patients to provide the care that cannot be delegated to the nursing assistant. Susan decides to assign the RN, because this patient requires the emotional and physical support best provided by an RN. During the shift, the RN spends time sitting with the patient. Close to the end of the shift, the patient dies. Was this a good decision with a bad outcome or a good decision with a good outcome?

Decision making is values-based, while problem solving was traditionally a more scientific process. With the introduction of evidence-based management, efforts to acquire evidence-based information as one is identifying alternative solutions to problems move the decision-making process into the scientific arena. Nurses will continue to make decisions on the basis of personal

TABLE 10-2 Problem Solving vs. Decision Making	
PROBLEM SOLVING	DECISION MAKING
Define problem	Set objective
Identify alternative solutions	Identify and evaluate alternative decisions
Select solution and implement	Make decision and implement
Evaluate outcome	Evaluate outcome

values, life experiences, perceptions of the situation, knowledge of risks associated with possible decisions and their individual ways of thinking but these factors will be influenced by the availability of information and solutions that have been scientifically tested. Because of these variables, that two individuals given the same information and using the same decision-making process would arrive at different decisions but the probability should be lower once evidence-based information is available.

In today's ever-changing health care environment, it is important for nurses and nurse managers to be effective in both problem solving and decision making. The good manager will evaluate the problem-solving or decision-making process on the basis of criteria that provide a view of the big picture. These criteria include the likely effects on the objective to be met, on the policies and resources of the organization, on the individuals involved, and on the product or service delivered.

The quality of patient care is dependent on the ability of the nurse to effectively combine problem solving with decision making. To do so, nurses must be attuned to their individual value systems and understand their effect on thinking and perceiving. The values associated with a particular situation will limit the alternatives generated and the final decision. For this reason, the fact that nurses typically work in groups is beneficial to the decision-making process. Although the process is the same, groups generally offer the benefits of a broader knowledge base for defining objectives and more creativity in identifying alternatives. The effectiveness of the group decision-making process is dependent on the dynamics of the group. It is therefore important for nurses to understand the roles of individuals within the group and the dynamics involved in working in groups to take full advantage of the group process. Chapter 11 focuses on communication, group process, and working with teams.

What Effect Does the Leader Have on the Group?

The leader's philosophy, personality, self-concept, and interpersonal skills all influence the functioning of the group. A leader is most effective if members are respected as individuals who have unique contributions to make to the group process. Can you remember our earlier discussion of the characteristics of a good leader? The ability to influence and motivate others is particularly important in the group process.

Whenever the combination of people in a group is altered, the dynamics are changed. If the group is in the working phase, it will revert to the initiating phase when a new person or persons are added and will remain there until they have been assimilated into the group and a new dynamic has been formulated. The most effective groups are those that have had consistent membership and are highly developed. These groups demonstrate friendly and trusting relationships; the ability to work toward goals of varying difficulty; flexible, stable, and reliable participation of members; and productivity with high-quality output. Leadership within these groups is democratic, and the members feel positive about their participation and the outcomes of the group process. Now let us apply these principles to a real situation!

When you graduate and accept a nursing position, you will become a new nurse in the work group, causing it to regress to the initiating phase. This is your opportunity to demonstrate to the members of the group that you are worthy of being included in the group. If this is your first nursing position, you will also demonstrate to the group that you are worthy of entering the nursing profession. During this time, you may experience feelings of loneliness, isolation, and distance that accompany the initiating phase. However, your feelings of pride, excitement, eagerness, and accomplishment should quickly eradicate those feelings of distance, because there is much to gain and much to offer when entering a new group with common goals.

Put your energy into forming supportive professional relationships, including the social aspects of these relationships. Seek and use feedback, and ask for help in areas that are not as familiar to you, such as priority setting. As you contribute your individual talents to the group, you will move from being a dependent new person to full group membership. It is important that you do not underestimate the length of time that may be needed to accomplish this task! Group processes proceed very slowly in some cases, and it may be six months or more before you are accepted as a full member of the work group. Do not be discouraged! Instead, use this opportunity to gain information regarding what you can offer to the next new member of the group and what you can do to make transitioning from school to practice a positive experience.

Management skills come with experience in nursing, so do not be too hard on yourself during the transition phase. Identify experienced staff nurses who are effective at managing the care of their assigned patients and identify nurse managers who have the skills you would like to incorporate into your management style. Look at the positive side of working with staff nurses and various nursing managers as a means to assist you in the development of your personal management style. Develop the ability to think like a manager as you carry out your assignments—always look at the big picture.

THE CHALLENGE OF CHANGE

How many times have you heard staff nurses complain about how powerless they feel about the lack of control they have over their work environment? They say they are frustrated that they cannot give the amount and quality of patient care they wish and that staffing patterns are placing undue stress on them. Do they talk about leaving the acute care environment and trying some other aspect of nursing (perhaps home health) as a less stressful option? Why do they run away from a situation, rather than thinking about how they can act to change it? Do they feel powerless to do so? Is it easier to withdraw and escape?

One thing we all know is that change is inevitable, particularly in today's health care delivery system. Economic factors have taken center stage, and cutbacks in all aspects of health care services are occurring. Change can be like a truck with no driver at the wheel: It moves slowly and steadily toward you (Figure 10-2). You have three options: you can move out of the situation and perhaps miss some opportunities; you can just stand there and withdraw, doing what you are told just to avoid conflict; or you can start to run with it, jump on, and try to steer it in a positive direction.

So, how do you begin to direct the change that is on the horizon? The first thing to know about the change process is that it, too, has similarities to problem solving and the nursing process. Let us lay them out and compare the two processes (Table 10-3).

Look familiar? Maybe it is not that hard to take control and be a change agent! The first thing you need to know about the change process is that resisting change is a natural response for most people. All of us are most comfortable in our state of equilibrium, where we feel in control of what we are doing. To deal effectively with change, it is important to understand that every change involves adaptation. It requires a period of transition in which the change can be understood, evaluated in light of its impact on the individual, and, one hopes, eventually be embraced.

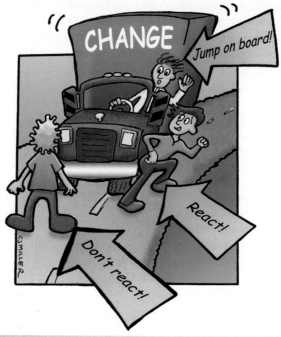

FIGURE 10-2

Change: react, don't react, or jump on board.

TABLE 10-3 Nursing Process vs. Change Process	
NURSING PROCESS	CHANGE PROCESS
Assessment	Recognition that a change is needed; collect data
Identification of possible nursing diagnoses	Identification of problem to be solved
Selection of nursing diagnosis	Selection of one of possible alternatives
Development of plan	Implementation of plan
Implementation of plan	Implementation of plan
Evaluation	Evaluation of effects of change
Reassessment	Stabilization of change in place

There are various reasons why people resist change, and understanding them will help you to implement the change process more effectively. Following are the most common factors that cause resistance to change:

- A perceived threat to self in how the change will affect the individual personally
- A lack of understanding regarding the nature of the change
- A limited ability to emotionally cope with change
- A disagreement about the potential benefits of the change
- A fear of the impact of the change on self-confidence and self-esteem

Kurt Lewin sought to incorporate these concepts in his Change Theory. He identified three phases in an effective change process: *unfreezing, moving,* and *refreezing.* In the unfreezing phase, all of the factors that may cause resistance to change are considered. Others who may be affected by the change are sought out to determine whether they recognize that a change is needed and to determine their interest in participating in the process. You will need to determine whether the environment of the institution is receptive to change and then convince others to work with you.

The *moving* phase occurs once a group of individuals has been recruited to take on responsibilities for implementing the change. The group begins to sort out what must be done and the sequence of actions that would be most effective. They identify individuals who have the *power* to assist in making the plan succeed. *(What types of power would be most effective?)* They also attempt to identify strategies to overcome the natural resistance to change—how to achieve a cooperative approach to implement the change. Once developed, the plan is then put into place.

The *refreezing* phase occurs when the plan is in place and everyone involved knows what is happening and what to expect. Publicizing the ongoing assessment of the pros and cons of the plan is an important part of its ultimate success. Be certain someone is responsible for continuing to work on the plan so that it does not lose momentum. Finally, make the changes stick—or *refreeze*. This will make the change a part of everyday life, and it will no longer be perceived as something new. Now let us apply this process to a real situation!

Patti is working in a medical-surgical unit at a 200-bed acute care hospital. She constantly hears her peers complaining about the lack of adequate nursing staff, and over the past 3 months, two full-time staff nurses have resigned. To cover the unit, part-time staff from temporary agencies and from the hospital staffing pool are being used to supplement the remaining regular staff. Because these staff members have little orientation to the unit and are frequently assigned where they are needed the most, the continuity of care and a potential for increased errors in patient care become a major concern.

Rather than continuing to complain about the situation or considering leaving, Patti decided to act and try to steer the change truck. She approached a few of the nurses and initiated a discussion about the changes in staffing and how scheduling had become a nightmare for the charge nurse. She enlisted the support of several members of the staff to begin problem-solving possible solutions. They agreed that increased staffing was probably not a possible immediate solution and determined to work within the constraints that they had.

Several of the pool nurses were receptive to requesting that their assignment be limited to this one unit and agreed to schedule their hours to complement each other. This, in essence, would add a shared full-time position, at no additional cost, and would also provide consistency of patient care. When the proposal was presented to administrators, they agreed to support the idea on the basis of its economic and patient-centered benefits.

The Change Truck—how will you respond?
- *React*—move out of the way. Let the truck (change) pass you by. However, opportunities may be missed.
- *Do not act*—just stand there and let the truck run over you. It will leave you behind and, more than likely, in worse shape than when you started.
- *Act*—start running when you see it coming. Pace with it until you can decide when to jump on and steer it in the direction you want to move.

Who Initiates Change and Why?

Another aspect to consider when evaluating change is to determine who wants the change and why. Is it the system? Is it management? Is it you, the nurse? Or is it the patient? There should be specific rationale for change and the identified change should be carefully planned, implemented, and evaluated to ensure the outcome is as anticipated. By identifying who is initiating the change and the reason for the change, the implementation plan can be better defined and understood, particularly regarding how implementation will affect the staff or the system.

System. The most common reason for change is that what you did before is no longer effective. For example, the handwritten medical record system is largely being replaced by the electronic medical record because the old system does not allow for the integration of the information in the record. The handwritten record generates volumes of paper, and is not adequate to keep pace with the number of patients and the need to access key information quickly from various individuals both inside and outside of the traditional hospital (home health nurse or hospice nurse at the patient's home).

Management. Change frequently occurs when new regulations are developed by agencies that license or approve the facility. This provides a new perspective and view regarding how the system currently operates and what part of the system needs to be changed for compliance with the new regulation. A significant change in almost all areas of the hospital occurred with the implementation of the HIPAA regulations. Employees at all levels needed to know "How will the implementation of HIPAA change my job? Do I know how to respond to a request for information?" (Critical Thinking Box 10-3.)

Patient. When customers are not happy, something within the system needs to change. What are the specific patient problems, and how can they be resolved? For example, patients are complaining about not receiving the information needed to make treatment decisions. Communicating effectively with the care team can help the nurse help the patient.

Yourself. Sometimes we impose change on ourselves. We may or may not like it, but we see a need for some aspect of change to occur (Table 10-4). Who has ever enjoyed being transferred to a different unit if the one we are working on is slated to close? Stop to consider how you are going to implement the change. How will your work environment be affected? If change involves other employees, include them as a part of that change. Gain the power that comes from working as a team.

Only when you feel threatened by a change will you go through the steps (i.e., resistance, uncertainty, assimilation, transference, integration) to conquer it (Wilson, 1996) (Figure 10-3). All change will elicit some type of resistance. It is up to you to increase the impetus for change while decreasing resistance. The decision to be involved with change will help steer you in a direction that will be most beneficial.

CRITICAL THINKING
BOX 10-3

- What changes have you made in your life?
- How long did one situation last before it changed again?
- You have just learned to deal successfully with the changes associated with being a student. Now you are facing the challenge of change again as you prepare for your role as a practicing registered nurse.

TABLE 10-4	Emotional Phases of the Change Process	
PHASE	CHARACTERISTICS	INTERVENTIONS
Equilibrium	High energy; feelings of balance, peace, and harmony	Explain how changes will affect the status quo
Denial	Denies reality that change will occur; experiences negative changes in physical health, emotional and cognitive behavior	Actively listen, be empathetic, and use reflective communication. Offer stress-management programs
Anger	Blames others; may demonstrate envy, rage, or resentment	Be assertive and assist with problem solving. Encourage employee to determine the source of his or her anger
Bargaining	Efforts made to try and eliminate the change; frequently talks in such terms as "If only"	Search for real needs and problems and explore ways to achieve outcomes through conflict management and win-win negotiation skills
Chaos	Diffused energy; feelings of powerlessness and insecurity and a sense of disorientation	Encourage quiet time for reflection as inner search for identity and meaning occur
Depression	No energy left; nothing seems to work; sorrow, self-pity, and feelings of emptiness	Encourage expression of sorrow and pain. Have lots of patience as employees learn to let go
Resignation	Lack of enthusiasm as change is accepted passively	Allow employees to move at own pace.
Openness	Some renewal of energy and willingness to take on new roles or assignments resulting from change	Patiently explain again, in detail, the desired change
Readiness	Willingly expends energy to explore new events that are occurring reunification of emotions and cognition	Assume a directive management style; assign tasks, provide direction
Reemergence	Feelings of empowerment as new project ideas are initiated	Mutually explore questions and develop an understanding of role and identity. Employees take actions based on own decisions

Adapted from Perlman D, Takacs GJ: The ten stages of change, *Nurs Manage* 21(4):34, 1990.

CONCLUSION

As a new graduate, you will be facing many transitions, including the transition from a "newbie" providing direct care for assigned patients, to managing the care for a group of patients, to a team leader role where you are managing the care of a group of patients through a team of staff. You may also be appointed to a formal management position or may assume the role of an

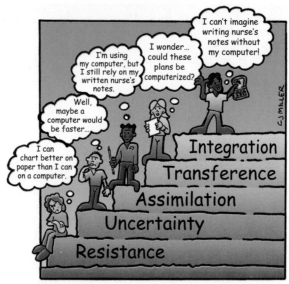

FIGURE 10-3

Five steps toward conquering change.

informal, but powerful, leader. All of these phases or roles require the characteristics of a leader who can influence others, including patients, to respond because they want to respond.

Think about the characteristics of your generation—will these influence your management style as you consider how you will positively engage with all the members of your staff? How will you contribute to the resolution of some of the differences in the nursing environment? Will you research the literature to find those actions that have been proven to be effective or will you do what has always been done? Understanding management and leadership along with your generational characteristics will facilitate the development of a leadership and management style that is a reflection of you. Improving your ability to reach out to those outside of the organization through communication and the use of the literature will provide you with the tools to build effective nursing management practices while also leading a successful team.

BIBLIOGRAPHY

Anderson RA, Crabtree BF, Steele DJ, McDaniel, Jr. RR: Case study research: the view from complexity science, *Qual Health Res* 15(5): 669-685, 2005.

Bass B: From transactional to transformational leadership: learning to share the vision, *Organizational Dynamics* Winter:19-31, 1990.

Blanchard K, Hersey P: *Management of organizational behavior: leading human resource*, New York, 1964, Morrow.

Boychuk-Duchscher J, Cowin L: Multigenerational nurses in the workplace, *J Nurs Admin* 34(11):493-501, 2004.

Burns J: Complexity science and leadership in healthcare, *J Nurse Admin* 31(10):474-482, 2001.

Clancy T: Managing organizational complexity, *JONA* 38:272-274, 2008.

Cordeniz J: Recruitment, retention, and management of generation X: a focus on nursing professionals, *J Healthcare Manage* 47(4):237-249, 2003.

Deming E: *Out of the crisis*, Cambridge, 2000, MIT Press.

Dyess S, Sherman R: Developing a leadership mindset in new graduates, *Nurse Leader* 8:29-33, 2010.

HCPro: *Magnet status: a guide for the nursing staff*, Marblehead, Mass, 2006, HCPro.

Hellriegel D, Jackson S, Slocum J: *Management*, ed 8, Reading, Mass, 1999. Addison-Wesley.

IMedia Connection (2006): *Talking to generation now.* Retrieved from *www.imediaconnection.com.*

Institute of Medicine: *Keeping patients safe: transforming the work environment of nurses*, Washington, DC, 2004, National Academies Press.

Malleo C (2010): Each generation brings strengths, knowledge to nursing field: A nurses journal. Retrieved from *http://www.cleveland.com/healthfit/index.ssf/2010/02/each_generation_brings_strengt.html.*

Mannion J: *From management to leadership*, Chicago, 1998, American Hospital Publishers.

Marquis BL, Huston CJ: *Leadership roles and management functions in nursing*, 4 ed, Philadelphia, 2003, Lippincott Williams and Wilkins.

Martin C: Bridging the generation gap, *Nursing* 34(12):62-63, 2004.

Mendez LC: Beverly Malone: an image of leadership, *Imprint* 53(5), 2006.

NAS: *Generation Y: the millennials. Ready or not, here they come,* NAS insights, NAS Recruitment Communications, 2006. Retrieved from

www.nasrecruitment.com/TalentTips/NASinsights/GenerationY.pdf.

Pfeffer P, Sutton R: Evidence-based management, *Harvard Business Review*, Jan. 1, 2006.

Porter-O'Grady T: A different age for leadership. Part 1: new context, new content, *J Nurs Admin* 33(2):105-110, 2003a.

Porter-O'Grady T: A different age for leadership. Part 2: new rules, new roles, *J Nurs Admin* 33(3):173-178, 2003b.

Porter O'Grady T: Researching shared governance: a futility of focus, *J Nurs Admin* 33(4):251-252, 2003c.

Rothbauer-Wanish H (2009): *Four functions of management.* Retrieved from *http://businessmanagement.suite101.com/article.cfm/four_functions_of_management.*

Scott D: The generations at work: a conversation with Phyllis Kritek, *Am Nurs* 39(3):7, 2007.

Stanley J, Gannon J, Gabuat J, et al: The clinical nurse leader: a catalyst for improving quality and patient safety, *J Nursing Manage* 16:614-622, 2008.

Sullivan E, Decker P: *Effective leadership and management in nursing*, Upper Saddle River, NJ, 2009, Pearson.

Tonges M, Baloga-Altieri B, Atzori M: Amplifying nursing's voice through a staff-management partnership, *J Nurs Admin* 34(3):134-139, 2004.

Tornabeni J, Miller J: The power of partnership to shape the future of nursing: the evolution of the clinical nurse leader, *J Nursing Manage* 16:608-613, 2008.

Trossman S: Talkin' 'bout my generation: gaining awareness of differences key to easing workplace tensions, *Am Nurse* 39(3):1-2, 2007.

Van Wagner K (2007): *Leadership theories: eight major leadership theories.* Retrieved from *http://psychology.about.com/od/leadership/p/leadtheories.htm.*

Verret C (2000): Generation Y: motivating and training a new generation of employees. *Hotel Online: Ideas and Trends.* Retrieved from *www.hotel-online.com/Trends/CarolVerret/GenerationY_Nov2000.html.*

Wertheim (n.d.): Historical background of organizational behavior, *College of Business Administration, Northeastern University.* Retrieved from *www.cba.neu.edu.*

Wilson P: *Change: coping with tomorrow today*, Shawnee Mission, Kan, 1996, National Press.

Additional resources are available online at *http://evolve.elsevier.com/Zerwekh/nsgtoday/.*

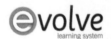

CHAPTER 11

Building Nursing Management Skills

Catherine Rosser, EdD, CNA-BC, RN, and Jessica Maack Rangel, MS, RN

We are what we repeatedly do. Excellence, then, is not an act, but a habit.
—ARISTOTLE

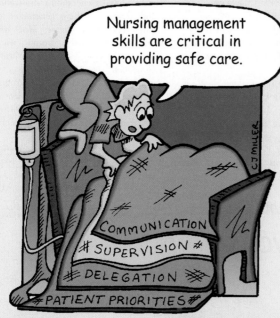

Communication should be clearly stated and directed to the appropriate, responsible individual.

After completing this chapter, you should be able to:

- Analyze effective communication as it relates to patient safety.

- Discuss TeamSTEPPS Tools as an evidence-based teamwork system to optimize patient outcomes.

- Identify current methods of transcribing physician's orders.

- Utilize a standardized hand-off communication tool (SBAR or I-SBAR-R) for receiving and giving change-of-shift report.

- Discuss strategies to manage and prioritize your time in the clinical setting.

- Define online bidding for nurse staffing and scheduling.

- Identify criteria for supervising and evaluating care provided by others.

*T*he entry level nurse is expected to demonstrate competence as a manager of patient care. The process of building nursing management skills encompasses effective communication, management of time in the clinical setting, and management of other members of the health care team. The topics in this chapter will be helpful in your development of management skills while you are a student, as well as during your transition period as a new graduate.

COMMUNICATION AND PATIENT SAFETY

We have all learned different ways of communicating. Our tone, inflections, and decibel level are all learned. Even gender plays a large part in how we communicate information. Consider asking a female colleague how her day was yesterday (or about a particular movie). Then ask a male colleague the same question. Chances are the information you receive will vary greatly in the amount of detail and the number of words it takes to tell the story.

The same is typically true in the medical field. Nurses and physicians are trained to communicate quite differently. Nurses are taught to be very broad in their narrative. They give a descriptive picture of the clinical situation. Physicians, on the other hand, learn to be very concise—they want the facts and the important points. Whether under stress or relaxed, nurses must find effective ways to communicate critical information in a very short period of time.

Communication failures are the leading cause of preventable patient deaths.

A 2003 study by The Joint Commission (TJC) reported that communication breakdown was the root cause of more than 60% of 2034 medication errors, of which 75% of those resulted in the death of the patient. In their Institute of Medicine Report, *To Err Is Human,* Kohn and colleagues (1999) recognized that medical errors in the health care delivery system had reached critical mass. These medical errors cause more than 98,000 deaths annually. Integrating teamwork and effective communication into day-to-day practice can help to reduce errors. Through exercises in teamwork, culture change, and self-awareness techniques, health care providers learn skill sets that promote expeditious and appropriate care. The Department of Defense (DoD) Patient Safety Program in collaboration with the Agency for Healthcare Research and Quality (AHRQ, 2007) developed an evidence-based teamwork system focused on improving communication and teamwork skills in the health care industry to improve patient outcomes. The result was TeamSTEPPS—Team Strategies and Tools to Enhance Performance and Patient Safety (Box 11-1). There is a multitude of other effective techniques to enhance team performance.

BOX 11-1   Goals of TeamSTEPPS

- Reduce clinical errors
- Improve patient outcomes
- Improve process outcomes
- Improve patient satisfaction
- Increase staff satisfaction
- Reduce malpractice claims

Communication challenges in practice were identified early by The Joint Commission. The National Patient Safety Goals were developed for implementation beginning in 2003 with the expectation of full implementation and compliance as a condition of accreditation. Ineffective communication was identified as the root cause for nearly 70% of all sentinel events reported. The majority of those untoward events involved communication failure. These failures involved incomplete communication among caregivers. The Joint Commission issued the National Patient Safety Goal #2: *Improve the effectiveness of communication among caregivers.* It is now a standard of expectation that facilities have a standardized approach to hand-off communication to include passing information regarding orders and test results.

How Can I Improve My Verbal Communication for Patient Safety?

Let us focus on a couple of areas. First, The Joint Commission notes that there is a big difference between verbal orders and telephone orders. Orders received verbally (with the physician present) should never be accepted except in an emergency or during a procedure where the physician is in a sterile procedural environment. There is too much opportunity for transcribing the order incorrectly. Telephone orders are acceptable because the physician is simply not present to input the orders themselves. To make this even safer, practice a "read back." In other words write down on input into the electronic health record the order or test results given to you and read it back to verify accuracy of the order and to confirm that it was understood correctly. As many as 50% of all medication errors have been directly attributed to the failure to communicate information at the point of transition (Institute for Healthcare Improvement, 2005). Specifically, any "handoff" of communication is a point of vulnerability, whether it is a telephone communication, a written communication, communication of a critical test result, or a shift-change report. All have been shown to be critical points in the patient's journey. Points of transition in communication encompass all disciplines.

Consider how often we misunderstand each other: You were supposed to bring home bread, eggs, and milk but you somehow forgot to pick up the milk. You got distracted. You had other things on your mind. You haven't been able to get much sleep lately because you have a new baby at home and you've become a bit forgetful.

These variables are called "human factors," and they often influence the communication transition between different parties. These are the very same factors that can and do affect your ability to recall information you just received.

How much more effective would it have been had you actually *written down* what you were told to bring home and then *read that list back* to the person who gave it to you? Cloudy-headed, distracted, worried, or sleepy—had you repeated the written list back to the other person, chances are the milk would have made it home too! This is precisely how to manage the verbal and telephone transmission of information from caregiver to caregiver (Box 11-2).

It's that simple! This process minimizes errors of omission and commission, and it eliminates the need to rely on memory to accurately recall an order. Your patients' lives depend on it!

How Can I Improve My Written Communication for Patient Safety?

The next natural communication concern is how we write to communicate. Legibility is a non-negotiable essential. Remember, the written word is another point of transmission that has

BOX 11-2	Safety Steps for Verbal and Phone Orders

Step 1: Order is communicated verbally.
Step 2: Order is written down verbatim or entered into the electronic health record.
Step 3: Written/entered order is read directly back to the person who gave it for confirmation that it is accurate and understood correctly.

CRITICAL THINKING
BOX 11-1

What happens when an "unsafe abbreviation" is found in a patient order?
• Step 1: Notify the author of the order containing an "unsafe abbreviation."
• Step 2: Ask for a clarifying order to clear any misinterpretation of the order.
• Step 3: Document the clarification.

proven to be a root cause of many catastrophic errors. How often has a medication ordered at 5.0 mg been mistaken for 50 mg because the pen used to mark the decimal point was too light to be noticed? Consider instead .5 mcg being mistaken for 5 mcg. The resultant overdose could have devastating consequences. When writing numbers, the trailing "0" *must be eliminated* to avoid the confusion between 5.0 mg and 50 mg. Likewise, the insertion of the "0" before the decimal is crucial to differentiate 0.5 mcg from 5 mcg.

Furthermore, many written abbreviations used to designate dosage frequency must be eliminated. Abbreviations such as Q.D. for "daily" have become targets for clarification because they can be easily misunderstood (Q.D. has been mistaken for Q.I.D. meaning "four times a day"). Many facilities have disallowed the use of these "unsafe" or "unapproved" abbreviations because of their potential for causing errors.

Organizations within the health care delivery system will have their own abbreviations, acronyms, and symbols that should not be used. These abbreviations and symbols may be in addition to the recommendations from The Joint Commission. It is imperative that you become familiar with what approved abbreviations, symbols, and acronyms that you can use. The Joint Commission has mandated that these dangerous abbreviations be eliminated from any documentation, printed or written, when communicating patient care issues (Critical Thinking Box 11-1, Table 11-1).

Once again, it's that simple! However, one more word of caution must be added for written communication. Cultural variances of the written word must be acknowledged and minimized. Consider a prescription written for a primarily Spanish-speaking patient that reads, "Take once daily for 5 days." The word *once* in Spanish means eleven! Whenever possible, interpretive services must be accessed if the language spoken and written is not the patient's primary language. Direct and succinct written and verbal communication in a language that is clearly understood by the patient is essential to appropriate and safe care. The Center for Medicare Services (CMS) requires organizations to provide language services for all patients who need it (Critical Thinking Box 11-2).

Health care literacy has become a focal point across the nation. It is staggering how many patients who are quite literate simply do not understand their discharge instructions or medication administration directions. The National Library of Medicine (n.d.) reported that reading

TABLE 11-1 The Joint Commission Official "Do Not Use" List of Abbreviations

OFFICIAL "DO NOT USE" LIST*

Do Not Use	Potential Problem	Use Instead
U (unit)	Mistaken for "0" (zero), the number "4" (four) or "cc"	Write "unit"
IU (International Unit)	Mistaken for IV (intravenous) or the number 10 (ten)	Write "International Unit"
Q.D.QD, q.d. qd (daily)	Mistaken for each other	Write "daily"
Q.O.D.QOD, q.o.d. qod (every other day)	Period after the Q mistaken for "I" and the "O" mistaken for "I"	Write "every other day"
Trailing zero (X.0 mg)†	Decimal point is missed	Write X mg
Lack of leading zero (.X mg)		Write 0.X mg
MS	Can mean morphine sulfate or magnesium sulfate	Write "morphine sulfate"
MSO₄ and MgSO₄	Confused for one another	Write "magnesium sulfate"

*Applies to all orders and all medication-related documentation that is handwritten (including free-text computer entry) or on preprinted forms.

†**Exception:** A "trailing zero" may be used only where required to demonstrate the level of precision of the value being reported, such as for laboratory results, imaging studies that report size of lesions, or catheter/tube sizes. It may not be used in medication orders or other medication-related documentation.

ADDITIONAL ABBREVIATIONS, ACRONYMS AND SYMBOLS (FOR POSSIBLE FUTURE INCLUSION IN THE OFFICIAL "DO NOT USE" LIST)

Do Not Use	Potential Problem	Use Instead
> (greater than)	Misinterpreted as the number "7" (seven) or the letter "L"	Write "greater than"
< (less than)	Confused for one another	Write "less than"
Abbreviations for drug names	Misinterpreted due to similar abbreviations for multiple drugs	Write drug names in full
Apothecary units	Unfamiliar to many practitioners Confused with metric units	Use metric units
@	Mistaken for the number "2" (two)	Write "at"
cc	Mistaken for U (units) when poorly written	Write "mL" or "milliliters"
μg	Mistaken for mg (milligrams) resulting in 1000-fold overdose	Write "mcg" or "micrograms"

From The Joint Commission: *Official 'Do Not Use' List.* Retrieved from *www.jointcommission.org/assets/1/18/dnu_list.pdf.*

CRITICAL THINKING BOX 11-2   Role-play with a partner transcribing verbal physician orders and reading back those orders for clarity and accuracy. Can you identify any "unsafe abbreviations?"

abilities of adults are typically three to four grade levels behind the last year of school completed. A high-school graduate typically has a seventh or eighth grade reading level. Therefore it is essential for the health care provider to have the patient repeat back what they understand about their condition, medications, education and discharge instructions. As a health care professional, you now speak a language that is quite unfamiliar to the public. Consider that you and the patient's physician may refer to their condition of high blood pressure as hypertension. Does the patient realize this is the same thing or do they think they have a hyper condition in which they cannot sit still? You might be surprised when you hear what the patient understands about their own condition!

Transcribing Written Orders. In the process of providing safe patient care, it is essential that physician or health care provider orders be communicated clearly and correctly to the health care team. The physician order must clearly indicate what is to be done, when it should be done, and how often it should be done. All orders must include the patient's identifying information and the current date and time. Table 11-2 provides a summary of the various types of orders. The process for transcribing orders may involve other health team members, such as the unit secretary, but it is the nurse's responsibility to verify that the orders are implemented correctly. This involves making sure that the order is clearly understood and legible. If any component of the order is not clear, the physician should be contacted for clarification (Box 11-3).

The computer prescriber order entry (CPOE) is an electronic means of entering a physician order. This system has the benefit of reducing errors by minimizing the ambiguity of handwritten orders, as well as intercepting errors when they most commonly occur—at the time the order is

---

TABLE 11-2   Types of Written Orders

Type	Description
One-time-only order	An order for a medication or procedure to be carried out only one time.
PRN order	An order to be carried out when the patient needs it, not on a scheduled basis. For example, a PRN pain medication order.
Standing order	A physician's routine set of orders for a specific procedure or condition. For example, a surgeon may have standing preoperative and/or postoperative orders for an abdominal surgery patient.
STAT order	An order that is to be implemented immediately. Usually, it is a one-time order. The term is derived from the Latin word statim, which means "immediately."

BOX 11-3   Steps in Transcribing Orders

1. Read all of the order(s).
2. Determine whether all request forms (laboratory, medication, diagnostic test) and/or phone calls have been initiated.
3. Review notes for order entries.
4. Follow institution policy for rechecking orders and signing off.

written. The CPOE system is integrated with other patient information, including laboratory, diagnostic results, and medication records.

COMMUNICATING WHEN IT IS CRITICAL—WHAT DO YOU NEED TO DO?

Critical Patient Tests

Communication of critical test results is yet another vulnerable time for errors to occur. Critical test results warrant expeditious communication to the responsible licensed caregiver without delay. This includes not only laboratory panic values, but also other diagnostic test results. The primary goal is to get the critical information to the person who can fix the problem in the quickest way. Documentation of how this was accomplished is essential to promoting and providing validation that the critical test result was communicated and if needed, acted upon.

Often, nurses are notified of a critical test result without passing that communication along to the physician who has the scope and authority to act upon that result. Assumptions are sometimes made that the physician is aware of the test result or that notifying the nurse is enough. The licensed caregiver in this case is the individual who is able to act on the result of the test. The nurse is often NOT that person. The physician who ordered the test IS.

> "When in doubt, call it out" to the physician and document the results of that conversation when clarifying ambiguous orders.

Managing critical information regarding a patient's test result is all about getting the information to the right person. What should be done if you cannot reach the physician who ordered a test with critical results? As a nurse, you may find it necessary to initiate the chain-of-command policy. Most institutions have a process that identifies a step-by-step method of whom to contact in case the physician cannot be reached The nurse continues to care for the patient, documenting the care that has been provided and all attempts that were made to contact the physician. Finally, the nurse is responsible for determining that resolution has occurred and documenting the resolution in the medical record. It is vital that you become aware of the chain-of-command policy at your place of employment and understand situations where it warrants being initiated. Merely documenting that you notified the physician in the patient's chart does not take responsibility of the patient's current health status off of you.

Critical Hand-Off Communication

The Joint Commission's National Patient Safety Goal #2 clearly states that health care facilities must implement a standardized approach to communications. The implementation of a hand-off communication tool helps to reinforce to clinicians that they have a responsibility to provide succinct, accurate information and safe quality care throughout the patient's hospitalization, thus making the patient's hospital journey a safe one.

One of the communication modalities that is often employed in the health care setting is called, "I-SBAR-R Communication." Originally, this tool was called SBAR, now it has been updated to I-SBAR-R to reinforce the importance of patient safety goal #2 (readback communication) and patient identification. Integrating I-SBAR-R techniques into your communication to other team members will organize your discussion and promote patient safety (Grbach, 2008).

I = Identification. Identify yourself and your patient (two identifiers to be used)

S = Situation. What is going on?

B = Background. What led to this? Patient's status prior to this?

A = Assessment. What do you think is happening?

R = Response or Request. What do you think should happen?

R = Readback or Response. Receiver acknowledges information given: What is their response?

Scenario: Mrs. Smith is an 84-year-old patient that was admitted with a diagnosis of uncontrolled diabetes. It's 2:00 AM and the nurse notices the patient in respiratory distress. She assesses Mrs. Smith and calls the physician:

"Dr. Brossett, I'm Nancy Jones, RN (I) and I've been caring for Mrs. Jane Smith, your 84-year-old patient in room 302 that you admitted tonight, who is experiencing increased shortness of breath and is very anxious. (S)

"She's not ever had an episode like this before. She has no history of respiratory distress, asthma, or COPD. She was sitting up in bed and had a sudden onset of shortness of breath. She does have a history of blood clots. (B)

"She is breathing 42 breaths a minute. Her pulse oximeter is showing an oxygen saturation of 82% on room air. She has bilateral breath sounds with some expiratory wheezes in all lobes. Her skin is pale, cool, and clammy. She is oriented but very anxious. She is afebrile, pulse of 120, and blood pressure of 92/60. Her glucose is 130. She is sitting up in bed; compression stockings are in place. (A)

"I've called a rapid response team. Would you like me to obtain arterial blood gases or administer some oxygen? Could you come in and see her?" (R)

Dr. Brossett states, "Thanks for the update on Mrs. Smith's condition. Please start the oxygen and call the laboratory to draw arterial blood gases. I'll be in within the next hour to see her." (R)

Imagine how differently this conversation could have gone had the nurse not had an organized manner to communicate this urgent situation, especially in the middle of the night when the physician may have been asleep!

I-SBAR-R provides a common and predictable structure and can be used in virtually any clinical setting. Use of I-SBAR-R also refines critical thinking skills—*before* communication is delivered, the person initiating the communication makes an assessment of the patient and gives a recommendation for ongoing care. I-SBAR-R is a communication strategy that helps organize and focus on critical information (Box 11-4). A recent initiative from The Joint Commission encourages the use of the acronym SHARE to promote effective handoff communication (Box 11-5).

Shift Change—So Much to Say ... So Little Time

Any time there is an exchange of information, there is a possibility of miscommunication either by omission (forgetting to share something important) or by simply focusing on the things that aren't as essential as others (the patient's sister's son who is coming to visit versus the pending critical test result). How can the nurse possibly begin to decide what is important to discuss in the short amount of time given to the change-of-shift report? With a standardized method to

| BOX 11-4 | Situation-Background-Assessment-Recommendation (I-SBAR-R) Tool |

I = Identification: Identify yourself and your patient (two identifiers to be used)
S = Situation: What is happening at the present time?
B = Background: What are the circumstances leading up to this situation?
A = Assessment: What do I think the problem is?
R = Recommendation: What should we do to correct the problem?
R = Readback or Response: Receiver acknowledges information given: What is their response?

Grbach W. (2008): Reformulating SBAR to "I-SBAR-R," *QSEN.* Retrieved from *www.qsen.org/teachingstrategy.php?id=33.*

| BOX 11-5 | The Joint Commission Handoff Communication Acronym: SHARE |

To improve effective patient hand-offs, The Joint Commission recommends following the "SHARE" acronym, which stands for:
• **S**tandardizing critical content: Make sure a patient's history and other key information is readily available and easy to comprehend.
• **H**ardwiring within your system: Identify new and existing technologies to aid in a patient's hand-off.
• **A**llowing opportunity to ask questions: Rather than take all information about a patient at face value, check and double check with others involved in the patient's care to ensure accuracy.
• **R**einforcing quality and measurement: Essentially, hold your colleagues (as well as yourself) accountable for actions taken and monitoring compliance.
• **E**ducating and coaching: Teach all colleagues the ins and outs of successful hand-offs.

From The Joint Commission (2010): Joint Commission Center for Transforming Healthcare tackles miscommunication among caregivers. Retrieved from *www.centerfortransforminghealthcare.org/news/display.aspx?newsid-23.*

"hand off" or communicate the care of the patient to another clinician, there is less likely to be a miscommunication of information. What this means for the nurse is that anytime a report is given to another, the adopted way of communicating information must be followed.

Here are some of the most critical elements of a change-of-shift report to include the following:
▪ Patient identifiers (typically name and date of birth)
▪ Diagnoses
▪ Physician/s on the case
▪ Pertinent medical/social history
▪ Current physical condition (review of systems)
▪ Resuscitation status (no resuscitation, full resuscitation)
▪ Nutritional status (nutritional intake, NPO, supplements)
▪ Pending or critical issues and tests

After the verbal report, a quick introduction with both off-going and oncoming caregivers is optimal. This provides the opportunity for the patient and the family to greet the oncoming caregiver and for both caregivers to assess the patient together, especially where there may be skin integrity issues or wounds involved. When I-SBAR-R guidelines are consistently used, the shift report and patient transfer are organized, thorough, and yet concise. Furthermore, important information is not forgotten, and the transition of care is smoother for everyone involved. The transition is then smoother.

How Can I Deal with All the Interruptions?

Interruptions are one of the major threats to effective time management. Not only is time taken away from goal-directed activities, but also additional time is needed to get refreshed and back on track. Of course, some interruptions are inevitable, but they can be minimized. Begin by recognizing when *you* are interrupting yourself. Do you start one task and then begin another rather than concentrating on completing the first? Do you respond to added distractions (television, ringing telephones, and chatty friends) at times when task completion is required? In these instances, you are cooperating with the interruption and allowing yourself to be interrupted. When possible, in non-emergency situations, use your time-management strategies and communication skills to remain focused on the task at hand. People will accept that you may need to get back to them when you have finished what you are doing. Write down when and where you can reach them and then follow through. Turn off your telephone's ringer and let the message service or answering machine pick up your calls, but check it every hour or so. This way you can return important calls when it is convenient.

Responding to interruptions can also mean you are doing your job. For example, when you are interrupted to answer a patient's call light or answer a physician's telephone call, you are doing your job. These activities are part of your nursing responsibilities. They may not be of an urgent nature and can be delayed a short time, or they may be urgent and necessitate immediate response—either way, you will need to deal with them eventually. Rather than feeling that you have been interrupted, remind yourself that what you are doing is accomplishing part of your job. There are many aspects of your job that you cannot control, but you can always choose how to respond.

Some facilities have identified medication administration and shift report as a critical time to minimize interruptions. To signify the need to not interrupt the caregiver engaging these critical tasks, some facilities have the staff wear orange vests until the task is complete. This way, everyone is aware from the physician to the families that the caregiver is engaged in a critical task that requires their full attention (Pape & Richards, 2010).

Everyone needs some totally uninterrupted time in which to relax, refocus, and reenergize. During clinical experience, at work, or at home, spend a few minutes in a quiet place by yourself (e.g., the nurses' lounge, the chapel, an empty patient room, a bedroom at home) to evaluate what is happening or what needs to happen next. Take several deep, slow breaths; read; meditate; relax; or get in touch with yourself. (Parents with small children can take turns watching their children so each adult can have some uninterrupted private time). Relaxing and taking a break from fast-paced activity will reenergize you and result in more productive use of your time. Self-care is the balance that helps you restore from a hard day at work!

What Skills Do I Need to Use the Telephone Effectively?

Many nurses spend time on the telephone talking with physicians, patients and their families, and other health care workers. Here are some tips for making telephone communication productive. It is always polite to ask the person you are calling if this is a convenient time to talk. You may encounter difficulties reaching people by telephone. If a game of "telephone tag" persists after two attempts, leave a message stating exactly when you will be available to talk (and then be there).

If you anticipate your conversation will involve complex information, make notes ahead of time so that you can keep your conversation as focused and brief as possible. Go ahead and try

> **BOX 11-6**   Tips for Communicating with Physicians on the Telephone
>
> 1. Say who you are right away.
> 2. Do not apologize for phoning.
> 3. State your business briefly but completely.
> 4. Ask for specific orders when appropriate.
> 5. If you want the doctor to assess the patient, say so.
> 6. If the doctor is coming, ask when to expect him or her.
> 7. If you get cut off, call back.
> 8. Document attempts to reach a doctor.
> 9. If a doctor is rude or abusive, tell him or her so.
> 10. If you cannot reach a doctor or get what you need, notify your chain of command.

CRITICAL THINKING BOX 11-3

Develop a flow sheet to organize your time and patient care for your clinical schedule. Obtain an assignment for an RN on one of the units to which you are assigned for clinical. Can you prioritize and delegate this RN's assignment appropriately?

organizing your conversation in the I-SBAR-R communication format. After discussing detailed, critical information over the telephone, it is wise to follow up with a written communication to the other person. Important telephone calls should also be followed up in writing. This helps clarify and confirm the information discussed. If your telephone conversation requires a follow-up action, you need to keep a written record of that action.

It is difficult to focus on a telephone conversation if you are doing something else at the same time. Your communication will be more effective if you do one thing at a time. (How many times have you been annoyed by a driver who is also talking on a cellular telephone or texting?) Once you have finished your discussion, get off the phone; do not stay on the phone to chitchat or gossip. Communicating with physicians on the telephone presents a challenge to recent graduates. Box 11-6 highlights some helpful tips.

MANAGING TIME IN THE CLINICAL SETTING

One of the main sources of job dissatisfaction reported by nurses is too little time. This "limited time" to provide patient care has been accelerated by the nursing shortage combined with cost-effective staffing, the increase in numbers of patients, and the higher acuity of these patients. In response to this issue, nurses must develop competent skills in time management and priority setting. Nurses can use several techniques to maximize their time spent providing patient care. Remember Pareto's 80/20 Rule. In this case, 20% of your patients will require 80% of your time! Those 20% should be the sickest patients. When their care and needs are met first, the rest of your assignment is much easier. It is important to determine which patients require the most time (80%). Then ask yourself—Do they require time that can be delegated to someone else, or do they require the time because they are the most unstable and ill patients? (Critical Thinking Box 11-3, Figure 11-1.)

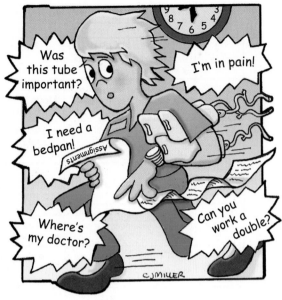

FIGURE 11-1
Can you work overtime?

Request consistent patient assignments whenever possible. This allows you to develop relationships with your patients and their families and promotes time management, because you become familiar with the special needs of these patients.

Get Organized Before the Shift Report

Develop your own work organization sheet or use one provided by the agency to write down information you need to begin coordinating care for a group of patients. Modify this form as you discover areas that need improvement. Make several copies so that you will always have one handy. Avoid gossiping and other distractions as you receive a report and begin to fill out your time management (or work organization) form. Get the information needed to plan the care for your patients and begin to organize your shift activities (Figure 11-2).

Prioritize Your Care

Setting priorities has become difficult in light of the dichotomy between the expected outcomes of efficiency and effectiveness and the perceived limitations of resources, including time. Priority setting is not only based on patient needs; it is also influenced by the needs of the organization and the accountability of the nurse. Priorities are established and reprioritized throughout the day according to patients' assessed needs and unscheduled interruptions, both minor and emergent. Plan your day around the patient you perceive to be the sickest. This is the patient who is at the greatest risk from harm if you do not address his or her needs first.

Name: *Susan*

Time	Activities	Room 416	Room 417	Room 418
7–8	✓ MAR Shift report ✓ vitals	✓ Bld sugar 7:30 insulin	I.V. @ 125/hr. turn ✓ pulses	7:45 pre-op NPO ✓ consent form
8–9	assessments meal trays	meds x3–9 up for meals	meds x2–9 If leg dsg. assist c̄ meal	To OR
9–10		shower chg bed ✓ pain meds	complete bath ✓ pulses turn	
10–11	Chart			Chg bed
11–12	meal trays lunch	up for meals ✓ Bld sugar insulin?	turn ✓ pulses assist c̄ meal	
12–13	Chart assessment	meds x2–12	IVPB–12	Return fm OR? N.G. suction I.V.
13–14		diabetic teaching	turn ✓ pulses If. leg dressing change	
14–15	I & O's IV's report info			

FIGURE 11-2

Work organization sheet.

Prioritize patients by using the ABCD system or Maslow's hierarchy of needs. Of highest priority are the patients with problems or potential problems related to the airway. Next are those having any difficulty with breathing, and then those with circulation problems. When using Maslow's hierarchy of needs to assist with prioritization, you need to meet physiological needs first: that is, resolve any difficulty with oxygenation first. Be flexible and reprioritize as emergencies occur.

Prioritize your patients after you receive report and immediately proceed to the patient whom you have placed highest on your priority list. Remember that this prioritization may change as you complete your initial assessments. Additional modifications will be made according to the placement of patients' rooms to avoid wasted time and movement. When you first enter a patient's room, introduce yourself, perform hand hygiene measures, and complete a quick environmental assessment. Think about any supplies you will need when returning to the room. Complete the focused assessment, validate the safety of your patient, and proceed to your next patient. Once you have completed your initial rounds, reassess your initial prioritization, modify according to your assessments, and plan your day.

CRITICAL THINKING BOX 11-4

How do the efficient nurses on your clinical unit prioritize their time and their patients?

For example, a characteristic assignment for the day could be:

A patient who is 1 day postoperative and wants something for pain

A geriatric patient who is vomiting

A patient with diabetes who is angry about the care from the last shift

A geriatric patient who has soiled the bed with urine

Which of these patients needs your immediate attention? Most likely the one who is vomiting because this patient is at increased risk for aspiration. Next is probably the patient who is in pain, then the geriatric patient who has soiled the bed with urine, and so on. With each patient, you may spend less than 5 minutes in the room before you move on to the next patient. But you will have a good idea of what each patient's immediate needs are.

Identify the busiest times on the unit; do not schedule a dressing change when medications need to be given. Plan on preparing medications at least 30 to 45 minutes before the hour they are due. This will provide time to research any medications with which you are unfamiliar. Do not procrastinate; start early. If you have dressing changes for several patients, start with the cleanest and progress to the more contaminated wounds (Critical Thinking Box 11-4).

Watch those nurses who always seem to get everything done, done well, and still enjoy nursing. Ask them about their "secrets" of time management, and try out some of their tips.

Organize Your Work by Patient

By organizing work by patient, the nurse maximizes the number of tasks that can be accomplished with each visit to the patient. The nurse thinks strategically: "How can I multitask or accomplish several objectives in one visit to the patient?" By using this technique, the nurse can combine assessment, administration of medications, and teaching during one patient visit (see Figure 11-2).

Another way to organize and coordinate the needs of the patient is by implementation of hourly rounds. This is where the caregivers (both nursing and ancillary help) can alternate visiting the patients every hour to verify the patients' needs are met proactively. This is often referred to as meeting the "three Ps": pain, position, and potty. Is the patient in pain? Does the patient need assistance in changing position? Does the patient need assistance in toileting needs? By implementing this strategy, patients use call bells less, have fewer falls, and have higher patient satisfaction. It also assists the nurse in attending to prioritized tasks with minimal interruptions (Figure 11-3).

MANAGING OTHERS

Communicating and getting along with other people are always challenging tasks. Most people are easygoing, straightforward, and supportive. They add to your energy and ability to function

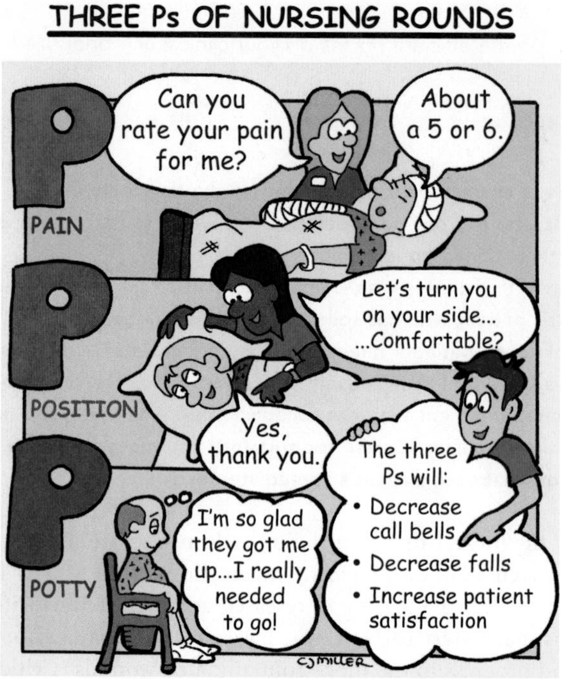

FIGURE 11-3
3Ps of hourly rounds.

effectively, and they contribute to your goal attainment. However, if you experience a phone call or visit from someone who just wants to talk when you are busy, you need to avoid being trapped. Tell them, "Now is not a good time. Could we discuss this later?" or even "I've got another appointment. Could we postpone this conversation until tomorrow?" Some individuals drain energy from others and from organizational accomplishment through their whining, criticizing, negative thinking, chronic lateness, poor crisis management, dependency, aggression, and similar unproductive behaviors. Occasional exhibitions of such behavior in relation to a personal crisis are understandable. However, when people use these behaviors as their everyday *modus operandi* (method of operating), they interfere with attainment of individual and organizational goals. Even in the best of human relationships, conflict and extreme emotions are inevitable. To protect your time and achieve your goals, it may be necessary to limit your time with such individuals. Avoidance is one strategy. Learning to say "no" and assertive communication can help as well.

What About Delegating and Time Management?

You may have observed nurses performing nonnursing activities during your clinical experience, which include but are not limited to cleaning, running errands, clerical duties, and stocking supplies. Appropriate delegation of non-nursing tasks can provide the nurse with additional time to dedicate to patient care. Even some patient care tasks can be delegated, once the training and competence of unlicensed personnel have been verified. These requirements vary in different states and institutions. Review Chapter 14 for more specifics on delegation.

Delegation includes more than asking someone to do something. Delegation has been defined by the American Nurses Association (ANA) as "the transfer of responsibility for the performance of an activity from one individual to another, with the former retaining accountability for the outcome" (ANA, 1995, p 4). This definition emphasizes that delegation increases the responsibility and accountability of the registered nurse (RN). Be sure you know the delegation rules and regulations of your state's nursing practice act. Additionally, you will need to know the delegation policies and job descriptions of nursing team members in your employing agency.

In general, most caregivers are by nature people-pleasers. We are even taught to anticipate and meet the needs of others. Because of this, we tend to have great difficulty in sharing and delegating the multitude of responsibilities given to us. Delegation is a learned skill and essential for us to adopt in order to be successful.

To increase delegation skills, it is sometimes necessary to overcome the myth of perfection. When you teach or train someone else to do a delegated task, initially that person may not be able to perform the activity perfectly or as well as you can. That is not important. What is important is that the person is able to meet the standards required to complete the task and to appropriately delegate to others. With experience, most people will improve (and may even surpass you) (Critical Thinking Box 11-5).

Determine which patients are the most stable and whose positive progress can be anticipated. The stable patients with predictable progress should be the first whose care is delegated. The care of unstable, unpredictable patients should only be delegated to an RN. An RN should also be assigned to any patient who is undergoing a procedure or treatment that may cause them to become unstable.

When you are dealing with unlicensed assistive personnel (UAP), you can delegate to them those activities that have specific guidelines that are unchanging. For example, feeding, dressing, bathing, obtaining equipment for the nursing staff, picking up meal trays, refilling water containers, straightening up cluttered rooms—all of these activities should have guidelines according to the institution policies, fit within the job description, and be followed by the unlicensed assistive personnel.

Patient teaching and discharge planning are also the responsibility of the RN. RNs are responsible for determining the patient's learning needs and establishing a teaching plan. It is also the RN's responsibility to coordinate and implement the discharge planning. The RN should request input from all nursing personnel who have assisted in providing care for the patient or who have been otherwise involved (e.g., dietary, physical therapy) in the patient's care. Once the RN implements the teaching plan, it is important that the other RNs, licensed practical nurses, vocational nurses, and unlicensed assistive personnel are aware of what the patient has been taught so that they may follow up and report any pertinent observations to the RN (Critical Thinking Box 11-6).

 CRITICAL THINKING BOX 11-5   On your clinical unit, how many levels of personnel provide patient care? How is the nursing care of patients delegated?

> **CRITICAL THINKING**
> **BOX 11-6**
>
> Determine how and to whom patient care is delegated on your current clinical unit. What guidelines are implemented?

Nursing care makes a difference in patient outcomes. This care is more than providing tasks. It incorporates assessment, care planning, and initiation of interventions, interdisciplinary collaboration, and outcome evaluations. It includes patient and family teaching, therapeutic communication, counseling, discharge planning, and teaching. To maximize the impact nursing care can have on patient outcomes, nurses must develop and integrate multiple strategies to promote effective time management.

Supervising and Evaluating the Care Provided by Others

To meet the demanding and complex needs of the public for safe quality patient care, it is imperative that the utilization of all nursing resources be maximized. The licensed practical nurse and other unlicensed personnel can function as an extension to the RN as a provider of care if definitive supervision and evaluative guidelines are established. State boards of nursing are responsible for articulating those guidelines.

> Unlicensed personnel: An individual not licensed as a health care provider; a nursing student providing care that is not a part of his or her nursing program.

Supervision entails providing direction, evaluation, and follow-up by the RN of nursing tasks that have been delegated to unlicensed personnel. The following criteria apply to the RN who functions in a supervisor capacity:

- Provide directions with clear expectations of how the task is to be performed.
- Verify the task is being performed according to standards of practice.
- Monitor the task being performed; intervene if necessary.
- Evaluate the status of the patient.
- Evaluate the performance of the task.
- Provide feedback as necessary.
- Reassess the plan of care and modify as needed.

These criteria apply to RNs who delegate nursing care for patients with acute conditions or those patients who are in an acute care environment. The continued growing need for unlicensed personnel, as well as the role of the practical nurse in providing care, will require the RN to serve in the supervisor and evaluator role and to be accountable and responsible for those assigned nursing tasks.

It is never easy to give constructive feedback regarding a deficiency or an area needing improvement; however, sandwiching the constructive feedback between layers of recognition and positive reinforcement makes the communication more palatable and more effective. Keep in mind that when providing constructive feedback, you are simply providing your evaluation of an individual's performance, not his or her character. Here's an example of how a supervisor effectively used the "sandwich" method of providing constructive feedback.

Carrie is a new graduate who has completed the first 6 weeks of employment. She is consistently tardy and delays shift report. When Carrie arrived in the supervisor's office for her evaluation, the supervisor was very nice in her approach to talking with her. The supervisor reviewed with Carrie the progress she has made in orienting to the unit and managing the care for a group of patients. Carrie was pleased with the recognition of her progress. Next, the supervisor addressed Carrie's tardiness on the unit and how it has affected the shift report. Carrie acknowledged this as a problem and discussed the situation, making some suggestions to alleviate the problem. The supervisor was supportive of Carrie's suggestions and her initiative to examine the tardiness issue.

When providing constructive feedback, do not:

- Argue with the staff person's perception of the event
- Reprimand, scold, or belittle the staff person
- Offer unsolicited personal advice (e.g., "This is what I think you should do …")
- Coerce or make intimidating statements to demonstrate your authority

CONCLUSION

Building nursing management skills is a new task for the graduate nurse. Implementing management skills in the clinical setting is challenging. By using effective communication, time management in the clinical setting, and managing other members of the health care team, the new graduate can begin to grow professionally and personally.

Once you get organized with your clinical schedule, you will become a more effective nurse and will begin to have the time to provide safe nursing care, which leads to positive patient outcomes.

BIBLIOGRAPHY

Agency for Healthcare Research and Quality (2007): TeamSTEPPS™: Strategies and Tools to Enhance Performance and Patient Safety. Retrieved from *www.ahrq.gov/qual/teamstepps.*

American Nurses Association: *The American Nurses Association basic guide to safe delegation*, Washington, DC, 1995, American Nurses Association. Retrieved from *www.safestaffingsaveslives.org/ WhatisSafeStaffing/ SafeStaffingPrinciples/ PrinciplesofDelegation.aspx.*

Grbach W (2008): Reformulating SBAR to "I-SBAR-R." Retrieved from QSEN *www.qsen.org/teachingstrategy.php? id=33.*

Institute for Healthcare Improvement (2005): IHI Saving Lives Web & Action Programs: Preventing adverse drug events through medication reconciliation. Retrieved from *www.IHI.org.*

Kohn L, Corrigan J, Donaldson M, eds: *Institute of Medicine Report: to err is human: building a safer health system*, Washington, DC, 1999, National Academy Press.

National Library of Medicine (n.d.): *Health literacy.* Retrieved from *http:// nnlm.gov/outreach/consumer/ hlthlit.html.*

Pape T, Richards BL: Stop "knowledge creep," *Nursing Management* 41(2):8, 2010.

The Joint Commission: *Patient safety: essentials for health care*, ed 4, Oakbrook Terrace, Ill, 2006, Joint Commission Resources.

The Joint Commission (2010): *Handoff Communication.* Retrieved from *www. centerfortransforminghealthcare.org.*

Additional resources are available online at *http://evolve.elsevier.com/Zerwekh/nsgtoday/.*

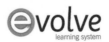

CHAPTER 12

Effective Communication and Team Building

JoAnn Zerwekh, MSN, EdD, RN

> *To effectively communicate, we must realize that we are all different in the way we perceive the world and use this understanding as a guide to our communication with others.*
> —ANTHONY ROBBINS

> *If you can laugh together, you can work together.*
> —ROBERT ORBEN

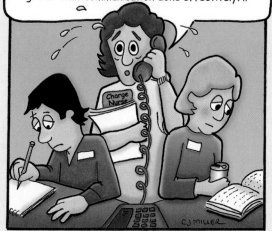

Communication should be clearly stated and directed to the appropriate, responsible individual.

After completing this chapter, you should be able to:

- Describe the basic components of communication.

- Identify effective ways of communicating with other health care workers.

- Describe an assertive communication style.

- Apply effective communication skills in common nursing activities.

- Identify different types of groups and explain group process.

- Discuss team building and group problem solving.

*C*ommunication is like breathing—we do it all the time, and the better we do it, the better we feel. At times communication can be so subtle; others are not able to comprehend the sender. Communication between people in everyday life is an exercise in subtleties and interpretations. The more personal the information, the more indirect and obscure the message becomes. In nursing, indirect communications and obscure terminology can be the difference between life and death. When you say, "I want to be clear when I communicate to others," it is no different from washing windows. The clearer the window, the better we see. Communicating what we see, what needs to be done, and teaching patients what they need to know is part of the foundation of nursing care (Critical Thinking Box 12-1).

COMMUNICATION IN THE WORKPLACE

Sharing information with the members of the health care team requires different approaches. This communication on a daily basis may involve delegation of a nursing procedure to nursing personnel, clarification of a physician's orders, reevaluation of a patient care assignment of another health care team member, or coordination of various hospital departments (e.g., radiology, dietary, pharmacy) to provide nursing care. Create role-playing situations with your peers by taking turns being in the supervisor and subordinate roles (Critical Thinking Box 12-2).

How Can I Communicate Effectively with My Supervisor?

Upward communication with supervisors takes on a formal nature. It is important to learn and then use the channels of communication. If you are a team member, this means you share information with your team leader. The team leader shares information with the supervisor, who shares information with the assistant vice president of nursing, who shares information with the vice president of nursing, and so on. From this example, you can see the communication approach taken with the appropriate chain of command.

Do you remember the game you played as a child in which someone whispers a secret to the next person, and each person repeats the secret down the line until the last person speaks the secret aloud? The secret may have started out as "Jenny was out picking berries today so she can bake a pie." By the end of the line, it may have become "Jenny is so allergic to cherries that she breaks out into hives." The point is that messages can get very distorted when they travel through the chain of command in the upward flow of communication. Arredondo (2000) says it is important in communicating with superiors to state needs clearly, explain the rationales for requests,

CRITICAL THINKING

BOX 12-1

TRY THIS ...

1. How many different ways can you communicate this sentence to change its meaning or tone? "I do not care how you've done that procedure before; do it my way now."
2. The instructor says to you, "Come to my office at 2:00. There's something I want to talk to you about." What are some possible interpretations of the message?
3. A patient's spouse says to you, "I do not need your help when we go home." How many possible explanations can you come up with regarding the meaning of the communication?

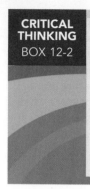

CRITICAL THINKING
BOX 12-2

TRY THIS...

Role-play these situations with your classmates. Try taking turns being the boss and subordinate roles.
1. The head nurse has asked the team leader and the nurse providing care to Mr. Smith to explain his progress.
2. You are the team leader giving reports to two nursing assistants and one LPN who will be working on your team today.
3. You are caring for a patient who has been newly diagnosed with insulin-dependent diabetes. You discuss the patient's care with the dietitian, the social worker, and the patient's wife.

and suggest the benefits to the larger unit. It is also important to listen objectively to the response of the supervisor because there may be good reasons for granting or not granting the request.

Arredondo (2000) gives the following tips for talking to your supervisor:
1. Keep your supervisor informed.
2. If a problem is developing, make an appointment to talk it over. Have specific information available, especially written documentation of facts. Focus on problem solving, not just the problems.
3. Show that you have important information to share and a sense of responsibility.
4. Be careful which words you use. Avoid blaming others, exaggeration, and overly dramatic expressions.
5. Do not talk to your supervisor when angry, and do not respond with anger. Use "I" statements, and explain what you think.
6. If you want to present a new idea, give your supervisor a written proposal, then meet to discuss it after the supervisor has read it.
7. Accept feedback, and learn from it.
8. Never go above or around your supervisor. Always communicate directly with your supervisor first before going further up the chain of command.

How Can I Communicate Effectively with Other Nursing Personnel?

When you speak with other professional nurses, you communicate in a lateral, or horizontal, flow of information. This flow is based on a concept of equality, in which no person holds more power than the other. This type of communication is best done in a work climate that promotes a sense of trust and respect among colleagues. When nurses work well together, their cohesiveness makes success more likely. This takes work and the deliberate use of facilitative messages (Northouse, 2001).

Ideally, professional nurses should view themselves as equals in their interactions with members of other health care disciplines, and their approach to communication should be a lateral one, even with physicians. At the basis of this communication is the ability of the nurse to see himself or herself as competent and worthy of being an equal to physicians, social workers, dietitians, and others. To gain this self-confidence is a major goal of every recent graduate. The use of effective communication practices, as described in this chapter, and communication reporting tools (see Chapter 11 for information on hands-off communication) will help you achieve that goal.

Even a recent graduate will soon be providing direction to licensed nursing personnel and unlicensed assistive nursing personnel (see Chapter 14 for further information on delegation). It is important to remember that these people have needs for satisfaction and self-esteem, too. Directions do not need to be given in the form of authoritative commands unless an emergency demands immediate action in a prescribed way. Marquis and Huston (2000) suggest that when you provide direction, you need to think through exactly what you want to be done, by whom, and when. You need to get the full attention of the other person so you know he or she hears you accurately. You should give clear, simple instructions in step-by-step order, using a supportive tone of voice. Before the other person goes to do the task, ask for feedback to verify that he or she has accurately heard your instructions. Follow-up is necessary to be sure your directions were carried out and to find out what happened, in case something more needs to be done. Involving personnel at other levels of nursing care in the planning and evaluation of the care will increase their sense of responsibility for the outcomes and will help you to seem less authoritarian. Refer to the checklist in Critical Thinking Box 12-3 to identify areas needed for growth.

CRITICAL THINKING BOX 12-3

FACILITATION SKILLS CHECKLIST

Directions: Periodically during the clinical experience, use this checklist to identify areas needed for growth and progress made. Think of your clinical patient experiences. Indicate the extent of your agreement with each of the following statements by marking the scale: **SA, strongly agree; A, agree; NS, not sure; D, disagree; SD, strongly disagree.**

1. I maintain good eye contact.	SA	A	NS	D	SD
2. Most of my verbal comments follow the lead of the other person.	SA	A	NS	D	SD
3. I encourage others to talk about feelings.	SA	A	NS	D	SD
4. I am able to ask open-ended questions.	SA	A	NS	D	SD
5. I can restate and clarify a person's ideas.	SA	A	NS	D	SD
6. I can summarize in a few words the basic ideas of a long statement made by a person.	SA	A	NS	D	SD
7. I can make statements that reflect the person's feelings.	SA	A	NS	D	SD
8. I can share my feelings relevant to the discussion when appropriate to do so.	SA	A	NS	D	SD
9. I am able to give feedback.	SA	A	NS	D	SD
10. At least 75% or more of my responses help enhance and facilitate communication.	SA	A	NS	D	SD
11. I can assist the person to list some alternatives available.	SA	A	NS	D	SD
12. I can assist the person to identify some goals that are specific and observable.	SA	A	NS	D	SD
13. I can assist the person to specify at least one next step that might be taken toward the goal.	SA	A	NS	D	SD

Adapted from Myrick D, Erney T: *Caring and sharing*, Minneapolis: Educational Media Corporation, 1984, p 154.

WHAT DOES MY IMAGE COMMUNICATE TO OTHERS?

Remember that old saying "Do not judge a book by its cover?"

Unfortunately, we know that most people do not follow that suggestion. People get impressions about us from the way we look, sound, talk, and act. Often we are less careful about the messages we send with our appearance and behavior than we are when we choose our words. But our image may speak louder than our words. Think about it. Would you feel comfortable accepting nutritional advice from a 300-pound nurse? How would you like it if your instructor criticized your professionalism while wearing dirty shoes, a wrinkled uniform, bright red nail polish, and four earrings in each earlobe? What would you think about a physician whose progress notes contain many misspelled words and poor grammar (Figure 12-1)?

Communication is enhanced by your credibility. And people listen more to people they respect. Your image will help you communicate your professional credibility. The place to start projecting a positive image is with the first impression your appearance creates (Vengel, 2000). Good personal hygiene is a must. Each day you have to pay attention to your grooming. This means a flattering, neat haircut; clean, well-fitting clothes; reasonable makeup if used; minimal jewelry; and clean, sensible shoes. Your image is improved greatly if your weight is appropriate for your height and bone structure. Your appearance at work should conform to the norms for professionals in your work setting; save your individuality for your personal time away from work.

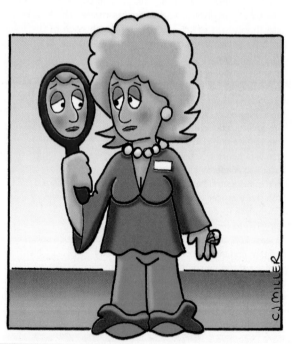

FIGURE 12-1
What does my image communicate to others?

Another aspect of your image is your depth and breadth of knowledge. You need to know your particular area of nursing thoroughly if you want the respect of others. However, you also need to know something about a wide variety of subjects so that you can have conversations with people beyond nursing. This means keeping up with current events, learning things about art or sports, and reading books. When people discover common interests, they are more willing to communicate with you.

Flexibility is necessary for effective communication with different kinds of people. This means that you are willing and able to adapt your behavior to relate more comfortably or effectively with others. Flexibility is part of a positive image and says to people that you are willing to accept responsibility for changing your behavior to meet the professional needs or requirements of others.

People who achieve success in their professional careers are enthusiastic. They let others know they are happy to be at work. They work harder, longer, and more accurately. They are pleasant to be around. They are sincere in their efforts to create a professional image that can be trusted.

Take an inventory of your appearance, knowledge, and attitude. If you are not sure what kind of image you are communicating, ask several trusted friends.

How Do Sex Differences Influence Communication Styles?

Men and women view their work environments from different perspectives (Vengel, 2000; Mindell, 2001). Men often see the world from a logical, sequential, focused perspective. Women often tend to see the big picture and to seek solutions based on what makes people feel comfortable rather than on logic. Subtle communication differences can create barriers to open, healthy communication between men and women in the workplace. Men may ask fewer questions in a public situation, especially if they feel that their questions might suggest ignorance. Women seem to be more comfortable asking questions (Mindell, 2001). In fact, there are times when a person can benefit from remaining silent and looking up information later in private so that others do not conclude that the asker lacks sufficient knowledge. At other times, a person must be assertive and ask questions so that he or she does not threaten the health of patients.

Within the workplace, the dominant communication style is direct, confident, and assertive. This style may be more familiar to men because they are often raised hearing more aggressive, direct language from their parents, whereas many women may be more used to a soft, supportive tone of voice and choice of words. Cultural values learned in childhood also play a role in the communication style a person chooses. This style may have to be modified to make interactions more successful. A woman who is communicating with a man may need to be more direct and assertive than usual, whereas a man may need to learn to be less aggressive in many situations.

Another sex difference in communication is related to childhood experiences with sports. Men often grow up with participation in team sports. They have worked toward a goal and have learned to strategize together for the good of the team, building a network of allies. Women have tended to be less involved with team sports than men. Women are more likely to have spent more time interacting with a few people they really like who share similar values and behaviors. Women are generally taught to be polite and to say nice things about and to others, whereas men are encouraged to do whatever it takes to help the team win. In the workplace, men and women need to understand their different points of view so that they can be team players and value cooperation and respectful relationships with each other.

To summarize, men and women have innately different communication styles, often developed from childhood experiences. To be successful in the workplace, we all have to learn as much as we can about communication differences, identify our own styles, and have the flexibility to use other communication techniques in situations that call for it.

What Should I Know About the "Grapevine?"

> The grapevine is like the tabloid papers. Would you bet your job on the accuracy of a rumor? So, when in doubt, check the facts out!

In addition to formal messages, communication can be informal. This type of communication flows upward, downward, and horizontally and is known as the *grapevine*. Whereas some people think of this kind of communication as gossip, others say it is the way things really get done. No matter how we describe the grapevine, we know it flourishes in all settings. People enjoy the satisfaction of the social interaction and recognition associated with the grapevine. It also provides information to employees that may not be easily obtained in any other way. It may be the quickest way to find out what the supervisor really values or what the new job openings are (Marquis & Huston, 2000) (Figure 12-2).

Mindell (2001) provides the following tips for controlling the grapevine:

1. Provide factual information to answer questions before they are asked. Few employees get all the information they feel they need.
2. Communicate face-to-face whenever possible. Do not trust the accuracy of messages through a third party.
3. Whenever rumors are running through the grapevine, hold a meeting to provide information and answer questions.

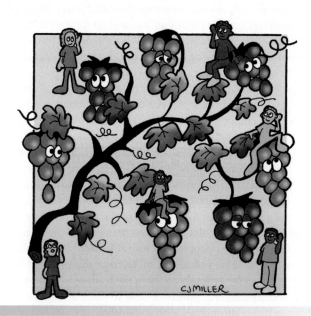

FIGURE 12-2

What should you know about the grapevine?

4. Do not spread rumors. Make sure you have all the facts from their source.
5. Enlist the support of respected leaders to spread the truth.
6. Address significant issues as soon as possible with your manager so that negative feelings can be defused.
7. Make sure what is put in writing is clear and accurately understood.

How Can I Deal with Cultural Diversity at Work?

Dochterman and Grace (2001) tell us that culture is a pattern of values and beliefs reflected in the behaviors we demonstrate. Whenever a group of people spend an extended period of time together, they develop a culture. Each of us comes from a cultural background, and we have beliefs, values, and behaviors that result from that background. In our workplaces, we will encounter many different types of people coming from diverse cultural backgrounds. To communicate effectively, we need to understand our own culture as well as the other person's culture. In addition, we must acknowledge and adhere to the cultural norms or rules that have developed in our workplace.

We must be aware of stereotypes that may interfere with our ability to see people as individuals. If we view people according to stereotypes, we might limit the way we perceive their communication. Even positive stereotypes make assumptions about people that may be inaccurate and thus may limit the nurse's ability to use all of his or her work skills effectively (Critical Thinking Box 12-4).

According to Arredondo (2000), communication goes through many filters when a person interacts with someone whom he or she perceives as different. Some of those filters are related to culture, sex, education level, age, and experience. When messages go through these filters, they may change because the actual communication symbols are interpreted according to a person's own cultural values and beliefs. This change may lead to misperceptions and misinterpretations. Communication is improved when we become more aware of the filters we use.

Within the work culture, people often communicate using jargon, inside jokes, or slang unique to the work setting. Acronyms are an example of jargon that health care workers understand but patients may not. It may seem to patients and their families that we are speaking in a code or foreign language. To interact effectively, we need to speak clearly, avoid jargon or slang, and keep our communication short and to the point. Long explanations can be confusing to people who are not familiar with the health care culture.

CRITICAL THINKING BOX 12-4

TRY THIS...

As you go about your work, take note of the various people you interact with and your reactions to them. Write these observations down so that you can reflect on them later. What kinds of thoughts come to mind when you see a female executive, an older woman, or a handsome man dressed in a suit? What kind of thoughts come to mind when you see people of ethnic origins that differ from your own? How do your initial impressions affect the way you communicate with each of these people?

Now picture yourself in the homes of five of your patients. Choose people from different cultural backgrounds. How are their homes different? In what ways do their homes reflect their culture? What do you need to know about each culture so that you can provide care effectively while avoiding any stereotyped beliefs?

Differences in the cultural backgrounds of workers can be a real asset. Sometimes we may have to provide care to patients who speak languages other than English, and we may need the skills of co-workers to translate or interpret, especially when cultural values influence the interpretation of the patient's behavior. We need to understand and respect cultural differences in patients. We can learn how to do this by learning about the differences among our co-workers. Respect and empathy enhance communication with people from other cultures, whether those people are patients or co-workers (Dochterman & Grace, 2001).

COMPONENTS OF EFFECTIVE COMMUNICATION

How Can I Communicate Effectively in Writing?

Communication takes place not only when words are spoken, but also when they are written and then read by someone else. A big part of a nurse's overall effectiveness depends on the ability to write effectively. This includes written treatment plans, progress notes, job descriptions, consultation requests, referrals, and memos. Some of you may even write articles for nursing journals or chapters for textbooks!

Mindell (2001) provides some guidelines for writing. First, determine whether you need to write in a formal way. Most upward communication needs to be formal, which means you should use proper titles, format, grammar, spelling, and punctuation. Never allow something you have written to be sent without careful proofreading. Nothing creates a negative impression faster than sloppy work, misspelled words, or poor grammar. If you need to, ask someone else to do this proofreading; be sure it is done well. Take the time to make necessary revisions before sending your written work on.

Also decide what your purpose is before you write (Marquis & Huston, 2000). This will help you to organize your thoughts so that everything you write helps to meet your purpose. Learn to write exactly what you mean. Choose words that are clear and specific. Often this means simple, small words. Be careful to use technical words only when you are sure you are choosing the correct words and your reader will understand you. Keep your sentences short and simple, with only one idea in each sentence.

Try using the KISS principle: Keep It Short and Simple.

When you learn to be clear and concise, you will write the essential information without many flowery phrases. Your readers will be very grateful if they can follow your thoughts easily. Make sure the first sentence in each paragraph identifies the key point for that paragraph. The reader should not have to guess what you are trying to say. Use a format that guides the reader. This means that visually on each page, main points are easy to locate, and concepts are identified by headings or titles. Remember, how well you write strongly influences how you are evaluated. What you put down on paper makes a lasting impression, and people will make judgments about your credibility and professionalism for a long time after you have actually written the words.

How Can I Learn to Speak Effectively?

From giving a change-of-shift report to another nurse to explaining your plans for a new approach on the unit to the organization's administration, you will have many opportunities to make presentations. Even now as a student, you may have the opportunity to conduct a presentation where you present to a group of people.

The first step in making effective presentations is to develop a positive attitude. ACCENTUATE the POSITIVE!

Many of us let our anxiety intimidate us. However, public speaking can be a great chance to show off our skills, our ability to be creative, and our willingness to be a star entertainer. Think of your presentation as a wonderful opportunity to have the attention of others on just you, even if only for a few minutes (Arredondo, 2000).

The second guiding principle in making good presentations is practice. PRACTICE makes PERFECT!

A well-planned rehearsal gives you a chance to see how long it will take you to say what you want, and it will help you feel more comfortable saying the words easily. Here are some tips on presentation preparation from Kushner (1997) and Peoples (1992).

Analyze Your Audience. What do they already know, and what do they need to know? Have an objective or two for what you want your audience to get out of your presentation.

Do Your Homework. Know enough about your subject to make your talk clear and believable. Make sure you can answer at least a few questions.

Plan the Presentation. This includes making an outline of the content and the teaching strategies you might use. Visual aids or activities may be used to involve the audience in active participation. Visual aids should keep the presentation focused and organized. They help you hold your audience's attention. (**Plus you are more likely to persuade with visual cues.**)

Add Spice to the Presentation. The more active your audience's participation, the longer they will pay attention. Choose at least one presentation strategy that involves them, such as question/answer, role playing, or small-group discussion. Highlight key points you want your audience to remember visually on slides or other types of media. **Use an attention grabber at the beginning** to make sure your audience is listening. This may be a friendly greeting, a stimulating question, a startling statistic, a relevant story, or a quote by an expert. Then tell your audience the purpose of the presentation and what it will cover in brief and concise words.

Create Cheat Sheets. Cheat sheets are your clues—the first couple of words around a topic to help you remember what to say or what questions to ask, or small pictures or drawings to jog your mind during the presentation in case you stumble and fumble with your thoughts and words. If the speech or presentation is an important one and fairly formal, you may want to prepare a script. This means you write out exactly what you will say and have it typed double-spaced, with a wide margin on the left side. Here you can write notes to yourself about when to use your visual aids or when to pass out materials for the audience. Even if you choose to write a script, **be sure to memorize the first 2 minutes of what you are going to say!**

The Closing. In your closing, review what you have said, summarize the benefits or implications of what you have said, and reiterate any action you want taken. (**Design your closing**

FIRST, since it is the most important part of the formal presentation. It may sound crazy to work backward, but the closing is what the audience will hear last and remember. Write it out and memorize it!)

Final Details. Be familiar with the room and equipment you will use. Determine that everything you need is there before you begin. Make sure the spelling is correct on your visual aids and handouts. Speak with confidence, energy, and enthusiasm. Make as much eye contact as you can. Use your hands and arms to make dramatic gestures. They add energy and interest.

What Listening Skills Do I Need to Develop?

Listening effectively is one of the most powerful communication tools you can have. It is more than just hearing the words of others. Listening involves concentrating all your energy on understanding and interpreting the message with the meaning the sender intended. Of the four verbal means of communication—writing, reading, speaking, and listening—listening requires most of our communication time. Yet we often pay the least attention to our listening skills (Mindell, 2001). It has been estimated that people actually remember only one-third of the messages they have heard, although they spend 70% of their time listening (Marquis & Huston, 2000).

> Did you know? People speak at 100 to 175 words per minute, but they can listen intelligently at 600 to 800 words per minute (Fowler, 2005).

There are reasons that people are not good listeners (Arredondo, 2000). We simply do not pay enough attention; we hear what we want to hear and filter out the rest. Listening requires concentration, and that means doing nothing else at the same time. Some people think of listening as a passive behavior; they want to be in control by talking more. We think a lot faster than people speak, so we often think way ahead or think about other things or daydream. Maybe too many distractions are interfering with listening, such as background noises or movements.

One of the most problematic reasons for ineffective listening is that people allow their emotions to dictate what they hear or do not hear. We pay more attention to people we like or respect and less attention to people or messages that make us feel uncomfortable. If the message is making demands on us to do more, change what we do, or do better, we may stop listening to deal with our own feelings of anger, guilt, or anxiety. We may start planning our own defensive response while the other person is still talking.

Think about situations you've been in where you've had difficulty listening, understanding, or remembering what was said. Consider these examples:

- A psychiatric patient who has recently been admitted displays acutely psychotic thought processes by talking rapidly in pressured speech, using words and phrases so loosely connected that the whole conversation is disorganized and incomprehensible.
- A head nurse spends 5 minutes screaming at her team leader, criticizing everything she has done that day, and then asks the team leader to carry out a very specific and detailed change in the physician's orders for a patient.
- Another nurse asks you to hang an intravenous solution for the patient in Room 1253 while you are writing some progress notes on a patient's chart. When you finish, you cannot remember the room number where you agreed to hang the intravenous solution.

It becomes essential to develop effective listening skills (Arredondo, 2000). Here are some tips:

Make Sure You Can Hear What Is Being Said. Move closer, eliminate distracting noises, and most of all, do not talk. You cannot hear someone else when you are talking.

Focus Your Attention on What Is Being Said. Actively concentrate by analyzing the key points as they are being said. Take notes. Do not do anything else while you are listening except to concentrate on hearing and understanding what is being said.

Recognize and Control Your Emotional Response to What Is Being Said. Focus on hearing and seeing accurately what is being communicated. You will have time to ask questions and explore feelings after the other person finishes.

Decide in the Beginning that You Will Listen and Accept the Other Person's Needs and Feelings, Whatever They Are. Improved understanding of the other person is gained through listening, and this understanding will help you to be more effective in solving problems and eliminating negative feelings.

Pay Attention to Nonverbal Communication as You Listen to the Words. Much of a message's meaning comes through in the sender's tone of voice, facial expressions, and body movements. You must listen with your eyes and your ears.

Fight Off Distractions. Do not let the speaker's style of communicating, his or her mannerisms, telephone calls, or other interruptions break your concentration.

Take Notes. If a lot of factual, important information is being given, take notes—but just jot down key words or numbers or the note-taking itself will become a distraction. You may also ask the speaker to put in writing what he or she has said.

Let the Speaker Tell the Whole Story. Make it a point not to interrupt. Try not to assume you know what is going to be said. Withhold formulating criticisms as you listen.

React to the Message, Not the Person. Ask yourself, "Are my feelings or biases interfering with my listening?" Seek feedback of your understanding by verifying what you have heard.

Respond Positively to the Feelings Being Communicated. Empathy and acceptance will make it easier for the communication to continue. Maintain a positive attitude about listening. Recognize that listening is necessary for success. Allow yourself to hear all sides of an issue.

Identify the characteristics of your listening skills in Critical Thinking Box 12-5.

How Can I Use Nonverbal Communication Effectively?

Nonverbal communication uses movements, gestures, body position, and voice tone to transmit messages (Arredondo, 2000). To convey confidence and leadership ability, it is necessary to learn to use certain nonverbal signals effectively. Here are some tips:

Make Eye Contact with the Person with Whom You Are Talking. This helps the person interpret your message more favorably and says that you are giving your full attention to the conversation.

Stand Up Straight, with Shoulders Back. You may want to lean slightly forward toward the other individual to convey your interest. Stand with your toes pointed slightly outward and slightly apart and approximately 18 inches to 4 feet from the person you are talking to so that you do not invade personal space. Avoid personal contact unless you know the person well and it is a casual conversation.

Use a Forceful Voice without Pauses to Suggest Confidence. Avoid a whining, nagging, or complaining tone. You may need to listen to your tape-recorded voice to get some insight into how you sound to others.

CRITICAL THINKING BOX 12-5	**TRY THIS ...** Develop a listening action plan. 1. I listen most effectively when ... 2. I have difficulty listening when ... 3. My best listening skills are ... 4. I need to improve on my skills at ... 5. In order to improve my listening skills, I will ...

Watch for Distracting Behaviors. Avoid negative behaviors that detract from your verbal messages: nodding constantly, yawning, playing with your hair, scratching yourself, cracking your knuckles, or twiddling your thumbs. When you use your hands in gestures, keep your forearm up and the palm of your hand open. Avoid making a fist or shaking a pointing finger at the other person.

How Can I Communicate Effectively by Using Technology?

Many of us are learning to use the technology that is changing our workplace and making communication easier. Although cellular telephones, email, text messaging, fax machines, portable personal computers, and voice mail may be conveniences, they must be used thoughtfully to make a positive contribution to your overall image as an effective communicator. Deep and Sussman (1995) give the following tips for the successful use of communications technology:

Do Not Misuse or Overuse Email, Text Messaging, or Fax Machines. Review the tips for effective use of email and text messaging. Although using a fax machine is not recent technology, remember that the person on the other end must read every page faxed to him or her, so be brief. If you need to send a long document, use either email or the mail.

Learn to Use Computer Software. Using technology can make not only your work, but communication easier and more effective. Integrated computer systems on hospital units, electronic health record systems, passive infrared tracking of patients and nurse location along with enhanced nurse-call systems, wireless inhouse telephone systems, and web-based electronic grease boards to track patients throughout the day of scheduled surgeries, diagnostics tests, etc., can be viewed on computer monitors in patient's room and/or from large display monitors strategically located throughout a department (Bahlman & Johnson, 2005).

Do Not Send an Emotional Outburst in an Email. These messages can seem more hostile than you intended, and you can alienate or anger many people. If you would not say these words in person, then do not send them by email (Box 12-1).

When You Leave Someone a Voicemail Message, Speak Slowly and Distinctly. This is especially important when you are leaving your telephone number so that the other person can return your call. It is frustrating to receive a message but not be able to understand the name or have to replay the message to get all of the digits in the phone number. Make your voicemail message brief but complete, saying when you called, what you want the other person to do, and when you can be reached.

Do Not Leave Callers on Hold If You Are Using Call Waiting. Explain to the first caller that you must briefly answer another call, then take the number of the second caller, with

BOX 12-1   Tips on Using Email Effectively

1. STOP, THINK ABOUT WHAT YOU WANT TO SAY, *THEN* WRITE.
   - Be sure to determine whether an email is the appropriate communication medium. Email is meant for quick, simple communication. Ask yourself whether a phone conversation would be more appropriate.
2. INCLUDE A DESCRIPTIVE SUBJECT LINE.
   - In the subject line of the email note, place a description of what the email is about. Be specific—for example, Quarterly QA Report or Case Study Assignment—Informatics.
3. MAKE YOUR EMAIL NOTE EASY TO READ.
   - Use short paragraphs, usually no more than four or five paragraphs at most—get to the point, quickly. Consider that most people have a limited attention span with email, especially if they are receiving a lot of messages.
   - Have ample white space on the page. Usually five to seven lines of text are best for a paragraph.
   - Use bullets or numbers to guide the reader.
   - Carefully choose your font size, type, and color. Using a bright color (such as purple) may not convey a professional tone like a standard black or navy font would. Very large fonts (14-point or more) might make your message seem "loud" and accusatory. A sans serif font, such as Arial or Tahoma 10-12 point, is easier to read on the computer screen than a serif font, such as Times Roman.
4. BE PRECISE, CONCISE, AND CLEAR.
   - Use a conversational writing style.
   - If responding to multiple questions embedded in a large email, copy the questions into your email and write your answers next to them.
   - When replying to a message, include enough of the original email note to provide context to your response.
   - If in doubt, spell it out—limit your use of jargon or abbreviations.
   - Always spell-check and proof your email before you send it out.
5. DEMONSTRATE "NETIQUETTE"—BE PROFESSIONAL AND MAINTAIN APPROPRIATE ONLINE TONE.
   - Do not type in all CAPS! Capitals can be used for emphasis, but ALL CAPS LOOKS LIKE YOU'RE YELLING AT THE PERSON. If you emphasize everything, then nothing is taken as important.
   - Do not type in all lower case—this violates the rules of English grammar and usage.
   - If a communication is upsetting to you, keep calm and collected. Your emotional state can slip into an email without notice, in the form of curt sentences, skipped pleasantries, and blunt comments.
   - Remember, unlike telephone and personal conversations that fade with time, impulsive email responses have "staying power"—meaning the email is readily available in e-mailboxes, can be printed out, distributed to others, and attain a level of importance that was never intended.
   - A word about flaming (which is the expression of extreme emotion or opinion in an email message, often derogatory)—be polite and pleasant and consider whether you want to respond to a "flaming" email.
6. BE CAREFUL WITH ATTACHMENTS.
   - Open attachments *only* if you trust the source, since attachments can contain executable files that can spread viruses and slow down processing.

Continued

BOX 12-1   Tips on Using Email Effectively—cont'd

- Consider the size of the attachments—large files (greater than 1000 KB or 1 MB) can clog up networks and rapidly fill your Inbox. Many servers prohibit the sending and receiving of large email file attachments.
- Use spam filters and delete chain emails or other scams—do not open the document or have the viewing pane open, because this can perpetuate the spam.

7. WATCH HUMOR.
   - Find different ways to express emotion, body language, and intonation. Use "smileys" (☺), also called Emoticons, to convey feelings in your message.
   - As in any setting, humor can be misconstrued, so be extra careful and use taste and discretion before transmitting any humor.

8. INCLUDE A SIGNATURE.
   - Include a signature with your email, usually no more than four to six lines of text. Remember, this part of your message is the last thing the receiver will read.
   - Include your name, title, contact information, and email address or URL. Many email programs can be set up to automatically attach a default signature or signature file to the end of all your outgoing messages (including replies).

9. REVIEW YOUR MESSAGE BEFORE SENDING.
   - Remember, email is not confidential—do not send personal or sensitive email, because there is no "secure" email system.
   - Review and proof your message before clicking "Send."

10. RESPOND TO EMAIL.
    - Make an effort to respond to email within 24 hours. Otherwise, use the auto-reply function to inform the person when you will respond.

11. TEXT MESSAGING
    - Keep in mind most agencies do not want you texting during you clinical experience. Check with faculty about using smart phone or PDA in the clinical area.

the assurance that you will call back as soon as you finish your first call. This interruption should take no more than 10 seconds. Be sure to write down the telephone number of the second caller so that you do not forget it by the time you finish the first call.

When You Call People, Ask If They Have Time to Talk and Offer to Call Back at a More Convenient Time If Necessary. People appreciate this courtesy and will be more likely to have a positive conversation with you if it is conveniently timed and is respectful of their busy schedules.

If You Are Conducting a Conversation or a Meeting with a Speaker Telephone or by Means of a Teleconference, Make Sure that Each Party to the Call Is Introduced to the Other People. Do not use the speaker telephone unless you are including a group in the conversation. Even with a conference call, there should be some structure to the discussion, including an agenda or a specified purpose and time for the call. Learn how to "mute" a conversation, especially when there is considerable background noise.

When You Have Business Cards Printed, Include Your Email Address and Your Fax Number. If you are sending messages by email, be sure to read your words carefully before sending them. Because you are sending words without the benefit of clarifying nonverbal communication, the likelihood of being misinterpreted is greater. Make sure your messages are as clear as they can be. Include your name and subject in the email note.

When You Need to Send a Personal Message, Especially a Reminder or a Thank-You Note, the Most Powerful Way is to Send a Handwritten Note. This conveys the importance you connect with the message and continues the interpersonal aspect of the communication. If you need to communicate something that you expect will have a significant emotional impact, do it face-to-face. This communication style also allows you an opportunity to read the other person's nonverbal communication and offers a chance to negotiate a comfortable understanding following your message delivery.

GROUP COMMUNICATION

What Is Group Process?

When we discuss the dynamics and communication patterns in groups, it is important to note that personality conflicts may develop during the different cyclical phases of the group. In **forming** the group, think back to orientation day for nursing school. There you sit surrounded by some people you have never seen before and some you have known from your prenursing classes. A common bond is that you are all there for well-defined reasons, including finding out who is in your clinical group and who the instructors will be. Of course, the orientation is mandatory. You sit in the auditorium or classroom talking, listening, and watching those around you, playing your part in a form of controlled pandemonium. The pandemonium can actually be considered the storming phase. In the **storming** phase, you begin to act out the roles you normally portray in the presence of your peers, as you discuss your fears, fantasies, and hopes for a successful outcome to your nursing program (Tuckman & Jensen, 1977).

Next, you are divided into clinical groups. You now begin to reevaluate the personality composition of the new groups. As you begin to react to your new relationships, you start to exhibit personality traits to establish the role you would like to be identified with in the group setting. Unfortunately, your unconscious defense mechanisms surface in the form of competitive conflict or one-upmanship within the group, with your hope that your response will secure the desired role in the group. It is at this time that **norming** begins to develop among members of the group, with the help of the clinical and lecture instructors. Norming occurs during the development of mutual goals and guidelines that help to redefine your behavioral roles in the group. This can allow agreement in performing activities to help establish a purposeful clinical experience that involves interdependence and flexibility.

During the **performing** phase, everyone knows one another, is able to work together, and trusts one another. The group works together and makes changes in a seamless way, because there is a high degree of comfort among the group members that funnels all of the energy of the group toward the tasks at hand—getting through nursing school. Later Tuckman and Jensen (1977) added the final stage, **adjourning,** which has been called *deforming* and *mourning* by others. This phase is about completion and disengagement, both from the tasks and the group members. Many of you have experienced or will experience the adjourning phase as you move from one clinical group to another or during the transition from student to graduate, as you are nearing completion of your nursing program.

Groups can be multipurpose and multidynamic, as are the basic role choices of each participant in a group. When working in a group, the real fun and excitement start when group members begin responding to and dealing with the unconscious and semiconscious defense mechanisms of the individuals who act them out through the roles they play in the group. The responses of the defensive individual tend to be unproductive, time-consuming, and inappropriate to the harmony and overall function of a group effort. Of course, they do give you something to talk and maybe laugh about later. In my years of nursing and group participation, the following tend to be my favorite dysfunctional group personalities.

The **self-servers** feel that the rules of the group do not apply to them. They show up late. They are usually unprepared to work. At times they will walk in and out of the group for superficial reasons, while appearing preoccupied with unrelated work or issues from outside of the group. When they do participate, their contributions are of little consequence. If they refuse to be functional members of the group, you may need to ask them to leave the group.

The first response of a **critical conservative** to a creative suggestion is, "No, it won't work" or "But it's always been done this way" and "How can you people succeed if you've never done this before?" They seem to have a criticism for any suggestion other than their own. If it is not done their way, it just is not right. They are obsessively negative and fearful of changes. It may be important to recognize the lessons of experiences and outcomes, but it is equally important to find new approaches to old problems.

The **motor mouths** talk just to hear themselves talk. They interrupt at any given moment to make statements or deliver a verbose response, possibly because they have been quiet for too long. Even when another person is talking, motor mouths will talk over the speaker's words just to be the center of attention. These people may begin to make a statement, only to ramble in and out of the group's issue, and end up talking about unrelated issues that are usually about themselves. I suggest keeping a cloth gag nearby or redirecting their conversation to focusing on the issue and periodically asking them for a short critical assessment of the issues in question.

The **mouse** is the silent observer who is fearful of voicing an opinion. Usually, the mouse sits transfixed, watching other individuals take risks and responsibility for their input to the group. The mouse nods his or her head at appropriate times and answers questions in one or two words. The mouse may be a real addition to the group, especially if others in the group are able to find ways to engage and encourage the mouse to voice opinions and feelings about the group issues. It is important to remember that these people may be some of the best observers and listeners; ask them for their input. You may find them to be a valuable asset to your team. Regardless of where you choose to work or the type of care delivery system you are in, these group members are always there!

How Can You Improve Communications in Group Meetings?

Nurses participate in many meetings, from patient care conferences to more formal committee meetings. Communication within a group of people can be an opportunity to influence the quality of care given to patients. When you participate as a member of a group, the following are positive behaviors that will help you to communicate effectively and will also help the group to accomplish its tasks more efficiently:

- Come prepared. Bring all the "stuff" you need.
- Listen. Be open to other viewpoints.
- Keep on track. Do not visit or chit-chat.
- Present your ideas or opinions. Ask other members for theirs.
- State disagreements. Be able to back them up.
- Clarify when needed. Do not assume.

All of us have been to and participated in meetings that were disorganized, confusing, and a waste of time. Critical Thinking Box 12-6 will help you to identify some unpleasant group meeting experiences and give you the opportunity to change future meetings.

CRITICAL THINKING
BOX 12-6

TRY THIS ...

Think of particularly unpleasant experiences you have had at meetings. You might think about meetings involving your clinical group or your class officers. Develop a list of ideas about what was wrong with those meetings.

What	Who	When	Completed
Schedule inservice on glucometer.	Janet & Linda	5/28/11	
Revise suction procedure.	Sue & Bill	4/23/11	5/8/11
Review charting, and report back to next unit meeting.	Tom & Amy	5/1/11	5/16/11

FIGURE 12-3

Action timeline for meetings.

The key to effective meetings is the planning and organization that occurs before the meeting is actually held. An effective technique using de Bono's (1999) Six Thinking Hats can spur a group meeting to better productivity and problem solving (Box 12-2). Planning should allow the leader to think through what the meeting is for, who should be there, and how it should run (Huber, 2000). There should be a clear purpose for every meeting and every item on the agenda. Every item should require some action by the group. If the purpose could be achieved in another way, such as by making a telephone call or sending a memo, there should be no meeting.

If you are making a formal presentation, some audiovisual equipment will be necessary, and chairs will need to be arranged so that everyone can see the presenter and the audiovisuals. If the meeting is for discussion and decision making, a table at which everyone can sit face-to-face is more effective. Look at Figure 12-3. This type of note-taking clarifies who is responsible for what activities. At the conclusion of the meeting, summarize the decisions, and identify the plan of action. At the end of the meeting, the time should be established for the next meeting. All members should receive a copy of the timeline information.

BOX 12-2	Edward de Bono's Six Thinking Hats: Looking at a Decision and Working Through a Problem Considering Six Points of View

Six Thinking Hats is an important and powerful technique created by Edward de Bono that can be used as an effective group process tool in meetings that get bogged down with diverse views and adamant positions. It offers a strategy to "think outside the box" by challenging the group to think or see all sides of an issue. Each "Thinking Hat" represents a perspective or way of thinking. During a meeting, a "different color hat" can be put on or taken off to indicate the type of thinking the person is using. By putting on a different hat in a particular sequence, problem solving is encouraged.

WHITE HAT: NEUTRAL, OBJECTIVE, CONCERNED WITH FACTS AND FIGURES, *THE FACT HAT*

Used to think about facts, figures, and other objective information (think of a scientist's white lab coat).

What facts and data are available?

What facts would help me further in making a decision?

How can I get those facts?

RED HAT: THE EMOTIONAL VIEW, *THE EMOTIONAL HAT*

Used to elicit the feelings, emotions, and other nonrational but potentially valuable senses, such as hunches and intuition (think of a red heart). Encourages people to express their feelings without the need for apology, explanation, or attempt to justify them.

How do I really feel?

What is my gut feeling about this problem?

BLACK HAT: CAREFUL, CAUTIOUS, *THE "DEVIL'S ADVOCATE" HAT*

Used to discover why some ideas will not work, this hat inspires logical negative arguments (think of a devil's advocate or judge robed in black). Helps you to see problems in advance (spot flaws in thinking), prepare for potential difficulties, and prepare contingency plans to counter the issues.

What are the possible downside risks and problems?

What is the worst-case scenario?

What are the weak points of the plan? It allows you to eliminate them, alter them, or prepare contingency plans to counter them.

YELLOW HAT: SUNNY AND POSITIVE, *THE OPTIMISTIC HAT*

Used to obtain a positive, optimistic outlook, this hat sees opportunities, possibilities, and benefits of a decision (think of the warming sun). Keeps you going when the going gets tough.

What are the advantages?

What would be the best possible outcome?

GREEN HAT: ASSOCIATED WITH FERTILE GROWTH, CREATIVITY, AND NEW IDEAS, *THE CREATIVE HAT*

Used to find creative new ideas (think of new shoots sprouting from seeds).

What completely new, fresh, innovative approaches can I generate?

What creative ideas can I dream up to help me see the problem in a new way?

Are there any additional alternatives or can we do this in a different way?

Could there be another explanation?

BLUE HAT: COOL, THE COLOR OF SKY, *THE ORGANIZING HAT*

Used as a master hat to control the thinking process (think of the overarching sky, or a "cool" character who's in control).

Review my thoughts—it suggests the next step for thinking.

Sum up what I have learned and think about what the next logical step is—asks for summaries, conclusions and decisions.

TEAM BUILDING

What Is Team Building?

Team building is a deliberate process of unifying a group of individuals into a functional working unit, accomplishing specific goals (Farley & Stoner, 1989). Another definition of a team is "a small number of people with complementary skills who are committed to a common purpose in performance of common goals, for which they hold themselves mutually accountable" (Katzenbach & Smith, 1993, p 45). Katzenbach and Smith state that there needs to be the right mix of attributes in three categories that help ensure a highly complementary and functional team. The three categories described are interpersonal skills, problem-solving and decision-making skills, and technical or functional expertise (Critical Thinking Box 12-7).

Teams are a formal way to actualize collaboration. Collaboration is at the heart of successful decision making. Collaboration among team members leverages skills, time, and resources for the benefit of the team and that of the organization. If you examine the word *collaboration*, you will see that "co-labor" is the core of the word—meaning "working together toward some meaningful end."

When Nurses Work as a True Team, Everyone Involved Benefits!

In health care, the imperative is in the quality of care and service-oriented teams, as seen by Sovie (1992). It is also clear that teamwork is essential in care delivery outcomes and cost-control (Figure 12-4). Sovie also says that nurse managers and supervisors need to learn how to function in their individual capacity while being effective as team players. It might be argued that there is a difference between the previous and current concepts of team nursing. The differences are not so much the personal mechanics of team nursing but more the constant updating of information in the fields of medicine and technology.

One of the most important ingredients in the team approach to nursing is a positive psychological and emotional bond between members of the team, which helps to develop more cohesiveness between the individuals of the team. Without a positive cohesive bond, there can and

---

CRITICAL THINKING
BOX 12-7

THINK ABOUT …

Try to assess and come to your own conclusion regarding the following hypothetical problem by picturing in your mind the *who, what,* and *why* before you read what the experts in the field would say:

You will be responsible for the care of your critically ill parent during his or her stay in the hospital over the next 2 months. Assemble a team of your nursing peers to deliver care to your parent. The care will be based on the highest level of difficulty because of the serious nature of the diagnosis.
• What nurses would you choose to help you?
• Why would you choose those specific nurses?
• What qualities would you want them to have when caring for your family member?
• What skill level would you want them to have to carry out the overall treatment plan?
• If some of them lacked the skill levels to meet the treatment plan criteria, what would be an appropriate approach to this inadequacy?

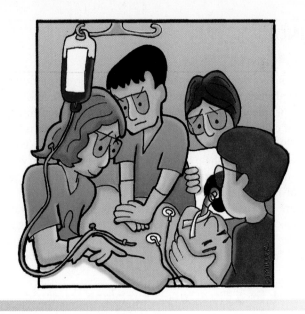

FIGURE 12-4

When nurses work as a team, everyone benefits.

will be limits to the overall quality and function of the team. You as nurses are the unknown intervening variables that either make or break the quality of the team nursing concept. You and your colleagues, as a professional collective group, have the skills necessary to handle the multitudes of problems associated with care delivery. You may want to ask yourselves:

- Are you as an individual mentally and emotionally prepared for real-world nursing?
- Do you have and can you maintain a strong positive self-image?
- Is your attitude about yourself and your peers conducive to support team-directed nursing?
- Are you willing to make difficult decisions in directing team care delivery?
- Are you willing to relinquish control of those under your direction when necessary?

You may also want to take the following into consideration:

- Does management actively and willingly support the nursing staff?
- Is the support constant, measurable, and appropriate to your needs?

Nurses read and do research to help formulate problem solving and innovative approaches in the establishment of functional care-delivery models. What is frequently left out of the equation is the extent of the role management is willing to play in helping to ensure the success of the new ideas. Is management willing to share control and leadership to help ensure a successful outcome in nurse-managed teams? I have been witness to the creation of nursing leadership roles—some consisting of team nursing care delivery, decentralization of authority, and shared governance—only to have them fail because of limitations and perceived liabilities placed on the nursing staff by management. At other times, failures were caused by the last-minute intervention of management, usurping the managerial authority of the nursing teams. Some other factors responsible for group or team failure are:

- Nursing staff being unprepared or lacking the intrapersonal skills needed to work with other staff members in a unified team setting.

- Nurses unwilling to move in and out of leadership roles to ensure the unity of the group and best possible outcomes.
- Management being pressured by upper management for faster adaptation to cost-cutting policies, which usually causes communication between management and nursing to consist of veiled threats, innuendoes, mixed messages, and other subtle negative forms that affect the morale of the nursing staff.
- Nursing supervisors and administrative staff who appear to support shared governance but are unwilling to relinquish actual control of the nursing staff.

Action always speaks louder than words. Work toward open and honest communication with administrators. Try to meet them halfway and find out what they are willing to do to support your teams or groups. How much interest do they have in the actual quality of health care delivery? Are they interested in learning the dynamics of your role as a nurse or the role of the nursing team? Let them know what type of support you need from them. Explain to them the importance of mutual respect and support in the overall quality of nursing care.

When forming teams, realize that perfection is an illusion created in the mind of a critic. All of us have different skill levels. To function as a unified team, you will need to work with peers whose skills may need enhancing. You can help your peers by working side by side with them to build confidence while sharing in learning situations. Find ways of making the learning situations enjoyable, show a sense of humor, and give positive reinforcement whenever possible. Fear and guilt undermine confidence and destroy the cohesiveness of a team or group.

In the forming of any team or group, the mental and emotional stability of the individuals who make up the team or group will be reflected in the quality of their work under stress and their ability to focus during care delivery and to establish a working rapport with the other team members. It is important for the stronger team members or group members to give support and guidance as needed. The attitude of the stronger members of the team can go a long way in building confidence in the other team members. The level of quality for any team is increased substantially by the level of comfort and camaraderie among the individuals who make up the team (see Evidence-Based Practice Box 12-1).

The mix of complementary skills and experience can also help to give strength to the overall group. Taking inventory of technical and communication skills helps identify where weakness and strengths need to be considered before assigning individual duties to the team members. The weaker team members should have learning opportunities, support, and guidance in order to strengthen the cohesiveness of the team.

Leadership roles in the team may be rotated to each member of the team. This allows the sharing of responsibilities and a chance for members to experience and test themselves in a leadership role. Most people will gravitate to their roles in a short period of time. It will be important for the team members to communicate with one another to ensure the quality and continuity of care to be delivered (Box 12-3 and Figure 12-5).

ASSERTIVE STYLES OF COMMUNICATION

All of us have a style or way of communicating with others that is often based on our own personality and self-concept. In other words, the kind of people we are and the way in which we see ourselves influence the process of communication. This style can be divided into three common

BOX 12-1   EVIDENCE-BASED PRACTICE

Team Member Knowledge

PRACTICE ISSUE

Institute for Healthcare Improvement (IHI) has identified the value of teams of health care workers when working with one another in order to improve health care outcomes. Previous research has established that team culture, team composition, communication, mutual respect, and trust increase the effectiveness of the team, thus resulting in positive outcomes of clinical care. Tacit knowledge is knowledge that is acquired without the intention to learn or even the awareness that something has been learned. This level of knowledge is strongly connected to individual skills. At the team level, tacit knowledge is related to the collective knowledge of the team members when they are working together for an extended period. The underlying shared experience that results in the ability to successfully anticipate the reaction of teammates is a characteristic of tacit knowledge.

Tacit knowledge and related characteristics as perceived by the members of a cardiothoracic surgery team was the focus of a research study.

IMPLICATIONS FOR NURSING PRACTICE

- The prominent theme that emerged from this study was the unscripted and unspoken knowledge and understanding of what it is that the other team members will do in a given set of circumstances. As one of the surgeons mentioned, the unspoken team performance reminded him of a dance where the partners knew what the other would do with no words being exchanged. Tacit knowledge requires all members of the team to be "in the moment" and be acutely aware of what all the other actors are doing at that time.
- A primary element of team performance was a theme of trust and communication.
- Tacit knowledge was an important attribute of high-performing health care teams.
- When team members have the experience of working with one another for extended periods, tacit knowledge is evident.
- Turnover of staff needs to be reduced so that tacit knowledge can be nurtured and shared. Shared decision making, building on individual strengths, open communication, and high levels of trust are all attributes that can help reduce staff turnover and, in many cases, may be more important than salary alone.
- Tacit knowledge cannot be consciously planned or deliberately constructed. It only occurs when all the members of the team can openly share with one another the accumulated experience and individual perspectives that each person contributes to the whole.

Considering This Information:

What can you do to promote the development of tacit knowledge within a team? During your clinical experience, what teams have you observed that exhibit the characteristics of tacit knowledge?

Reference for the Evidence

Friedman L, Bernell S: The importance of team level tacit knowledge and related characteristics of high-performing health care teams, *Health Care Management Review* 31(3):223-230, 2006.

types: passive or avoidant, aggressive, and assertive (Marquis & Huston, 2000). The following are some characteristics of each style:

People who tend toward **passive or avoidant behavior** let others push them around. These people do not stand up for themselves; do what they are told regardless of how they feel about it; are not able to share their feelings or needs with others; have difficulty asking for help; and feel hurt, anxious, or angry at others for taking advantage of them.

BOX 12-3   Basic Roles of Group Members

The following are some roles that individuals adopt when participating in a group. Each member may adopt more than one role.
- Opinion giver—states beliefs or values
- Opinion seeker—asks for clarification of beliefs or values
- Information giver—offers facts or personal experience
- Information seeker—asks for facts pertinent to what is being discussed
- Initiator—proposes new ideas on how the goal can be reached or how to view the problem
- Elaborator—expands on the idea of another; takes the idea and works out what would happen if it were adopted
- Coordinator—brings together ideas and suggestions
- Orientor—keeps the group focused on goals or questions the direction taken by the group
- Evaluator or critic—examines possible group solutions against group standards and goals
- Clarifier—checks out what someone said by restating or questioning
- Recorder—acts as the groups memory (e.g., takes notes)
- Summarizer—pulls together related ideas, restates suggestions, and offers decisions or conclusions

From Sullivan EJ, Decker P: *Effective leadership and management in nursing*, ed 4, Menlo Park, Calif, 1997, Addison-Wesley, p 144.

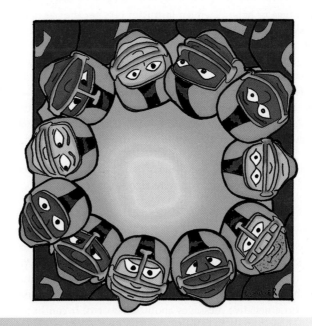

FIGURE 12-5
We win as a team!

Aggressive behavior means that a person puts his or her own needs, rights, and feelings first and communicates that in an angry, dominating way; attempts to humiliate or "put down" other people; conveys a righteous, superior attitude; works at controlling or manipulating others; is seen by others as punishing, threatening, demanding, or hostile; and shows no concern for anyone else's feelings.

Assertive behavior means that a person stands up for himself or herself in a way that does not violate the basic rights of another person; expresses true feelings in an honest, direct manner; does not let others take advantage of him or her; shows respect for other's rights, needs, and feelings; sets goals and acts on those goals in a clear and consistent manner and takes responsibility for the consequences of those actions; is able to accept compliments and criticism; and acts in a way that enhances self-respect.

See if you can match the person with his or her style by using the descriptions you have read.

■ JANE

Jane is a very shy, quiet senior nursing student who can't think straight when her instructor asks her questions in the clinical area. She wishes she could be more like her classmates, who seem to find it easy to talk about their experiences during clinical conference. During her evaluation, her instructor says she doesn't know enough theory and can't handle the pressures of the clinical unit. Jane says nothing and signs her evaluation. When she gets back to her room alone, she cries uncontrollably.

■ SUSAN

Susan is a senior nursing student who is highly verbal with her classmates. She is known to be opinionated and in every conference with her clinical group finds a chance to criticize someone. She blames the nursing staff on the clinical unit for making her look bad by giving her too much work to do and not enough time or help. When her instructor tells her she has not integrated sufficient theory in her written assignments, she says, "It's not my fault; you should have told me sooner."

■ MARK

Mark is a senior nursing student who is described by his clinical group as goal-oriented and confident. He wrote learning objectives for himself at the beginning of the last clinical experience and brought them with him, along with a self-evaluation for his final evaluation conference. He listened to his instructor's suggestions, thanked her, and said, "I appreciate your concern for the quality of my nursing skills. I'm aware now of what I need to pay attention to in my first few months in my new job."

If you decided that Jane used a passive or avoidant style, Susan used an aggressive style, and Mark used an assertive style, you were right. Congratulations!

Why Are Nurses Not More Assertive?

It seems as though many nurses do not consistently act or communicate in an assertive way. Some have a hard time believing in their own rights, feelings, or needs. This difficulty may have gotten its start in childhood through exposure to many negative statements or experiences. It is important to recognize that communication style is learned and reinforced over time. While in nursing school and working in the nursing profession, additional experiences or comments may reinforce those negative messages about self-worth. It can be very difficult to change behavior, especially when risk taking is necessary. The first step is to recognize what the barriers are. What is it that prevents you from being more assertive? Is it previously learned behavior, or are you afraid of the repercussions of assertive communication? Check the list in Box 12-4. If this list includes statements you feel are true, then you have identified some roadblocks to your ability to develop more assertive communication.

Look over this list of barriers to assertive communication and think about yourself. Do any of these explain your feelings? Assertiveness takes self-awareness and practice. It will help you to

---

BOX 12-4   Barriers to Assertiveness

Barriers to assertiveness include the following beliefs:
- Assertive communication should not threaten others.
- If you do not have anything nice to say, do not say anything at all.
- If you feel uncomfortable when presenting your position or stating your feelings, then you are nonassertive.
- Assertiveness should come easily and spontaneously.
- Health care facilities do not promote or support assertive behavior.
- You cannot be assertive and consider another person's feelings and behavior.
- Assertive behavior is just another way of complaining.
- If I am assertive, I will lose my job.
- There is no difference between assertiveness and aggressiveness.

---

identify and accept your position right now with regard to assertiveness so that you can make a plan to develop this skill.

What Are the Benefits of Assertiveness?

Assertive communication is the most effective way to let other people know what you feel, what you need, and what you are thinking. It helps you to feel good about yourself and allows you to treat others with respect. Being assertive helps you to avoid feeling guilty, angry, resentful, confused, or lonely. You have a greater chance to get your rights acknowledged and your needs met, which leads to a more satisfying life.

What Are My Basic Rights as a Person and as a Nurse?

As an adult human being, you have some legitimate rights. You may have to do some work to allow yourself to believe in your rights. You may have learned other values that make it difficult to accept the validity of these rights. But belief in your own value as a separate individual and confidence in the positive concepts associated with assertiveness as a communication style will help you to believe in your rights.

Consider the rights and responsibilities of the nurse. The issue of rights can become one-sided. When nurses consider rights, responsibilities must also be included. These rights are yours as a registered nurse; acquiring them and holding them are your responsibility (Chenevert, 1988).

How Can I Begin to Practice Assertive Communication?

There are a variety of ways to learn to be more assertive in your communication style, but they all involve self-awareness and practice. It may not feel totally comfortable at first, but as you work at it, assertive communication will come more naturally.

Changing one's behavior requires a conscious decision.

You should practice being assertive in a situation in which there is minimal risk to you, so that you can experience success. If sharing your feelings with your instructor or head nurse makes you extremely uncomfortable, set the situation aside. You can work on it after you are more confident. Share your feelings and practice being assertive with someone with whom you are comfortable. Personal risk should be at a minimum.

It is helpful to practice being assertive by yourself at first. Rehearse what you might say by talking to yourself while looking in a mirror. Once you feel more comfortable, ask a friend to help you practice. The two of you can role-play some assertive conversations. You may even want to videotape or audiotape your practice so you can get an idea of how you look and how you sound. When you are ready, try out your new assertive communication skills in a mildly uncomfortable situation you would like to change. Pay attention to how you feel. Ask for feedback from the other person. You will then be able to evaluate your progress and decide what other information you want to practice.

What Are the Components of Assertive Communication?

Assertive communication is a technique used to get one's needs met without purposely hurting others. It incorporates the principles of therapeutic communication, active listening skills, and a willingness to compromise. When you use these skills, you will be able to express yourself more effectively during challenging situations and handle confrontation in a professional manner. When you are confronted by a situation that provokes anger, take a deep breath, pull yourself away, get your emotions under control, and then approach the individual privately in a non-threatening manner. Following are some hints for using assertive communication:

- Use "I" statements: "I am really upset about …"
- Describe the behavior that has upset you and focus on the present: "You have been having excessive personal telephone calls over the past 2 days."
- Discuss the consequences of the behavior: "This behavior is contrary to the agency policy and could result in …"
- State how the behavior needs to be modified and the time for this change: "You must immediately stop this interruption to your work and request that people not call you at work unless it's an emergency."

The following strategy is a way to think about expressing your feelings and needs that will assist you to communicate assertively:

I feel … about … because …

Let us look at an example:
- I feel tired and cranky because I'm not paying enough attention to my family's needs.
- I feel hurt and angry about Dr. Jones yelling at me in front of you because I need to feel competent and respected at work.

These statements are most successful when you maintain direct eye contact, stand up straight, and speak in a clear, audible, firm tone of voice. After expressing your own feelings and needs, it is helpful to seek clarification of the other person's feelings or needs. This can be done with the following questions:

"How do you feel about that?"

"What were you thinking and feeling at that time?"

"How would that affect you?"

With skillful listening and clear communication, the problem can be defined without placing blame or "putting down" the other person. Notice the use of "I" messages—that indicates willingness to accept responsibility for the process of defining the problem and negotiating a workable solution. To find a compromise, you have to be willing to meet the other person halfway. You may agree to try it your way one time and the other person's the next. Or you may both agree to change or give up something. You may do something for him or her if she does something else for you. Remember that in the work setting you cannot always have things exactly as you want them. You must be willing to change and compromise (Elgin, 2000).

When to Use Assertive Communication

Here are some examples of situations in which assertive communication would be helpful.

■ COMMUNICATING EXPECTATIONS

Supervisor: "You're being pulled to the orthopedic unit today because they're short-staffed."

　Nurse: "I expect to be oriented into the unit and the equipment before I give nursing care because I haven't worked on that unit in more than a year."

■ SAYING NO

Physician: "Come with me right now. I need some help doing a procedure on Mr. Smith."

　Nurse: "I can't come with you right now. Let me have the nursing assistant get Mrs. Anderson back to bed and I'll help you then."

■ ACCEPTING CRITICISM

Head Nurse: "It seems to me that you are having difficulty updating your nursing care plans and getting them on the patient record before the end of the shift."

　Nurse: "I have been falling behind on my care plans. I would like to look at some examples of good care plans. Do you think you could help me with that? I'd be willing to spend some time at home reviewing them."

■ ACCEPTING COMPLIMENTS

Home care patient's spouse: "My wife feels very comfortable when you are here taking care of her. It's obvious you know what you're doing."

　Nurse: "Thank you. Your feedback is important to me."

■ GIVING CRITICISM

Nurse: "I want to talk with you about your care of Mrs. Samuelson. I found her sitting in a wheelchair alone in the hallway. It is your responsibility to make sure that she is not left alone, so that nothing happens to her."

　Aide: "I do not think that's my job."

　Nurse: "We talked about your responsibilities of caring for Mrs. Samuelson this morning when you received your assignment. If you have difficulty in carrying out this assignment, I expect you to ask for help."

■ ACCEPTING FEEDBACK

Head Nurse: "I wanted to tell you that I have noticed an improvement in your communication with Dr. Turner. He has not complained about his patient's care for 2 weeks, and yesterday he told me that he had a positive discussion with you about home health care options for Mrs. Atkins."

Nurse: "Thank you. I have been working very hard at not responding angrily to his sarcastic comments and criticisms."

■ ASKING FOR HELP

Nurse: "I am having a hard time with Mr. Jones. He seems to have a way of pushing my buttons, so I get angry. It is hard for me to ask for help, because I expect myself to care for all patients without difficulty."

Community Health Nurse Supervisor: "Mr. Jones can be a difficult patient. Can I help you?"

Nurse: "Yes. I need help in understanding why I get so angry at him, and I want to know how to handle him in a more positive way."

Remember that you need to evaluate how your assertive communication feels to you and to seek feedback from others about how you are being interpreted. You need to know whether people perceive you as aggressive rather than assertive. It may mean modifying your communication to make sure you are standing up for yourself without violating the rights of others.

It should also be noted that some situations will not get resolved just because you communicated assertively. Finding a workable solution is a process involving other people who must take responsibility for their own feelings and needs. When others are unable to acknowledge their feelings, to listen, or to negotiate a compromise, your assertive communication may make you feel better about yourself but may not produce an immediate solution. But keep trying. Persistence pays off.

CRITICAL THINKING
BOX 12-8

COMMUNICATION EXERCISE

Directions: Use the following situations to reflect on key points covered in this chapter. Think of a way to communicate effectively in each situation. You may want to consider your own individual solutions and then role-play or discuss your ideas with a group of your classmates.

1. Develop a list of 10 patients who are hospitalized on your unit. For each patient, provide some personal information, a diagnosis, and some data about his or her progress during the last 24 hours. Use the information you have listed to give a change-of-shift report to the four staff members who will be caring for these patients during the next 8 hours.

2. You have asked to speak to Dr. Sanders about your concerns in caring for one of her patients who has required much physical care since she has gone home from the hospital. Dr. Sanders has a reputation for being cold, aloof, and sarcastic. You have never spoken directly to her alone before.

3. You are a member of the home health care agency's procedures committee. After attending the last meeting, you have been given the responsibility for drafting a revision to the procedure used when administering controlled substances. You know that you need more information before you can begin your work. Send a memo to at least three different members of the agency staff identifying what information you would like them to provide for you. Make a follow-up phone call to make sure they received the memo.

Remember, too, that there are some situations in which you must simply follow orders. You cannot always meet your own needs; you must do what a physician or your head nurse tells you to do. Sometimes you must put aside your own needs to meet the needs of the patients you are caring for. However, your judgment will increase as you gain experience, and you will recognize ways to communicate your needs and feelings, with the goal of improving the processes and procedures used in your work setting.

CONCLUSION

Interpersonal skills, effective communication, group process, and team building are important for the nurse, because they form the foundation for creating an effective working environment. Well-planned, well-executed, and well-validated communication, along with caring and a positive attitude, will foster motivation, success, and satisfaction for the nurse in both the student role and as a new graduate.

Now that you have learned more about communicating effectively, try doing the student exercise in Critical Thinking Box 12-8. And happy communicating!

BIBLIOGRAPHY

Arredondo L: *Communicating effectively*, New York, 2000, McGraw-Hill.

Bahlman DT, Johnson FC: Using technology to improve and support communication and workflow processes, *AORN J* 82(1):65-73, 2005.

Chenevert M: *Pro-nurse handbook*, ed 3, St. Louis, 1988, Mosby.

Deep S, Sussman L: *Smart moves for people in charge*, Reading, Mass, 1995, Addison-Wesley.

Dochterman J, Grace H: *Current issues in nursing*, ed 6, St. Louis, 2001, Mosby.

Elgin S: *The gentle art of verbal self-defense at work*, Paramus, NJ, 2000, Prentice Hall.

Farley MJ, Stoner MH: The nurse executive and interdisciplinary team building, *Nurs Adm Q* 13(2):24-30, 1989.

Fowler K (2005): Active listening, *Mind-Tools*. Retrieved from *www.mindtools.com/CommSkll/ActiveListening.htm*.

Huber D: *Leadership and nursing care management*, Philadelphia, 2000, Saunders.

Katzenbach JR, Smith DK: *Wisdom of teams*, New York, 1993, Harper Business.

Kushner M: *Successful presentations for dummies*, Foster City, Calif, 1997, IDG.

Marquis B, Huston C: *Leadership roles and management functions in nursing: theory and application*, ed 3, Philadelphia, 2000, JB Lippincott.

Mindell P: *How to say it for women: communicating with confidence and power using the language of success*, Paramus, NJ, 2001, Prentice Hall.

Northouse P: *Leadership theory and practice*, ed 2, Thousand Oaks, Calif, 2001, Sage.

Peoples DA: *Presentations plus*, New York, 1992, John Wiley & Sons.

Sovie MD: Care and service teams: a new imperative, *Nurs Econ* 10(2):94-100, 125, 1992.

Tuckman B , Jensen M: Stage of small group development revisited, *Group Organiz Stud* 2:419-427, 1977.

Vengel A: The influence edge: how to persuade others to help you achieve your goals, San Francisco, 2000, Berrett-Koehler Communications.

Additional resources are available online at *http://evolve.elsevier.com/Zerwekh/nsgtoday/.*

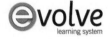

CHAPTER 13

Conflict Management

JoAnn Zerwekh, MSN, EdD, RN

> *Everything that irritates us about others can lead us to an understanding of ourselves.*
> —CARL JUNG

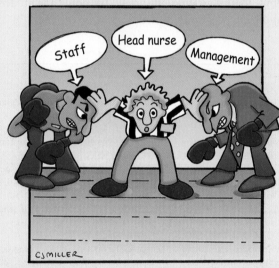

There is a better approach to conflict resolution than fighting it out.

After completing this chapter, you should be able to:

- Identify common factors that lead to conflict.

- Discuss five methods to resolve conflict.

- Discuss techniques to use in dealing with difficult people.

- Discuss solutions and alternatives in dealing with anger.

- Identify situations of sexual harassment in the workplace and discuss possible solutions.

an you imagine a world without conflict? Why, it would be a world without change! Conflict is inevitable wherever there are people with differing backgrounds, needs, values, and priorities.

A stereotypical perspective of conflict related to nursing is that "nice" nurses avoid conflict. According to Beauregard and colleagues (2003), although caricatured images of the nurse may encompass the "old" battleaxe, the control freak, the naughty nurse, or the doctor's handmaiden, the primary perception of the nurse by the public is one of the caring angel who is gentle and kind. Conflict within the nursing profession has traditionally generated negative feelings to the extent that many nurses use avoidance as a coping mechanism, because of their feeling that the "public's stereotypical image of them demanded that they be 'nice,' self-sacrificing, and submissive nurses and that if they engaged in conflict they would be branded emotional or unfeminine women" (Kelly, 2006, p 27).

The presence of conflict in a situation is not necessarily negative but may, in fact, have some positive results. As a process, conflict is neutral. Following are some possible outcomes of conflict:

- Disturbing issues are brought out into the open, which may avert a more serious conflict.
- Group cohesiveness may increase as individuals resolve issues.
- New leadership may develop as a consequence of resolution.
- The results of conflict can be constructive (this occurs when productive outcomes are achieved) or destructive, leading to poor communication and creating dissatisfaction.

CONFLICT

What Causes Conflict?

Let us look at some common factors of conflict as they relate to nursing.

Role Conflict. When two people have the same or related responsibilities with ambiguous boundaries, the potential for conflict exists. For example, a nurse on the 11 PM to 7 AM shift may be uncertain whether he or the nurse on the 7 AM to 3 PM shift is responsible for weighing a patient.

Communication Conflict. Failing to discuss differences with one another can lead to problems with communication. Communication is a two-way process; when one person is unclear in a communication, the process falls apart. A recent graduate may find that with a busy schedule, numerous patient demands, and a shortage of time, it is easy to forget to notify a patient's family of a change in visiting hours—a great annoyance to the family members who cannot visit when they arrive.

Goal Conflict. We all have unique goals and objectives for what we hope to achieve in our places of employment. When one nurse places his or her personal achievement and advancement above everyone else's, conflict can occur. An example of this can be seen in the newly graduated nurse who pursues an advanced nursing degree immediately following undergraduate education; the experienced nurse in the unit may feel that the new graduate nurse requires a minimum length of time at the bedside before advancing his or her education.

Personality Conflict. Wouldn't it be great if we got along with everyone? Of course, we all know that there are just some people with whom we have a difficult time. The situation is all too familiar, and many times we may find ourselves with such thoughts as "I'll try and overlook her negative, lousy behavior; after all, she doesn't have much of a family life." Trying to change another person's personality is like guaranteeing an unhappy ending to a story.

Ethical or Values Conflict. During a cardiac arrest, a young graduate nurse has a conflict with the physician's order of "No Code," on a young adolescent patient. She has difficulty taking care of the adolescent because he reminds her of her younger brother who died tragically in an automobile accident.

Conflicts in nursing may fit into one or more of the aforementioned categories. Consider some common areas of conflict among nursing staff, including scheduling days off, determining vacation leave, assigning committees, patient care assignments, and performance appraisal, to name just a few.

What Are Common Areas of Conflict Between Nurses and Patients— and Between Nurses and Patients' Families?

Guttenberg (1983) identifies five common areas of conflict among nurses and their patients and families.

1. **Quality of care.** This is by far the most common area of conflict and the easiest to remedy. Families typically are concerned with how well their loved one is being attended to, how friendly the nurses are, how well the hospital or home health services are provided and coordinated, and how flexible the hospital is with visiting hours and meeting their special needs.
2. **Treatment decisions.** This area of conflict often arises between the family of an older adult and the nurse. A physician may order a treatment with which the family does not agree. In this situation it is very important that the nurse not defend the physician's orders or attempt to persuade or convince the family that the physician or nurse knows what's best for the patient. In these situations the issue is rarely the treatment itself but rather the family's desire to decide what is right for their loved one. Be sure to clarify the orders and explain to the family that you are supposed to carry them out unless the family negotiates directly with the physician to change them. Conflict may also exist between the nurse and physician regarding care of older adults. For example, a physician may decline performing a medical procedure on an older patient secondary to advanced age or preexisting comorbidities.
3. **Family involvement.** For example, when a young adult is diagnosed with cancer, numerous issues may arise concerning the presence of family members during procedures and the extent of their involvement in the overall care. Such issues are based on the family's real need to feel significant and adequate in meeting the young adult's needs.
4. **Quality of parental care.** This can become an issue when nurses are unhappy with how parents are participating in their child's care. It is helpful to offer parenting classes, to encourage parents to meet other parents, and to model positive parenting techniques. Fear of being a bad parent by not responding to every cry an infant makes is a good example of where the nurse can educate the parents on responding to their infant's physical and emotional needs.
5. **Staff inconsistency.** This is another easily preventable issue. Make sure that staff members on each shift are consistent in enforcing hospital policies and that they notify other shifts of any attempts at manipulation by family members or patients.

CONFLICT RESOLUTION

What Are Ways to Resolve Conflict?

Unresolved conflicts waste time and energy and reduce productivity and cooperation among the people with whom you work. In contrast, when conflicts are resolved, they strengthen relationships and improve the performance of everyone involved. The key to successfully managing conflict is tailoring your response to fit each conflict situation instead of just relying on one particular technique. Each technique represents a different way to achieve the outcome you want and to help the other person achieve at least part of the outcome that he or she wants. How do you know which technique to use? That depends on the following:

- How much power do you have in this situation compared with the other person?
- How much do you value your relationship with the person with whom you are in conflict?
- How much time is available to resolve the conflict?

An example of a model for conflict resolution can be found in Figure 13-1. This model incorporates several views on conflict resolution. Filley (1975) described three basic strategies for dealing with conflict, according to outcome: win-win, lose-lose, and win-lose. Various others have identified the following five responses to resolve conflict: competition, accommodation, avoidance, compromise, and cooperation. In a recent study, the prevalent style for conflict resolution of nursing students was compromise, followed by avoidance (Hamilton, 2008). As noted in this research study, compromise attempts to meet the needs of individuals on both sides of a conflict, while collaboration, which may take more time offers the best avenue or approach to settling the conflict that will satisfy both (win-win solution).

Let us look at an example and apply the model.

Suppose the head nurse on your unit has posted the vacation schedule for the month of December. You, as a recent graduate, have requested to be off during the week of Christmas. You notice on the schedule that none of the recent graduates has received the Christmas holidays off. You feel that this is unfair because you will not have an opportunity to be with your family during the Christmas holidays. How can you resolve this conflict?

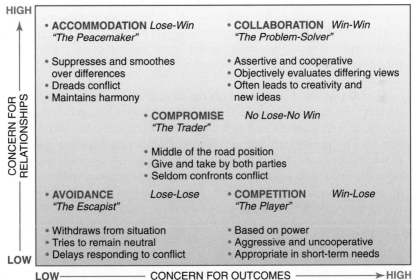

FIGURE 13-1

Model for conflict resolution. *(Modified from Douglas E, Bushardt W: Interpersonal conflict: strategies and guidelines for resolution, J AMRA 56(18), 1988; and Sullivan E, Decker P: Effective management in nursing, Menlo Park, Calif, 1988 Addison-Wesley.)*

Competition. This is an example of the *win-lose* situation. In this situation, force—or the use of power—occurs. It sets up a type of competition between you and your head nurse. Typically, competition is used to resolve conflict when one person has more power in a situation than the other. *In the given situation, the head nurse refuses your request for Christmas vacation, explaining that the staff members with more seniority have priority for vacation at Christmas time.*

Avoidance. Avoidance is unassertive and uncooperative, and leads to a *lose-lose* situation. In some situations, avoidance is not considered a true form of conflict resolution because the conflict is not resolved and neither party is satisfied. *In the given situation, you would not have approached the head nurse with the Christmas schedule issue.* Usually, both persons involved feel frustrated and angry. There are some situations in which avoiding the issue might be appropriate, such as when tempers are flaring or when strong anger is present. However, this is only a short-term strategy; it is important to get back to the problem after emotions have cooled.

Accommodation. Accommodation is the *lose-win* situation, in which one person accommodates the other at his or her own expense but often ends up feeling resentful and angry. *In the given situation, the head nurse would basically put her own concern aside and let you have your way, possibly even working in the scheduled slot for you. The head nurse loses and the graduate nurse wins in this situation, which may set up conflict among staff and other recent graduates.* When is accommodation the best response? Is it when conflict would create serious disruption, such as arguing, or when the person you are in conflict with has the power to resolve the conflict unilaterally? Basically, in this response to conflict, differences are suppressed or played down while agreement is emphasized.

Compromise. Compromise or bargaining is the strategy that recognizes the importance of both the resolution of the problem and the relationship between the two people. Compromise is a moderately assertive and cooperative step in the right direction in which one creates a *modified win-lose* outcome. *In the given situation, the head nurse compromises with you by allowing you to have Christmas Eve off with your family, but not the entire week.* The problem lies in the reduced staffing that will occur for a short period of time. The compromise may not be totally satisfactory for either party, but it may be offered as a temporary solution until more options become available.

Collaboration. Collaboration is the strategy that involves a high level of concern for the problem, the outcome, and the relationship. It deals with confrontation and problem solving. The needs, feelings, and desires of both parties are taken into consideration and reexamined while searching for proper ways to agree on goals. Collaboration is a *win-win* solution, a commitment to resolve the issues at the base of the conflict. It is fully assertive and cooperative. *In the given situation, you and the head nurse discuss the week of Christmas vacation and the staffing needs and agree that you will work the first three days of that week and the head nurse will work the second half of that week. You also agree to be there the first part of the week to complete the audit on the charts from the previous week for the head nurse. In this situation both persons are satisfied, and there is no compromising what is most important to each person. That is, the head nurse gets her audit completed and the recent graduate gets to spend half of the Christmas week with her family.* What is your particular style for resolving conflict? (Critical Thinking Box 13-1.)

What Are Some Basic Guidelines for Which Technique to Use?

In some situations, certain techniques and responses work best. You may have to use accommodation or avoidance when you lack the power to change the situation. When you have conflict

CONFLICT QUESTIONNAIRE

Directions: Consider situations in which you find your wishes differing from those of another person. For each of the following statements, think how likely you are to respond in that way to such a situation. Check the rating that best corresponds to your response.

	Very Unlikely	Unlikely	Very Likely	Likely
1. I am usually firm in pursuing my goals.	_____	_____	_____	_____
2. I try to win my position.	_____	_____	_____	_____
3. I give up some points in exchange for others.	_____	_____	_____	_____
4. I feel that differences are not always worth worrying about.	_____	_____	_____	_____
5. I try to find a position that is between others and mine.	_____	_____	_____	_____
6. In approaching a negotiation, I try to consider the other person's wishes.	_____	_____	_____	_____
7. I try to show the logic and benefits of my position.	_____	_____	_____	_____
8. I always lean toward a direct discussion of the problem.	_____	_____	_____	_____
9. I try to find a fair combination of gains and losses for both of us.	_____	_____	_____	_____
10. I attempt to work through our differences immediately.	_____	_____	_____	_____
11. I try to avoid creating unpleasantness for myself.	_____	_____	_____	_____
12. I might try to soothe other's feelings and preserve our relationship.	_____	_____	_____	_____
13. I attempt to get all concerns and issues immediately out.	_____	_____	_____	_____
14. I sometimes avoid taking positions that create controversy.	_____	_____	_____	_____
15. I try not to hurt the other's feelings.	_____	_____	_____	_____

CRITICAL

SCORING: Very Unlikely = 1; Unlikely = 2; Likely = 3; Very Likely = 4.

	Item:	Item:	Item:	
COMPETING:	1 _____	2 _____	7 _____	TOTAL _____
COLLABORATING:	8 _____	10 _____	13 _____	TOTAL _____
COMPROMISING:	3 _____	5 _____	9 _____	TOTAL _____
AVOIDING:	4 _____	11 _____	14 _____	TOTAL _____
ACCOMMODATING:	6 _____	12 _____	15 _____	TOTAL _____

From Thomas KW: Toward multidimensional values in teaching: the example of conflict behaviors, *Acad Manage Rev* 2:487, 1977.

in a relationship that you value, it might be more helpful to use accommodation, compromise, or collaboration. When there is no immediate, pressing sense of time to solve an issue, then any of the five techniques can be used. However, when you are facing an emergency situation or a rapidly approaching deadline, your best bet is to use competition or accommodation. Just remember the following key behaviors in managing conflict:

- Deal with issues, not personalities.
- Take responsibility for yourself and your participation.
- Communicate openly.
- Listen actively.
- Sort out the issues.
- Identify key themes in the discussion.
- Weigh the consequences.

Suppose that you follow all of these suggestions and you still are confronted with that difficult situation or that difficult person. Read on.

DEALING WITH DIFFICULT PEOPLE

What Are Some Techniques for Handling Difficult People?

Now that we have discussed types of conflict management techniques, we are ready to look at techniques for handling difficult people. How do you deal with an abusive physician or supervisor? How do you react when someone constantly complains and gripes about something? How do you deal with the know-it-all who will not even listen to your thoughts on an issue? (See Evidence-Based Practice Box 13-1 for suggestions on managing difficult employees.)

I am sure, if you have not by now, you will in the near future run into a Sherman tank (Figure 13-2). According to Bramson (1981), Sherman tanks are the *attackers*. They come out charging and are often abusive, abrupt, and intimidating. But more important, they tend to be downright overwhelming.

Remember Dr. Smith, who flew into a tirade because you forgot to have a suture removal set at his patient's bedside at 8 AM sharp? Remember how you felt? "My heart was beating so loud I could hear it, and I was sure everyone else around could hear it, too. I was so furious at him for the comments he made."

In understanding Sherman tanks, it is important to realize that they have a strong need to prove to themselves and to others that their view of the situation is right. They have a very strong sense of what others ought to do but often lack the caring and the trust that would be helpful in getting something done. They usually achieve what they want, but to do so causes them a lot of disagreements, lost friendships, and uncomfortable relationships with their co-workers. Sherman tanks are often very confident and tend to devalue those whom they feel are not confident. Unfortunately, they demean others in a way that makes them look very self-important and superior. How do you cope with a Sherman tank? The most important thing is to keep your fear and anger under control and avoid an outright confrontation about who is right and who is wrong. Following are some specific things you should do:

- Do not allow yourself to be run over; step aside.
- Stand up for yourself. Defend yourself, but without fighting. Seek support when warranted.

BOX 13-1   EVIDENCE-BASED PRACTICE

Managing Difficult Employees

PRACTICE ISSUE

Nurse managers are often faced with the difficult employee. The difficult employee's negative conflict behavior affects team performance effectiveness, job satisfaction, and turnover intention.

In an environment of team collegiality, there is less negative conflict and increased commitment to the organization and greater satisfaction, autonomy, and control over practice. In professional practice environments, nurses experience constructive conflict approaches, and effectiveness is enhanced in the workplace.

It is part of the nurse manager role to create an environment that facilitates professional practice. This type of environment requires that employees are socialized to their nursing role. In these professional practice environments, the unique preferences, perspectives, opinions, concerns, and choices of the individuals are recognized and valued. During nursing school, professional role socialization ("think like a nurse") is initiated and later solidified during the early years of practice when the new graduate incorporates knowledge, skills, attitude, and affective behavior associated with carrying out the expectations of the nursing role.

IMPLICATIONS FOR NURSING PRACTICE

Effective role socialization occurs when the nurse engages in actions that benefit other nurses and/or patients and families by helping, supporting, and encouraging mutual goal accomplishment and/or well-being.

There needs to be positive interdependence among the nursing staff.

- Nurses need to understand and use constructive conflict management skills.
- There is high trust among the nursing staff.
- Prosocial behavior is noted among staff with the feeling of "sink or swim together" versus "you sink and I swim."
- A high, basic self-esteem is noted among nursing staff in an empowering, healthy workplace environment.
- The conflict negotiation strategy used is collaboration (win/win) or it is "no deal."

Considering this Information:

How might you employ some of the strategies listed in this chapter to deal with a difficult employee? What types of activities are you involved as a student that promotes a positive professional practice environment?

Reference for the Evidence

Cornett PA, O'Rourke M: Building organizational capacity for a healthy work environment through role based professional practice, *Crit Care Nurs Q* 32(3):208-220, 2009.

Cornett, PA: Managing the difficult employee: a reframed perspective, *Crit Care Nurs Q* 32(4):314, 2009.

Hader R: Workplace violence survey 2008: unsettling findings, *Nurs Manag* 39(7):13-19, 326, 2008.

Siu H, Laschinger HKS, Finegan J: Nursing professional practice environments: setting the stage for constructive conflict resolution and work effectiveness, *J Nurs Adm* 38(5):250-257, 2008.

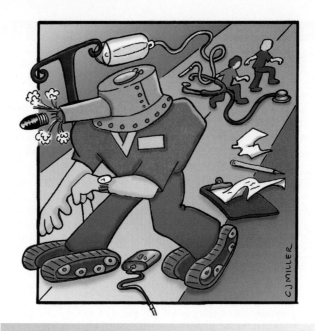

FIGURE 13-2
Sherman tank.

- Give them a little time to run down and express what they might be ranting about.
- Sometimes, it is necessary to be rude; get your word in any way that you can.
- If possible, try to get them to sit down. Be sure to maintain eye contact with them while you are stating your opinions and perceptions very forcefully.
- Do not argue with them or try to cut them down.
- When they finally hear you, be ready to be friendly.

Next to the Sherman tanks are the *snipers* (Figure 13-3). The snipers are the pot-shot artists. They are not as openly aggressive as the Sherman tanks. Their weapons are their innuendoes, their digs, and their nonplayful teasing, which is definitely aimed to hurt you. Snipers tend to choose a hidden rather than a frontal attack. They prefer to undercut you and make you look ridiculous. So, when you are dealing with a sniper, remember to expose the attack, that is, "smoke them out." Ask them very calmly:

"That sounded like a put-down. Did you really mean it that way?" Or you might say, "Do I understand that you don't like what I'm saying? It sounds as if you are making fun of me. Are you?"

When a sniper is giving you criticism, be sure to get group confirmation or denial. Ask questions or make statements such as, "Does anyone else see the issue this way?" "It seems as though we have a difference of opinion," or "Exactly what is the issue here? What is it that you don't like about what occurred?" One way to prevent sniping is by setting up regular problem-solving meetings with that person.

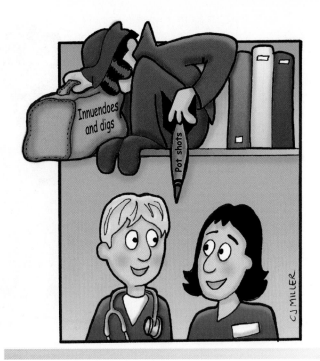

FIGURE 13-3
The sniper.

Also difficult to cope with are the *constant complainers*. These people often feel as though they are powerless and get attention—but seldom action—on their problem. A complainer points out real problems but does it from a very nonconstructive stance. Coping with a complainer can be a challenge. First, it is important to listen to the complaints, acknowledge them, and make sure you understand what the person said by paraphrasing it or checking out your perception of how the person feels. Do not necessarily agree with the person; with a complainer, it is important to move into a problem-solving mode by asking very specific, informative questions and encouraging him or her to submit complaints in writing. For example, try communicating with the constant complainer in the following manner:

"Did I understand you to say that you are having difficulty with your patient assignment?"

"Would it be helpful if I went to the pharmacy for you, so that you could complete your chart on your preoperative patient?"

Next are the maddening ones: the *clams* (Figure 13-4). The clams have an entirely different tactic from the previous three. They just refuse to respond when you need an answer or want to have a discussion. It might be helpful to try to read a clam's nonverbal communication. Watch out for wrinkled brows, a frown, or a sigh. How to deal with a clam? Try to get them to open up by using open-ended questions and waiting very quietly for a response. Do not fill in their silence with your own conversation. Give yourself enough time to wait with composure. Sometimes a little "clamming" on your own part might be helpful by using the technique called the "friendly,

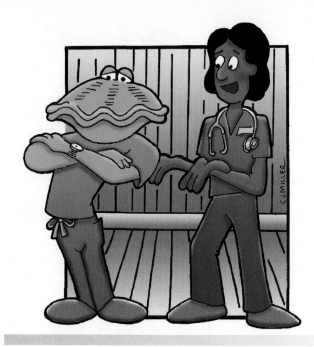

FIGURE 13-4

The clam.

silent stare," or FSS. The way to set up the FSS is to have a very inquisitive, expectant expression on your face with raised eyebrows, wide eyes, and maybe a slight smile—all nonverbal cues to the clam that you are waiting for a response. When clams finally open up, be very attentive. Watch your own impulses—do not bubble over with happiness just because they have finally given you two moments of their time. Avoid the polite ending; in other words, get up and say, for example:

"This was important to me. I'm not going to let this issue drop. I'll be back to talk to you tomorrow at 2 o'clock." Do not be the nice guy and say, "Thanks for coming in. Have a nice weekend. I'll see you tomorrow."

Be very direct and inform the clam what you are going to do, especially if the desired discussion did not occur.

What Is Anger?

Anger is something that we feel. Usually when we get angry, we assume it is because we are upset about what someone has done to us. Often we want to pay them back or take out our rage on them. Usually when anger occurs, it is hard to see beyond the moment because most people are consumed with thoughts of revenge or the wrongdoing that has occurred to them. Weiss and Cain (1991) state that "Anger is often a cover-up emotion … that disguises what is really going on inside you." But, anger is a signal, and according to Lerner (1997), it is "one worth listening to" (p 1). She goes on further to say that:

Our anger may be a message that we are being hurt, that our rights are being violated, that our needs or wants are not being adequately met, or simply that something is not right. Our anger may tell us that we are not addressing an important emotional issue in our lives, or that too much of ourselves—our beliefs, values, desires, or ambitions—are being compromised in a relationship. Our anger may be a signal that we are doing more and giving more than we can comfortably do or give. Or our anger may warn us that others are doing too much for us, at the expense of our own competence and growth. Just as physical pain tells us to take our hand off the hot stove, the pain of our anger preserves the very integrity of our self. Our anger can motivate us to say "no" to the ways in which we are defined by others and "yes" to the dictates of our inner self. (p 1)

No matter what, when feelings of frustration, disappointment, or powerlessness take over, there is no doubt anger is in the making. Anger seems to begin in situations fraught with threats and anxiety.

Anger has two faces. One is *guilt,* which is anger aimed inward at what we did or did not do, and the other is *resentment,* which is anger directed toward others at what they did or did not do.

> The following is true about both guilt and resentment: They both accumulate over time and lead to a cycle of negative energy that poisons our relationships and stifles our personal growth.

However, there is another side of the coin. If feeling angry signifies a problem, then ventilating anger does not necessarily solve it. Actually, ventilating anger may serve to maintain it if change and successful resolution do not occur. Tavris (1984) suggests that we teach two things about dealing with anger: first, how to think about anger, and second, how to reduce the tension. More about this later in the chapter.

Lerner (1997) gives some helpful advice on how to determine your characteristic style of managing anger. Box 13-1 has a summary of five different anger styles. Just think about anger from a cardiovascular point of view. Most authorities consider anger one of the most damaging and dangerous emotions because your pulse and blood pressure become elevated, sometimes to dangerous heights.

What Is the Solution for Dealing with Anger?

> Change the image of it!

Stop. Appraise the situation. Do not do a thing. You are at a pivotal point. You have two ways to go: One is to get angry; the other is to reappraise the situation. Try to look at a way to reinterpret the annoying comment. Consider the following example:

"Who does that head nurse think he is to treat me like I'm a dummy!" or "How could someone be so thoughtless as to not remember my birthday!" You can reinterpret these and say to yourself, "Maybe if they weren't so unhappy, they wouldn't have considered doing such a thing" or "Maybe that person's having a rough day." The important thing here is to empathize with the person and to try to find justifications for the behavior that was so annoying to you.

BOX 13-1   Characteristic Styles of Managing Anger

PURSUERS

- React to anxiety by seeking greater togetherness in a relationship.
- Place a high value on talking things out and expressing feelings.
- Alone or away from the relationship.
- Tend to pursue harder and then coldly withdraw when an important person seeks distance.
- May negatively label themselves as "too dependent" or "too demanding" in a relationship.
- Tend to criticize their partner as someone who cannot handle feelings or tolerate closeness.

DISTANCERS

- Seek emotional distance or physical space when stress is high.
- Consider themselves to be self-reliant and private persons-more "do-it-yourselfers" than help-seekers.
- Have difficulty showing their needy, vulnerable, and dependent sides.
- Receive such labels as "emotionally unavailable," "withholding," and "unable to deal with feeling" from significant others.
- Manage anxiety in personal relationships by intensifying work-related projects.
- May cut off a relationship entirely when things get intense.
- Open up most freely when they are not pushed or pursued.

UNDERFUNCTIONERS

- Tend to have several areas in which they just cannot get organized.
- Become less competent under stress, thus inviting others to take over.
- Tend to develop physical or emotional symptoms when stress is high in either the family or the work situation.
- May become the focus of family gossip.
- Earn such labels as the "patient," the "fragile one," "the sick one," the "problem," or the "irresponsible one."
- Have difficulty showing their strong, competent side to intimate others.

OVERFUNCTIONERS

- Know what is best not only for themselves but for others as well.
- Move in quickly to advise, rescue, and take over when stress hits.
- Have difficulty staying out and allowing others to struggle with their own problems.
- Avoid worrying about their own personal goals and problems by focusing on others.
- Have difficulty sharing their own vulnerable, underfunctioning side, especially with those people who are viewed as having problems.
- May be labeled the person who is "always reliable" or "always together."

BLAMERS

- Respond to anxiety with emotional intensity and fighting.
- Have a short fuse.
- Expend high levels of energy trying to change someone who does not want to change.
- Engage in repetitive cycles of fighting that relieve tension but perpetuate the old pattern.
- Hold another person responsible for one's own feelings and actions.
- See others as the sole obstacle to making changes.

Modified from Lerner H: *The dance of anger: a woman's guide to changing the patterns of intimate relationships*, New York, HarperCollins, 1997.

Look. What image about yourself or another is about to be or has been breached—what *should*'s, *must*'s, or *need to*'s have been violated? In other words, what has just occurred that has led you to feel angry at yourself or another?

After receiving the end-of-shift report and making rounds to her patients, a recent graduate goes into a patient's room to take vital signs. Within moments the patient has a cardiac arrest. Two hours later while completing her chart, the recent graduate states guiltily, "I should have taken those vital signs earlier. It just needs to be the first thing I do when I get on the unit. I should have been on top of this. I must do better." Notice the self-criticism in the recent graduate's comments. Guilt, like resentment, can be a habit. It demonstrates—too clearly—how we respond to a situation in a negative manner. To help you get in touch with these feelings, try eliminating the words "must" and "should" from your vocabulary for just an hour. It is quite surprising to find out how frequently we use these terms.

Change. How do you change the image? One of the ways is to use humor. Humor makes the anger (guilt and resentment) tolerable. Remember that it is difficult to laugh and frown at the same time. (It only takes 15 facial muscles to laugh, but twice that many to frown.) If reappraising the situation and humor both fail as ways to deal with your anger, some suggest venting the anger—for example, by getting mad, yelling, shouting, telling someone off, or breaking things. Although this might make us feel better momentarily, in the long run such outbursts make us feel worse.

Why does this method of venting anger, that is, letting it all hang out, make us feel worse? First, think of all the physiological changes that are occurring in your body: blood pressure, pulse, and respirations increase; the muscles contract; and adrenalin is released. Sound familiar? It is the "fight or flight" adrenal response. Can it be healthy to maintain a constant state of stress and readiness to respond? Another disadvantage of an uninhibited outburst of anger is that it may lead the other person to retaliate.

It might be important to recognize the difference between venting and acknowledging our anger. A typical expression of anger might be something such as the following:

"Hey, you turkey, what do you think you're doing? Don't you know how to put that catheter in? Are you stupid or something? Either you figure it out, or you get out of here. You hear me?"

This approach is insulting, demeaning, and accusatory. It is also likely to lead to some type of provoking response. In contrast, when we acknowledge our feelings, we make statements such as *"I feel angry about …"* or *"I feel hurt about …"* or *"I feel guilty about …"* The use of "I" statements is our first step toward taking responsibility for ourselves by owning up to our own feelings instead of blaming others.

Venting anger simply does not work unless you want to intimidate those around you, coerce them into submission with a hot temper, or, better yet, look childish while ranting, raving, and beating the floor or each other with foam bats. So, what does work? *Face it, embrace it, and erase it!*

First, acknowledge the anger *(face it):* Ask "What am I feeling? Anger? Guilt? Rage? Resentment?"

Second, identify the provoking or triggering situation *(embrace it):* Ask "What caused this feeling? Whose problem is it?"

Third, determine what changes need to occur *(erase it):* Ask "What can I change? Can I accept what I cannot change?" Then take action and let go of the rest. Other ways to deal with anger and get out of the vicious cycle of guilt and resentment include the following:

Move.

Get Active. Try exercise or anything involving physical activity, such as walking, aerobics, and running. Clean out the garage or a kitchen drawer. If you are sitting, get up. If you are in bed, move your arms around. Just get up and do something!

Focus.

Refocus on Something Positive. Think of your cup as half full, not half empty. Look at the provoking situation: "My head nurse won't give me Christmas off. However, I am not scheduled to work either Christmas Eve or New Year's Eve. So, by working Christmas Day, I'm assured the other days off."

Breathe.

Pay Attention to Your Breathing. Slow it down. Take deep, slow breaths, feeling the air move through your nose and down into your lungs. Check out your body for areas of tenseness. Often anger can be felt as tightness in the chest and abdomen.

Conflict is an inevitable part of our day-to-day experience. How we negotiate and handle conflict and anger may not always be easy. You might be thinking right now "This looks good on paper, but in real life, it is not that easy to put into practice." If you are feeling this way, take a risk at changing your approach and viewpoint.

The important thing is learning about yourself.

How do you deal with conflict? How do you handle difficult people? How do you respond when angry?

SEXUAL HARASSMENT IN THE WORKPLACE

In today's world, sexual harassment as a source of conflict has been taken seriously, as evidenced by the widespread visibility and increased recognition of the issue. The potential impact of harassment on nursing students both in the classroom and in the practice area is significant.

According to Dowell (1992), nursing administrators and educators must be proactive in writing and implementing policies regarding sexual harassment. In a study by Libbus and Bowman (1994), 70% of female staff nurses surveyed reported sexual harassment by male patients and co-workers, with the most common complaint being sexual remarks and inappropriate touching. In addition, in a survey of nursing administrators, 68.8% of those who responded reported sexist attitudes among employees in their organizations, and 47.7% reported observing instances of sexual harassment (Blancett & Sullivan, 1993). These studies reflect the prevalence of sexual harassment in health care settings.

The issue of sexual harassment came to the forefront during the 1991 confirmation hearings of Supreme Court Justice Clarence Thomas (Allen, 1992). Now a once-secretive problem is openly discussed in newspapers and by the media. As awareness about sexual harassment increased, we all realized how little we knew about it and what we could do about it. The majority of cases involve women who report being harassed by men. In nursing, the stereotypical situation of sexual harassment involves a nurse (i.e., a woman) and a doctor (i.e., a man) because of the large number of nurses who are women. However, with the increase in the number of men entering the nursing profession, there is the potential for men to experience sexual harassment in the workplace. Roth and Coleman (2008) agree that actual and perceived barriers exist that prevent men from entering the nursing profession. In an effort to remove existing barriers and attract more men into the nursing profession, the authors recommend that the image of male nursing and the media's depiction of male nurses be showcased as positive and that increasing diversity by recruiting men within the nursing workforce be embraced by both the public and nursing profession (Figure 13-5).

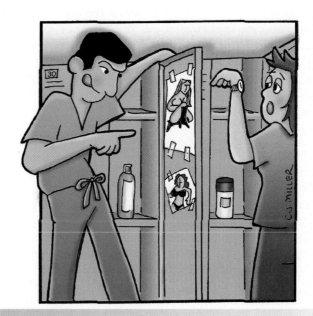

FIGURE 13-5
Sexual harassment.

What Is Sexual Harassment?

According to Friedman, "sexual harassment refers to conduct, typically experienced as offensive in nature, in which unwanted sexual advances are made in the context of a relationship of unequal power or authority" (1992, p 9). He goes on to explain that victims of sexual harassment are subjected to sexually oriented verbal comments, unwanted touching, and requests for sexual favors. The typical problem, known as quid pro quo harassment, arises when unwelcome sexual advances have been made and an employee is required to submit to those demands as a condition either of employment or of promotion. "Hostile work environment" has been used as a legal claim to show that "the atmosphere in the work (or other) environment is so uncomfortable or offensive by virtue of sexual advances, sexual requests, or sexual innuendoes that it amounts to a hostile environment" (Friedman, 1992, p 16). Let us look at hypothetical examples of how sexual harassment can affect nursing.

Samantha, a recent graduate, was receiving continued requests from a male patient to provide him with a complete bed bath. However, when a male nurse was assigned to this patient the following day, the patient reported to the male nurse that he was capable of bathing himself and proceeded to take a shower.

Lisa, the evening charge nurse, was quite excited that Tom, a recent graduate, was going to work on her unit. Lisa pursued Tom by repeatedly asking him for assistance with patient care and when she called him into her office, she would touch him inappropriately.

What Can I Do About It?

There are two ways to deal with this type of workplace conflict: informally and formally through a grievance procedure. Start with the most direct measure. Ask the person to STOP! Tell the harasser in clear terms that the behavior makes you uncomfortable and that you want it to stop immediately. Also, you might want to put your statement in writing to the person, keeping a copy for yourself. Tell other people, such as family, friends, personal physician, or minister, what is happening and how you are dealing with it. Friedman (1992) suggests keeping a written journal of harassing events, including all attempts used to try to stop the harassment. The need to exercise power and control, rather than sexual desire, is frequently the motive of the sexual harasser (perpetrator). If sexual harassment is occurring as a result of miscommunication and misinterpretation of actions and is primarily sexually driven, not power-driven, then telling the perpetrator to stop will often clear up any misconceptions. However, if the perpetrator is power-driven, the harassment will continue as long as he or she views the victim as passive, powerless, and frightened. What may be most difficult for the recent graduate is facing the fear that surrounds threats of job insecurity or public embarrassment (Friedman, 1992).

If a direct request to the perpetrator to stop does not work, then an informal complaint may be effective, especially if both parties realize a problem exists and want it to be solved. The goal of the informal method is to stop the harassment but not punish the perpetrator. This method assists the person filing the complaint in maintaining some type of harmonious relationship with the perpetrator. According to Friedman, "a formal grievance usually requires filing a written complaint with an official group such as a hearing" (1992, p 65). This is a legal procedure that is guided and regulated by federal and state laws specific to this type of grievance. Before a 1991 amendment to the Civil Rights Act (Title VII), the means of correcting this bad situation—making it right or compensating the victim for difficulty encountered—were quite restricted.

What has occurred as a result of this act is that victims of intentional discrimination may now seek compensatory and punitive damages. Each state has an Equal Employment Opportunity Commission, which has as its specific charge the enforcement of Title VII.

Unfortunately, sexual harassment may be a form of conflict you are faced with in the workplace. It is important to learn to deal with your feelings and be aware of actions to take in case this happens to you. When this type of situation is resolved in a constructive, positive manner, it allows you an opportunity to feel better about your ability to deal with conflict.

CONCLUSION

Most of us have experienced conflict. Building effective conflict management skills is key to dealing with patients, staff, and physicians. Various models exist to provide a framework for effective conflict resolution; the "win-win" model of *collaboration* is the strategy that aims for the highest level of resolution and is fully assertive and cooperative in approach. It takes creative nursing management and understanding to recognize and acknowledge that conflict will exist whenever human relationships are involved. This needs to be tempered with open, accurate communication and active listening by maintaining an objective, not emotional, stance as conflict resolution strategies are utilized.

BIBLIOGRAPHY

Allen A: Equal opportunity in the workplace, *J Post Anesth Nurs* 7(2):132-134, 1992.

Beauregard M, et al: Improving our image a nurse at a time, *J Nurs Adm* 10:510-511, 2003.

Blancett SS, Sullivan PA: Ethics survey results, *J Nurs Admin* 23(3):9-13, 1993.

Bramson R: *Coping with difficult people*, New York, 1981, National Press Publications.

Dowell M: Sexual harassment in academia: legal and administrative challenges, *J Nurs Educ* 31(1):5-9, 1992.

Filley AC: *Interpersonal conflict resolution*, Glenview, Ill, 1975, Scott Foresman.

Friedman J: *Sexual harassment: what it is, what it isn't, what it does to you, and what you can do about it*, Deerfield Beach, Fla, 1992, Health Communications.

Guttenberg RM: How to stay cool in a conflict and turn it into cooperation, *Nurs Life* 3(3):25-29, 1983.

Hamilton, P: Conflict management styles in the health professions, *Southern Online Journal of Nursing Research* 8(2):2p, 2008.

Kelly J: An overview of conflict, *Dimens Crit Care Nurs* 25(1):22-28, 2006.

Lerner H: *The dance of anger: a woman's guide to changing the patterns of intimate relationships*, New York, 1997, Harper & Row.

Libbus MK, Bowman KG: Sexual harassment of female registered nurses in hospitals, *J Nurs Admin* 24(6):26-31, 1994.

Roth J, Coleman C: Perceived and real barriers for men entering nursing: implications for gender diversity, *J Cult Divers* 15(3):148-152, 2008.

Tavris C: Feeling angry? Letting off steam may not help, *Nurs Life* 4(5):59-61, 1984.

Weiss L, Cain L: *Power lines: what to say in problem situations*, Dallas, 1991, Taylor.

Additional resources are available online at *http://evolve.elsevier.com/Zerwekh/nsgtoday/*.

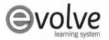

CHAPTER 14

Delegation in the Clinical Setting

Ruth I. Hansten, RN, MBA, PhD, FACHE, and Marilynn Jackson, RN, PhD, CHTP, CCA

Let whoever is in charge keep this simple question in her head (NOT how can I always do the right thing myself but) how can I provide for this right thing always to be done?
—FLORENCE NIGHTINGALE

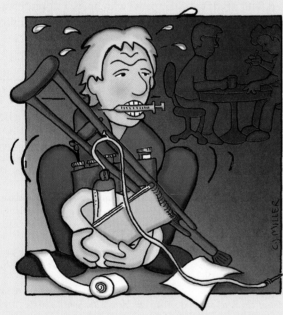

Nurses need to recognize when to delegate.

After completing this chapter, you should be able to:

- Define the operational terms delegation, supervision, and accountability.

- Delegate tasks successfully on the basis of outcomes.

- Select the right person for the right task.

- Apply the "four Cs" of initial direction for a clear understanding of your expectations.

- Provide reciprocal feedback for the effective evaluation of the delegate's performance.

*U*nless you are practicing on a deserted island with only one patient and you are the health care provider, chances are great that you will be working with other members of the health care team. How do you make best use of the resources they have to offer? What is your role as the registered nurse (RN) on the team in terms of making these decisions? Your ability to effectively delegate tasks that need to be done, on the basis of desired outcomes will go a long way in determining the success of the efforts of your work.

WHAT DOES DELEGATION MEAN?

We begin where we always must, with an understanding of the terms under discussion. Fortunately, there have been many people hard at work for years, creating operational definitions of the term *delegation* to assist us in standardizing our approach. It helps if everyone is talking about the same thing when in the heat of controversy! Clinical delegation has been with us since the dawn of team nursing, but in past years it has taken on new meaning, as we have seen the addition of many types of assistive personnel in our care delivery models. Many RNs are uncomfortable with the idea of someone "practicing on their license," or at the very least, taking away the tasks they like to do best. Current evidence would lead us to the conclusion that inappropriate delegation and supervision may be leading to missed care and untoward clinical outcomes (Bittner & Gravelin, 2009; Kalisch et al, 2009). Research reviewing failures to rescue (FTR), a situation in which patients are deteriorating but the symptoms are not noted before death, indicates that vital signs, neurological status, and urine output changes may occur up to 3 days before the final events. The RN's choice of nursing assistants, how carefully they are supervised, and how well the RN interprets patient data provided by assistive personnel, may be life-threatening or life-saving to patients (Bobay et al, 2008.) Let us take a look at delegation and accountability to clarify RNs' confusion about their roles. It helps to clear the air by beginning with the vocabulary and achieving an understanding of the basic concepts.

Delegation: "… the process for a nurse to direct another person to perform nursing tasks and activities. National Council of State Boards of Nursing (NCSBN) describes this as the nurse transferring authority while ANA calls this a transfer of responsibility. Both mean that a registered nurse (RN) can direct another individual to do something that that person would not normally be allowed to do. Both papers stress that the nurse retains accountability for the delegation" (NCSBN, 2005, p 1).

Assignments: "… the distribution of work that each staff member is responsible for during a given work period. The NCSBN uses the verb 'assign' to describe those situations when a nurse directs an individual to do something the individual is already authorized to do, e.g., when an RN directs another RN to assess a patient, the RN is already authorized to assess patients in the RN scope of practice" (NCSBN, 2005, p 1).

As you can see, these are very generic definitions, used as a standard across the country; most states have incorporated similar definitions into their nurse practice acts. (Have you reviewed your state nurse practice act lately?) A good deal of decision making is left to you as the RN and is dictated by your state's nursing practice act. You will be selecting what task and in what situation to delegate. You will make a decision to delegate on the basis of your assessment of the desired outcome and the competency of the individual delegate. This is certainly more involved than a simple process for time management! In the pages ahead, we discuss steps that use the "five rights" that will assist you in this practice, making it easier for you to maximize the work of your team in a safe manner.

Supervision: "... the provision of guidance or direction, oversight, evaluation and follow-up by the licensed nurse for accomplishment of a delegated nursing task by assistive personnel" (NCSBN, 2005, p 1).

Nurses are often confused regarding supervision. This responsibility does not belong to only the one with the title of manager or house supervisor; rather, the expectation by law is that any time you delegate a task to someone else, you will be held accountable for the initial direction you give and the timely follow-up (periodic inspection) to evaluate the performance of the task. See Figure 14-1 for the Delegation Decision Tree, which was prepared and adopted by ANA and NCSBN. There are four steps in the Delegation Decision Tree.

Step 1—Assessment and Planning: The visual representation is noted in Figure 14-1.

Step 2—Communication: Must be a two-way process involving the nurse who assesses the nursing assistive personnel's understanding of the delegated task and the nursing assistive person who asks questions regarding the delegation and seeks clarification of expectations if needed.

Step 3—Surveillance and Supervision: The purpose of surveillance and monitoring is related to nurse's responsibility for patient care within the context of a patient population. The nurse supervises the delegation by monitoring the performance of the task or function and assures compliance with standards of practice, policies, and procedures. Frequency, level, and nature of monitoring vary with needs of patient and experience of assistant.

Step 4—Evaluation and Feedback: Evaluation is often the forgotten step in delegation and should include a determination if the delegation was successful and discussion of parameters to determine the effectiveness of the delegation (ANA & NCSBN, 2006, pp 7-9).

Delegation and supervision are integrated processes: Once you delegate, you must supervise.

WHO IS ACCOUNTABLE HERE?

One of the biggest questions concerning teamwork and delegation is the issue of personal accountability. The definition of delegation already notes that the nurse is accountable for the total nursing care of the individuals. What does this really mean?

Accountability: "Being answerable for what one has done, and standing behind that decision and/or action" (Hansten & Jackson, 2009, p 79).

Accountability: "Being responsible and answerable for actions or inactions of self or others in the context of delegation" (NCSBN, 1995, p 1).

Accountability has gotten a lot of bad press, and many nurses feel that being accountable means "I am the one to blame." With that kind of attitude, no wonder there is reluctance to delegate! What is the point of delegating if someone else is going to make a mistake and you are going to be taking the blame? (Notice how we focus on the negative and forget that accountability

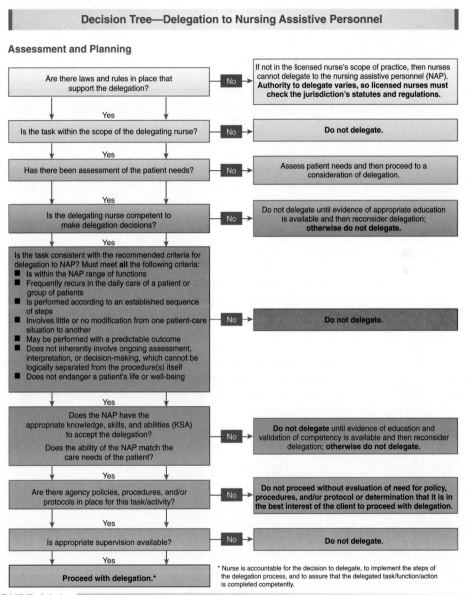

FIGURE 14-1

Delegation Decision Tree. *(From National Council of State Boards of Nursing: Appendix B: National Council of State Boards of Nursing Decision Tree for Delegation to Nursing Assistive Personnel, 2005, pp 7-9. Retrieved from www.ncsbn.org/Joint_statement.pdf.)*

also means taking the credit for the positive results we achieve through the actions and decisions we make, as well as our freedom to act because of our licensure.) Our individual choice to take actions (personal accountability) is based on our professional knowledge and judgment, unleashing the art and science of nursing as applied to a real-time individual patient and family situations, and the gifts and skills of team members each day (Samuel, 2006). Here is an important reminder about accountability before you take the weight of the world on your shoulders:

> "The delegatee is accountable for accepting the delegation and for his/her own actions in carrying out the task" (NCSBN, 1995, p 3).

It is important to focus on what you are accountable for in this process and to let the delegate also assume his or her own level of accountability. Remember, you are accountable for the following:

- Making the decision to delegate in the first place.
- Assessing the patient's needs.
- Planning the desired outcome.
- Assessing the competency of the delegate.
- Giving clear directions and obtaining acceptance from the delegate.
- Following up on the completion of the task, providing feedback to the delegate.

What if the delegate makes a mistake doing the task? What are you accountable for? Let us consider the following example:

> It is 7 AM on your busy medical-surgical unit. You scan your assignment quickly, reviewing the high points with your nursing assistant before going into report. With trays coming at 7:30, you remind your assistant that your patient in Room 210 will be going to surgery this morning and is to have nothing to eat or drink. Coming out of report, you make brief rounds, only to find that (you guessed it!) your patient in Room 210 is happily drinking her morning coffee and eating a bagel.
> What are you accountable for?
> Did you delegate correctly?
> What do you do now?

Based on a review of the previous guidelines, we can say that you did indeed delegate appropriately. Your communication may or may not have been as complete as it needed to be (more about that later). You are accountable for correcting the clinical effects of this error: Did the patient eat or drink too much, requiring that surgery be canceled or delayed? If so, you will call the operating room and make the appropriate adjustments in this patient's care on the basis of the decision regarding her surgery time. What about the nursing assistant? You are also accountable for following up with her regarding her performance, giving the appropriate feedback so that she understands her level of personal accountability as well. For more on the "how-to's," read on as we discuss the five rights of clinical delegation.

THE FIVE RIGHTS OF CLINICAL DELEGATION
1. The right task
2. Under the right circumstances
3. To the right person
4. With the right directions and communication and
5. Under the right supervision and evaluation (NCSBN, 2005, p 2).

THE RIGHT TASK

The first part of any decision regarding delegation is the determination of what needs to be done and then the assessment of whether this is a task that can be delegated to someone else. Many nurses, unfortunately, suffer from "supernurse syndrome" and believe that no task should be delegated because no one can do it better, faster, or easier than they can (Figure 14-2). In comparison, other nurses may be all too eager to delegate the least desirable tasks to someone else. A word of caution is necessary here: If we focus only on making task lists for people to do, we eliminate the very core of our purpose. Remember, your role as the RN on the team involves the coordination and planning of care, with your primary focus on identifying with the patient and the physician the desired outcomes for your patients. Once determined, interventions will be readily apparent, and the decision regarding possible delegation of these tasks must be made.

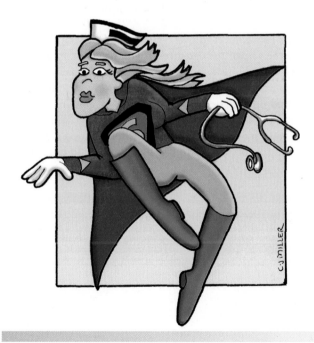

FIGURE 14-2

Many nurses suffer from "supernurse syndrome."

What Can I Delegate?

Fortunately, there are several references to assist you in making this determination. The first place we recommend looking is in the nurse practice act for your state. Each state board of nursing has a nursing practice act that dictates what a nurse can and cannot delegate to other nursing assistive personnel. Be sure you become familiar with the state nursing practice act where you are working!

At this point, the majority of state boards have addressed the issue of delegation and have developed rules that may offer specific guidelines regarding who can do what. The scope of practice for each level of care provider usually includes a description of the tasks that may be performed at that level.

The next place to look is in your organization, getting a copy of the job description, nursing responsibilities, and the skills checklist for each care provider. This will give you a very specific list of tasks to work from, but remember, there are other considerations. Simply because the skills checklist includes ambulation of patients, it may not be advisable to delegate the first ambulation of a postoperative total hip replacement patient to the new patient care assistant (Critical Thinking Box 14-1).

If you have questions and need clarification for your state, call the board of nursing for assistance (see *www.ncsbn.org*). Be aware that your state may have introduced or passed a bill that may affect your practice with residents of neighboring states. As of November 2009, 24 states had passed or were in the process of approving interstate compact licensure regulation legislation designed to allow nurses to practice across state lines because of Internet consultation, telenursing, or other technology that would broadcast nursing practice across state borders (NCSBN, 2009). If you have questions and need clarification in your state, call the board of nursing for assistance.

Beyond the law, your employer will have job descriptions and skills checklists that should clearly define the role of the caregiver. If you have not seen these items, be sure to review them soon. This is the baseline for determining "who does what" and selecting the right task to delegate. As many organizations develop creative assistant roles to leverage the professional judgment of scarce registered nursing personnel, the scope of practice of each role is defined first by law. If the organization extends the role of a patient care technician to include preoperative teaching, you want to be aware that this is clearly an RN function and not allowed by law to be delegated to the technician. A job description and a policy would not override the legal limits of the scope of practice.

CRITICAL THINKING BOX 14-1

IN YOUR ORGANIZATION, CAN YOU DELEGATE THE FOLLOWING TASKS?

YES	NO	
_____	_____	Bladder retention catheter insertion
_____	_____	Taking vital signs
_____	_____	Feeding a patient
_____	_____	Hygienic care
_____	_____	Medication administration
_____	_____	Discontinuing an intravenous line
_____	_____	Teaching insulin administration

Is There Anything I Cannot Delegate?

Again, your first resource is the law. Many states are very specific in their description of what duty cannot be delegated and belongs only to the RN's scope of practice. The NCSBN reminds us that:

Nursing is a knowledge-based process discipline and cannot be reduced solely to a list of tasks. The licensed nurse's specialized education, professional judgment, and discretion are essential for quality nursing care. ... While nursing tasks may be delegated, the licensed nurse's generalist knowledge of client care indicates that the practice-pervasive functions of assessment, evaluation and nursing judgment must not be delegated (NCSBN, 1995, p 2).

According to nurse-attorney Joanne P. Sheehan, nurses cannot delegate the following:

- Assessments that identify needs and problems and diagnose human responses.
- Any aspect of planning, including the development of comprehensive approaches to the total care plan.
- Any provision of health counseling, teaching, or referrals to other health care providers.
- Therapeutic nursing techniques and comprehensive care planning (Sheehan, 2001, p 22) (Critical Thinking Box 14-2).

With the right task selected according to the scope of practice, the policies in your agency, and your assessment of the situation, there is still work to be done.

THE RIGHT CIRCUMSTANCES

Next, "Right Circumstances—appropriate patient setting, available resources, and consideration of other relevant factors" (NCSBN, 1995, p 2) suggests that the staffing mix, community needs, teaching obligations, and the type of patients being cared for should also be considered. Different rules for delegation may apply regarding what and how an RN must delegate in home care, long-term care, or in community homes for the developmentally disabled or group boarding homes for assisted living (Hansten et al, 1999, Hansten & Jackson, 2009) (Evidence-Based Practice Box 14-1).

How Can I Determine the Strengths and Weaknesses of Team Members?

Often motivated by the fear that a delegate may make a mistake in an assigned task, nurses' focus on the potential weaknesses of their team members. As nurses, we are educated to anticipate the worst so that we can prevent accidents, adverse drug reactions, and negative sequelae to disease processes and treatments alike. As prudent as this approach may be for the safety of all

---

CRITICAL THINKING BOX 14-2

WHERE TO LOOK FOR DETERMINATION OF THE RIGHT TASK

State nurse practice act
Employee job description
Skills checklist
Demonstrated competency

BOX 14-1 EVIDENCE-BASED PRACTICE

Delegation and Supervision

PRACTICE ISSUE

With health care personnel shortages and changes in health care reimbursement nurses are dreaming if they believe they will be able to practice effectively without expert delegation skills in the future. Compounding the fractures that can occur in teamwork when multiple individuals must communicate in a complex situation, early discharges, advances in technology, increased RN autonomy, better informed consumers, and expanded legal definitions of liability all increase the need to use the best delegation and supervision techniques (Croke, 2003).

A study geared to understand the critical thinking processes of nurses in delegation showed that nurses often expected assistive personnel to have a higher degree of knowledge and skill than they possessed or were licensed to perform, such as the nursing process, prioritizing, and assessment (Bittner & Gravelin, 2009). Nurses report difficulty with delegating because of the structure of care delivery with multiple assistive personnel reporting to multiple RNs, and challenges in how to communicate what needs to be done as well as how to follow up without offending coworkers (Standing & Anthony, 2008). However, difficulties with delegating appropriately means that there is missed care, leaving hospitalized patients in jeopardy of the consequences of omissions, such as hospital acquired pressure ulcers, infections, and errors, as well as failures to rescue deteriorating patients (Kalisch et al, 2009). These hospital acquired conditions and errors will not be reimbursed by many insurers and cost the patient/family and health care organizations billions per year nationally (Virkstis et al, 2009).

Review of care issues involving cases in which the five rights of delegation and supervision were not followed showed that problems were related to RNs not providing the right direction or communication (13.9%) or with lack of supervision (12.4%). 60.6% of deficiencies were related to the UAP not following through with a task that was delegated or not following unit/department procedures (Standing and Hertz, 2001).

In order to help nurses learn how to work effectively within teams at their worksite, organizations have provided in-depth education, application of the principles of delegation at work, and combined the training with a consistent care delivery structure. At the end of 16 weeks of instructor-guided self-study, professional practice skills have improved up to 37%, and the use of supervision checkpoints by RNs with team members has doubled in frequency (Hansten, 2008a).

IMPLICATIONS FOR NURSING PRACTICE

- There is a need for ongoing education for nurses in team leadership skills and unit practices that create care delivery models supporting nurses in delegating and supervising effectively in highly complex work (Hansten, 2005; Hansten & Jackson, 2009; Standing & Anthony 2008).
- Each health care team must create a care delivery model that includes a clear plan for the day and proper times for initial direction and ongoing supervision and updating of clinical and performance information (Hansten, 2008a, 2008b).
- There is patient safety evidence that communication lapses were a root cause of approximately 65% of sentinel events from 1995 to 2006. The Joint Commission's (TJC) National Patient Safety Goals for 2008 included a need to develop a standardized approach to hand-off communication. Although many hospitals have interpreted the term *hand-off* to consist of the information shared between shifts and at patient transfer, the need for accurate ongoing updating of patient data *during* a team's shift or episode of care would also apply. TJC continues to incorporate improved patient/family and care provider communication in their standards.

Missed care from poor quality delegation and supervision skills and unclear assignments can result in health care acquired conditions that will no longer be paid for by insurers. These conditions cost the

BOX 14-1   EVIDENCE-BASED PRACTICE—cont'd

patients and their families more than dollars, including untoward pain and suffering. The reimbursement losses and costs from poor quality can provide the motivation to sink scarce funds into delegation and teamwork skill development.

Considering This Information:

What education and orientation processes are in place in your organization to promote effective delegation and supervision? If these processes are not present now, how can you be involved in their development? What unit processes could be created that would help teams collaborate throughout the shift?

References for the Evidence

Alfaro-LeFevre R (2008): Critical thinking indicators. Retrieved from *www.alfaroteachsmart.com/2008_2009CTI.pdf*.

Bittner N, Gravlin G: Critical thinking, delegation, and missed care in nursing practice, *JONA* 39(3):142-146, 2009.

Croke E: Nurses, negligence, and malpractice, *AJN* 103(9):9, 2003.

Hansten R: Relationship and results oriented healthcare: evaluate the basics, *JONA* 35(12):522-525, 2005.

Hansten R: *Relationship & results oriented healthcare planning & implementation manual*, Port Ludlow, WA, 2008a, Hansten Healthcare PLLC.

Hansten R: Why nurses still must learn to delegate, *Nurse Leader* October:19-25, 2008b.

Kalisch B, Landstrom G, Williams R: Missed care: errors of omission, *Nursing Outlook* 57:3-9, 2009.

Standing T, Anthony M: Delegation: what it means to acute care nurses, *Applied Nsg Research* 21:8-14, 2008.

Standing T, Anthony M, Hertz J: Nurses' narratives of outcomes after delegation to unlicensed assistive personnel, *Outcomes Manage Nurs Pract* 5(1):18-23, 2001.

The Joint Commission (2010): 2010 Patient Safety Goals. Retrieved from *www.jointcommission.org/PatientSafety/NationalPatient SafetyGoals*.

The Joint Commission (2010): 2010 Patient Safety Goals—Sentinel Events. Retrieved from *www.jointcommission.org/SentinelEvents/ Statistics*.

Virkstis ND, Westheim J, Boston-Fleischhauer C: Safeguarding quality: building the business case to prevent nursing-sensitive hospital-acquired conditions, *JONA* 39(7/8):350-355, 2009.

concerned, it is worthwhile to discuss the need to be clear on the strengths of the team members as well.

Recall the last time you were given specific, positive feedback about your performance as an RN. (We hope this occurs often!) How did you feel? Most of us are energized and restored by the reinforcement that our hard work has been recognized. When working with assistive personnel or any other colleague, the recognition of strengths will begin to get us on the right track in our relationship.

Assigning tasks on the basis of the strengths of the person will allow the patient to experience the very best care—and allow the delegate to provide the very best care. Now, as a supervising RN, you are in a new position with respect to the long-term performance of delegates. If assistive personnel are assigned only those tasks they are good at, they may not grow in their abilities and skills. This mistake is exemplified by a hospital that had created a new multiskilled patient care assistant (PCA) role with certified nursing assistants (CNAs). These CNAs had been trained to do phlebotomies as well, as authorized by the state board. Phlebotomists had been eliminated but were given the option of training for the new PCA role. When all of the PCAs worked together, the lab tests were drawn by those who had been phlebotomists because they were more comfortable with that skill. You can certainly imagine the chagrin of the supervising nurses when all the PCAs who were former phlebotomists were off on vacation and maternity leave. None of the PCAs who were formerly CNAs had become proficient at this skill! Recognize strengths, and encourage the best patient care possible by using them, but challenge delegates to grow too.

The dreaded weaknesses in performance of team members can often be prevented by asking the right questions before delegating. Nurses can be reticent about asking personnel such as float personnel or agency replacement staff about whether they feel comfortable in completing the assignment they have received. Float and temporary personnel tell us that they would prefer being asked about their competency at the beginning of a shift or assignment, with the offer of help and clarification, rather than having to locate an RN later to request information. The American Nurses Association (ANA) Code of Ethics states, "The nurse is responsible and accountable for individual nursing practice and determines the appropriate delegation of tasks consistent with the nurse's obligation to provide optimum patient care" (ANA, 2001). Be assured that although it is the responsibility of the RN to assess the competency of those they supervise, the delegate must be "accountable for accepting the delegation and for his/her own actions in carrying out the task" (NCSBN, 1995, p 1). The RN who is familiar with the situation, however, must ask the correct questions to determine whether the person is competent.

For example, if an RN were planning to ask a nursing assistant to feed a baby with respiratory difficulties, based on the outcome that the baby would be able to ingest 12 ounces of formula this shift, what questions might the RN ask to determine the potential strengths and weaknesses? If the individual has not had experience in this procedure, how could the nurse ensure future competency? In this situation, an RN would certainly ask questions about past experiences with feeding babies who had difficulty swallowing. If the delegate assures the RN that she or he is competent, the RN may go further in asking what the CNA would do if coughing or choking occurred. Depending on the situation, the RN would probably want to demonstrate feeding techniques and observe the skills to ensure the competency of the delegate.

What Are the Causes of Performance Weaknesses?

Let us take a look at an example of a performance weakness and try to determine what the potential causes may be.

In this scenario, you are an RN working a night shift on a hematology-oncology unit, and an agency nursing assistant, Pam, comes to work with you this shift. Pam is excited about the possibilities of interviewing for a regular night shift position and would love to work extra on holidays and weekends. As you begin to discuss her assignment for the night, she states, "Oh, I forgot to tell you, I do not ever take patients who are HIV-positive! Ever!"

There are some potential costs and benefits to your response to this statement. As the nurse, you could ignore this statement and continue with your work. You may decide this person has problems, and you may elect to deny her request for an interview. Or, you may determine there is something behind her refusal. How you respond may cost you a potentially valuable staff member and could upset the other members of your staff and the patients. Avoiding the problem or accommodating her refusal could become a terrible headache for making assignments and would be contrary to the mission of your organization.

Experience has shown that there are several potential causes of performance inadequacies (Critical Thinking Box 14-3). One of the most common causes is that employees are not aware of what is expected of them. Does Pam know that at this facility it is part of your policy that

CRITICAL
THINKING
BOX 14-3

POTENTIAL SOURCES OF PERFORMANCE WEAKNESS
- Unclear expectations
- Lack of performance feedback
- Educational needs
- Need for additional supervision and direction
- Individual characteristics: past experiences, motivational or personal issues

everyone takes care of all patients, whether or not they are known to be HIV-positive? Perhaps being aware of this expectation would assist Pam in making her decision about whether to apply for work on this unit.

Often, being clear about expectations is not enough. All of us have some blind spots in our own performance. Perhaps we think we are doing just fine, meeting performance competencies and beyond, but colleagues have noted that we are not performing procedures according to policy. If these observations are not shared, we will blithely believe we are doing great. Another common cause of performance difficulties is that others have not shared their perceptions of our performance with us. Pam may have adopted this attitude regarding HIV-positive patients in other work settings, but because of the desperation for her help, no one had shared the fact that this behavior falls short of competencies in her job description.

Another common origin of performance weakness is an educational need. Does Pam need more education about how HIV infection is transmitted and how it is prevented? Surely, she had to complete some content regarding this in her CNA certification course, but it seems she did not internalize this content. Or is there a personal problem? She may have just witnessed the death of a loved one from AIDS and feels unable to cope with seeing others with this disease at this time.

The amount of supervision needed can be another source of performance problems. As an RN, you must determine the degree of "periodic inspection" needed by the delegate. Some people require additional direction but are still able to do the job competently. In the absence of that direction, they will be unable to create positive patient outcomes. Nurses tell us they wish that the assistive personnel on their staff would be self-directed and take initiative without being told. We question whether an RN's hope that all will do their jobs without interaction or supervision on his or her part fits with the definition of supervision! Again, as leader, the RN must determine how much supervision is needed for the individual delegate, just as we determine the degree of observation needed for each patient on the basis of our assessment of their needs. In Pam's case, her reluctance to work with patients with HIV may have nothing to do with supervision but may reflect a need for guidance, education, or a frank discussion of expectations.

As the RN who is supervising Pam, what steps would you take to determine the cause of her performance weakness—her assertion that she refuses to care for patients with HIV? What questions would you ask? How would you respond so that you could continue to use Pam's services this shift, maintain the integrity of your mission, and preserve the potential for hiring a new employee?

Matching the right person with the right task is the third step in the circular process of delegation. This process includes planning and articulating priority patient outcomes, assessing the competency of the delegate to perform the task, determining the potential strengths and weaknesses of the assistive personnel, and planning how much supervision is needed. To ensure that the right task will be done by the right person, additional clarification of expectations, performance feedback, and planning for education needs may be necessary; these steps will promote the long-term success of the team.

THE RIGHT PERSON

Once you have determined that a task can be delegated, matching the task to the right person involves the definition of delegation once again. Nurses must select the right task for a competent person in a *selected* situation. We have already discussed how you would determine the correct task. But how do we select the right person in the right situation (Figure 14-3)?

How Can I Use Outcomes in Delegating?

In planning for the right person to do a task, focusing on outcomes is essential (Critical Thinking Box 14-4). According to the Alfaro-LeFevre's (2008) evidence-based critical thinking indicators, which are outcome focused guides appropriate delegation as well as critical thinking in nursing (p 8).

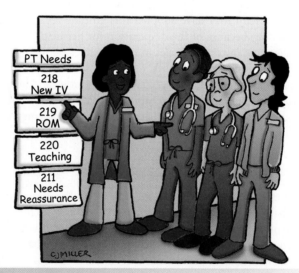

FIGURE 14-3

It can be difficult to know who the best person is to handle a given situation.

TALKING ABOUT OUTCOMES: WHAT'S IN IT FOR ME?
- Provides a method to decide appropriate assignments: who should be doing what task
- Gives you a sense of purpose for the shift (short term) and long term
- Enhances your ability to motivate coworkers along a track to achieving the outcomes
- Clarifies your role as leader of the team
- Verifies and clarifies patient/family expectations when outcomes are discussed and planned with them
- Promotes job satisfaction and collaboration for the whole team

For example, two patients are admitted to a hospital. Each of these individuals will need a bath today (task), but who will give the baths is related to the outcome you are trying to achieve. For Mr. Peterson, who has been homeless and is in dire need of hygienic care so that you can perform a complete and accurate skin assessment, the priority outcome you and your patient desire is that Mr. Peterson will be clean. With Ms. Ibutu, who is a paraplegic, today is the day that her caregivers and she will demonstrate how they will assess her skin for areas of breakdown and how to perform range of motion to her lower extremities. The RN's decision about who will do which task is dependent on the plan of care and the goals that the team has established in the discussion with the patient or family (Table 14-1).

This same logic applies when you have heard in report that a patient, Mr. Handelsky, is unstable. In your current care delivery system on your unit, the licensed practical (or vocational) nurse (LPN or LVN) may carry out the initial gathering of vital sign data in your postoperative intensive care unit (ICU). Suppose, for example, that the report you received stated that there had been increasing cherry-red drainage in the chest tube and that the patient's cardiac monitor showed supraventricular tachycardia, with increasing respiratory rate. On the basis of the outcome for the shift, Mr. Handelsky will maintain cardiorespiratory homeostasis and continue on critical path for the first day post-thoracotomy. Using your insight that his condition may be deteriorating, you may make a different decision regarding who will be there for initial patient contact. If the assistant working with you today is an experienced team member, you may choose to send him in to see the patient immediately while you check on another critical patient. Or if the assistant is a "float" from an agency, known to you only by initial questioning, you may immediately make a visit to see Mr. Handelsky and begin to set up the plan for the data gathering and schedule for reporting that you will expect from your assistant. This would be a very different process if the outcome you wanted to achieve was pain relief and comfort for a terminal patient.

TABLE 14-1 Using Outcomes in Delegating			
PATIENT	OUTCOME	TASK/PROCESS	WHO WILL PERFORM IT?
Mr. Peterson	Patient will be clean.	Bath	Nursing assistant or other care associate
Ms. Ibutu	Patient and caregivers will know how to perform skin assessment and range of motion.	Bath with education regarding home care	RN: teaching plan; OT, PT, or rehabilitation aide may also assist
Mr. Handelsky	Patient will maintain cardiorespiratory homeostasis and continue on care path day 1. Patient will be free of pain and comfortable for this shift. Long-term outcome: pain-free death.	Initial baseline vital signs and assessment, close monitoring Pain assessment and treatment, comfort measures (repositioning skin care)	RN: assessment and interpretation of data LPN: data-gathering and reporting RN: initial plan for comfort measures and pain assessment Assistant: comfort measures, report of progress

LPN, Licensed practical nurse; *OT*, occupational therapist; *PT*, physical therapist; *RN*, registered nurse.

Take a moment to consider the outcomes for a particularly difficult patient you have been dealing with lately. Were you clear on outcomes? If so, have you shared them with colleagues? Focusing on outcomes takes time, but remember, "If you fail to plan, you plan to fail." Why should an RN focus on outcomes? Discussion of goals not only establishes who should be doing what task, but also allows RNs to motivate others. How many of us jump on a train if we do not know where it is going? A purpose and a destination allow all team members to function more effectively. When assistive personnel are given the same assignment daily, without variation, without any understanding of why they are doing what they are doing, it is similar to being an assembly line worker putting widgets in a machine. Satisfaction and motivation of coworkers generally come from the feeling that they are making a difference in the lives of their patients.

In a similar manner, you as the leader of the team would feel much better at the end of your shift or assignment if you could feel comfortable with the outcomes you have assisted the patient in achieving. You could actually verify the outcomes and plan with the patients, much as you were always told to do by the teachers in your nursing program! Much time is saved by streamlining the care to the patient's expectations.

Again, the RN is accountable for the patient, for determining the situation in which delegation will be used, and for the selection of the right person to do the right task, in addition to the periodic inspection and follow-up of those they supervise. The right communication will begin that clarification process, bringing us to the next step in the five rights of delegation.

THE RIGHT DIRECTION AND COMMUNICATION

How Can I Get the Delegate to Understand What I Want?

No matter what, it always comes back to communication. How clear you make your initial direction will be the cornerstone in determining the success of your delegated task and, ultimately, the performance of your team. The bottom line, whether the patient outcome was achieved, hinges on your ability to give initial direction that clearly defines your expectations of the delegate in performing the assigned task. It is not surprising that this is a step that is often done poorly or left out entirely because the assumption is made that the individual "knows what the job is and should just do it."

The first component of supervision, according to its definition, is the provision of initial direction. Achieving a balance in which we provide enough information for the person to understand the request without overstating the case and risking confusion or condescension requires that we tread a fine line. The use of the "four Cs" of initial direction will help you to plan your communication (Critical Thinking Box 14-5). Many hospitals are now performing shift reports or handovers at the bedside, engaging the patients in the discussion of their priorities, the plan for care, and what each person will do for them during the shift (Hansten, 2008a).

Let us assume that you are working in a home health agency and you are planning the care for a patient with heart failure (HF). You have made your initial visit, assessing the patient and planning the outcomes you and the team will work toward in the next 3 weeks. Your patient is taking diuretics, antihypertensives, heart medications, and potassium supplements, in addition to being on a restricted diet. She is frequently short of breath and requires an assistant three times per week for hygienic care. In addition to providing hygienic care, you would like that assistant to monitor the blood pressure and check the patient's weight on the days you are not

CRITICAL THINKING
BOX 14-5

THE FOUR Cs OF INITIAL DIRECTION

CLEAR: Does the team member understand what I am saying?
CONCISE: Have I confused the direction by giving too much unnecessary information?
CORRECT: Is the direction according to policy, procedure, job description, and the law?
COMPLETE: Does the delegate have all the information necessary to complete the task?

(Hansten R, Jackson M: *Clinical delegation skills: A handbook for professional practice,* ed 4, Sudbury, Mass: Jones & Bartlett, 2009, pp 287-288; LaCharity L, Kumagai C, Bartz B: *Prioritization, delegation, assignment,* ed 3, St. Louis: Mosby, Elsevier, 2011, p 6.)

making a visit and to notify you if the blood pressure is outside of the range of 120 to 170 systolic and 50 to 90 diastolic or for any weight fluctuation. Using the four Cs listed, you can evaluate your communication.

Mrs. Jones has a heart condition and high blood pressure that requires medication and constant monitoring. One of our goals is to help Mrs. Jones have a stable blood pressure, in a range that is normal for her. On the days that you are visiting and giving the patient her bath, I would also like you to take her blood pressure. If it is outside the range of 120 to 170 systolic and 50 to 90 diastolic, I would like you to let me know. We may need to adjust her medication, change her diet, and call her physician or the HF clinic for different orders. I would also like you to check her weight and let me know about any changes of more than 2 pounds from her home health admission weight of 185, so if she weighs 187 or more. This will help us determine if she is retaining fluid.

Clear: Does the home health aide understand what is being asked of her? This direction is fairly straightforward—an easily understood instruction of taking the blood pressure. Is it clear that the aide is to determine and report the patient's weight?

Concise: Have you confused the assistant by giving too much information? Or is it enough for her to complete the task? Only the assistant can help you with this determination. You will need to ask directly, "Am I confusing you?" or "Do you have enough information to do the job?" Every individual has different needs. However, you will want to make certain to check this out; some people will not be honest or accurate in their assessments of their understanding or abilities, leading to trouble later. Many of us are reluctant to ask questions, being afraid to admit our need for additional information. (We do not want to look like we do not know what we are doing!) This reluctance can ultimately result in harm to the patient because assumptions are made that the direction was understood when, in fact, it was not.

Correct: Is a home health aide able and allowed to monitor blood pressures? Where would you look for additional information if you were not sure? Is the location of the scale identified? Does the time of day of the visit make any difference?

Complete: Does the assistant have enough information to fulfill your expectations? Once again, you will need to ask the delegate for clarification of his or her understanding of what you are asking. If you expect this assistant to also note the respirations and alert you to increased effort of breathing, have you shared that in your initial direction? Or did you assume she would naturally observe all vital signs because you alerted her to the patient's condition (and besides, she is a good assistant)? In our attempts not to appear condescending (I do not want to insult this assistant by reminding her to note the respirations—she might think I do not trust her to think!), we may often choose not to be as complete as we should be in giving initial direction. What about lost weight? Is that significant to report?

Another common pitfall is the rationale that comes from working with someone over a period of time. A working relationship develops, and a routine or pattern of performance is established. When this happens, we start talking less and less to the other individual, believing that "she knows what I expect her to do." Consider the following situation:

You are working on a surgical unit in a partnership with Sam, an LPN you have been working with for the past year. Your easygoing style has led to a comfortable reliance on each other and the feeling that each knows what the other expects. On this particular evening shift, you are traveling down the hall, intent on administering medication to one of your patients. You also know a patient from the postanesthesia care unit (PACU) will soon be coming back from surgery. Seeing Sam coming your way, you state, "Sam, the postop is coming back in Room 103." Evaluate your initial direction.

Did you believe that Sam just knew you wanted him to check on the patient, get the first set of vital signs, position the patient, check the dressing and the drains, note the status of the IV, degree of pain, and report the patient's status to you as soon as possible, until you can see the patient yourself?

Fifteen minutes later, you see Sam at the portable computer in the hallway. You ask him, "Sam, is the new post-op patient in Room 103 here?" Expecting a brief report, you are surprised when Sam says, "I don't know. Is he here? I thought you were going to assess him when he got here." What went wrong?

No matter how long you have been working with someone, the right communication is essential to ensure the success of teamwork. Sam did not *accept* the delegated task (remember what the delegate is accountable for?) because he did not understand what you meant. Be sure that you check the delegate's understanding of what you are saying. Failing to do this may result in unmet expectations, which lead to anger and frustration. More important, the patient will not receive the optimal care that both you and the delegate want to provide In this case a new postoperative patient was not fully assessed during a critical period.

You have carefully assessed the patient, determined your plan on the basis of outcomes, and selected the right task to delegate to the right person. You have even given clear initial direction as part of the right communication. Now what? The final right of delegation is also a part of supervision: the periodic inspection of the actual act. Read on as we continue with a discussion of the right feedback.

THE RIGHT SUPERVISION AND EVALUATION

How Can I Effectively Give and Receive Feedback?

Many nurses have shared their discomfort with giving and receiving feedback from coworkers. Few of us enjoy telling colleagues how they are doing or hearing about how we may have missed the mark; however, when you are supervising others, it is absolutely necessary to give feedback

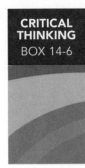

CRITICAL THINKING
BOX 14-6

FEEDBACK FORMULA
- Ask for the other individual's input first!
- Give credit for effort.
- Share your perceptions with each other.
- Explore differing points of view, focusing on shared outcomes.
- Ask for the other individual's input to determine what steps may be necessary to make certain desired outcomes are achieved.
- Agree on a plan for the future, including timeline for follow-up.
- Revisit the plan and results achieved.

Modified from Hansten R, Jackson M: *Clinical delegation skills: A handbook for nurses*, 4 ed, Sudbury, Mass, Jones & Bartlett, 2009.

during your "periodic inspection." By following a formula for giving and receiving feedback and practicing it daily, RNs are assisted in the difficult job of correcting the performance of others. The reciprocal feedback process also permits you, as supervising RN, to hear how your own supervisory performance and communication affected the outcomes of the team (Critical Thinking Box 14-6).

Let's look at how this process can be used in a situation in which positive feedback is intended.

An RN (Pat) is working with a float RN (Julia) for the first time. Julia is new in the pool but is an experienced nurse. Pat is so pleased with Julia's experience and performance that she has gone off to have a nice long break and lunch with an old friend from the third floor. She has also taken time to meet with a colleague from the evening shift regarding a unit problem. Unfortunately, she has not been present on the unit much today. When Pat is having lunch with her friend, she exclaims, "That new float Julia is just excellent! If it weren't for her, I couldn't be here having lunch with you. I hope that she knows how organized and valuable she is!" Her friend, Alex, states, "Well, you know you should tell her, not just me, about this." When Pat returns to the floor, flushed with good intentions of making Julia's day with effusive praise, she tells Julia about how lucky she has been to work with her today.

Because all of us crave positive feedback, and Julia is new to your organization, will Julia tell Pat that she's been trying to find her for hours? Probably not. But she *may* tell others, "Pat is one of those 'dump and run' nurses. I don't want to work on that floor again!" What if Pat asked *first*, "How have things been going for you today, Julia? I know this is your first day on the unit." Julia may have determined it was possible (and expected) to give reciprocal feedback: "I've been trying to find you! I have completed everything, but it hasn't been easy. Where have you been?" The best intentions can be destroyed by not asking the other individual for input first.

If you plan to give some negative feedback to an individual, you will also need to ask for her or his input first. For example:

You have just noted that the night shift CNA did not record the intakes and outputs (I & Os) on three patients on your telemetry unit. You have called him and are thinking about how to discuss this with him in a positive manner; yet you know that he is not going to want to chat because it is about time for him to get some rest.

If you said, "Why didn't you record the I & Os in the electronic medical record (EMR)!?," the CNA would probably react defensively. If you state, "How was your night? I noticed that the I & Os are not in the EMR," you have allowed the person to respond with what happened. If this CNA went home early with the flu or the unit experienced three codes, it would not be an effective or popular action for you to pounce on the team member for missing data entry.

This brings us to the next step in the process—giving credit for what has been accomplished. Let us return to Pat and Julia. At this point, Julia's input has been received. Pat can state, "Well, I can see I didn't help you as much as I should have, and I forgot to give you my beeper number. But I do want you to know that I've checked on all of our patients, and they are very happy with their care today." After hearing input and giving credit where it is due, exploration of the gaps in the relationship and their communication and initial direction at the beginning of the shift can now be undertaken with open and frank discussion.

The discussion of differences will progress most smoothly if both parties recognize that they share common objectives: safe, effective care of the patients on their unit, as reflected in the fulfillment of shared, planned outcomes or goals determined by collaborative discussion among patients and care team members. When difficulties or conflicts occur, remember the reason you are both there: the patients.

Julia and Pat may clarify what happened and what actions each may take to ensure that the missed communication does not happen again in the future. Do not try to "fix" the situation for the other individual or prescribe what you will do for them. The other individual will know what he or she needs to do to achieve your shared outcomes. For example, Pat may have decided that what would fix it for Julia would be to convene an hour before shift tomorrow and go through the unit manuals and read procedures. However, the most Julia may need is a beeper number and some more discussion and planning about assignments at the beginning of the shift.

Too often we may think, "Why wait for the others to come up with ideas when we can solve the problem for them?" RNs who lead teams throughout the nation tell us that their work lives would be much better if everyone were behaving in an accountable manner. When we ask others for their step-by-step plan to prevent the problem in the future, it helps them determine that they are accountable for their own performance. In our scene with the missing I & O data, the RN will ask, "How can you make sure those I & Os are charted before you leave in the future? What will work for you?" This type of statement confers the necessary respect for the delegate's ability to determine how to adapt his work performance.

Do not miss the final steps in the formula. The individuals must agree on how they will proceed in the future and when they will revisit the problem or issue again. Julia may determine that she'll remind Pat in the future when she gets to the unit that she will need her beeper number and a plan for the day. When the next shift is completed, they will want to compare notes about how the shift has proceeded and whether patient outcomes have been achieved. The CNA may decide to ask the RN next week whether she has noted any missing I & Os. The pair will be able to evaluate whether the CNA's charting plan has been effective and can proceed to celebrate the success of the plan or to try other interventions.

Practice using the feedback formula. Remember the following three most important points:

ASSESSING YOUR DELEGATION SKILLS

Assemble these documents:

- Your state nurse practice act
- Your job description and those of coworkers and delegates
- Skills checklists
- The patient list or assignment form from your unit
- A list of the usual staffing complement for your shift

1. Using the above, determine the short-term outcomes for an average patient assignment based on the information you have been given in a report. What tasks could be delegated to the individuals you have on staff? When will you complete further assessment of the patient situations?
2. Based on the outcomes and job descriptions, how will you determine the competency of individuals to complete the tasks you have determined could be delegated?
3. How will you communicate the team's plan using outcomes in your discussion?
4. How often will you communicate with the delegates, based on their need for supervision and patient complexity and dynamics? Have you used the four Cs?
5. How will you evaluate the effectiveness of your plan? How will you give positive feedback to the team?
6. A mistake was made by a delegate. You determined the person was competent, but the procedure was done improperly. For what are you accountable? How will you give feedback to the individual, encouraging his or her growth and accountability?
7. Have you implemented the five rights of delegation?

- Ask for the other person's input first.
- Give credit for accomplishments and efforts.
- Ask the other individual to come up with steps for resolving the issue.

How would you use this formula to tell a supervisor that you are concerned about how long it has been since you have heard about your intershift transfer and you are getting worried about whether it will take place? How would you give positive feedback to an individual on your team who has been improving his ability to get out on time? What about a delegate who is "missing in action"—the person you cannot seem to locate when you need her?

CONCLUSION

We often hope for an exact prescription for what to delegate—as well as when and how. Because nursing assessment and professional judgment are necessary for clinical delegation, each situation will be different. Whether you work in an intensive care unit in a large tertiary hospital or a rural long-term care facility, the template of the delegation process—*in the right circumstances, matching the right task with the right delegate, communicating effectively, and offering and receiving feedback*—will be similar. To judge your comfort and assess your ability to integrate this process in your daily work life, complete the exercise in Critical Thinking Box 14-7. Good luck!

BIBLIOGRAPHY

Alfaro-LeFevre R (2008): Critical thinking indicators. Retrieved from *www.alfaroteachsmart.com/2008_2009 CTI.pdf*.

American Nurses Association (2001): Code of ethics for nurses. Retrieved from *www.ana.org/ethics/chcode.htm*.

Bittner N, Gravlin G: Critical thinking, delegation, and missed care in nursing practice, *JONA* 39(3):142-146, 2009.

Bobay K, Fiorelli K, Anderson A: Failure to rescue. A preliminary study of patient-level factors, *J Nurs Care Qual* 23(3):211-215, 2008.

Hansten R: Relationship and results oriented healthcare: evaluate the basics, *JONA* 35(12):522-525, 2005.

Hansten R: *Relationship & results oriented healthcare planning & implementation manual*, Port Ludlow, WA, 2008a, Hansten Healthcare PLLC.

Hansten R: Why nurses still must learn to delegate, *Nurse Leader* 6(5):19-25, 2008b.

Hansten R, Jackson M: *Clinical delegation skills: a handbook for professional practice*, ed 4, Sudbury, Mass, 2009, Jones & Bartlett.

Hansten R, Washburn M, Kenyon V: *Home care nursing delegation skills: a handbook for practice*, Gaithersburg, MD, 1999, Aspen.

Kalisch B, Landstrom G, Williams R: Missed care: errors of omission, *Nursing Outlook* 57:3-9, 2009.

National Council of State Boards of Nursing: *Concept paper on delegation*, Chicago, 1990, NCSBN.

National Council of State Boards of Nursing: *Concepts and decision-making process*, National Council position paper, Chicago, 1995, NCSBN. Retrieved from *www.ncsbn.org/ 323.htm/definitions#definitions*.

National Council of State Boards of Nursing (2009): Participating states in the nurse licensure compact implementation. Retrieved from *www.ncsbn.org/ 158.htm*.

National Council of State Boards of Nursing (2006): Joint statement on delegation, American Nurses Association (ANA) and National Council of State Boards of Nursing (NCSBN). Retrieved from *www.ncsbn.org/joint_statement. pdf*.

National Council of State Boards of Nursing (2005): Joint statement on delegation, American Nurses Association (ANA) and National Council of State Boards of Nursing (NCSBN). Retrieved from *www.ncsbn.org/Joint_statement. pdf*.

Samuel M: *Creating the accountable organization*, Katonah, NY, 2006, Xephor Press.

Sheehan JP: UAP delegation: a step-by-step process, *Nurs Manag* 32(4):22-24, 2001.

Additional resources are available online at *http://evolve.elsevier.com/Zerwekh/nsgtoday/*.

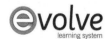

CHAPTER 15

The Health Care Organization and Patterns of Nursing Care Delivery

Susan Sportsman, RN, PhD

Every patient needs a nurse.
—AMERICAN NURSES ASSOCIATION

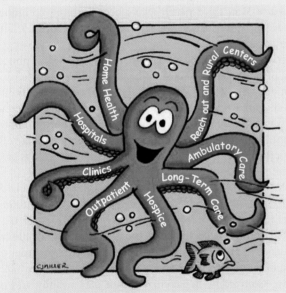

Health care should be within reach of everyone.

After completing this chapter, you should be able to:

- Describe challenges facing health care that impact the delivery of nursing care, including:

  - Reduction of costs

  - Evidence-based care

  - Shortage of health care professionals

  - Patient safety

- Trace the history of the use of nursing care delivery models.

- Consider ways to structure nursing services to improve care while reducing costs.

he U. S. health care delivery system has been changing dramatically over the last 35 years. The first decade of the new millennium is over, and these changes seem to be escalating, making the health care environment even more complex. Nurses practicing in such an environment must be comfortable with change and be willing to embrace the challenges that change brings. A first step to ensuring that your nursing practice evolves in a positive direction is to be knowledgeable about these changes.

WHAT ARE SOME IMPORTANT CHALLENGES CURRENTLY FACING HEALTH CARE?

Cost of Health Care

Health care costs have been on the rise for many years. Health care spending surpassed $2.2 trillion in 2007, more than 3 times the $714 billion spent in 1990 and more than 8 times the $253 billion spent in 1980. In 2007, the U.S. health care spending was about $7421 per resident, accounting for 16.2% of the nation's Gross Domestic Product (GDP). According to the Kaiser Family Foundation, factors that are driving the escalation of health care costs are prescription drugs and technology, chronic disease, aging of the population, and administrative costs (Kaiser Family Foundation, 2007).

Managed Care

In an effort to reduce health care costs, while maintaining or improving access and quality, many payers (insurance companies and U.S. or state governments) have changed the way they pay hospitals and providers for services. In the early 1900s, patients or their families paid the physician or the hospital directly for the care they received. As health care insurance became an employment benefit after the Second World War, third-party payers became more common. These third-party payers paid the provider an agreed-upon fee for each service provided. The more the provider charged, the more the payer paid.

In the early 1980s, Medicare introduced the prospective payment system as a way of reimbursing hospitals. This marked the beginning of a movement to control health care costs. Under this system, which insurance companies soon adopted, a fixed fee was paid to the hospital according to a preset reimbursement rate for the diagnosis given at discharge. A hospital could treat a patient so that a shorter length of stay was necessary, reducing the consumption of resources. This would allow the hospital to show a greater profit or smaller loss for caring for a patient with a particular diagnosis. This practice began the trend of managed care in which health care is paid at a prearranged rate rather than as billed.

In the most extreme type of managed care, called *capitation*, employers pay a set fee each month to an insurance company for each covered employee and dependent. This amount does NOT vary based on the care given. Potential patients may never need any health care, or they may require extensive hospitalizations. Regardless, the costs of care must be taken out of the set fee. Under this arrangement, there is incentive for the insurance company and the provider to work aggressively to keep patients healthy, because prevention and/or early intervention are likely to be less expensive than hospitalization. Conversely, if patients do not stay healthy and/or overuse hospitalization, the health care provider may actually lose money.

As a part of the managed care trend, health maintenance organization (HMO) plans have become very popular as a form of insurance. In HMOs, an annual payment is made on behalf of the members to a group of providers who deliver all of the health services covered under the plan, including physician and hospital services. HMOs have grown because they provide a strong incentive to avoid hospitalization, which consequently reduces costs. HMO members often like the ease of utilizing health care with an HMO, because there are fewer uncovered services and forms to fill out. However, the choice of providers is limited; members must use physicians that are part of the HMO, and they may not see specialty physicians without a referral from their primary care provider.

The preferred provider organization (PPO) is another type of insurance plan designed to meet the goals of managed care. To avoid out-of-pocket expenses, members must use physicians who have agreed to provide services at a lower price to the insurer. However, members may use an "out-of-network" provider without a referral, if they are willing to pay more for that service.

What Has the Impact of Managed Care Been on Costs?

Initially, managed care reduced the cost of health care. However, costs have increased sharply in response to the backlash from restrictive managed care policies. Since 1999, employer-sponsored health insurance premiums have increased by 199%, placing cost burdens on both the employers and the workers (Kaiser Family Foundation, 2007). Currently, there are various proposals to reform the U.S. health care system to reduce cost while increasing access to care for those who do not have insurance. The proposals are divided between a stronger role for government negotiation and market-based models which rely on competitive forces. Despite the variety in policy views, the areas which seem most likely to be implemented as strategies to reduce costs include (1) investment in information technology, (2) improving quality and efficiency of care delivery, (3) adjusting provider compensation, (4) prevention, (5) increasing consumer involvement in purchasing, and (5) altering the tax benefits for employer-sponsored insurance (Kaiser Family Foundation, 2007). The American Nurses Association (2009) issued a similar statement on reducing associated health care costs by focusing on health promotion and disease prevention, cultural competency, health education, chronic disease management, coordination of patient care, and community-based nursing care. These strategies are important for nurses to consider in reducing health care costs.

STRATEGIES TO CONTROL COSTS

Hospital care accounts for the largest share (31%) of the health care expenditures and physician services are second, accounting for 21%. Reducing costs in these areas has the greatest impact on reducing total costs (Kaiser Family Foundation, 2007). Specific efforts to reduce hospital costs include case management, evidence-based practice, appropriate staffing, improving retention of staff, use of the electronic health record (EHR), and reducing patient care errors.

CASE MANAGEMENT

Case management is one of the strategies suggested to reduce costs while ensuring coordination of care. Central to any case management program are (1) coordination of care; (2) communication and collaboration between health care providers, payers, and patients; and (3) attention to the continuum of care for continuity of services provided (Thomas, 2009). Registered nurses (RNs), social workers, and therapists may all be case managers; although how they perform their role depends on the scope of practice of their discipline. All case managers must be skilled at communication, critical thinking, negotiation, and collaboration. They must be knowledgeable about resources available to patients. The case manager not only collaborates with individual patients, but also with family and other support systems of the patient.

Case management is effective in providing care, but all patients do not need this intensity of interaction. To provide such care to all patients would be wastefully expensive. Patients should be assigned a case manager only if they:

- Have complicated health care needs
- Are receiving care that is expensive as well as complicated
- Pose discharge planning problems
- Receive care from multiple providers
- Are likely to have significant physical or psychosocial problems

There are two types of case management generally used in an acute care hospital. The first is the traditional model, which focuses on discharge planning and determining if the care planned throughout the patient's hospital stay is necessary and appropriate (utilization review), so that the insurer will pay for the services. In this approach, the case manager reviews the chart every 3 to 7 days and may carry a case load of between 16 and 28 patients per day. The full immersion model of case management requires the case manager to review the chart and communicate with physicians and nurses caring for the patients on his/her case load daily. The increased level of interaction is designed to minimize the likelihood that insurers will not pay because of untimely communications to insurers and perhaps reduce the likelihood of treatment delays. Because of the increased intensity of the workload of the case manager in this system, caseloads are usually 12 to 14 patients on medical and neurology specialty units and 16 to 18 patients on surgical and cardiology units (Thomas, 2009).

What Tools Are Used to Support Case Management?

Clinical pathways and **disease-management protocols** are similar strategies that support the work of the case manager to reduce expensive variations in care.

> Clinical pathways, also known as care maps, are multidisciplinary plans of "best" clinical practice for groups of patients with a specific medical diagnosis.

These pathways support the coordination and delivery of high-quality care. There are four essential elements of a clinical pathway:

- A timeline outlining when specific care will be given
- The categories of care or activities and their interventions
- Intermediate and long-term outcomes to be achieved
- A variance record

The variance record allows caregivers to document when and why the progress of individual patients varies from that outlined in the pathway. Clinical pathways differ from practice guidelines, protocols, and algorithms, because they are used by the multidisciplinary team and have a focus on quality and coordination of care for individual patients. A sample of a clinical pathway can be found in the Evolve resources.

> Disease management is a system of coordinated health care interventions and communications for persons with conditions in which self-care is important in controlling the disease.

According to the Disease Management Association of America (DMAA), disease management:

- Supports the physician or practitioner/patient relationship and plan of care
- Emphasizes prevention of exacerbations and complications by using evidence-based practice guidelines and patient empowerment strategies
- Evaluates clinical, humanistic, and economic outcomes on an ongoing basis, with the goal of improving overall health (DMAA, 2005).

Managed care organizations often enroll members who have a specific disease, such as diabetes, in a program tailored for the needs of patients with that condition. The program focuses on prevention and educational activities when members are NOT in the acute stage of the disease, so that they will be prepared to understand and manage symptoms throughout their lives. Nurses, often employed by health plans, are frequently involved in this component of disease management. Disease-management protocols also outline standard interventions to be implemented during the acute stage of the illness, although physicians or other providers may make modifications to provide individualized care.

According to the Congressional Budget Office (Holtz-Eakin, 2004), a disease management intervention includes selection of types of patients and providing them with education, monitoring, feedback, and coordination of care. The success of disease management interventions can be measured by process outcomes, such as the extent to which the patient follows through with the evidence-based guidelines established for the particular disease. Over a longer period of time, it is possible to measure whether the patient's condition is improved or whether there is a reduction in negative outcomes which negatively impact patients' quality of life or increase the cost of providing care. The Congressional Budget Office reviewed research related to disease management protocols in congestive heart failure, coronary artery disease, and diabetes to determine whether disease management programs can reduce the overall cost of health care. They concluded that that these programs may improve the quality of care, but there was insufficient evidence to conclude that disease management can generally reduce overall health spending (Holtz-Eakin, 2004).

Both critical pathways and disease-management protocols are generally based on clinical guidelines that incorporate nationally acceptable ways to care for a specific disease. Clinical guidelines are specific practice recommendations that come from a rigorous review of the best evidence on a specific topic (Melnyk & Fineout-Overholt, 2005). These guidelines are typically developed by government agencies, such as the Agency for Healthcare Research and Quality (AHRQ), or an organization devoted to health promotion and disease prevention, such as the American Public Health Association and the Center for Disease Control. A website developed by AHRQ, in collaboration with the American Medical Association (AMA) and the American Association of Health Plans, provides a resource for clinical practice guidelines at *www.guideline.gov*.

A new approach to reduce costs and improve quality is the pay for performance (P4P) payment system. Physicians, hospitals, medical groups, and other health care providers are rewarded for meeting certain performance measures for quality and efficiencies. Disincentives, such as eliminating payments for negative consequences of care (medical errors) or increase costs have also been proposed. An example of such disincentives includes hospitals not receiving reimbursement for care given to treat hospital-acquired problems, such as pressure ulcers. The 2006 Institute of Medicine report, "Preventing Medication Errors" "recommends this type of incentives so that the profitability of hospitals, clinics, pharmacies, insurance companies, and manufacturers (are) aligned with safety goals." There are a number of pilot programs from the government or other payers currently in process to evaluate the effectiveness of such approach (Thomas & Caldis, 2007).

EVIDENCE-BASED PRACTICE

How Do We Know that Critical Pathways and Disease-Management Protocols Reflect the Latest and Best Practice?

In 2000, the Institute of Medicine (IOM) released a report, "Crossing the Quality Chasm: A New Health System for the 21st Century" (IOM, 2000). This report noted that it takes 17 years for the results of research in health care to be transmitted consistently into practice.

> Evidence-based practice is one strategy to reduce the amount of time required to integrate new health care findings into practice.

Evidence-based practice is the use of current best evidence in making decisions about patient care. It flows from clinicians asking, "What is the best way to manage a particular situation?" Melnyk and Fineout-Overholt (2005) believe that evidence-based practice uses the following steps to answer clinical questions:

- A systematic search for the most relevant evidence to the question
- Critical evaluation of the evidence found (Is the evidence logical and valid?)
- Your own clinical experience (Does your experience fit with the evidence?)
- Patient preferences and values (Will your patients accept the recommendations drawn from the evidence?)

The answer to these questions can then be implemented in practice or incorporated into critical pathways and disease-management processes.

In 1997, 2002, and again in 2007, AHRQ promoted evidence-based practice in everyday care through establishment and funding of 14 evidence-based practice centers (EPCs). These centers develop evidence reports on topics relevant to clinical, behavioral, economic, or other health organization and delivery issues—specifically those that are common, expensive, and/or significant to the Medicare and Medicaid populations. Some of the EPCs specialize in conducting technology assessments for the Centers for Medicare and Medicaid Services (CMS). One EPC concentrates on supporting the work of the U.S. Prevention Task Force (AHRQ, 2007b).

Most nurses use their own clinical experience and patient preferences and values in planning nursing care. However, searching for the evidence to the question at hand and critically evaluating it may be more difficult. Table 15-1 outlines a rating system to help you know how strong the evidence from research or other sources might be. There are at least five centers in schools of nursing in the United States that can serve as resources regarding evidence-based practice in nursing:

- The Academic Center for Evidence-Based Nursing (ACE) at the University of Texas Health Science Center at San Antonio *(www.acestar.uthscsa.edu)*
- The Indiana Center for Evidence-Based Nursing Practice—a collaborative of the Joanna Briggs Institute *(www.joannabriggs.edu.au/about/home.php)*

TABLE 15-1 Evaluation Criteria for Evidence for Clinical Questions

LEVEL	DEFINITION
Level I	Evidence comes from a review of a number of randomized controlled trials (RCTs) or from clinical practice guidelines that are based on such a review.
Level II	Evidence comes from at least one well-designed RCT.
Level III	Evidence comes from well-designed controlled studies that are not randomized.
Level IV	Evidence comes from well-designed case-controlled and cohort studies.
Level V	Evidence comes from a number of descriptive or qualitative studies.
Level VI	Evidence comes from a single descriptive or qualitative study.
Level VII	Evidence comes from the opinion of authorities and/or reports of expert committees.

From Sackett D, et al: *Evidence-based medicine: how to practice and teach EBM,* London: Churchill Livingstone, 2000.

CRITICAL THINKING BOX 15-1

What are the advantages to using evidence-based nursing care? What are the barriers? How might these barriers be overcome?

- The Sara Cole Hirsch Institute for Best Nursing Practice Based on Evidence at Case Western Reserve School of Nursing *(http://fpb.case.edu/HirshInstitute/index.shtm)*
- The Center for the Advancement of Evidence-Based Practice-Arizona State University *(http://nursingandhealth.asu.edu/evidence-based-practice/index.htm)*
- New Jersey Center for Evidenced Based Practice—in collaboration with the Joanna Briggs Institute *(http://sn.umdj.edu/research/jbicenter.htn)*

See Critical Thinking Box 15-1. Also see Chapter 24 for more information on how evidence-based practice affects economics.

SHORTAGE OF NURSES

Although hospitals and other health care organizations have experienced nursing shortages over the past 50 years, the most recent shortage, which began in 1998, seems to be the most persistent (Buerhaus, 2009). On July 2, 2009, the U.S. Bureau of Labor Statistics reported that the health care sector of the economy is continuing to grow despite significant job losses in nearly all industries. In September 2009, the Bureau of Labor Statistics confirmed that 544,000 jobs have been added to the health care sector since the 2009 recession began. In addition, in 2009, Buerhaus and colleagues found that despite the current easing of the nursing shortage due to the recession, the U.S. nursing shortage is projected to grow to 260,000 RNs by 2025. A shortage of this magnitude would be twice as large as any nursing shortage experienced in this country since the mid-1960s (American Association of Colleges of Nursing, 2009).

What Can Be Done to Recruit Nurses to the Profession?

Since 1999, several groups have focused on nursing recruiting. For example, Johnson & Johnson has launched a new public awareness campaign to generate interest in careers as nurse educators *(www.discovernursing.com)*. In addition, Nurses for a Healthier Tomorrow is a coalition of 43 nursing and health care organizations working together to raise interest in nursing careers. The coalition has launched a website, created a televised public service announcement, and designed print ads that can be downloaded for free online *(www.nursesource.org)*.

How Can Health Care Organizations Retain Nurses?

Retention of nurses is as important as recruitment. Kovner, Brewer, et al. (2009) found that when nurses leave for another position or retire early, the effects on the hospital's bottom line is significant. The authors suggest that as much as 5% of a hospital's budget may go to paying for nursing turnover. Factors which positively influence nurses' intent to stay on their job included autonomy, variety, supervisory support, workgroup cohesion, procedural justice (rights are applied universally to all employees), collegial nurse/doctor's relations, and opportunity for promotions (Kovner et al, 2009) (Box 15-1).

Negative influences included high workload, organizational constraints, and mandatory overtime (Kovner et al, 2009). In addition, Wieck and colleagues (2009) found that the effectiveness of incentives to remain employed varied with the age of the nurse.

Magnet Hospitals

Recognizing the characteristics that influence a positive work environment upon nurse retention is not new. In the early 1980s, during a previous nursing shortage, the American Academy of Nursing conducted research to identify organizational attributes of hospitals successful in recruiting and retaining nurses. American Academy of Nursing Fellows nominated 165 hospitals throughout the nation that had reputations for successfully attracting and retaining nurses and delivering high-quality nursing care. Ultimately, 41 hospitals were distinguished by high nurse satisfaction, low job turnover, and low nurse vacancy rates, even when hospitals located in the same area were experiencing nursing shortages. These hospitals were called "magnet" hospitals, because of their successes in attracting and keeping nurses.

BOX 15-1	Forces of Magnetism

Force 1: Quality of nursing leadership
Force 2: Organizational structure
Force 3: Management style
Force 4: Personnel policies and programs
Force 5: Professional models of care
Force 6: Quality of care
Force 7: Quality improvement
Force 8: Consultation and Resources
Force 9: Autonomy
Force 10: Relationships between the community and the health care organization
Force 11: Nurses as teachers
Force 12: Image of nursing

From American Nurses Credentialing Center (2004): *Forces of magnetism*. Retrieved from *www.nursecredentialing.org/magnet/forces.html*.

CRITICAL THINKING BOX 15-2

What are the factors that YOU think result in a great working environment? What factors result in an unacceptable environment?

The Magnet Recognition Program identifies characteristics or outcomes, known as "Forces of Magnetism," which exemplify excellence in nursing (see Box 15-1). Ten years after the identification of the original magnet hospitals, the American Nurses Credentialing Center (ANCC) established a new magnet hospital designation process, similar to accreditation by The Joint Commission (TJC). Recently, the recognition program has been expanded to provide national recognition for excellence in long-term care nursing facilities and smaller community hospitals. In the current competitive environment, receiving the magnet status may serve as a recruiting and marketing tool for hospitals, attesting to a professional work environment and quality nursing (Critical Thinking Box 15-2).

There appears to be a relationship between the effects of the hospital care environment and patient mortality and nurse outcomes. For example, Aiken and associates (2009) studied 10,184 nurses and 232,343 surgical patients in 168 Pennsylvania hospitals to determine the net effects of nurse practice environments on nurse and patient outcomes, after accounting for nurse staffing and education. Nurses evaluated their practice environment, using the practice environment scales of the Nursing Work Index. Outcomes included nurse job satisfaction, burnout, intent to leave, and reports of quality of care, as well as mortality and failure to rescue in patients. The results of this study suggested that nurses reported more positive job experiences and fewer concerns with care quality, and patients had significantly lower risk for death and failure to rescue in hospitals with better care environment (Aiken et al, 2009).

PATIENT SAFETY

Patient safety remains an important issue in the current health care environment. In 1996, the IOM initiated a concerted, ongoing effort to assess and improve the quality of care in the United States. The first phase documented the seriousness of the quality problems. In the second phase (1999-2001), two reports were released. "To Err Is Human: Building a Safer Health System" (IOM, 1999) focused on how tens of thousands of Americans die each year because of medical errors. "Crossing the Quality Chasm: A New Health System for the 21st Century" (IOM, 2000) defined six aims to improve health care quality, including that care is:

- Safe
- Effective
- Patient-centered
- Timely
- Efficient
- Equitable

The third phase, which is going on now, focuses on determining ways that the future health care delivery system described in earlier reports can be realized. Box 15-2 outlines some of the more recent IOM reports from this initiative. Visit *www.iom.edu* for more information.

BOX 15-2	Recent Reports of Health Care Quality from the Institute of Medicine

- Preventing Medical Errors: Quality Chasm Series
- Hospital Based Emergency Care: At the Breaking Point
- Leadership by Example: Coordinating Government Roles in Improving Health Care
- Crossing the Quality Chasm: A New Health System for the 21st Century
- Ensuring Quality Cancer Care
- Envisioning the National Health Care Quality Report
- To Err Is Human: Building a Safer Health System
- Fostering Rapid Advances in Health Care
- Health Professions Education: A Bridge to Quality
- Priority Areas for National Action: Transforming Health Care Quality
- Key Capabilities of an Electronic Health Record System
- Patient Safety: Achieving a New Standard for Care
- Keeping Patients Safe: Transforming the Work Environment of Nurses
- 1st Annual Crossing the Quality Chasm Summit: A Focus on Communities
- The Healthcare Imperative: Lowering Costs and Improving Outcomes: Workshop Summary
- Value in Health Care Accounting for Cost, Quality, Safety, Outcomes, and Innovation: Workshop Summary
- Redesign Continuing Education in the Health Professions

From *www.iom.edu.*

One of the IOM reports, "Keeping Patients Safe: Transforming the Work Environment of Nurses," suggests that the work environment of nurses needs to be changed to better protect patients. The report makes recommendations in the areas of (1) nursing management, (2) workforce deployment, and (3) work design and organizational culture (IOM, 2003). For example, restructuring of hospital organizations in response to managed care often has undermined the trust between nurses and administration. The report urged health care organizations to involve nurse leaders in all levels of management in decision making and to ask nursing staff their opinions about care design, because nurses are very effective in detecting processes that contribute to errors.

A report, "Health Care at the Crossroads: Strategies for Addressing the Evolving Nursing Crisis," released by TJC in 2002, concurs with the IOM recommendations. This report suggested that nurse executives should delegate decision-making authority to nurse managers and other nursing unit leaders about how units should be run and how scarce resources should be spent. This demonstrates the confidence that the nurse executive has in the competency of the managers. In turn, the authority to make real-time, critical decisions at the point of care should be delegated from the unit leaders to the nursing staff. In the middle of the night, when administrators are not present, the decisions of nurses control patient outcomes (TJC, 2002).

In 2008, TJC published another report, "Guiding Principles for the Development of the Hospital of the Future." This report outlines principles to (1) support economic viability, (2) guide technology adoption, (3) guide achievement of patient-centered care, (4) guide design of hospitals of the future, and (5) address staffing challenges. Table 15-2 outlines the principles in this report related to patient-centered care.

TABLE 15-2   The Joint Commission Principles to Guide Patient-Centered Care

- Make adoption of patient-centered care values a priority for improving patient safety and patient and staff satisfaction
- Incorporate patient-centered care principles into the activities of hospital oversight bodies and transparency initiatives
- Address barriers to patient and family engagement, such as low health literacy and personal and cultural preferences
- Eliminate disparities in the quality of care for minorities, the poor, the aged, and the mentally ill
- Improve the quality of care for the chronically ill through adoption of care models that encourage coordinated, multi-disciplinary care
- Use robust process improvement tools to improve quality and safety, and support achievement of patient-centered care

From The Joint Commission (2008): *Guiding principles for the development of the hospital of the future.* Retrieved from *www.jointcommission.org/assets/1/18/Hosptal_Future.pdf.*

The concern about patient safety extends to other areas within TJC. In 2004, TJC established its National Patient Safety Goals, which have been revised each year since then. The goals and related implementation expectations are identified by program—ambulatory care, assisted living, behavioral health care, critical access hospitals, disease-specific care, home care, hospital, laboratory, long-term care, networks, and office-based surgeries *(www.jointcommission.org/ PatientSafety/NationalPatientSafetyGoals).* See Table 22-1 for a complete list of the 2010 TJC Hospital National Patient Safety Goals.

One of TJC goals is to improve the effectiveness of communication among caregivers. Although the requirements of this goal deal with clear communication regarding physician orders and test results, there are other issues surrounding communication that may reduce patient safety and job satisfaction of nurses. A national study, "Silence Kills," sponsored in part by the American Association of Critical-Care Nurses describes interviews with more than 1,700 nurses, physicians, clinical care staff, and administrators. This report found that fewer than 10% of those interviewed speak to colleagues about behaviors that could result in errors or other types of harm to patients. These behaviors may include trouble following directions, demonstration of poor clinical judgment, or taking dangerous shortcuts. The results are often broken rules, mistakes, lack of support, incompetence, poor teamwork, disrespect, and micromanagement. When clinicians speak up, these conversations are called "crucial conversations" (American Association of Critical-Care Nurses, 2005).

The authors believe that having these "crucial conversations" should result in significant reductions in errors, improved quality of care, reduction in nursing turnover, and marked improvement in productivity (Patterson et al, 2005). (See Chapter 11 for additional information on communication and patient safety.) In an effort to address the issues identified in "Silence Kills," the American Association of Critical-Care Nurses has established Standards for Establishing and Sustaining Healthy Work Environments. Table 15-3 identifies these standards. (Also see Critical Thinking Box 15-3.)

TABLE 15-3	American Association of Critical-Care Nurses Standards for Establishing and Sustaining Healthy Work Environments	
CATEGORY	STANDARD
Skilled communication	Nurses must be as proficient in communication skills as they are in clinical skills.
True collaboration	Nurses must be relentless in pursuing and fostering true collaboration.
Effective decision making	Nurses must be valued and committed partners in making policy, directing and evaluating clinical care, and leading organizational operations.
Appropriate staffing	Staffing must ensure the effective match between patient needs and nurse competencies.
Meaningful recognition	Nurses must be recognized and must recognize others for the value each brings to the work of the organization.
Authentic leadership	Nurse leaders must fully embrace the imperative of a health work environment, authentically live it, and engage others in its achievement.

From American Association of Critical-Care Nurses (2005): *AACN standards for establishing and sustaining healthy work environments: a journey to excellence.* Retrieved from *www.aacn.org.*

CRITICAL THINKING BOX 15-3

WHAT DO YOU THINK?
- How many hours are too long to work?
- Is there an increase in errors made by nurses working 12 hours or longer?
- How would you handle it if the supervisor asked you to work 6 more hours after your 12-hour shift because the floor is short?
- What is your responsibility as a professional when it comes to overtime?

The Institute for Healthcare Improvement (IHI), a not-for-profit organization founded in 1991, is also focused on improving the quality of health care. The IHI goal is to aim for health care for all with:
- No needless deaths
- No needless pain or suffering
- No helplessness in those served or serving
- No unwanted waiting
- No waste (IHI, 2006)

An IHI initiative which embodied these goals was the 100,000 Lives Campaign, which began in 2004 and ended in June 2006. This project was designed to engage thousands of U.S. hospitals in an effort to prevent 100,000 needless inpatient deaths by implementing improvements in care. At the end of the campaign, IHI announced that more than 3100 participating hospitals had saved an estimated 122,343 lives. Building on this success, in December 2006, IHI launched the

5 Million Lives Campaign. The focus was expanded beyond mortality to also include harm, introducing high-impact interventions that build on those of the 100,000 Lives Campaign. These concerns include:

- Hospital-acquired infection, starting with methicillin-resistant *Staphylococcus aureus*
- High-alert medications
- Surgical complications
- Pressure ulcers
- Congestive heart failure
- Governance structures that can have enormous impact on a facility's ability to drive change (IHI, 2006)

Another IHI effort to improve safety and quality in hospitals began in 2003, when IHI, in collaboration with the Robert Wood Johnson Foundation, developed a process for transforming care in hospitals in medical surgical units. The initiative, known as Transforming Care at the Bedside (TCAB), involves a 4-point framework design theme and six core values of work redesign. Front-line staff, with the full support of the executive team, create, design, test, and implement patient care improvements (called tests of change). The improvement efforts are centered on a patient's or an employee's need. Small rapid tests of change provide a mechanism for avoiding delays, discussions, debates, meetings, and layers of administrative sign-offs that often occur in improvement efforts. The TCAB process includes a series of steps to create a replicable approach that can be done in a short period of time:

- Clarify the current state by observations—include those involved.
- Understand the root problem to solve.
- Select a process to focus on.
- Design a prototype (plan, do, check, act).
- Begin small (one patient, one nurse, one idea, one try) and rapidly move/test.
- Identify failures quickly and reject them.
- Determine possible improvements and quickly broaden the test of change.
- Determine definite "just do its" and quickly implement (Martin et al, 2007).

The emphasis on safety has not only resulted in the initiation of specific programs to improve patient care, but has also stimulated evaluation of those measures. For example, Donaldson and colleagues (2009) evaluated the efforts of nine multihospital organizations that used rapid response teams. This evaluation determined the impact of rapid response teams through the eyes of the nurse. Nurses surveyed identified four categories of assistance which resulted from calling the team, including (1) physical assistance in the form of "extra hands, eyes, brains, and bodies"; (2) one-call mobilization of urgent assistance; (3) clinical and communication competences of critical care nurses; and (4) the ability to expedite transfer to a more intensive level of care.

Similarly Sharpnack-Elganzouri and colleagues (2009) assessed 151 nurses during 980 unique medication administrations in medical-surgical units at a rural hospital, an urban community hospital, and an academic medical center. The study evaluated the nursing effort and work-flow in the medication administration process. Nurses averaged more than 15 minutes on each medication pass and were at risk of an interruption or distraction with each one. The authors concluded that systems challenges during medication administration lead to threats to patient safety, work-arounds, workflow inefficiencies, and distractions during a time when focus is most needed to prevent error.

WHAT ARE THE EFFECTS OF VARIOUS PATTERNS OF NURSING CARE DELIVERY?

Over the years, nursing care has been delivered in many ways, including total patient (private duty model), functional, team, primary, and relationship-based care (Figure 15-1). Although we often talk about these systems as distinct from one another, in the real world, you seldom find pure forms of these systems. Consequently, you must be prepared to work in systems that may be a combination, tailor-made to fit the needs of a specific organization.

What Is the Total Patient Care or Private Duty Model?

Originally, nursing was organized around the total patient care or private duty model. RNs were hired by the patient and provided care to one patient, typically in the patient's home. In the 1920s, 1930s, and again in the 1980s, this approach was used in which one nurse assumes responsibilities for the complete care of a group of patients on a 1:1 basis, providing total patient care during the shift.

The quality of care in the total patient care model is considered to be high, because all activities are carried out by RNs, who can focus their complete attention on one patient. Tiedeman and Lookinland (2004) suggest that this model is efficient because it (1) decreases communication time between staff caring for a patient, (2) reduces the need for supervision, and (3) allows one person to perform more than one task simultaneously. Some nurses prefer this model because they can focus on patients' needs without the work of supervising others; others feel that their skills and time are wasted doing patient care activities that could be done by others with

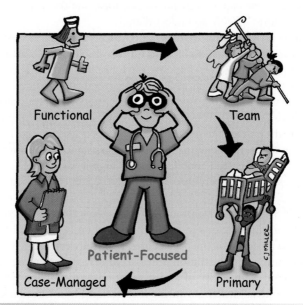

FIGURE 15-1
Evolving patterns of nursing care delivery.

less skill and education. Patient satisfaction tends to be high with this model if continuity of care and communication are maintained among nurses (Tiedeman & Lookinland, 2004).

What Is Functional Nursing?

The movement to use RNs as employees of hospitals came with the outbreak of World War II. RNs took over the work in the hospital and that, coupled with the war effort, stimulated the nursing shortage of that period. This forced hospitals to develop alternative models of nursing. The positions of aides and licensed vocational/practical nurses came into being, and in some states, they were allowed to perform functions such as administration of medications and treatments. This functional kind of nursing, which broke nursing care into a series of tasks performed by many people, resulted in a fragmented, impersonal kind of care (Figure 15-2). Fragmentation of care caused patient problems to be overlooked, because they did not fit into a defined assignment.

Tiedeman and Lookinland (2004) note that this assembly line approach provided little time for the nurse to address psychosocial or spiritual needs. They cite a number of studies, which found that errors and omissions increased when functional nursing was used. This approach would seem to be cost-efficient, because it can be implemented with fewer RNs. However, there are studies that suggest that the functional method, in fact, costs more than primary nursing care. In addition, patients, nurses, and physicians have been critical of this approach because of the fragmentation and the lack of accountability for the total patients (Tiedeman & Lookinland, 2004).

What Is Team Nursing?

In the 1950s, team nursing evolved as a way to address the problems with the functional approach. In this type of nursing, groups of patients were assigned to a team headed by a team leader,

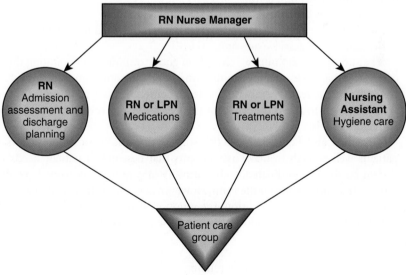

FIGURE 15-2

Lines of authority: functional nursing.

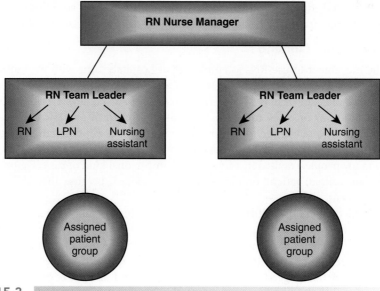

FIGURE 15-3

Lines of authority: team nursing.

usually an RN, who coordinated the care for a designated group of patients (Figure 15-3). The team leader determines work assignments for the team on the basis of the acuity level of the group of patients and the ability of the individual team members. The following is an example of the components of a team:

- An RN who is the team leader
- Two licensed vocational nurses/practical nurses assigned to patient care
- Two unlicensed assistive personnel (UAP)

The success of team nursing centers on good communication among the team members. It is imperative that the team leader continuously evaluates and communicates changes in the patient's condition to the team members. The team conference is a vital part of this approach, allowing team members to assess the needs of their patients and revise their individual plans of care on an ongoing basis.

Tiedeman and Lookinland (2004) suggest that the team model allows the nurse to know patients well enough to make assignments that best match patient needs with staff strengths. Patient needs are coordinated, and continuity of care may improve, depending on the length of time each member stays on the team. However, care can be fragmented and the model ineffective when staff is limited. In addition, the amount of time required to communicate among team members may decrease productivity (Tiedeman & Lookinland, 2004).

What Is Primary Nursing?

In the 1960s and 1970s, primary nursing evolved. In this system, a nurse plans and directs the care of a patient over a 24-hour period. This approach is designed to reduce or eliminate the fragmentation of care between shifts and nurses, because one nurse is accountable for planning

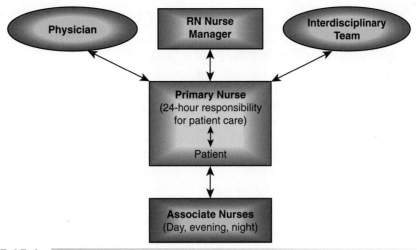

FIGURE 15-4
Lines of authority: primary nursing.

the care of the patient around the clock. Progress reports, referrals, and discharge planning are usually the responsibility of the primary nurse. When the primary nurse is off duty, an associate nurse continues the plan of care. An RN may be the primary caregiver for some of the assigned patients, whereas an associate nurse is the primary caregiver for others. Some forms of primary nursing evolved into an all-RN staff (Figure 15-4). You may also find primary nursing being mixed and modified with nurse extenders, such as paired partners, or partners in care. Although team nursing took the RN away from bedside care, primary and modified primary nursing puts the nurse back in close contact with the patient.

Relationship-based practice is the new name for primary nursing. The RN, who may be called the care coordinator, the responsible nurse, the principal responsible nurse, the case manager, or the care manager, manages and coordinates patient's care in the hospital and the discharge plan. This nurse develops a relationship and can be identified by the patient, the patient's family, and the health care team as having the responsibility and authority for planning the nursing care the patient is to receive.

What Is Patient-Focused Care?

Patient-focused care is another delivery system that has evolved during the last 15 years. Because of earlier nursing shortages, some traditional nursing interventions, such as phlebotomy and diet instruction, have been given to members of departments that do not report to nursing. These ancillary workers spend a great deal of time in transit from one unit to another. Time is also lost when there is not work for this single-function member to do. These tasks can be centralized on the unit under the direction of the RN. UAP are cross-trained to perform more than one function, thus increasing the level of productivity. In this system, the patient comes into contact with fewer people, and the RN, who is familiar with the patient's plan of care, supervises the delivery of care. This model also moves RNs to a higher level of functioning, because they are now accountable for a fuller range of services for the patient. Tasks that do not require an RN can be delegated to UAP under the supervision of the RN.

What Is the Most Effective Model of Nursing Care?

In the past, there has been a great deal of literature about models of care delivery. However, there is a lack of systematic evaluation regarding the use of the various models, often because of the lack of similarity in staffing and patient populations on comparison units (Tiedeman & Lookinland, 2004). As a result, it is impossible to determine the impact that models of nursing care have on patient outcomes, costs, or job satisfaction. It may be that the model of nursing care delivery is less important than other factors, including the nurse-to-patient ratios, use of over-time, and the organizational culture in which the nurse works, in influencing outcomes (Critical Thinking Box 15-4).

However, the current emphasis on quality and safety of patient care has had an impact on care delivery models. Kimball and colleagues (2007) evaluated new innovative care delivery modules that have the potential to change or reinvent care delivery. Of the 45 models identified, 30 were selected for further research, including telephone interviews and review of supporting information. Each of the models needed to (1) serve primarily adult patients; (2) rely on nurses to play a primary role in care delivery; (3) include an acute care hospital component; (4) integrate technology, support systems, and new roles; and (5) improve quality, efficiency, and cost. The models were ranked based upon (1) the model's match with the criteria, (2) the degree of inno-vation, (3) the level of integration with other settings and providers of care, (4) the existence of measurable results, and (5) the potential for sustainable outcomes.

Each of these models had some common elements. The first is an *elevated RN role,* which moves from traditional care delivery to serving as a "primary care manager." The second element is a *sharpened focus on the patient.* The care is nurse-managed, but patient-directed, which results in greater patient and family involvement, increasing compliance and speedy recovery. The third common element includes *specialized tools for assessment, teaching, and measurement,* which ensures smooth transitions from one level of care to another. The fourth element involves *the leveraging of technology* (e.g., electronic medical records, pharmacy robots, cell phones, or walkie-talkies) to enhance communication, reduce labor-intensive documentation, improve access to information, or reduce wasted time. The fifth includes the *measurement of a broad range of clini-cal, quality, financial, and satisfaction indicators* to drive the redesign and indicate viability and sustainability. The development of each of these models also involved the early and regular involvement of caregivers. Five of the models evaluated by Kimball and colleagues (2007) are described in Table 15-4.

What Is the Impact of Staffing Patterns on the Quality of Care?

Regardless of the model of care used, nursing staffing must be addressed, particularly in hospitals, which require 24-hour coverage. In 2004, the AHRQ released a report that summarized the latest

CRITICAL THINKING BOX 15-4   What factors influence the patterns of nursing care delivery?

TABLE 15-4 Innovative Nursing Models

Name	Description	Role of the Nurse	Advantages
The 12-Bed Hospital	Large hospital segmented itself into 12- to 16-bed unit	RN is designated a patient care facilitator who serves as a CEO of the unit. Assumes 24/7 accountability for directing and managing individualized care for each patient. Primary contact for physicians, social workers, and other members of the interdisciplinary team. Serves as a liaison for patients and families. Mentors other RNs and team members.	Improved care, decreased nursing care fragmentation, improved communication and quality of patient care
Primary Care Team	Differentiated nursing practice team composed of an RN case manager, an RN or LVN/LPN, and a clinical assistant	Designed to increase the value of the experienced RN in patient care. Principles include: Team involves patient in planning, by asking on each shift, "What is the most important thing I can do for you this shift?" Twice each shift, have a "Take 5 for Safety" huddle—a quick team update on patients. RN care manager is supported by a unit manager and a case manager.	Decreased nursing vacancy, turnover rates; improved physician satisfaction with nursing knowledge and communication
Collaborative Patient Care Model	A multidisciplinary, population-based case management model, targeting high-volume, high-risk, and high-cost patients in disease-specific or population-based groups	RN patient care coordinators and physicians co-chair multidisciplinary practice groups.	Reduction of average acute length of stay and reduced care-giver turnover

Continued

TABLE 15-4 Innovative Nursing Models—cont'd			
NAME	DESCRIPTION	ROLE OF THE NURSE	ADVANTAGES
Transitional Care Model	Provides comprehensive in-hospital planning, care coordination and home follow-up of high-risk older adults by an interdisciplinary team	APRNs conduct assessments and with physicians, design and coordinate patient care and discharge plans. APRN implements the plan of care in the home for 1 to 3 months.	Decreased total number of hospital readmissions and total health care costs
Hospital at Home	An acute home-based program of older patients with COPD, heart failure, cellulitis and pneumonia; provides hospital-level care at home	RN is the coordinator of care for a team consisting of a physician, RN, and nursing assistant. RN observes the patient in the home during the first 24 hours—level of care is determined. Physician visits daily.	Aims to avoid many complications, including delirium resulting from the hospital admission of older patients

APRN, Advanced practice master's degree prepared nurse.
Adapted from Kimball B, et al: The quest for new innovative care delivery models, *J Nurs Admin* 37:392-398, 2007.

findings of AHRQ-funded and other research on the relationship between nurse staffing levels and adverse patient outcomes. This report concluded that:
- Lower levels of hospital nurse staffing are associated with more adverse outcomes.
- Patients in hospitals today are more acutely ill than in the past, but the skill levels of the nursing staff have declined.
- Higher acuity patients have added responsibilities that have increased the nurse workload.
- Avoidable adverse outcomes, such as pneumonia, can raise treatment costs by up to $28,000.
- Hiring more RNs does not decrease profit.
- Higher levels of nurse staffing could have positive impact on both quality of care and nurse satisfaction (AHRQ, 2004).

The largest of these studies found significant associations between too few nurses on a unit and higher rates of pneumonia, upper gastrointestinal bleeding, shock/cardiac arrest, urinary tract infections, and failure to rescue. Other studies in the review found associations between lower staffing levels and pneumonia, lung collapse, falls, pressure ulcers, thrombosis after major surgery, pulmonary compromise after surgery, longer hospital stays, and 30-day mortalities (AHRQ, 2004).

In 2007, the AHRQ funded research to review studies from 11 databases to assess how nurse-to-patient ratios and nurse work hours were associated with patient outcomes in acute care hospitals, factors that influence nurse staffing policies, and nurse staffing strategies that improved patient outcomes. They found that higher RN nurse staffing was associated with less hospital related mortality, failure to rescue and other patient outcomes, but the higher RN staff might not be the cause of these outcomes, since hospitals that invest in adequate nursing staff may also invest in other initiatives to improve quality. They also found that the effect of increased RN staffing on patient safety was strong and consistent in ICUs and in surgical patients. Greater RN hours spent on direct patient care were associated with decreased risk of hospital-related death and shorter lengths of stay (AHRQ, 2007a).

Determination of the number of nursing staff needed relative to the number and acuity of patients on a unit is the challenge of staffing. In the past 20 years, patient classification systems (or acuity systems) have been used to determine the number of nurses needed on a unit at any one time. Patient acuity is the measure of categorizing patients based upon their nursing care requirements. Patient classification systems, particularly with increased computerization and the ability to access the system online, provide many benefits. Specifically they can be used to (1) improve patient care outcomes, (2) identify appropriate staffing, (3) track budget compliance and costs, and (4) maintain nurse retention through their ability to impact staffing through assessment of patients' conditions (Harper & McCully, 2007).

How Are Nursing Work Assignments Determined?

Once appropriate staffing levels for a unit are determined, specific nurses must be scheduled. How work assignments are given varies with individual institutions and is related to the model of care delivery, condition of the patient, the architecture of the unit, and the expertise of the staff.

> A major problem in scheduling nurses is the fact that patient acuity fluctuates dramatically from day to day and from season to season.

For example, over the Christmas holidays there is often a significant decrease in the number of elective surgeries. In response, some hospitals may close units or reduce the number of staff on any given unit. By contrast, in the middle of the influenza season, the hospital might be full and understaffed.

Nursing has tried a variety of approaches to anticipate the number and qualifications of nurses that will be needed for a specific period of time for a specific group of patients. Regulatory agencies such as The Joint Commission require that staffing be based on some sort of organized system. Staffing in organizations may be based on budgeted nursing hours per patient per day. Hours per patient per day are calculated by the number of patient care staff working during a 24-hour period and divided by the number of patients served in a day.

Whether nursing resource requirements are defined by nursing hours per patient days or as nurse-patient ratios, the underlying assumption is that all patients, patient days, and nursing staff are equal. In fact, the nursing resource requirement is also influenced by the intensity of patient care needed, the length of stay of the patient, and the competency of the staff. There are three approaches to document that the organization has a minimum number of nurses to ensure safety in any given acute care unit: (1) identifying and mandating fixed staffing ratios and (2) establishing a hospital-specific written staffing plan, which typically uses computerized patient acuity systems; or (3) reporting/public disclosure of staffing plans.

In 1999, California was the first state to pass comprehensive legislation to establish minimum nurse-to-patient ratios for RNs and LPN/LVNs in acute care, acute psychiatric, and specialty hospitals. Once the bill was passed, the California Department of Health Services (CDHS) was charged with determining what the ratios in various patient care areas should be. In 2005, the governor suspended the law scheduled to take effect on January 1, 2005, which required one nurse for every five patients in medical-surgical units, which was a change from the ratio of one nurse for every six patients. A judge ruled that the governor's administration overstepped its authority and barred the administration from delaying the implementation of the staffing rations. Although a few states have regulated the ratios in specialty areas, such as intensive care units or labor and delivery rooms, California is the only state to mandate ratios in every patient care unit in every hospital in the state (DeVandry & Cooper, 2009). Aiken and colleagues (2009) conclude that patient mortality rates have decreased and nursing retention rates have steadily increased since implementation of the mandated nurse staffing ratios in California.

In contrast to fixed nurse-patient ratios, a written plan includes the following critical factors:

- Establishing initial staffing levels that are recalculated at least annually or more often as necessary
- Setting staffing levels on a unit-by-unit basis
- Identifying ways to adjust staffing levels from shift to shift, based on intensity of patient care
- Using outcomes and nurse-sensitive indicators to evaluate the adequacy of the plan

Written staffing plans should be developed by an advisory committee composed of a number of RNs, a significant portion of whom are involved in direct patient care at least part of the time (Critical Thinking Box 15-5). Nevada, Ohio, Connecticut, Washington, Illinois, Oregon, and Texas use staffing plans/committees. In addition, New York, Vermont, New Jersey, Rhode Island, and Illinois require reporting and/or public disclosure related to nursing staffing. The reporting of staffing may be made readily available to the public or reported to a state agency (DeVandry & Cooper, 2009).

The research regarding the effectiveness of the three approaches has not been conclusive and the optimal nurse to patient ratio has not been determined (DeVandry & Cooper, 2009). Until the evidence regarding staffing becomes clearer, the judgment of the competent RN is critical in making decisions regarding the necessary staff. At this point, recommendations regarding staffing remain at a broad level. For example, the TJC report "Guiding Principles for the Development of the Hospital for the Future" identifies principles to address the staffing challenge:

CRITICAL THINKING BOX 15-5

How might you handle a staffing crisis? What are the advantages and disadvantages to each of the following:

- What are the unit census, acuity, and patient-classification systems?
- Does your organization have a float pool within the staff or an agency or outside staff available?
- Check on your part-time staff to work an extra shift.
- Will another staff member cover the extra shift for a day off later in the schedule?
- Can you do with partial-shift coverage during the "peak" shift hours?
- Ask a staff member to work a double shift—either stay late or come in early.
- Work the shift yourself.
- What other solutions can you think of?

- Address the misdistribution of health care workers across the globe by instilling fair migration and compensation policies for affected countries.
- Expand health professional education and training capacity to accommodate the growing demand for health care workers.
- Create work place cultures that can attract and retain health care workers.
- Support the development of health professional knowledge and skills required to care for patients in an increasingly complex environment.
- Educate health professionals to deliver team-based care and promote teamwork in the hospital environment.
- Develop the competence of health professionals to care for geriatric patients.

These principles emphasize the need to ensure a positive work environment for employees, which includes encouraging team work. Kalisch and Lee (2009) explored staff characteristics, staffing and scheduling variables associated with the level of teamwork in nursing staff on acute care hospital patient units. A sample of 1758 nursing staff members from two different hospitals on 38 patient care units completed the Nursing Teamwork Survey. The researchers found that staff with less than 6 months of experience, those working 8- or 10-hour shifts (as opposed to 12 hours or a combination of 8 and 12 hours), part-time staff (as opposed to full time), and those working on night shift had higher team scores. The higher team work scores were also associated with no or little overtime. The higher the perception of the adequacy of staffing and the fewer patients cared for on a previous shift, the higher the teamwork scores.

What About Scheduling Patterns?

Nursing has also been concerned about scheduling practices and options because in many health care environments, nursing care must be provided 24 hours a day, 365 days per year. That is why there are numerous scheduling patterns other than the typical 8-hour shift 5 days a week. From working 10-hour days 4 days a week to the weekend alternative (known as the Baylor plan) of two 12-hour weekend shifts for 36 hours of pay, nurses have tried numerous patterns and combinations of shifts.

What About the Use of Overtime?

With the current shortage of health professionals, employees are also encouraged and sometimes required to work overtime. In fact, Trinkoff and colleagues (2006), in a study of more than 2000 nurses across multiple care settings, found that at least one fourth of the respondents reported working 12 hours or more per shift, one third of the sample reported working more than 40 hours per week, and one third reported working 6 days or more in a row at least once in the previous 6 months. Similarly, the landmark study of nurses by Rogers and associates (2004) found that 14% of nurses in the study reported working shifts of 16 hours or longer in the previous 4 weeks; 81% of shifts ran more than their scheduled limit. This work pattern results in fatigue, which can produce performance similar to someone who is intoxicated from alcohol. Fatigue can also produce physical performance effects that inhibit critical cognitive functions, including lapses of attention, irritability, memory lapses, decreased ability to detect and react to subtle changes, slowed information processing, difficulties dealing with unexpected situations, and communication difficulties (Graves & Simmons, 2009).

The negative effects of fatigue can have serious consequences on the provision of nursing care. Yet, only limited action has been taken on a state-by-state level to eliminate mandatory overtime

BOX 15-1 **EVIDENCE-BASED PRACTICE**

Creating Healthy Work Environments to Retain Nurses

PRACTICE ISSUE

Kramer and colleagues (2009) reviewed literature from seven professional organizations/regulatory bodies to identify structures and leadership practices, which influence a healthy working environment likely to retain nurses. They also analyzed 88 additional studies to identify structures most helpful in supporting nurses to provide high-quality patient care. Creating healthy nursing environments improves quality patient care and employee retention.

IMPLICATIONS FOR NURSING PRACTICE

Structures most frequently cited that influence a healthy working environment are:
- Management style of the nurse leader is visionary, visible, open and rich, and includes skilled communications.
- Opportunities for education, professional growth, development, and advancement are available, including tuition reimbursement, continuing education, and certification.
- Nurse staffing structures provide adequate numbers and flexible scheduling.
- Flat, decentralized organizational structure promote unit-based and shared decision-making.
- Collaborative, interdisciplinary relationships are demonstrated through evidence such as committee membership and minutes.
- A culture of interdisciplinary collaboration, teamwork, and safety exists and is nurtured.
- Personnel policies include salary and benefits competitive for geographical area and advancement, such as career ladders.
- Quality improvement infrastructure and environment are in place, including research and evidence-based practice initiatives.
- Meaningful recognition structures are operative, including recognition of nurses' contributions and the value of these contributions; reward/pay for performance.

Structures most helpful in supporting nurses to provide high-quality patient care are:
- Nurse-managers who share power; request evidence used to make autonomous decisions; hold staff accountable in positive, constructive ways for decisions made; promote group cohesion and teamwork; and resolve conflicts constructively
- Structures that support EBP teams
- Approval from administration for nurses to make autonomous decisions, interdisciplinary collaboration, and for leadership/participation in council activities
- Programs that help develop effective team work
- Staffing structures that consider RN competence, level of patient acuity, flexible scheduling, and flexible care delivery systems
- Availability and support for educational programs
- Regular, interdisciplinary patient care rounds, review and critique sessions, and critical pathway and protocol development
- Structure for regulation and determination of nursing practice by nurses at all levels of the organization
- Development of and "living" a patient-centered culture in which values are known, subscribed to, and transmitted to newcomers

Considering This Information:

What can you do as a nursing leader to promote a healthy work environment?

Reference for the Evidence

Kramer M, Schmalenberg B, Maguire P: Nine structures and leadership practices essential for a magnetic (healthy) work environment, *Nursing Administrative Quarterly* 34:4-17, 2009.

for nurses. In addition, there are no regulations that prevent nurses from voluntarily electing to work overtime. The Texas Nurses Association (2009) has published a booklet, "Tired Is Trouble; A Nurse Leader's Guide to Managing Fatigue in the Workplace" which helps nurses to assess organizational systems and practices, staffing and scheduling practices. It also provides suggestions for developing an organizational strategic plan for fatigue management *(www.texasnurses.org)* (Evidence-Based Practice Box 15-1).

CONCLUSION

The emphasis on cost control and managed care has changed the way that nursing care is delivered. New models of health care delivery are being developed in which we look at the desired outcome and "manage backward" to achieve that outcome at the lowest level of expenses. Because of some of the unexpected negative consequences of managed care, there is a renewed emphasis on evidenced-based care to enhance patient safety. We are continually challenged to develop more innovative and creative ways to ensure excellence in patient care with limited dollars. Nurses can meet this challenge.

BIBLIOGRAPHY

Agency for Healthcare Research and Quality (2004): Hospital nurse staffing and quality of care: research in action. Retrieved from *www.ahrq.gov*.

Agency for Healthcare Research and Quality (2007a): Nurse staffing and quality of patient care. Retrieved from *www.ahrq.gov/clinictp/nursesttp.htm*.

Agency for Healthcare Research and Quality (2007b): Evidence based practice center. Retrieved from *www.ahrq.gov/clinic/epc*.

Aiken L, Sloane D, Cimiotti J, et al (2009): Implications of the California nurse staffing mandate for other states, *Health Services Research*. Retrieved from *www.nationalnursesunited.org/assets/pdf/hsr_ratios_study_042010.pdf*.

Aiken L, Clarke S, Sloane D, et al: Effects of hospital care environment on patient mortality and nurse outcomes, *JONA* 39(7/8):S45-S51, 2009.

American Association of Colleges of Nursing (2009): Nursing faculty shortage fact sheet. Retrieved from *www.aacn.nche.edu/Media/FactSheets/NursingShortage.htm*.

American Association of Critical-Care Nurses (2005): AACN standards for establishing and sustaining healthy

work environments: a journey to excellence. Retrieved from *www.aacn.org*.

American Association of Critical-Care Nurses and VitalSmarts (2005): Silence kills: the seven crucial conversations for healthcare. Retrieved from *www.silencekills.com/UPDL/PressRelease.pdf*.

American Nurses Association (2009): ANA on reducing healthcare costs. Retrieved from *www.nursingworld.org/MainMenuCategories/Healthcareand PolicyIssues/HealthSystemReform/What-ANA-is-Doing/ANA-on-Reducing-Health-Care-Costs.aspx*.

American Nurses Credentialing Center (2004): Forces of magnetism. Retrieved from *www.nursecredentialing.org/magnet/ProgramOverview/Forcesof Magnetism.aspx*.

Buerhaus P: *The future of the nursing workforce in the United States: data, trends and implications*, Sudbury, MA, 2009, Jones and Bartlett.

DeVandry S, Cooper J: Mandating nurse staffing in Pennsylvania: more than a numbers game, *JONA* 39:470-478, 2009.

Disease Management Association of America (2005): Definition of DM.

Retrieved from *www.dmaa.org/index.asp*.

Donaldson N, Shapiro S, Scott M, et al: Leading successful rapid response teams: a multisite implementation evaluation, *JONA* 39:176-181, 2009.

Graves K, Simmons D: Reexamining fatigue: implications for nursing practice, *Crit Care Nursing Q* 32:112-115, 2009.

Harper K, McCully C: Acuity systems dialogue and patient classification system essentials, *Nursing Administration Quarterly* 3:284-299, 2007.

Holtz-Eakin D (2004): An analysis of the literature on disease management programs, *Congressional Budget Office*. Retrieved from *www.cbo.gov/doc.cfm?index=5909&type=0*.

Institute for Healthcare Improvement (2006): Protecting 5 million lives from harm. Retrieved from *www.ihi.org/IHI/Programs/Campaign*.

Institute of Medicine (2000): Crossing the quality chasm: a new health system for the 21st century. Retrieved from *www.iom.edu*.

Institute of Medicine (2003): Keeping patients safe: transforming the work environment of nurses. Retrieved from *www.iom.edu.*

Institute of Medicine (1999): To err is human: building a safer health system. Retrieved from *www.iom.edu.*

Kaiser Family Foundation (2007): U.S. health care costs: background brief. Retrieved from *www.kaiseredu.org/ topics_im.asp?1&parentID=61&id=358.*

Kalisch B, Lee H: Nursing teamwork, staff characteristics, work schedules, and staffing, *Health Care Management Review* 34:323-333, 2009.

Kimball B, et al: The quest for new innovative care delivery models, *JONA* 37:1-11, 2007.

Kovner C, Brewer C, Greene W, Fairchild W: Understanding new registered nurses' intent to stay at their job, *Nursing Economics* 27(2), 2009.

Kramer M, Schmalenberg B, Maguire P: Nine structures and leadership practices essential for a magnetic (healthy) work environment, *Nursing Administrative Quarterly* 34:4-17, 2009.

Martin S, et al: Transforming care at the bedside: implementation and spread model of single-hospital and multihospital systems, *JONA* 37:444-451, 2007.

Melnyk B, Fineout-Overholt E: *Evidence-based practice in nursing and health care: a guide to best practice*, Philadelphia, 2005, Lippincott Williams & Wilkins.

Patterson K, et al: *Crucial conversations: tools for talking when stakes are high*, New York, 2005, McGraw-Hill.

Rogers AE, et al: The working hours of hospital staff nurse and patient safety, *Health Affairs* 23:202-212, 2004.

Sharpnack-Elganzouri ES, Standish C, Androwich I: Medication Administration Time Study (MATS): nursing staff performance of medication administration, *JONA* 39:204-210, 2009.

Sportsman S: Human resource practices and management in hospitals. In: Leiyu S, ed: *Human resources practice and management in the health care sector*, Sudbury, MA, 2005, Jones and Bartlett.

Thomas F, Caldis T (2007): Emerging issues of pay-for-performance in health care, *Health Care Financing Review*. Retrieved from *www.allbusiness.com/ health-care/health-care-facilities-nursing/8919708-1.html.*

Thomas P: Case management delivery models, *JONA* 39:30-37, 2009.

The Joint Commission (2005): Facts about the sentinel event policy. Retrieved from *www.jointcommission. org/aboutUs/Fact_sheets/sep_facts.htm.*

The Joint Commission (2002): Health care at the crossroads: strategies for addressing the evolving nursing shortage. Retrieved from *www. jointcommission.org/NR/rdonlyres/ 5C138711-ED76-4D6F-909F-B06E0309F36D/0/health_care_at_the_ crossroads.pdf.*

The Joint Commission (n.d.): National patient safety goals. Retrieved from *www.jointcommission.org/PatientSafety/ NationalPatientSafetyGoals.*

Tiedeman M, Lookinland S: Traditional models of care delivery: what have we learned? *JONA* 34:291-297, 2004.

Trinkoff A, Geiger-Brown J, Brady B, et al: How long and how much are nurses now working, *Am J Nursing* 106:60-67, 2006.

Wieck L, Dols J, Northam S: What nurses want: the nurse incentives project. *Nursing Economics* 27:169-201, 2009.

Additional resources are available online at *http://evolve.elsevier.com/Zerwekh/nsgtoday/.*

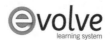

CHAPTER 16

Economics of the Health Care Delivery System

Mary Ellen Murray, PhD, RN

> *Of all the forms of inequality, injustice in health care is the most shocking and inhuman.*
> —MARTIN LUTHER KING JR

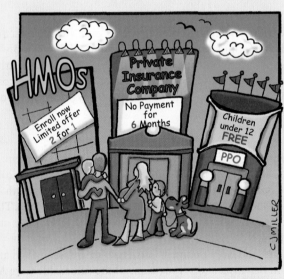

Value is the intersection of cost and quality in health care.

After completing this chapter, you should be able to:

- Define economics and health care economics.

- Compare the market for health care to a normal market for goods and services.

- Use a basic knowledge of health care economics to analyze trends in the health care delivery system.

- Describe what is meant by operating budget, personnel budget, and capital budget.

- Define economic research strategies.

- Describe what is meant by the term fiscal responsibility in clinical practice.

- Discuss strategies you will use to achieve fiscal responsibility in your clinical practice.

he rate of increase in national health care spending slowed to 4.4% in 2008—the slowest rate of increase in 48 years (Hartman et al, 2010). However, it may not be time to celebrate! In 1995, national health care expenditures (NHCE) topped $1 trillion dollars for the first time. The 2008 figure represents NHCE of $2.3 trillion, more than doubling the 1995 figure in 3 years. By the year 2018, those expenditures are projected to exceed $4.3 trillion dollars. In 2008, the national health care expenditures consumed 16.2% of the gross domestic product (GDP, the value of all the goods and services produced in the United States annually). The percentage of the GDP devoted to health care is predicted to be 20.3% by 2018 (NHCE projections, 2008-2018). The outcome of this investment, in terms of the public health of the population, is a nation lagging behind many comparable industrialized nations. In 2010, an estimated 45 million persons were without health insurance. Prescription drug coverage under Medicare is limited. Great disparities in access to health care exist among racial and ethnic populations. There are vast differences in the reimbursement for the treatment and care of physical and mental illness (Murray, 2002). All of these statistics have implications for the clinical practice of nursing.

WHAT ARE THE TRENDS AFFECTING THE RISING COSTS OF HEALTH CARE?

Both intrinsic and extrinsic factors contribute to rising costs of health care. Intrinsic factors include characteristics of the population (the population is getting older and requiring more of the health care system), the demand for health care, and employer-paid health insurance. Extrinsic factors include the availability of technology, prescription drug costs, and workforce costs (Figure 16-1). The recession facing the United States, and the world, in 2009 to present has both intrinsic and extrinsic effects.

Intrinsic Factors

The U.S. population grew by 32.7 million people from 1990 to 2000, the largest increment in American history (U.S. Census Bureau, 2006). Population estimates for the years 2008 to 2009 projected a 9% increase. Population projections for the years 2000-2010 predict a growth of almost 27 million people, with the greatest increase among the 45- to 64-year-old age group. This is important information because older people typically use increased health care resources and may not have the income to purchase them.

Over the projection period of 2009-2019, the Baby Boomers (citizens born between 1946 and 1964) will become eligible for Medicare health insurance. "Provisions of the Affordable Care Act are projected to result in a lower average annual Medicare spending growth rate for 2012 through 2019 (6.2%), 1.3 percentage points lower than pre-reform estimates" (Centers for Medicare & Medicaid Services, 2010, p 2). There is also an increasing demand for health care in the United States. Demand, in the economic sense, is the amount of health care services that a consumer wishes to purchase. Another aspect of increased demand for health care has to do with the widespread availability of health insurance. This has the effect of lowering the cost of health care to individuals who have health insurance. In contrast with demand for health insurance, the need for health care is defined as the amount of health care that the experts believe a person should have to remain as healthy as possible, based on current medical knowledge (Feldstein, 2004). The question then arises: Should the amount of health care provided be based on need or demand?

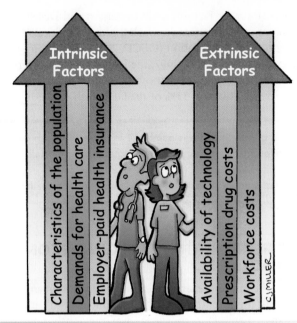

FIGURE 16-1

Trends affecting the rising cost of health care.

Extrinsic Factors

The availability of new medical technology has contributed to the rising costs of health care. If an institution does not offer technology that a competitor offers, it is likely that the market share (percentage of persons in an area selecting that institution) of the institution will decline. To attain a competitive edge, an institution needs to be an early adopter of expensive, new technology. Then, thinking sequentially, someone has to pay for the technology, and this cost will be passed on to consumers in the form of higher health care costs.

Prescription drug care costs are projected to rise from a projected $219 billion (2006) to $299 billion in 2010, to $446 billion in 2015 (Borger et al, 2006). The major impact of the Medicare prescription drug program is a shift in payment for the drugs from private sources to the government.

A final factor driving health care costs is the increase in hospital care expenditures, which were projected to be $663 billion in 2006 and $882 in 2010 (Borger et al, 2006). One of the main factors contributing to these increases is rising labor costs. Although this is good news for the nursing profession, it is part of a national problem.

The current recession in the United States has decreased private health spending and increased in Medicaid enrollment and expenditures. Similarly, economists project a decrease in hospital prices due to a weakening demand for hospital services, again related to the recession. There is also a projected decrease in the private insurance sector in prescription drug growth, as many consumers either fill fewer prescriptions or become more willing to use lower cost generic drugs. However, Medicare and Medicaid prescription drug spending will offset the private sector recession related decrease.

The Organization for Economic Co-operation and Development (OECD) is a forum where the governments of 30 democracies work together to address the economic, social, and environmental challenges of globalization (OECD, 2007). This group reports statistics related to health expenditures and outcomes. In 2007, the United States was reported to spend 16% of the GDP for health care for every man, woman, and child in the country. The country nearest to the United States that year was France at 11% of the GDP.

> "In 2006, the United States was number 1 in terms of health care spending per capita, but ranked 39th for infant mortality, 43rd for adult female mortality, 42nd for adult male mortality, and 36th for life expectancy" (Murray et al, 2010).
>
> This has led some to question whether the United States has the best health care system in the world or just the most expensive.

WHAT IS THE EFFECT OF THE CHANGING ECONOMIC ENVIRONMENT ON CLINICAL PRACTICE?

Because nurses belong to the largest health care profession and are thus in a position to influence health care costs, it is essential that all nurses understand basic concepts of economics and fiscal (money) management. This knowledge was previously taught in graduate courses for nurse managers or nurse executives. However, the world has changed! One nurse author (Hunt, 2001) states, "Clinical competency is not the only tool needed in an era when economics dominates the health care arena" (p 11).

> Today all nurses need to couple their clinical skills with business skills that enable them to be full participants in designing and delivering health care.

INTRODUCTION TO ECONOMICS

A simple definition of economics is the allocation of scarce resources. An analogy might be made to the income that an individual earns. The paycheck is a limited, finite amount of money, and choices must be made about how to spend, or allocate, the money. Such choices might include rent, a car payment, food, clothing, and health insurance payments. Individuals may not be able to pay for all of the goods or services that they wish to have, so decisions must be made and priorities established.

Similarly, health care is a limited resource, and choices have to be made. The choices about health care that concern economists are made at the national level. Questions to answer include these: How much does the country wish to spend on health care, what services does the country wish to provide, what is the best method for producing health care, and how will health care be distributed (Feldstein, 2004)?

What Are the Choices About Amount of Spending?

Currently, the United States is spending slightly more than 16% of its income on health care. As the payer for Medicare (the national health insurance program for people aged 65 years or older, some people younger than age 65 with disabilities, and people with end-stage renal disease) and Medicaid (a joint federal and state program that pays for medical assistance for certain individuals and families with low incomes and resources), the federal government is the nation's largest purchaser of health care. Yet this amount does not fully meet the needs of the populations served under these programs, let alone provide for the health care needs of persons without insurance.

The Affordable Care Act of 2010

Congress and President Obama signed into law the Affordable Care Act of 2010. This type of health care reform is anticipated to provide health care coverage at an affordable cost for all Americans.

> *To help lower costs, the Affordable Care Act:*
> - *Sets up a new competitive private health insurance market—through state Exchanges—giving millions of Americans and small businesses access to affordable coverage, and the same choices of insurance that members of Congress will have.*
> - *Holds insurance companies accountable by keeping premiums down and preventing many types of insurance industry abuses and denials of care, and ending discrimination against Americans with pre-existing conditions.*
> - *Puts our budget and economy on a more stable path, since it is expected to reduce the deficit by more than $100 billion over the next ten years—and by more than $1 trillion over the second decade—by cutting government overspending and reining in waste, fraud and abuse*
> —(U.S. DEPARTMENT OF HEALTH AND HUMAN SERVICES, 2010, PARA 5).

What Are the Choices About Services to Provide?

Oregon State passed legislation between the years 1989 and 1995 that provides an example of choices about the services provided to persons with Medicaid coverage. Consumers and providers of health and social services were charged with developing a ranked list of health care services in order of their benefit to the entire population being served and to reflect community values. Coverage for all conditions at a certain level would be set by the state legislature dependent on budget constraints. In the listing of services, treatment of, for example, premature infants, cleft palate, hip fracture, or stroke was covered, whereas radial keratotomy, cosmetic dentistry, and treatment of varicose veins were not included (Oregon Health Policy and Research, 2004). Although this is one type of rationing of health care and Americans are typically opposed to any type of rationing system, it must be noted that the services denied under the Oregon plan are consistent with those denied reimbursement under other private and public insurance plans (Critical Thinking Box 16-1).

Like physicians, rationing of care is an important issue facing the nursing profession. The International Hospital Outcomes Study considered rationing of nursing care. Researchers in

CRITICAL THINKING BOX 16-1

What implications does the Oregon plan have on the health care industry? Have you encountered this type of "rationing system" in your own state's programs?

Switzerland (Schubert et al, 2008) explored the association between the implicit rationing of nursing care and patients outcomes in Swiss hospitals. They found that despite low levels of rationing of nursing care, it was a significant predictor on all six patient outcomes that were studied.

What Are the Choices About Methods to Produce Health Care?

One informal definition of managed care is this: the right care, in the right amount, by the right provider, in the right setting. This definition implies that there are several ways to produce health care. For example, a woman may choose to have an annual physical examination by a nurse practitioner, a certified nurse-midwife, a gynecologist, or a family practice physician. Each provides care from a different perspective and at a different price. In another example, certain procedures that were once done only in hospitals are now done in an outpatient setting, many with the addition of home health nursing. Lumpectomy and simple mastectomies are surgical procedures that are now done in an outpatient setting and that illustrate a different method of producing health care. Deciding the best method is subject to research and must include an analysis of the costs.

What Are the Choices About Allocation?

These decisions involve "who gets what." The underlying question is this: Is health care a right or a commodity (like cars or clothing) to be allocated by the market place? The World Health Organization (WHO) states in its constitution that the enjoyment of the highest attainable standard of health is one of the fundamental rights of every human being (WHO, 2004). The American Nurses Association Health System Reform Agenda (2008) also affirms that health care is a basic human right and that a health care system that ensures universal access to essential health care services is essential. In another document, the ANA (*Code for Nurses,* 2001) states that nurses should provide care without consideration of the patient's social or economic status. However, even if one believes that health care is a right, challenging questions remain. How much health care is a right? Who pays for the health care of people who cannot afford it? Let us assume that an instructor is teaching senior nursing students who all agree that health care is a right. The instructor then asks the students how much of their paycheck they would be willing to forfeit in taxes so that everyone could have this right of health care. It is rare that students are willing to subsidize others' health care at a cost of more than one-third of their own salary.

Even beyond the costs of care is the question of allocation decisions—that is, who decides who gets what health care. Several responses are possible: the government, payers of health care, individuals, the market place, and rationing systems.

Government Allocation Decisions. Through its funding of Medicare, the government has made multiple allocation decisions. The U.S. government has decided it will pay for inpatient health care and some outpatient care for patients older than 65 years of age and selected others. Unfortunately, many of the persons covered by Medicare have come to believe that Medicare covers "everything," and this is not so. It is particularly challenging to nurses when elderly patients assume that they "have Medicare" and thus "nursing home care is paid for." This is a frequent misinterpretation of Medicare coverage. There are many limits to the services reimbursed by Medicare and many requirements that must be met before the government will make payment (Critical Thinking Box 16-2).

Hospice is reimbursed $75 per visit by Medicare B for home visits. For one particular group of patients, it costs hospice an average of $98 per day to provide care.
- What are the implications for hospice?
- What options should the hospice nurse manager and nurses consider?

Payer Allocation Decisions. All insurance companies have rules about the services that will be covered and the requirements that must be met under their policies. One rule involves the presence of preexisting conditions. If, for example, a patient has been diagnosed with AIDS or has been treated for mental illness, that person may be denied coverage for treatment of that particular condition—or denied coverage altogether. When the insurance is a benefit of employment, this is less likely to occur. At other times, if an individual is applying for insurance, she or he may be required to fill out a lengthy questionnaire about health history or submit to a physical examination. The findings of these resources may be used to deny or limit coverage.

Once an insurance policy is in effect, there are additional rules regarding the services that will be covered. Most policies require preauthorization (pre-approval) of services before the patient receives care, except in cases of emergency. For example, a physician's office will typically communicate the need for a surgical procedure to the insurance company and obtain this approval. If the patient is admitted to the hospital in an emergency, however, this requirement is normally waived and the hospital has a limited amount of time to gain the approval or reimbursement for the care may be denied.

Another restriction on resource allocation involves the process of concurrent utilization review (UR). This is a strategy used by managed care companies to control both costs and quality. The process requires that hospital staff, typically registered nurses, communicate the plan of care for a hospitalized patient to the payer or their representative. The payer then determines whether the care is appropriate, medically necessary, and covered under the terms of the policy or the contract with the provider (Murray & Henriques, 2003). For example, if a patient is admitted to the hospital the day before elective surgery, that day's cost will almost certainly be denied reimbursement. Preoperative patient teaching and surgical preparation can be done on an outpatient basis at a much lower cost than a day in the hospital.

Marketplace Allocation Decisions. A final alternative for the allocation of resources is the marketplace. This decision making implies that health care is a normal good, like a car or a piece of clothing, where an increase in income leads to an increase in demand for the good, and the rules of supply and demand apply. However, the market for health care has some significant differences from the market for normal goods.

Unpredictability of Demand. The first difference in the market for health care is the unpredictability of demand. When a person is well, there is little demand for health care services. There is a great demand for health care when a person is ill, and the timing of illness is, of course, uncertain. Consider for example, the case of a patient needing a heart transplant. A patient does not wait until the price comes down. Rather, the surgery is purchased at any price if a donor heart is available.

Consumer Knowledge. Another difference in the health care market involves the knowledge of the consumer. If an individual is purchasing a coat or a car, the person usually knows a good deal about the item being purchased or consults *Consumer Reports* for further data. This is not the case in health care, about which patients tend to have limited knowledge and limited ability to interpret the available knowledge.

Barriers to Entry to the Market. Even if patients had sufficient knowledge to treat their own illnesses, the health care market is fraught with barriers. All providers must pass examinations and be licensed by appropriate boards. Prescriptive authority is heavily regulated and closely controlled.

Lack of Price Competition. The health care market, unlike the market for clothing and automobiles, does not engage in price competition. When, for example, have you heard of a sale on appendectomies or "2 for the price of 1" hip replacements? Of course, it does not happen. But more problematic is the fact that health care consumers frequently do not know the cost of their care—especially if it is being paid for by an insurance provider. In fact, many consumers indicate that they "never saw a bill" for their hospitalization. This is considered to be a measure of the quality of their insurance. Is there any other product that would be routinely purchased without knowledge of its price? The lack of this knowledge leads to predictable consumer health care purchasing behavior.

The classic Rand Health Insurance Experiment (Keeler & Rolph, 1983) was a controlled research study that examined the effect of different co-payments on the utilization of health care. Participants in the study either received free care or paid co-payments of 25%, 50%, or 95%. Economic theory would predict that as price increases, the purchase of goods or services would decline. That is exactly what happened. With a co-payment of 25%, there was a decline in utilization of health care of 19% compared with a free plan. There were even greater declines in utilization of health care services at the higher rates of co-payments. This consumer behavior is so predictable that health care economists have a term for it: *moral hazard*. It refers to a situation in which a person uses more health care services because the presence of insurance has lowered the price to the person.

A final method of allocating health care resources is some system of rationing. Rationing is a type of allocation decision that suggests a need-based system. One author defines rationing as a decision to "(1) withhold, withdraw, or fail to recommend an intervention; (2) informed by a judgment that the intervention has common sense value to the patient; (3) made with the belief that the limitation of health care resources is acute and seriously threatens some members of the economic community; and (4) motivated by a plan of promoting the health care needs of unidentified others in the economic community to which the patient belongs" (Sulmasy, 2007, p 19). Americans find this inherently distasteful. One example of a rationing decision is to not perform heart transplants on patients over 65 years of age with the rationale that the money could be spent on, for example, well-child immunization programs. The major ethical questions (Sulmasy, 2007) involved in rationing decisions include (1) Who makes the decision and (2) using what criteria? However, most Americans find the concept of rationing inherently unacceptable. The counterargument to this position is that rationing occurs every day in the U.S. health care system, but the decision is currently made on the basis of the individual's ability to pay for care.

BUDGETS

A *budget* is a tool that helps to make allocation decisions and to plan for expenditures. It is important that staff nurses understand budget processes because these decisions directly impact their clinical practice. For example, staff nurses working on a patient care unit may feel that there

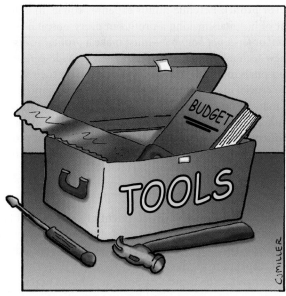

FIGURE 16-2

Budget—a tool that helps make allocation decisions.

is not enough time to care for acutely ill patients on the unit. A clinical manager may respond that the "budget will not allow" additional staff. The reality is that the budget is a human made planning tool and must be flexible in order to be useful. Savvy staff nurses will understand the budget process and be able to relate patient acuity to staffing needs. To engage in these discussions, all nurses need to understand basic concepts of budgets as well as different types of budgets: capital budgets, operating budgets, and personnel budgets (Figure 16-2).

What Are the Basic Concepts of Budgets?

When preparing a budget, one must first consider the unit that the document or budget will serve. It could be an entire hospital, a department, or an individual patient care unit. This discussion will focus on the budget of a patient care unit, because that is the work environment of most registered nurses.

Here are the basic terms that nurses must know:

Revenue: All the money brought into the unit as payment for a good or service. Some departments in the hospital are defined as revenue centers. Examples might include radiology or surgery. Typically, these departments generate a great deal of income for the larger organization.

Expense: All the costs of producing a product. Nursing care units are typically labeled as cost centers; that is, they do not directly generate revenue. Most hospitals have a fixed room rate that includes nursing care. Nurse leaders have questioned the appropriateness of nursing care being lumped into the room rate, but few have been able to effect a change. Some exceptions to this include nursing care to patients in the recovery room, intensive care, or labor and delivery, where there is a separate charge for nursing care.

Margin (or profit): Revenue minus expenses equals margin or profit. Nurses may cringe at the thought of hospitals making a profit but every hospital—whether it is defined as a *not-for-profit hospital* or *for-profit hospital*—must make a profit. Profits are needed to replace equipment, purchase new technology, and, in some cases, provide care for indigent patients. In addition, for-profit hospitals must pay stockholders a return on their investment. The necessity of making a profit is so crucial to the continued existence of an organization, that there is an old adage that states, "No margin, no mission." This means that if an organization does not make a profit, it is unable to fulfill the purpose or mission of the organization, no matter what it might be. The lay public will often describe hospitals as "for profit" or "not for profit." Often faith-based institutions are included in the latter category. In reality, all hospitals must make a profit. It is more significant how the profit is used.

What Are the Types of Budgets?

The budget process involves the development of three budget types that are combined to make an overall budget for the patient care unit: the capital budget, the operating budget, and the personnel budget. The budget covers a 12-month time period that may begin January 1, July 1, or October 1, depending on the institution.

Capital Budget. The beginning point of a budget cycle is usually the *capital budget.* Hospital administrators usually ask departments or patient care units for a list of items that their area will need to purchase in the coming year. These items are usually restricted to equipment costing more than $5000 and lasting more than 1 year. Each manager must rank such requests for the unit and write a justification of why the item is necessary. At a unit level, for example, the nurse manager may request replacement beds, telemetry equipment, or computers. Most managers will discuss unit needs with staff nurses and seek their input. Staff nurses do the work of the organization and are in the best position to know what is needed for patient care. Next, all of the organization's needs are summarized and prioritized according to the funds available. Rarely is there sufficient capital to fund all the requests, and difficult allocation decisions and choices must be made.

Operating Budgets. This budget includes a statement of the expected expenses of the unit for a time period, usually 1 year. The budget process begins with a statement of volume projections. The nurse manager projects how much patient care will be given in the coming year. The volume that nurses are concerned with is measured in patient days, and thus the question is, "How many patient days of care will be provided in the coming year?" The manager would first look at past data to examine how many days were given in the previous year. It is also helpful to look at monthly data, so that it can be determined whether there was a month that exceeded projections, perhaps a month in which there was a flu epidemic or one that had a very low number of patient days due to vacations of medical staff who admit patients. Knowledge of these trends helps the manager to project volume for the next year. The manager would next consider any changes in the patient care unit that might affect volume projections. For example, if two new surgeons are added to the staff, if the unit would begin to provide care for a new clinical population of patients, or if the unit is to be designated as the overflow unit for same-day surgery patients, all of these would increase the volume projections.

In an outpatient setting, the nurse manager of a clinic considers the volume of patient care visits. The manager carefully considers anything that might increase or decrease that volume in the coming year. This might include adding more clinic exam rooms, retirement or addition of

In most hospitals, nursing care is "lumped" in with the room charge and thus nursing care is an expense in the budget and not a revenue center. Most patients (except ICU, step-down, labor and delivery, recovery room) pay the same amount for nursing care. What are the advantages/disadvantages of this for nursing?

professional providers, or events and changes within the provision for and competition of health care dollars in the geographic area.

In addition to projecting the patient day volume, nurse managers also examine the activity of the unit and the acuity (the intensity of care required) of patients. The activity is usually described as *admissions, discharges, and transfers* (ADTs). One measure of activity is the average daily census—that is, how many patients are occupying beds on the unit at midnight. However, this measure by itself results in underestimating the work of the unit. A more accurate picture is gained by the addition of the ADT data, because even though these patients may not be counted in a midnight census, they require many hours of care by registered nurses (Critical Thinking Box 16-3).

Managers must also consider the acuity of the patients on the unit. In an intensive care unit, patients are extremely ill and require many hours of care per day. The number of care hours decreases as patients are moved to general patient care units. Each institution considers the acuity of patients but may use different methods of arriving at measurements. There are several computerized software packages available, whereby nurses enter patient data and the software program produces estimates of the staffing needs of the unit. Programs are designed for each clinical population of patients, obstetrics, pediatrics, psychiatry, and the like. Nurses enter data concerning many factors, including numbers of patients, functional abilities, telemetry monitoring, and postoperative day. These factors help to define how much care patients need and thus can be used to project staffing needs. At the time the budget is created, the nurse manager can review the data to see whether the staffing planned for the unit was adequate to meet patient care needs.

On a daily basis, there may be vacant beds on a patient care unit. However, if there are not sufficient registered nurses available to provide care for the patients who *could potentially* occupy these beds, the unit would not be able to accept additional admissions. Therefore, the nurse manager frequently reports "available staffed beds" rather than "vacant beds." When there are no available staffed beds, it is a critical situation. The manager may be asked to work on increasing the supply of nurses by calling in additional staff. Another strategy might be to identify patients that could be safely discharged early if required. In the worst case scenario, the emergency department may divert potential patients to another hospital, a situation that hospital administration executives deplore! The nurse manager must be prepared to advocate for safe patient care in these situations.

The *operating budget* also includes all of the items necessary for care on the unit. These are called *line items* in a budget and include such things as supplies, telephones, small equipment (e.g., wheelchairs, nurse pagers, and fax machines), postage, and copying costs. Some of these are *variable costs*—that is, costs that change with the volume of patients cared for in a year. Some institutions would include a factor for the variable costs of housekeeping or laundry. There may be a line item for travel for staff nurses to attend clinical conferences or to pay for specialty

CRITICAL THINKING BOX 16-4

As a staff nurse, you have been asked to serve on your unit's financial management committee. You have been told to reduce expenses by 3% overall—in any way you choose to do it.

Given the definitions of fixed and variable costs, where do you think you could begin to look for cost reductions? Develop some ideas of possible cost reductions. Remember that your commitment is to preserve the high quality of patient care.

certification of nurses. These are expenses frequently paid by employing institutions. Other costs, such as heat and electricity, are considered *fixed costs*, and do not change with volume of patients. A nurse manager considers all these things when planning an operating budget (Critical Thinking Box 16-4).

Personnel Budget. The *personnel budget* for a nursing unit is the largest part of unit expenses, and nursing is the largest part of personnel expense. In most hospitals, nursing costs represent at least 50% of hospital expense budgets (Pappas, 2008). This has caused some hospital administrators, who need to reduce expenses to state:

"Follow the dollars, and they will lead to nursing."

Staff nurses need to understand how a nurse manager determines the number of nurses required to care for patients. As discussed, beginning considerations are acuity of patients and the volume or number of patients. The manager must also consider the clinical expertise of the nursing staff. If a unit has a high percentage of new graduates, there will be a decreased ability to safely care for a higher volume of acutely ill patients on the unit. Next, the manager engages in a series of calculations, all of which are easily understood by staff nurses.

Hours Per Patient Day (HPPD). Each patient-care unit will have a designated number of hours of care per patient day. In an intensive care unit, this might be as high as 22 hours per day; on a general surgical unit, it might be 6 to 8 hours. However, nurses need to be aware that these hours must be spread over three shifts (if the institution uses 8-hour shifts) or two shifts (in the case of 12-hour shifts). Nurse managers typically derive *staffing patterns*, that is, combinations of staff (RN, LPN, nursing assistants), that are needed for each shift. These may vary for weekends, nights, and even days of the week. For example, if Monday is a day when many surgical procedures are performed, staffing must include higher numbers of registered nurses to assess and monitor postoperative patients.

Full-Time Equivalent (FTE). An FTE represents the number of hours that a nurse employed full-time is available to perform all of the employment activities. This is calculated to be 2080 hours (52 weeks times 40 hours), but is usually split into productive and nonproductive time (Hunt, 2001).

Productive Time. This figure reflects the amount of time the nurse is available to give care to patients. One work day (8 hours) is usually considered to be 7.5 productive hours.

Nonproductive Time. This time reflects the amount of time that is not available for direct care. Some examples of nonproductive time include vacations, days off, holidays, time at educational seminars, time for committee work (e.g., quality improvement), breaks, and lunch. If these factors are not calculated into the budget, staffing needs may be seriously underestimated. Skilled nurse managers know their staff and can project nonproductive time. For example, if a unit has a very senior staff that accrues annual vacations of 4 to 6 weeks, this must be considered in the budgeting process.

What Are the Economics of Caring? As clinicians, many nurses are reluctant to incorporate knowledge of health care economics into their clinical practice, feeling that it makes them somehow less compassionate or less caring. However, it can be argued that the reason nurses must understand health care economics is that they can bring the values of nursing to the decision-making process for patient care. They can become advocates for patient in the budget process. For example, an administrator with a master of business administration degree may examine the budget of a nursing care unit and make a decision to decrease staffing. A nurse who understands the budgeting process and the research evidence about nurse staffing and patient outcomes can argue persuasively against reductions in nursing HPPD.

It is also important that the nurse is able to evaluate the research that provides the evidence for clinical practice change. Many nurses report that their goal is to give "cost-effective care." However, they use this term loosely and do not understand the economic analysis strategy of cost effectiveness analysis (CEA). This strategy provides information about the cost of an intervention and the effectiveness of an intervention.

At the level of providing care for individual patients, staff nurses must understand fiscal responsibility for clinical practice. *Fiscal responsibility* concerns a threefold responsibility: first to the patient, second to the employing institution, and finally to the payer of health care. It is defined as the duty/obligation of the nurse to allocate (1) financial resources of the patient to maximize health benefit to the patient and (2) financial resources of the employer to maximize organizational cost-effectiveness, and (3) financial resources of the payer with knowledge and efficiency (Figure 16-3).

Fiscal Responsibility to the Patient

The primary fiscal responsibility the nurse has is always, and most importantly, to the patient. This means that a nurse uses the most cost-efficient combination of resources to maximize the health benefit to the patient. A nurse needs to understand the costs of care and different reimbursement systems because this will affect the development of a plan of care. It is important that nurses assess the resources that a patient has available to dedicate to health care. These may include not only insurance coverage, but also the availability of family members or community resources to aid in care.

For example, many churches team up to provide transportation to treatment for patients receiving chemotherapy. Communities vary widely in the resources they offer to patients and families. There may be free support groups, online chat rooms, or Meals on Wheels services available. All of these are valuable community health care resources that are not monetary.

In another example, when creating a discharge plan for a patient, it is essential that a nurse understand the health care resources the patient requires and how they will be paid for. A physician may write orders for prescription medications that are not covered by the patient's insurance. Often patients are reluctant to admit that they cannot afford these medications, and they may either not have the prescription filled or go without other necessities to purchase the medication. Sometimes patients even resort to cutting medications in half to make them "last longer," thereby

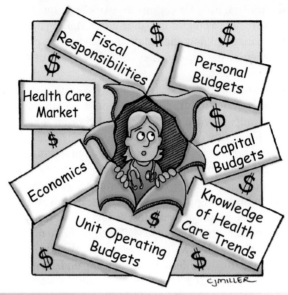

FIGURE 16-3

Nurses play an important role in the economics of health care.

receiving only a partial dose of the medication. If nurses understand patients' insurance coverage and include this in assessment data, they can make better plans of care. It is especially important that nurses understand Medicare coverage, because in some hospitals more than 50% of patients have this coverage. Table 16-1 summarizes the basics of Medicare insurance. Nurses need to be aware that the coverage for Medicare is very complex and the complete documentation for coverage is available online.

It is also important that nurses engage in early discharge planning, beginning the process on admission or even before admission. For example, if a patient is to have a scheduled surgery for hip replacement, the nurse in the orthopedic surgery clinic may talk with the patient about convalescence and continued physical therapy in the rehabilitation unit of a skilled nursing facility. If this process is done before admission, the patient and the family will have the opportunity to visit several facilities and make a selection.

It is important to understand that this does not mean that patients will not receive care or medications if the patient cannot afford to pay for it. It does mean that the nurse will work to ensure that patients get the care they need, regardless of their ability to pay. In the example of a patient who is to be discharged with a prescription that he or she cannot afford, there may be programs within the hospital that provide low-cost medications. Another alternative is to determine whether a generic drug is available at a lower cost. Some patients even choose to order their prescriptions by mail from Canada to obtain medication at lower costs. This practice is legal in some states and illegal in others.

It is also important that nurses understand that fiscal responsibility for clinical practice is a responsibility shared with all other health care disciplines. Nurse practitioners and physicians write orders requiring medications, diagnostic procedures, and laboratory tests. Therefore, they

TABLE 16-1   The Basics of Medicare Insurance Coverage

WHICH PART OF MEDICARE	COST	DESCRIPTION OF COVERAGE	DOES NOT COVER
Medicare Part A	Usually no premium if you or your spouse paid Medicare taxes while working.	Hospital care, hospice care, home health care. Some skilled nursing facility following 3 day inpatient stay.	Long-term care in nursing home
Medicare Part B	Standard amount $96.40 unless exceed the income limits in which case the fee is income determined.	Medically necessary services like doctors' services, outpatient care. Preventive services like pap tests, flu shots.	Routine dental care, dentures, hearing aids, cosmetic surgery
Medicare Part C	Medicare Advantage Plans (MAP) —a plan like an HMO. Medicare will pay a fixed amount each month to the company providing the MAP.	The MAP covers all of Part A and Part B but there may be requirements to get care from selected providers. May offer additional benefits such as hearing, vision, and dental as well as health and wellness programs.	May not cover if you go outside of the selected provider network. You must follow plan rules, like getting a referral to see a specialist. You may only join a plan at certain times during the year and are expected to stay in the plan for a year.
Medicare Part D	Medicare Drug Coverage Individual must have Part A and/or B. Costs will vary with the plan the individual chooses.	There is a yearly deductible—before plan begins to pay. Co-pay—amounts the individual pays at the pharmacy after the deductible. Coverage gap—After the individual and the plan pays a certain amount, the individual pays all of the cost out-of-pocket until a yearly limit is reached. Then the individual receives "catastrophic" insurance whereby the individual again pays the co-pay.	Limits on how much medication the individual can get at one time. Step therapy—the individual must try one or more lower cost drugs that are similar to a higher cost drug.

Centers for Medicare & Medicaid Services: *Medicare & you, 2010.* Retrieved from *www.cms.hhs.gov/medicare/*.

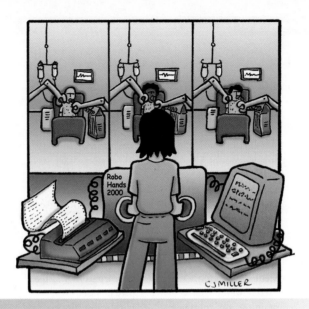

FIGURE 16-4

Advances in computer technology continue to assist the nurse, but technology cannot replace the humanistic aspect of nursing care.

share fiscal responsibility. Clinical social workers have a great knowledge of health care resources available to patients both in the hospital and in the community. All members of the interdisciplinary team share this responsibility and contribute to the goal of maximizing the benefit of health care resources for patients (Figure 16-4).

Nurses also need to advocate for staffing levels that will permit them the time they need to monitor and assess their patients, that is, time to exercise their clinical judgment. Research has demonstrated that nursing care makes a difference in preventing patient deaths and complications (Needleman et al, 2006). Using this evidence to support requests for additional nursing hours to care for acutely ill patients is a rational and respectful way to communicate.

Fiscal Responsibility to the Employing Institution

Nurses also have a responsibility to the institution or agency where they are employed. The most important way for a nurse to demonstrate fiscal responsibility is by providing quality patient care. For example, thorough hand hygiene and the use of sanitizing gels prevent infections that may increase patient costs. Similarly, the prevention of falls and pressure ulcers are clinical practices that have significant cost implications. (See Evidence-Based Practice Boxes 16-1 and 16-2.)

Nurses who continually improve their clinical practice by using evidence-based practice or "best practice" guidelines are also engaging in quality practice that is cost-effective.

BOX 16-1   EVIDENCE-BASED PRACTICE

The Cost of Nurse-Sensitive Adverse Events

PRACTICE ISSUE

In a time of increasing health care costs and an emphasis on providing safe and quality care to patients, nurses need to understand the cost of complications that were effected by nursing care.

IMPLICATIONS FOR NURSING PRACTICE

- Six adverse events were studied: medication error, falls, urinary tract infection, pneumonia, and pressure ulcer.
- For patients with congestive health failure, the cost of an adverse event was $1,029.
- For surgical patients, the cost of an adverse event was $903.
- The odds of pneumonia occurring in surgical patients decreased with additional registered nurse hours per patient day.

Considering This Information:

What is an evidence-based argument that you can make to assure that quality (remember this is the consideration of cost and quality) care is provided to patients?

Reference for the Evidence

Pappas SH: The cost of nurse-sensitive adverse events, *JONA* 38:230-236, 2008.

BOX 16-2   EVIDENCE-BASED PRACTICE

Preventing Pressure Ulcers on the Heel: A Canadian Cost Study

PRACTICE ISSUE

The heel is an area that is especially at risk for the development of pressure ulcers.

IMPLICATIONS FOR NURSING PRACTICE

- Two methods of preventing pressure ulcers on the heel were compared:
  - Method A involved protective bandaging plus usual care.
  - Method B received a hydrocellular dressing for protection of the heel in addition to usual care.
- 44% of patients in Method A group developed pressure ulcers on the heel compared with 3.3% in Method B group.
- Method B group cost $11.67 more than method A group.

Considering This Information:

What is an evidence-based argument that you can make for the more expensive treatment?

Reference for the Evidence

Bou JETI, et al: Preventing pressure ulcers on the heel: a Canadian cost study, *Dermatology Nursing*, 21:268-272, 2009.

Nurses also have an obligation to use the resources of the institution wisely. The most costly health care resource that nurses allocate is their time. The nurse considers patient care needs and prioritizes how professional nursing time shall be allocated. Although it would be ideal for nurses to have unlimited time with each patient, it is rarely possible. As a beginning point, the nurse knows that the most important reason that a patient is hospitalized is to receive assessment and monitoring by a registered nurse. If a patient does not need this assessment, it is likely that they can be safely cared for in a less expensive health care setting, such as a skilled nursing facility. The care plan the nurse develops and implements includes prioritizing the needs of unstable patients. At other times, the nurse may decide that the patient and family require teaching from a professional nurse. It may also be that the patient and family require psychosocial support, a nursing intervention that requires a high level of nursing expertise.

Nurses also need to understand the *prospective payment system*. Under this system, the hospital is paid a set amount for the care of a patient with a certain condition or surgery. If the hospital engages in efficient clinical care practices, the organization makes a profit. If the hospital is not efficient, it may lose money. Medicare reimburses under this prospective system—called *diagnostic-related groups (DRGs)*—as do many private insurance companies. This system has had a large impact on nursing practice. For example, if the nurse does not have a discharge plan in place on the day a discharge decision is made, perhaps due to the lack of planning for transportation for a patient, it may be that the patient will remain in the hospital for an additional day while arrangements are made. This incurs unnecessary costs for the hospital. From another perspective, an unnecessary hospital day is a quality issue. Patients in the hospital are subject to the possibility of infection, the hazards of immobility and bed rest, and even the potential for malnutrition.

Another way that nurses practice fiscal responsibility is by accurately documenting the patient's condition. This must include the severity of the patient's illness as well as the plan of care. If this is not documented, it may be that insurance companies will not reimburse for the care. For example, if the nurse documents "up and about with no complaints," it is very likely that the hospital day will not be covered by insurance. However, if the nurse documents the assessments and monitoring that are being done at frequent intervals, the care will likely be reimbursed.

There are other ways in which nurses recognize institutional fiscal responsibility. For example, the nurse should be aware of bringing only the needed supplies into a patient room, because any unused supplies cannot be returned to stock. Some supplies are to be charged to patients upon use. The fiscally responsible nurse makes this a part of practice, if required.

Another example involves breaks and meal times. The nurse takes breaks and meal times as scheduled, to remain healthy and fully functioning on the job. An occasional shift may be hectic, and it may not be possible to take breaks, but if this is the norm, it is a situation that creates burnout and should be resolved.

Fiscal Responsibility to the Payer of Care

At present, the United States government is the largest single payer of health care. For government funded care such as Medicare and Medicaid, the ultimate payer then is the tax payer. For private insurance, the payer may be the insurance company selected by an employer. In all cases, the nurse has the obligation to efficiently and effectively use resources. The nurse needs to provide documentation that the patient requires care in the appropriate setting. This includes communicating the severity of illness of the patient as well as the plan of care. Without this documentation, the payer may determine that a particular level of care is not necessary and may not reimburse for that care. It is also clear that the application of evidenced-based practice guidelines will enable the nurse to select interventions that are cost effective and that result in the best outcomes.

Box 16-1 summarizes some strategies to help achieve fiscally responsible clinical practice. Box 16-2 summarizes some questions that a new graduate of a nursing program might want to ask during a job interview to assess how a prospective employer views fiscal responsibility.

BOX 16-1   Strategies for Fiscally Responsible Clinical Practice

The nurse:
- Provides quality nursing care that prevents complications
- Makes conscious decisions about the allocation of professional nursing time
- Understands Medicare and Medicaid insurance coverage
- Engages in evidence-based practice and follows best practice guidelines
- Shares information with patients and families about the costs of care and alternatives
- Assigns assistive personnel (nurse aides, certified medical assistants) appropriately to help with care
- Works with the members of other health care professions to promote fiscal responsibility for clinical practice
- Documents patient condition accurately
- Begins discharge planning on admission
- Completes charge slips for patient supplies, if required
- Avoids burnout by taking scheduled breaks, meal times, and vacations
- Engages in safe clinical practice that will avoid personal injuries

---

BOX 16-2   Questions for the New Graduate to Consider Asking During Interviews

- How are financial concerns of patients dealt with? For example, if a patient is unable to afford needed medications on discharge, what resources are available to nurses to help the patient?
- How is acuity of patients assessed and factored into staffing?
- What are the budgeted hours per patient day for the unit?
- What is the turnover rate on this unit? Why do nurses stay/leave this unit?
- How do staff nurses have input into capital budget requests for the unit?
- How are data about unit financial indicators communicated to the staff?
- What percentage of salary is used as an estimate of fringe benefits?
- What is the overtime rate on this unit?
- Can you tell me about the discharge planning process for patients on this unit?
- What is the staff development plan for professional nurses on this unit?

CONCLUSION

Given the dire predictions about health care costs being forecast for the next 10 years, it is imperative that nurses consider the economics of clinical practice. Throughout most of nursing history, nurses have not wanted to learn about the costs of care, considering such concerns about as important or appealing as unnecessary paper work. Nurses proclaim that they want to be caregivers, not accountants. However, nurses humanize health care institutions. They bring the values of caring and compassion to the workplace. In the turbulent years to come, incorporating fiscal responsibility into clinical practice will be seen as another way of caring (Murray, 2002).

BIBLIOGRAPHY

American Nurses Association: *Code of ethics for nurses with interpretive statements*, Washington, DC, 2001, American Nurses Publishing.

American Nurses Association: *Health care reform agenda*, Washington, DC, 2008, American Nurses Publishing.

Borger C, et al: Health spending projections through 2015: changes on the horizon, *Health Affairs Web Exclusive* 25:61-71, 2006. Retrieved from *www.content.healthaffairs.org/cgi/content/full/25/2/w61.*

Centers for Medicare & Medicaid Services (2010): *National health care expenditure projections: 2009-2019.* Retrieved from *www.cms.gov/NationalHealthExpend Data/Downloads/NHEProjections2009 to2019.pdf.*

Centers for Medicare & Medicaid Services (2010): *Welcome to Medicaid.* Retrieved from *www.cms.hhs.gov/medicaid/ whatismedicaid.asp.*

Feldstein PJ: *Health care economics*, ed 6, New York, 2004, Delmar.

Hartman M et al: The National Health Care Expenditure Accounts Team. Health spending growth at a historic low in 2008, *N Engl J Med* 29:147-155, 2010.

Hunt PS: Speaking the language of finance, *AORN J* 73:774-787, 2001.

Keeler EB, Rolph JE: How cost sharing reduced medical spending of participants in the health insurance experiment, *JAMA* 249:2220-2222, 1983.

Murray CJL, Phil D, Frenk J: Ranking 37th—measuring the performance of the U.S. health care system, *N Engl J Med* 362:98-99, 2010.

Murray ME: Another way of caring, *RN Newsletter Madison District Nurses' Association* 4:2-3, 2002.

Murray ME, Henriques JB: Denials of reimbursement under managed care, *Manag Care Interface* 16:22-27, 2003.

Needleman J, et al: Nursing staffing in hospitals: Is there a business care for quality? *Health Affairs* 25:204-211, 2006.

Oregon Health Policy and Research (OHPR) (2004): *Prioritized list.* Retrieved from *www.ohppr.state.or.us/ index.html.*

Organization for Economic Co-operation and Development (2007): *OECD in figures 2006-2006—health spending and resources.* Retrieved from *www.oecd. org/topicstatsportal/0,3398, en_2825_495642_1_1_1_1,00.html.*

Pappas SH: The cost of nurse-sensitive adverse events, *JONA* 38:230-236, 2008.

Schubert M, et al: Rationing of nursing care and its relationship to patient outcomes: the Swiss extension of the International Outcome Study, *Int J Health Care Quality* 20:227-237, 2008.

Sulmasy DP: Cancer care, money, and the value of life: Whose justice? Which rationality? *J Clin Oncol* 25:217-222, 2007.

U.S. Census Bureau (2006): *Population and housing narrative profile.* Retrieved from *www.census.gov/popest/states/ tables/NST-EST2009-02.csv.*

U.S. Department of Health and Human Services: Understanding the affordable care act: About the law, 2010. Retrieved from *www.healthcare.gov/law/about/ index.html.*

World Health Organization: *Basic texts,* ed 44, 2004. Retrieved from *www.who.int/ governance/en/.*

Additional resources are available online at *http://evolve.elsevier.com/Zerwekh/nsgtoday/.*

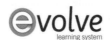

CHAPTER 17

Political Action in Nursing

Michael L. Evans, PhD, RN, NEA-BC, FAAN

> *One of the penalties for refusing to participate in politics is that you end up being governed by your inferiors.*
> —PLATO

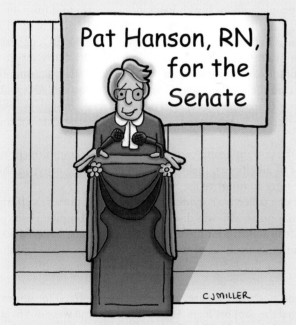

Pat Hanson, RN, for the Senate

CJMILLER

Nurses are playing a major role in the political process for planning the future of health care.

After completing this chapter, you should be able to:

- Define politics and political involvement.

- State the rationale for individual nurse's involvement in the political process.

- List specific strategies needed to begin to affect the laws that govern the practice of nursing and the health care system.

- Discuss different types of power and how each is obtained.

- Describe the function of a political action committee.

- Discuss selected issues affecting nursing: multistate licensure, nursing and collective bargaining, and equal pay for work of comparable value.

oo often nurses feel the legislative process is associated with wheeling and dealing, smoke-filled rooms, and the exchange of money, favors, and influence. Many believe politics to be a world that excludes people with ethics and sincerity—especially given the controversies in presidential administrations and political party ideologies that so often result in gridlock. Others think only the wealthy, ruthless, or very brave play the game of politics. It seems that most nurses feel that the messy business of politicking should be left to others while they (nurses) do what they do best and enjoy most: take care of patients.

Today, however, nurses are coming to realize that politics is not a one-dimensional arena, but a complex struggle with strict rules and serious outcomes. In a typical modern-day political struggle, a rural health care center may be pitted for funding against a major interstate highway. Certainly, both projects have merit, but in times of limited resources not everyone can be victorious. Nurses are now aware that in order to influence the development of public policy in ways that affect how we are able to deliver care, we must be engaged in the political process.

Leavitt and colleagues (2002) wrote that "the future of nursing and health care may well depend on nurses' skills in moving a vision. Without a vision, politics becomes an end in itself—a game that is often corrupt and empty" (p 86). To demonstrate these skills, nurses must elect the decision makers, testify before legislative committee hearings, compromise, and get themselves elected to decision-making positions. Nurses realize that involvement in the political process is a vital tool that they must learn to use if they are to carry out their mission (providing quality patient care) with maximum impact.

Based on research, "the number of people without health insurance coverage rose from 46.3 million in 2008 to 50.7 million in 2009, while the percentage increased from 15.4 percent to 16.7 percent over the same period" (U.S. Census Bureau, 2009). These uninsured individuals (approximately 51 million) receive virtually no health care while countless other inadequately insured individuals receive health care only sporadically. Rural and inner-city residents have alarmingly high morbidity and mortality. Health care for rural citizens is virtually nonexistent. Although the situation is improving in some ways with managed care, even those fortunate enough to have insurance often experience problems accessing the care they need because of cost-cutting strategies.

Nurses' recognition of problems in the current health care system, and their commitment to the principle that health care is a *right* of all citizens, fuel their desire to become active in the political arena and to form a collective force to improve the health care system.

An example of the power of the nursing collective is evidenced in organized nursing's efforts to provide support and defense of a Texas nurse who was discharged from her hospital position for reporting a physician to the Texas Medical Board for medical care that the nurse believed was unsafe patient care (ANA, 2010). The nurse, a member of the Texas Nurses Association and the American Nurses Association, also faced a third-degree felony charge for "misuse of official information."

The Texas Nurses Association became aware of the case and immediately offered to support the nurse involved in the case and enlisted the support from ANA as well. The call went out from ANA to all nurses and more than $45,000 was donated by both individuals and organizations from across the United States to support the defense of this nurse. ANA and the Texas Nurses Association strongly criticized the criminal charges and the fact that this case could have a long-term negative impact on nurses advocating for their patients as whistle blowers.

The case went to trial and the nurse was found not guilty by a jury. ANA President Rebecca M. Patton, RN, MSN, CNOR, said of the outcome, "ANA is relieved and satisfied that Anne Mitchell (RN) was vindicated and found not guilty on these outrageous criminal charges—today's verdict is a resounding win on behalf of patient safety in the U.S. Nurses play a critical, duty-bound role in acting as patient safety watch guards in our nation's health care system. The message the jury sent is clear: the freedom for nurses to report a physician's unsafe medical practices is non-negotiable. However, ANA remains shocked and deeply disappointed that this sort of blatant retaliation was allowed to take place and reach the trial stage—a different outcome could have endangered patient safety across the U.S. having a potential chilling effect that would make nurses think twice before reporting shoddy medical practice. Nurse whistle blowers should never be fired and criminally charged for reporting questionable medical care" (ANA, 2010, para 5).

It is important for nurses to join and to support nursing organizations that advocate and lobby on behalf of nurses, nursing, and quality health care. Not all nursing organizations have a governmental affairs division for lobbying. The American Nurses Association has lobbyists in Washington, DC, to advocate for the concerns of the profession. In addition, most of the constituent state nurses associations have legislative activities at the state level. (Several nursing associations, including the ANA, are described in Chapter 9.) Before joining a nursing association, you should ask whether the association lobbies on behalf of the interests of its members. The future power of nurses depends on nurses joining and supporting such associations.

> Nursing will continue to lobby for new federal and state legislation that improves the quality and availability of nursing and health care.

WHAT EXACTLY IS POLITICS?

Politics, described by Mason and colleagues as "the process of influencing the allocation of scarce resources" (2007, p 4), is a vital tool that enables the nurse to "nurse smarter." Involvement in the political process gives an individual nurse a tool that augments his or her power, or clout, to improve the care provided to patients. Whether on the community, hospital, or nursing unit level, political skills and understanding how laws are enacted enable the nurse to identify needed resources, gain access to those resources, work with legislative bodies to lobby for changes in the health care system and overcome obstacles, thus facilitating the movement of the patient to higher levels of health or function (Figure 17-1).

Let us look first at the nursing unit level:

Your hospital is in the process of selecting a new supplier of IV pumps. You and the other nurses on your unit want to have input into that decision, because IV pumps are essential to the care of your patients and you have a definite opinion about the type of IV pump that works best. But the intensive care unit nurses, who are thought to be more important and valuable because the nursing shortage has made them as rare as hen's teeth, have the only nurse position on the review committee (and therefore, the director's ear!). You and the nurses on your unit strategize to secure input into this important decision.

Your plan might look like this:
- Gather data about IV pumps—cost, suppliers, possible substitutes, and so on.
- Communicate to the head nurse and supervisor your concern about this issue and your plans to get involved in the decision (by using appropriate channels of communication).
- State clearly what you want—perhaps request a seat on the committee when the opportunity arises.
- Summarize in writing your request and the rationale, submitting it to the appropriate people.
- Establish a coalition with the intensive care unit nurses and other concerned individuals.

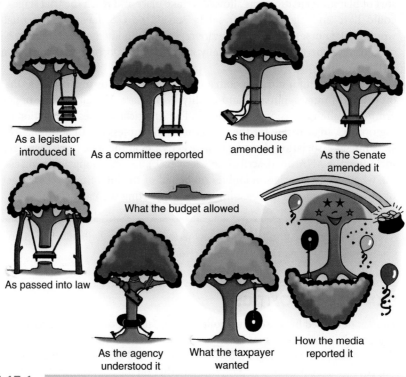

As a legislator introduced it

As a committee reported

As the House amended it

As the Senate amended it

As passed into law

What the budget allowed

As the agency understood it

What the taxpayer wanted

How the media reported it

FIGURE 17-1
How laws grow.

- Recall that the mother of the Vice President of Purchasing was a patient on your unit and needed an IV pump in her care and be sure to include this example in your written request.
- Get involved with other hospital issues and contribute in a credible fashion (i.e., do not be a single-issue person).

What Other Strategies Would You Suggest?

The scenario above illustrates what a politically astute nurse would do in this situation. Although the example applies to a hospital setting, the strategies are comparable to those necessary for getting involved on a community, state, or even federal level. Practicing at the local level will provide good experience for larger issues—one has to start somewhere. Furthermore, a nurse involved on the local level will be able to hone her or his skills, thus gaining confidence in her or his ability to handle similar "exercises" in larger forums.

In the above example, the nurse was able to formulate several "political" actions to influence the outcome of the IV pump decision (Critical Thinking Box 17-1).

What Are the Skills That Make Up a Nurse's Political Savvy?

Ability to Analyze an Issue (Those Assessment Skills Again!). The individual who expects to "influence the allocation of scarce resources" must do the homework necessary to be

What are some issues in your school or hospital that are examples of political issues or the result of politics?

well informed. She or he must know all the facts relevant to the issue, how the issue looks from all angles, and how it fits into the larger picture.

Ability to Present a Possible Resolution in Clear and Concise Terms. The nurse must be prepared to frame and present coherent arguments in support of the recommendation. Preparation includes anticipating questions and objections so that a rebuttal will be logical and well developed.

Ability to Participate in a Constructive Way. Too often, a person disagrees with a proposal being suggested to a hospital unit (or city council), but only gripes about it. The displeased individual seldom takes the time to study the problem or to understand its connection with other hospital departments (or city programs in a broader issue). Most important, the displeased person seldom suggests an alternate solution.

In short, if an individual's concern is not directed toward solving the problem, that person will not be seen as a team player, but as a troublemaker. Constructive responses, perhaps something as simple as posing a single question such as "What solution would you suggest?" may help those involved think in positive terms and redirect energy to a more productive mode. Positive action can produce the kind of creative brainstorming that results in a solution.

> Only complaining about something does not usually change anything. Proposing a solution is a source of power, because that solution may be chosen as the course of action.

Ability to Voice One's Opinion (Understand the System). Once the homework is done, let the *right* person know the determined opinion or solution. For example, the nurse might communicate concern and knowledge about the issue to the nurse manager and supervisor. Of course, it is important to make an intelligent and well-informed decision about the person to whom it is best to voice one's opinion.

Having a confidant or mentor who knows the environment is one way to acquire this information as he or she can provide you insight regarding the appropriate person to express your opinion and suggestions. Another strategy is to use your listening skills. Simply standing back and listening are assets that will come in handy! Whatever the technique, studying the dynamics of the institution with all senses will help the nurse decide on the best person and the most appropriate way to communicate the proposed solution.

Ability to Analyze and Use Power Bases. While discussing issues with colleagues and studying the organization, be alert to the various power brokers. In the previous IV pump vignette, the nurse notes the VP of Purchasing is an obvious source of power in the hospital. This VP will certainly concur with, if not make, the final decision. However, be aware that power does not always follow the lines on the organizational chart. The power of the nurse aide on the oncology unit who just happens to be the niece of the newly appointed member of the Board of Trustees may escape the notice of some. This person could be used to influence a decision if necessary. Similarly, the fact that the VP of Purchasing's mother was on the unit should be filed in your memory for future use.

Facts may be facts, but *where* one gets information can sometimes make a statement as powerful as the information itself. Having the ability to use many different channels of information will give the nurse the power to choose among them.

WHAT IS POWER, AND WHERE DOES IT COME FROM?

Sanford (1979) describes five laws of power. She recommends that these laws be studied to identify strategies to develop power in nursing. The laws are as follows:

Law 1: Power Invariably Fills Any Vacuum

When a problem or issue arises, the prevailing desire is for peace and order. People are willing to give power to someone interested in restoring order to situations of discomfort. Therefore someone will eventually step forward to handle the dilemma. It may be some time before the discomfort or unrest grows to heights sufficient for someone to take the lead.

Nonetheless, a person exerting power will step forward to offer a solution. In some situations, this person may be the previously identified leader, the nurse manager, or the department chair. More often there is an official power broker influencing the action. Know that there are opportunities to exert influence—for example, by taking the leadership role (i.e., stepping forward to fill the vacuum).

Law 2: Power Is Invariably Personal

In most instances, programs are attributed to an organization. For example, a fictitious program, ImmunEYEs, was proposed by the state and national children's and health associations. If one investigated, however, it might be found that the program began with a small group of friends talking over a pizza one evening, lamenting the number of infants still not immunized. In the course of their conversation, one might have said, "If we were to create a media blitz that would get the need for immunizations in the consciousness of parents—get the need for immunizations in their face!" And the next person might have said, "In their *eyes!* Yea, ImmunEYEs. Let's do it!"

Initiatives such as this start with one person creating a new approach to a problem. That person exercises power by providing the leadership or spark to create the strategy to carry out such an initiative, thus inspiring and motivating people to contribute to the effort.

Law 3: Power Is Based on a System of Ideas and Philosophy

Behaviors demonstrated by an individual as she or he exerts power reflect a personal belief system or a philosophy of life. That philosophy or ideal must be one that attracts followers, gains their respect, and rallies them to join the effort. Nurses have the opportunity to ensure that a patient's right to health care (versus privilege), access to preventive care, and similar values are reflected in policies and procedures.

Law 4: Power Is Exercised Through and Depends on Institutions

As an individual, one can easily feel powerless and unable to deal with the complex problems facing a hospital, community, or state. But through a nursing service organization, a state nurses association, or a similar organization, that individual can garner the resources needed to magnify her or his power. The person-to-person network, the communication vehicle (usually an organization's newsletter or journal), and the organizational structure are established for precisely this function—to support and foster changes in the health care system.

Law 5: Power Is Invariably Confronted with and Acts in the Presence of a Field of Responsibility

Actions taken create a rippling effect by speaking to the other nurses for whom nurses act and, most important, the patients for whom nurses advocate. The individual in the power position is acting on behalf of the group. Power is communicated to observers and is reinforced by positive responses. If the group thinks that its ideals are not being honored, the vacuum will be filled with the next candidate capable of the role and supported by the organization.

Another Way to Look at Power and Where to Get It

In a classic, much-referenced work, French and Raven (1959) describe five sources of power. They are (in order of importance): reward power, coercive power, legitimate power, referent or mentor power, and expert or informational power. These descriptions of power were presented in the discussion of nursing management in Chapter 10. The discussion there described the use of power within the ranks of nursing. Here, the use of power is presented as it applies to the political process, especially through political action in nursing.

The strongest source of power is the ability to *reward*. The best example of making use of the reward power base is the giving of money. If, for example, one gives a decision maker financial support for a future political campaign, the recipient will feel obligated to the donor and may, from time to time, "adjust opinions" to repay these obligations! Today, because caps have been placed on campaign contributions, the misuse of this type of reward has been reduced.

An additional source of reward-based political power is the ability to commit voters to a candidate through endorsements. This illustrates the importance of having a large number of members in an organization—in other words, a large voting bloc. This reinforces the imperative for nurses to join and support nursing organizations that advocate on behalf of nurses, nursing and quality health care.

Second in importance is the power to *coerce* or "punish" a decision-maker for going against the wishes of an organization. The best example of this power, the opposite of *reward*, is the ability to remove the person from office at election time.

Third in importance is *legitimate* power, or the influence that comes with role and position. Influence derives from the status that society assigns individuals as a result of, for instance, old family money, membership in a respected profession, or a prominent position in the community. The dean in a school of nursing has a certain amount of influence just because of who he or she is. Right? A nurse's commitment to enhancing nursing's influence explains why we encourage and assist each other to achieve key decision-making positions—to build nursing's legitimate power base.

The fourth power base is that of *referent* or *mentor* power. This is the power that "rubs off" of influential persons. When representatives of the student body talk with a faculty member about a problem they are having with a course and receive her or his support, the curriculum committee or dean is more likely to listen sympathetically than if the students were arguing only for themselves. The faculty member, joining with the students to solve their problem, adds to the

CRITICAL THINKING BOX 17-2

Who are the people in positions that reflect the different power levels in your school, hospital, and community?

students' power. The wish to build this type of power encourages nurses to join coalitions, especially those including organizations with greater power than our own.

The last and weakest of the power bases is that of *expert* or *informational* power. Nurses know about health and nursing care and are thus able to impart knowledge in this area with great confidence and style. Typically, nurses communicate this authority through letters written to legislators, testimonies presented in hearings, and through other contacts made on behalf of nursing and patients. In summary, power is derived from various sources. Nurses use, with the greatest frequency and ease, the weakest of the power bases—that deriving from their expertise. Although this is an important power base, we must develop and exercise the other types as well. Only then will nurses realize the full extent of our potential (Critical Thinking Box 17-2).

NETWORKING AMONG COLLEAGUES

It has been said that one should never be more than two telephone calls away from a needed resource, whether it be a piece of information, a contact in a hospital in another city, or input into a decision one is about to make. The key to successful networking is consciously building and nurturing a pool of associates whose skills and connections augment your own.

As a nursing graduate, one should begin the important task of networking by selecting an instructor from nursing school, one who is able to speak to your performance during nursing school. Ask this person if they would be willing to write a letter of reference for your first job. If she or he agrees, nurture this contact from now on. Keep this individual apprised of your whereabouts, your successes, and your plans for the future. This person will be an important link not only to your school, but also to your future educational and career undertakings. Then, at each future work site, find a head nurse or supervisor willing to write a reference and with whom to maintain contact. Keep building the network over your career.

Remember that this network must be nourished. Constant use of one's resources without reciprocation will exhaust them and make them unreliable sources of assistance in the future. But if properly cared for, this network will provide support for the rest of your career.

BUILDING COALITIONS

A *coalition* is a group of individuals or organizations who share a common interest in a single issue. Groups with whom nurses might form coalitions are as diverse as the topics about which nurses are concerned. For example, nurses are concerned about and lobby for adequate, safe childcare, a safe environment, and women's issues. The numerous organizations interested in these diverse issues are potential candidates for a coalition with nursing organizations. It is not unusual, however, for two organizations to be in a coalition on one issue but adversaries on another. Indeed, this is common in the political arena, where negotiations and compromises are the norm.

CRITICAL THINKING
BOX 17-3

What are examples of nursing coalitions in your community or state?

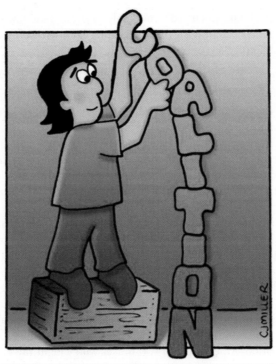

FIGURE 17-2

How do we build a coalition?

A warning: *the selection of coalition partners should strengthen your cause or organization.* Forming coalitions is a strategy to empower oneself. Therefore, build coalitions with people more powerful than you and build coalitions with organizations enjoying greater power than nursing, not less (Critical Thinking Box 17-3 and Figure 17-2).

What About Trade-Offs, Compromises, Negotiations, and Other Tricks of the Trade?

Politics is not a perfect art or science. In the heat of battle, nurses are often called on to compromise, but if they are unwilling to bend on some principle, they sacrifice all. To hold out for the ideal typically means that no progress toward the ideal will be realized. Often, changes in health care policies are achieved in incremental steps. However, the decision to compromise a value or principle must be carefully made with full realization of the implications—not an easy decision!

| CRITICAL THINKING BOX 17-4 | Who in your state government supports legislation that is pro nursing and pro health care? |

The political skills discussed so far apply to any situation, whether in a family, a hospital unit, or a community. The next part of the chapter is focused on skills that apply specifically to the governmental process.

How Do I Go About Participating in the Election Process?

One key to successful political activity is involvement in the election process. This is the stage where one can get to know the candidates; they also get to know you. In addition, it is a time when one makes important contacts for that network.

Getting involved in a candidate's campaign is simple. First, study the positions to be filled. Then, with the help of the local nurses' association, the local newspaper, or the county or state Democratic or Republican Party, select the candidate whose views on health care most closely match yours. Next, find the candidate's campaign headquarters. After this, contact the candidate's volunteer coordinator and see when volunteer help is needed. Most campaigns are crying for assistance with folding letters and stuffing envelopes, looking up addresses, and preparing bulk mailings. They will welcome you with great enthusiasm! Be sure to tell the campaign staff that you are a nurse and would be more than willing to contribute to the candidate's understanding of health care issues and to assist in drafting the candidate's positions on these issues (Critical Thinking Box 17-4).

Beware: *Involvement in campaigns and party organizations can lead to catching the political "bug."* Victims of the political bug are overcome by a powerful desire to make changes in the system and see a multitude of opportunities to educate people about the health needs of a county, state, and nation. An example of two nurses who caught the bug: During a past national presidential election, the nurses at a state caucus volunteered to write the resolution for the party's position on health care, which, if passed, would become a plank in the platform. After much work drafting the statement and bringing it before various committees, they were ecstatic when it passed and became the health statement for their party! (Review Evolve Resources for an example of the effectiveness of political action by nurses.)

What Is a Political Action Committee?

Another way that nurses can influence the elective process is through involvement in an organization's political action committee (Box 17-1). Political action committees, or PACs, grew out of the Nixon/Watergate era, when Congress decided that candidates for public office were becoming too dependent on money supplied by special interests—individuals who give large political contributions and thereby exert undue influence over the elected official's decisions.

As a result, Congress limited the amount of money an individual may contribute to a candidate, established strict reporting requirements, and created a mechanism whereby individuals can pool their resources and collectively support a candidate.

The ANA National Political Action Committee is called ANA-PAC. Through this vehicle, nurses across the country organize to collectively endorse and support candidates for national offices. Likewise, state nurses associations have state-level PACs to influence statewide elections.

BOX 17-1   An RN's Activist Toolkit

How can you become more involved? What does it take to initiate action on the issues that are important to you? The following is a listing of information about what programs ANA has to offer that unifies nurse's political voices.

ANA-PAC ENDORSEMENT PROCESS

As a part of each election cycle, ANA-PAC endorses candidates who have demonstrated strong support for nursing and health care issues. "During the 2005-2006 election cycle, ANA-PAC endorsed 112 candidates for Federal Office—this endorsement represents the ANA's highest seal of approval. Out of the 112 candidates who were endorsed, 100 won, 10 lost, 1 withdrew. This 89% win rate is ANA's highest ever!" (ANA, 2007, p 1)

NURSES STRATEGIC ACTION TEAM (N-STAT)

ANA's Nurses Strategic Action Team (N-STAT) is a program that unites thousands of nurses across the nation to inform lawmakers how nurses feel about key bills as they move through Congress by letting you know when your e-mails, phone calls, and letter will make the most impact via action alerts. N-STAT is involved in grassroots lobbying by sending notices (usually e-mail) about key legislation and providing specific information about whom to contact to have their voice heard (ANA, 2007).

NURSE POLITICAL ACTION LEADERS (N-PAL)

ANA's Nurse Political Action Leaders (N-PAL) program is another grassroots effort to reach out to nurse's elected officials on issues of concern to the profession. N-PAL relies heavily on online communication, e-mails, and electronic media rather than on more conventional means to communicate with elected officials, so information is passed expediently. The goal of the N-PAL program is to ultimately advance legislation that promotes excellent patient care, a safe workplace, and a successful, productive workforce by the work of ANA members who are chosen as Nurse Political Action Leaders that work as liaisons to legislators and legislative staff in assigned legislative districts. The ANA and the Constituent Member Associations (CMAs) collaborate to appoint an N-PAL for each Congressional District and for each Senator (ANA, 2007).

From American Nurses Association: ANA-PAC, 2007. Retrieved from *www.nursingworld.org/MainMenuCategories/ANAPoliticalPower/Election2008/ToolKit.aspx*.

There may be PACs in your area that endorse candidates in city elections. All PACs must comply with the state or federal election codes and report financial support given to candidates for public office.

Today, PACs play an important role in the political process, because they provide a mechanism whereby small contributors can act as a collective, participating in the electoral process when otherwise they would feel outmaneuvered by the bigger players.

The ANA's Endorsement Handbook stresses four points regarding PACs:

1. **Political focus.** The only purpose of any PAC is to endorse candidates for public office and then supply them with the political and financial support they need to win an election.
2. **No legislative activities.** A PAC does not lobby elected officials; that is the job of the ANA or the state nurses association and its government-relations arm. A PAC simply provides financial and campaign support for candidates whose views are generally consistent with those of its contributors.
3. **Not "dirty."** A PAC does not "buy" a candidate or a vote. However, the very nature of political life suggests that candidates who recognize an organization's ability to affect their electoral prospects will be inclined to listen to the group's views when considering specific pieces of legislation.
4. **Health concerns only.** Nursing PACs evaluate the candidates on nursing and health concerns only. In other words, ANA-PAC might solicit the candidates' ideas about how Congress might address the problem of older adult abuse in long-term care facilities or expanding health care

ANA-PAC, The American Nurses Association's Political Action Committee.

insurance coverage to cover the uninsured. But the organization as a nursing PAC should not include questions, for instance, about the source of funding for the new cabinet on foreign commerce. The organization speaks for members only on issues covered in its philosophical statements, resolutions, position statements, legislative platforms, or other documents that its members as an organization have accepted (Critical Thinking Box 17-5).

After Getting Them Elected, Then What?

Lobbying is the attempt to influence or sway a public official to take a desired action. Lobbying is also characterized as the education of the legislator about nursing and its issues. Educating officials, like educating patients, is an important part of the nurse's role.

As nurses, we can lobby in several different ways. The first and best opportunity to lobby comes when the nurse first meets the candidate and evaluates her or him as a potential office-holder. This is the time to assess the candidate's knowledge of health care issues. Take the time to teach and to learn.

A second opportunity comes when the official needs information to decide how to vote on an issue. Depending on time constraints, the issue, and other considerations, a nurse might decide to lobby the official in person or in writing. If time and financial resources permit, the most powerful type of contact is a face-to-face visit. The only way to ensure time with your senator or representative is to make an appointment. Even then, you may not be successful.

If an unscheduled visit to the Capitol precludes an appointment, the best time to catch your senator or representative is early in the day, before the legislative sessions or committee meetings start; they rarely start before 10 or 11 AM. Contact with the legislator's aid or assistant can be just as effective as time with the official. Busy federal and state officials depend heavily on their staff. Treat staff members with the respect they deserve! Be sure to leave a business card or your name and contact information in writing, including an e-mail address. Make sure that they know how to contact you if they should have any questions.

Finally, remember that contact should be made between legislative sessions and during holidays when the official is in her or his home district. The structure and content of the visit should be similar to that of a written contact. That is, know your issue, keep it short, identify the issue by its bill number and title, and communicate exactly what action you want the senator or representative to take. Box 17-2 is a list of specific "Dos and Don'ts When Lobbying." As you begin lobbying, add your recommendations to the list.

If you cannot visit your representative because of time or travel restrictions, a well-written letter, e-mail, or telephone call can communicate your message. Examine the sample letter in Box 17-3. Note that some pointers are listed at the foot of the page. Examples of the proper way to address a public official can be found in Box 17-4.

Letters are common methods of communicating with elected officials; however, a telephone call, fax, or e-mail is often necessary to relay your opinion when time is limited before an

BOX 17-2   Dos and *Don't*s When Lobbying

DO:

- Make sure your legislator knows constituents who are affected by the bill; suggest visits to programs in his or her area.
- Clearly identify the bill, using title and number, if possible.
- Be specific and know about the issue or bill before you write or talk.
- Identify yourself (occupation, hometown, member of ANA).
- Use your own words; if writing, use your own stationery. No form letters!
- Be courteous, brief, and to the point.
- Provide pertinent reasons for your stand.
- Show your legislator how the issue relates to his or her district.
- Respect your legislator's right to form an opinion different from yours.
- Present a united front. Keep our internal problems at home.
- Write letters of appreciation to your legislators when appropriate.
- Write letters at appropriate times; for example, when a bill is in committee, request action that is appropriate for that stage in the legislative process.
- Establish an ongoing relationship with the public official.
- Know issues or problems your legislator is concerned about and express your interest in assisting him or her.
- Attend functions sponsored by coalition members. Be seen!
- Get involved in your legislator's campaign for reelection—or his or her opponent's, if necessary!

DON'T:

- Write a long letter or one letter dealing with multiple points; deal with a single bill or concern per letter or contact.
- Use threats or promises.
- Berate your legislator.
- Be offended in the event of a canceled appointment. Things are unpredictable during a legislative session.
- Demand a commitment before the legislator has had time to consider the measure.
- Pretend to have vast influence in the political area.
- Be vague.
- Hesitate to admit you do not know all the facts, but indicate you will find out—and do!

important vote. The suggested format and content of the electronic message and telephone message are similar to that of a letter or face-to-face interview.

Deciding on the type of contact to make with the decision-maker will vary depending on the situation. For example, if the bill is coming up for the first time in committee, the strategy may be that 10 to 15 people write letters or e-mail messages or call the members of the committee. At this point, the *number* of contacts with the office is important. The reason is that the legislator's assistant typically answers the telephone or opens the mail, tallies the subject of the contact, and puts a hash mark in the "Pro HB 23" or "Con HB 23" column, for instance. Therefore a greater impact will be realized if multiple contacts pertain to one bill. Bags of form letters, however, may have a negative impact on a lobbying effort. Make sure your callers/writers understand the issue and are able to individualize their contact with the elected official. People who contact the legislator's office with a script that they do not understand will not further the lobbying efforts of an organization.

The aforementioned efforts are sufficient early in the process; however, if a major, controversial bill is coming up for a final vote in the Senate, activating a statewide network and bombarding the senators with letters, e-mail messages, telephone calls, faxes and telegrams—as many as possible—is a typical strategy. The bigger the issue, the bigger the campaign should be.

BOX 17-3 Example of a Letter to a Public Official

Ima Nurse, RN
123 Main Street
Any Town, USA 12345-6789
The Honorable Y. R. Important, Jr.
United States Senate
Washington, DC 20510
Dear Senator Important:

I request your support of SB 101 regarding appropriations for nursing education and research. This bill is vital to the country's efforts to improve the number and quality of registered nurses. As you recall, the 2010 Verimportant Nursing Study demonstrated the growing demand for Advanced Nurse Practitioners to work with the increasing numbers of people older than 65 years of age. This bill will provide funding to increase the number of faculty and student slots in the country's schools of nursing and to support nursing research in gerontological nursing. The expanding numbers of older people in our area of the country are not able to get the health care they deserve. During a trip home, I would like to take you to the Main Street Senior's Clinic. I know that you would be pleased with this service, as are the health care providers and the patients.

Will you support this bill? Do you have any questions about it? If so, please call me or the State Nurses' Association Headquarters.

Thank you for your concern with this issue and your continuing support of health care issues.

Sincerely yours,

Ima Nurse, RN

POINTS TO NOTE

1. Neat, without typos or grammatical errors
2. Correctly addressed
3. Professional letterhead
4. Covering single topic
5. Refers to the bill by number and content
6. States request in first sentence
7. Brief rationale for request
8. Uses RN in inside address and salutation

BOX 17-4 How to Address Public Officials

THE PRESIDENT*: THE HONORABLE (FULL NAME)

President of the United States
The White House
Washington, DC 20500
Dear Mr./Madam President:
Speaking:
"Mr./Madam President"
"President (Last Name)"

THE VICE PRESIDENT

Writing: The Honorable (Full Name)
Vice President of the United States
Executive Office Building
Washington, DC 20501
Dear Mr./Madam Vice President:
Speaking:
"Mr./Madam Vice President"
"Vice President (Last Name)"

A SENATOR

Writing: The Honorable (Full Name)
United States Senate
(will have office building and room address)
Washington, DC 20510
Dear Senator (Full Name):
Speaking: "Senator (Last Name)"

A REPRESENTATIVE

Writing: The Honorable (Full Name)
U.S. House of Representatives
(will have office building and room address)
Washington, DC 20515
Dear Mr./Ms. (Full Name):
Speaking: "Representative (Last Name)"
"Mr./Ms. (Last Name)"

A MEMBER OF THE CABINET

Writing: The Honorable (Full Name)
Secretary of (Cabinet Agency)
(will have office building and room address)
Washington, DC 20520
Dear Mr./Madam Secretary:
Speaking: "Mr./Madam Secretary"
"Secretary (Last Name)"

*The correct closing for a letter to the president is "Very respectfully yours." The correct closing for all other federal officials noted here is "Sincerely yours."

CRITICAL THINKING BOX 17-6   When are the bills that affect nursing and health care going to be presented to your state legislature? Is safe staffing on the legislative agenda?

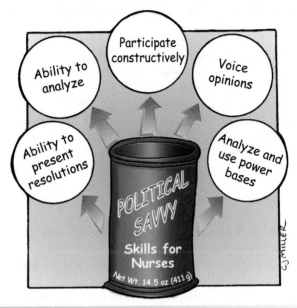

FIGURE 17-3
Skills to make a nurse politically savvy.

At several points in a lobbying season, but certainly after contacting the elected official for a major vote, a follow-up thank-you letter will strengthen your contact with the legislator and help establish you in her or his political network. In addition to reinforcing the reason for your original contact, thank the official for her or his concern with the issue and work in solving the problem by writing the bill or voting for it (or whatever) and for paying attention to your concern (Critical Thinking Box 17-6).

In summary, there are specific skills to learn for effective political involvement. But remember that many of the skills needed to be politically savvy are the very ones that will serve you well in everyday professional negotiations (Figure 17-3).

As a recent graduate getting oriented to your first job and beginning to look around at what you and your colleagues need to improve, you will agree that political involvement is necessary to reach your goals.

This author implores you not to wait to be "allowed" to make a difference, not to wait to be invited to join, and not to let someone else do the job. Please step forward! Act like the powerful, informed, influential nurse that you are. There is much that needs to be done; be a part of the action to achieve solutions!

Margaret Mead said, "Never doubt that a small group of thoughtful, committed citizens can change the world. Indeed, it's the only thing that ever has." The nursing profession has much to accomplish to address the problems with affordable, readily available health care for all. Make sure you are a part of the solutions to be discovered in the future!

CONTROVERSIAL POLITICAL ISSUES AFFECTING NURSING

Uniform Core Licensure Requirements

What Is It? The Nursing Practice and Education Committee, formed by the National Council of State Boards of Nursing (NCSBN), proposed the development of core licensure requirements. This was in response to an increasing concern regarding the mobility of nurses and the maintenance of licensure standards to protect the public health, safety, and welfare. With the implementation of Mutual Recognition, it is important that health care consumers have access to nursing services that are provided by a nurse who meets consistent standards, regardless where the consumer lives. NCSBN (1999) defines competence as "the application of knowledge and the interpersonal, decision making, and psychomotor skills expected for the nurse's practice role, within the context of public health, welfare and safety" (p 3).

The competence framework is based on the recommendations from the 1996 Continued Competence Subcommittee. This framework consists of the three following primary areas:

- Competence development: the method by which a nurse gains nursing knowledge, skills, and abilities.
- Competence assessment: the means by which a nurse's knowledge, skills, and abilities are validated.
- Competence conduct: refers to health and conduct expectations, including assurance that licensees possess the functional abilities to perform the essential functions of the nursing role.

An interesting question proposed by the committee was this: *Do you really think nursing is that much different, that much safer on your side of the state boundary line?* (NCSBN, 1999, p 3). The summary of the proposed competencies and the *2005 Continued Competence Concept* paper may be found at the National Council's website *(www.ncsbn.org)*, which includes the rationales for the proposed requirements and discussion of how the committee developed the recommendations.

Agreements, known as *nurse licensure compacts (NLC)*, specify the rights and responsibilities of nurses who choose or who are required to work across state boundaries and the governing body responsible for protecting the recipients of nursing care. At press time, Arizona, Arkansas, Colorado, Delaware, Idaho, Iowa, Kentucky, Maine, Maryland, Mississippi, Missouri, Nebraska, New Hampshire, New Mexico, North Carolina, North Dakota, Rhode Island, South Carolina, South Dakota, Tennessee, Texas, Utah, Virginia, and Wisconsin have enacted nurse licensure compacts (NCSBN, 2010). Visit the NCSBN website for a map of the enacted and pending NLC states *(www.ncsbn.org/158.htm)*.

States entering into NLC agree to mutually recognize a nursing license issued by any of the participating states. To join the compact, states must enact legislation adopting the compact. The nurse will hold a single license issued by her or his state of residence. This license will include a "multistate licensure privilege" to practice in any of the other compact states (both physical and electronic). Each state will continue to set its own licensing and practice standards. A nurse will have to comply only with the license and license renewal requirements of her or his state of

CRITICAL THINKING BOX 17-7	How will interstate licensure compacts affect the licensure and practice of nursing in your state?

residence (the one issuing the license), but she or he must know and comply with the practice standards of each state in which she or he practices (NCSBN, 2009) (Critical Thinking Box 17-7).

As these agreements are established, experience with additional problems arising from the multistate practice of nursing will be identified and solved in amendments to state practice acts.

Nursing and Collective Bargaining

March! There are no bunkers, no sidelines for nursing today. We find ourselves the center of attention. As the government and corporate America fight escalating health care costs, AIDS is wreaking havoc and technology swells unchecked. Underpaid, overworked, and overstressed nurses are in the midst of a conflagration. Nursing is in greater demand than ever before. Remember Scutari. We must organize, unite, go on the offensive.
—Margretta Madden Styles, 1988, quoted in Hansten and Washburn, 1990, p 53.

The National Labor Relations Act is a federal law regulating labor relations in the private business sector (extended to voluntary, nonprofit health care institutions in 1974). This law grants employees the right to form, to join, or to participate in a labor organization. Furthermore, the law gives employees the right to organize and bargain with their employer through a representative of their own choosing.

Collective bargaining continues to be a point of debate among nurses. Those supporting collective bargaining argue that it is a tool to force positive changes in the practice setting, a method of controlling the practice setting. Many positive changes in the clinical setting are attributed to advances made during contract negotiations.

Opponents feel that as a profession, nurses should not use collective bargaining but instead should influence the practice setting in ways that mean employee and employer working as a team and not as adversaries. They contend that a strike, the ultimate tool of any labor dispute, should not be used. Opponents further argue that practice standards are not negotiable. The points of disagreement between employer and employee are almost always economic: pay, vacation, sick leave, and similar issues. Chapter 18 presents a more detailed discussion of collective bargaining issues. Regardless of your opinion on collective bargaining, the process will involve political action.

What do you think? A paragraph in the ANA's publication *What You Need to Know About Today's Workplace: A Survival Guide for Nurses* summarizes the challenge for us, which is still accurate today:

In a work environment that is constantly changing, it is imperative that nurses are able to assess the true merits of various labor-management structures, to evaluate the real value of proposals to upgrade compensation packages, to determine appropriate levels of participation in workplace decision-making bodies, and to distinguish between long-range solutions and "quick fixes" to workplace problems (Flanagan, 1995, p 5).

Equal Pay for Work of Comparable Value or Comparable Worth?

The concept of comparable worth or pay equity holds that jobs equal in value to an organization ought to be equally compensated, whether or not the work content of those jobs is similar. Pay equity relates to the goal of equitable compensation as outlined in the Equal Pay Act of 1963, and "sex-based wage discrimination" is a phrase that refers to the basis of the problems defined by Title VII of the Civil Rights Act of 1964.

As long ago as World War II, the War Labor Board suggested that discrimination probably exists whenever jobs traditionally relegated to women are paid below the rate of common-labor jobs such as janitor or floor sweeper. One of the first cases was that of the *International Union of Electrical Workers v. Westinghouse*. The union proved that male-female wage disparity existed and uncovered a policy in a manual that stated women were to be paid less because they were women. Back pay and increased wages were given in an out-of-court settlement in an appellate-level decision.

It was nurses who initiated the action in *Lemons v. the City and County of Denver*. Nurses employed by the city of Denver claimed under the Civil Rights Act that they were the victims of salary discrimination, because their jobs were of a value equal to various better-paid positions throughout the city's diverse workforce. The court ruled that the city was justified in the use of a market pricing system (a form of pay based on supply and demand) even though it acknowledged the general discrimination against women. The court said that the case (and the comparable-worth concept) had the potential to disrupt the entire economic system of the United States. Because of this judgment and the fact that the nurses were unable to prepare a job evaluation program to substantiate their claim, the judge dismissed the case.

Legislative Campaign for Safe Staffing

The ANA has launched a campaign for legislative changes to address safe staffing. Safe Staffing Saves Lives is a national campaign to advocate for safe staffing legislation. As stated on ANA's website *(www.safestaffingsaveslives.org)*, "ANA believes that staffing ratios should be required by legislation, but the number itself must be set at the unit level with RN input, rather than by the terms of the legislation" (ANA, 2008, p 1). The position of ANA is not to demand fixed nurse-patient ratios, but to develop a system that takes into account the variables that are present and to determine a safe staffing ratio. Principles that address patient safety, quality control, and patient access to care are necessary to establish a foundation for national legislation (Trossman, 2008).

In March 2008, ANA conducted a Safe Staffing Saves Lives Summit: Conversation and Listening Session. Representatives of state associations, nursing specialty, and other health care organizations, as well as representatives from health care facilities, were present. The purpose of the session was to address the issue of preventing peaks in patient flow as a method of improving the RN workload. Hospitals cannot afford to provide peak staffing 24 hours a day, 7 days a week. At Boston Medical Center (BMC), elective surgeries were scheduled to avoid peaks in patient census and to maintain a more predictable census. According to a representative from the BMC, this approach had a very positive impact on predicting and maintaining safe staffing on the nursing units (Trossman, 2008).

From the ANA website on safe staffing: "ANA's proposal is not a 'one size fits all' approach to staffing. Instead, it tailors nurse staffing to the specific needs of each unit, based on factors including patient acuity, the experience of the nursing staff, the skill mix of the staff, available technology, and the support services available to the nurses. Most importantly, this approach treats nurses as professionals and empowers them at last to have a decision-making role in the care they provide" (2008, p 1).

Much work still needs to be done in the area of safe staffing. Nurses are very concerned regarding staffing issues—mandatory overtime, increased numbers of assistive personnel replacing licensed personnel, and increased patient acuity are factors contributing to the problem. Changes will be achieved as we educate the public as well as legislative representatives, and nurses take the primary role to initiate changes in the workplace environment.

CONCLUSION

Politics, policy making, and advocating for patients are key processes for nurses to claim their "power" as a driving force in health care. Participating in ANA-PAC activities provides an opportunity to be at the grassroots level of lobbying. Shaping policy and becoming active in the legislative area are practice roles for nurses. By having an understanding of the political process, nurses can and will make significant strides in promoting legislation that will positively affect the health of the nation.

BIBLIOGRAPHY

American Nurses Association (2008): *Safe staffing.* Retrieved from *www.safestaffingsaveslives.org.*

American Nurses Association (2010): *Not guilty—Texas jury acquits Winkler County Nurse.* Retrieved from *www.nursingworld.org/FunctionalMenu Categories/MediaResources/Press Releases/2010-PR/Texas-Jury-Acquits-Winkler-County-Nurse.aspx.*

Flanagan L: What you need to know about today's workplace: a survival guide for nurses, Kansas City, Mo: American Nurses Association, 1995.

French JRP, Raven B: The bases of social power. In Cartwright D, editors: *Studies in social power,* Ann Arbor, Mich, 1959, University of Michigan.

Hansten RI, Washburn M: *I light the lamp.* Vancouver, Wash, 1990, Applied Therapeutics.

Leavitt JK, Cohen SS, Mason DJ: Political analysis and strategies. In Mason DJ, Leavitt JK, Chaffee MW, editors: *Policy and politics in nursing and health care,* 2002, St. Louis, Saunders.

Mason DJ, Leavitt JK, Chaffee MW: Policy and politics: a framework for action. In Mason DJ, Leavitt JK, Chaffee MW, editors: *Policy and politics in nursing and health care,* 2007, St. Louis, Saunders.

National Council of State Boards of Nursing (1999): *Uniform core licensure requirements: a supporting paper.* Retrieved from *www.ncsbn.org/667.htm.*

National Council of State Boards of Nursing (2005): *Continued Competence Concept paper.* Retrieved from *www.ncsbn.org/919.htm.*

National Council of State Boards of Nursing (2009): *Nurse licensure compact.* Retrieved from *www.ncsbn.org/nlc.htm.*

National Council of State Boards of Nursing (2010): *Participating states in the NLC.* Retrieved from *www.ncsbn.org/158.htm.*

Sanford ND: *Identification and explanation of strategies to develop power for nursing in power: nursing's challenge for change.* Kansas City, Mo, 1979, American Nurses Association.

Trossman S: ANA's campaign to promote patient safety and quality health care. *Am Nurse* 40:1, 2008.

U.S. Census Bureau (2009): *Income, poverty and health insurance coverage in the United States.* Retrieved from *www.census.gov/newsroom/releases/archives/income_wealth/cb10-144.html.*

Additional resources are available online at *http://evolve.elsevier.com/Zerwekh/nsgtoday/.*

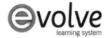

CHAPTER 18

Collective Bargaining: Traditional (Union) and Nontraditional Approaches

Joann Wilcox, RN, MSN, LNC

It is time for a new generation of leadership to cope with new problems and new opportunities. For there is a new world to be won.
—JOHN F. KENNEDY

Difficulties are meant to rouse, not discourage. The human spirit is to grow strong by conflict.
—WILLIAM ELLERY CHANNING

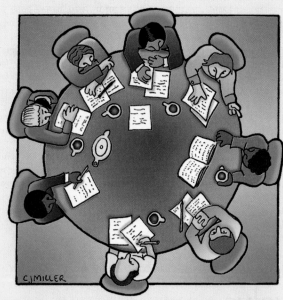

Is there a place for collective bargaining in nursing?

After completing this chapter, you should be able to:

- Identify the milestones in the history of collective bargaining.

- Compare traditional and nontraditional collective bargaining.

- Identify conditions that may lead nurses to seek traditional or nontraditional collective bargaining.

- Identify the positive and negative aspects of traditional and nontraditional collective bargaining.

- Discuss the impact of the silence of nurses in public communications and the perception of nurses by the public

ou will soon be accepting your first position as a registered nurse (RN). You will be adjusting not only to a new role, but also to a new workplace. Even in these times of dramatic change in health care, many of you will start your career in a hospital. In fact, the demographics about nurses show that:

- Approximately 60% of nurses in practice are providing care in hospitals (Bureau of Labor Statistics, 2010-2011).
- The hospital is also the most common employer of graduate nurses in their first year of practice; more than 85% of new graduates were working in a hospital in their first year of employment (Wendt & O'Neill, 2006).

As you begin to interview for your first position in your career as a professional RN, there is no doubt you will find yourself both excited and anxious. Your prospective employer will assess your ability to think critically and to perform at a professional level in the health care setting. The potential employer will ask, "Is this applicant a person who will be able to contribute to the mission of the organization and to the quality of health care offered at this organization?"

While the employer assesses your potential to make a contribution, it is equally important that you remember that an interview is a *complex two-way* process. You will, of course, be eager to know about compensation, benefits, hours, and responsibilities. These are very tangible and immediate interests. However, these are not likely to be the best predictors of satisfaction with your practice over time as the ability to practice your profession as defined by licensure and education will be the foundation leading to job satisfaction and professional fulfillment.

You should be prepared to assess the potential employer's mission and ability to support your professional practice and growth. It is extremely important that you gain essential information about the organization, its mission and its culture. It is easy to overlook very significant organizational issues that will ultimately affect your everyday practice of nursing when your primary focus is on becoming employed and in wondering if you will succeed in this first professional role. Williams (2004) identifies these questions to keep in mind: Who does the potential employer include in developing solutions and making decisions in the dynamic environment of health care and how are selections made for this activity? How will you voice your expertise and the challenges you repeatedly encounter? Will your ideas for process improvement be encouraged?

Hospital structures and governance policies can have a dramatic influence on the effectiveness of a registered nurse and how he or she can fulfill their obligation to patients and families. Nurses have defined the discipline of nursing as a profession, and as members of this profession, they must have a voice in and control over the practice of nursing. When that voice and control are not supported by the work setting, conflicts most likely will arise. In some states, nurses have made a choice to gain that voice and assume control of their practice by using a traditional collective bargaining model, commonly known as a labor union. Other states (Center for American Nurses [CAN], 2008) have elected to control practice through interest-based bargaining (IBB) or a nontraditional approach to collective bargaining to accomplish having that voice and control over practice (Budd et al, 2004) (Box 18-1). Some states use both models to meet the needs of the diverse membership.

| BOX 18-1　Terms |

Traditional collective bargaining—A legally regulated collective bargaining unit or a union that assists members to gain control over practice, economics in the health care industry, and other health care issues that threaten the quality of patient care

　National Nurses United (NNU)—The new RN SuperUnion formalized in December 2009

　Nontraditional collective bargaining—Shared governance, or interest-based bargaining (IBB); a collaborative-based, problem-solving approach to assist nurses to have a voice in the workplace and control over issues that affect their practice

　Center for American Nurses (CAN)—An organization that represents the interests of nurses who are not formally represented by a collective bargaining unit or union (Budd et al, 2004)

WHEN DID THE ISSUES LEADING TO COLLECTIVE BARGAINING BEGIN?

Since World War II, there have been phenomenal advances in medical research and the subsequent development of life-saving drugs and technologies. The introduction of Medicare and Medicaid programs in 1965 provided the driving force and the continued resources for this growth. This initiative opened access to health care for millions of Americans who were previously disenfranchised from the health care system.

The explosion in knowledge and technology, coupled with an expanded population able to access health care quickly, increased the demands on the health care system and many of the providers in that system. These advances have required nursing to adapt as the complexity and volume of patients accessing health care continue to increase. For example, at the time when the acuity of hospitalized patients increased due to shorter lengths of stay, organizations were responding to cost containment demands by downsizing numbers of staff. As more patients have access to all services in the health care system, the number of care hours available for each patient has declined because fewer staff per patient are being hired. Overall, patients are sicker when they enter the system. Yet they are moved more quickly through the acute care setting because of such innovations as same-day surgery, same-day admissions, and early discharge. Add to these changes the periodic shortages of nurses prepared for all levels of care, the increased use of unlicensed assistive personnel to provide defined, delegated nursing care, and growing financial pressures on the health system, and tensions are understandably high.

Enormous financial challenges confront health care institutions. As a registered nurse working in the health care industry, you will encounter and use newly developed and very costly health care technologies. At the same time, you will experience, first-hand, the impact of public and private forces that are focused on placing restraints on cost and reimbursement for a patient's care.

As a professional RN, you are at the intersection of these potentially conflicting forces. For you, these forces will be less abstract; they are not just important concepts and issues facing a very large industry. As a nurse, these concepts and forces are patients with names, faces, and lives valued and loved within a family and a community. You are responsible for the care you provide and for advocating on these patients' behalf and—as you will soon discover—the health of the health care industry.

As a nurse, you will become familiar with how, when, and why events occur that adversely or positively affect the patient and the health of the organization. This places you in a unique position to take an active lead in developing solutions. These solutions must be good for patients and for your organization. During your interview, while you are assessing the potential employer's mission and support of your practice and growth, it is easy to overlook those significant organizational attributes that will ultimately affect your everyday practice of nursing. Therefore during your interview, it would be important for you to ask those questions identified in the beginning of this chapter.

THE EVOLUTION OF COLLECTIVE BARGAINING IN NURSING

In the early 1940s, most registered nurses working in hospitals were subject to arbitrary schedules, uncompensated overtime, no health or pension benefits, and no sick days or personal time. During this era, 75% of all hospital-employed nurses worked 50 to 60 hours a week meeting these arbitrary schedules and uncompensated overtime (Meier, 2000).

In 1946 the American Nurses Association House of Delegates unanimously approved a resolution that formally initiated the journey of RNs down the road of collective bargaining. Activist nurses within the American Nurses Association (ANA) founded the United American Nurse (UAN) in 1999. They believed in the creation of a powerful, national, independent, and unified voice for union nurses. In 2000 the UAN held its first National Labor Assembly annual meeting. The participants in this meeting were staff nurse delegates (UAN, 2008).

Many formally organized unions have competed for the right to represent nurses. It was the opinion of many nurses supporting this precedent that the state nurses associations were the proper and legal bargaining agents and were also the preferred representatives for nurses in this country for purposes of collective bargaining. During the late 1980s, the demand among nurses for representation continued to grow; yet efforts to organize nurses for collective bargaining were being stymied by a decision from the National Labor Relations Board (NLRB) that stopped approving all-RN bargaining units. A legal battle then ensued with the American Nurses Association (ANA) and other labor unions against the American Hospital Association (AHA). The NLRB issued a ruling that reaffirmed the right of nurses to be represented in all-RN bargaining units.

WHO REPRESENTS NURSES FOR COLLECTIVE BARGAINING?

Traditional and Nontraditional Collective Bargaining

The national professional organization for nursing is the ANA, with its constituent units, the state, and territorial nursing associations. Through its economic security programs, the ANA recognizes state nursing associations as the logical bargaining agents for professional nurses and the states have been the premier representatives for nurses since 1946! These professional associations are indeed multipurpose; their activities include economic analyses, provision of related education, addressing nursing practice, conducting needed research, and providing traditional as well as nontraditional collective bargaining, lobbying, and political action.

The creation of the UAN by the ANA, strengthened their collective bargaining capacity at a time when competition to represent nurses for collective bargaining was growing. The UAN was established in 1999 as the union arm of the ANA with the responsibility of representing the traditional collective bargaining needs of nurses (UAN, 2008). At this same time, a relatively new approach to collective bargaining was being developed and introduced into the labor market. This approach is a nontraditional process referred to as interest-based bargaining (IBB) or shared governance (Brommer et al, 2003; Budd et al, 2004). This is a nontraditional style of bargaining that attempts to problem-solve differences between labor and management. Although this style of bargaining and mediation will not always eliminate the need for the more traditional and adversarial collective bargaining, many believe this non-adversarial approach of negotiation may be closer to the basic fabric of the discipline of nursing and its ethical code.

The organization that represents IBB, or the nontraditional collective voice in nursing, is the Center for American Nurses (CAN). This is a professional association established in 2003, replacing the ANA's Commission on Workplace Advocacy, which was created in 2000 to represent the needs of individual nurses in the workplace who were not represented by collective bargaining. CAN defines its role in workplace advocacy as providing a multitude of services designed to address the products and programs necessary to support the professional nurse in negotiating and dealing with the challenges of the workplace and in enhancing the quality of patient care (Critical Thinking Box 18-1, Box 18-2) (CAN, 2008).

CRITICAL THINKING BOX 18-1   What is the status of your state nursing association in regard to workplace issues? Is your state a member of the NNU or CAN or both? What is being done on a local basis that reflects the activities of your state association?

BOX 18-2   Center for American Nurses (CAN)

MISSION

To create healthy work environments through advocacy, education, and research

VISION

The leader in workforce advocacy for professional nurses

PURPOSE

To articulate, advocate, and provide workforce advocacy solutions to equip nurses in shaping their work environment

VALUES

- **Leadership:** Resolve professional workforce issues; act as professional resource; provide role models for the balance between personal and professional life
- **Personal and Professional Development:** Encourage individual nurse initiative in creating a healthy work environment and advocating for change in a positive yet persistent manner
- **Partnership:** Build collaborative organizational and individual relationships beneficial to The Center and its professional work
- **Stewardship:** Manage and develop The Center's human and financial resource

Reprinted with permission from Center for American Nurses, 2008.

In June 2008, the American Nurses Association Board of Directors voted to "not renew either affiliation agreement with the UAN and the CAN and proposed significant bylaw changes to be debated at the June House of Delegates" (*Nursing World*, 2008, p. 3). The changes to the bylaws were approved by the delegates. The rationale for these changes was to "strengthen and provide additional choices for our state nursing associations" (*Nursing World*, 2008, p 3).

In 2009, the largest union and professional organization of registered nurses was officially formalized. This organization is the National Nurses United (NNU) and is an outgrowth of the joining of three individual organizations-the California Nurses Association, the Massachusetts Nursing Association, and the United American Nurses (the former UAN) (Nations, 2009). The Michigan state association joined the NNU in early 2010 and there are 27 states, which have an affiliation agreement with NNU (National Nurses United, 2010). This union (NNU) has 150,000 members and is only a few months old (*Michigan Nurse*, 2010).

In 2010, the CAN exists as an independent organization, following the original mission of the organization while continuing to have a relationship with ANA as both are focused on addressing the issues that impact the profession of nursing and the health of the population served.

Whether your state is a member of CAN or NNU, or both, it is necessary to recognize that workplace advocacy is a concern that directly affects every practicing nurse. It is critical that nurses support the organizational efforts to address the growing problems regarding the safety of the workplace, as well as safe and competent nursing care.

CAN and NNU: What Are the Common Issues?

Staffing Issues. Staffing issues and policies related to nurse staffing are among the most prevalent topics discussed in any type of negotiations. There is much discussion in both the national and state legislatures regarding proposals aimed at addressing the way in which nurses should be staffed to be able to provide safe patient care. There is also much objection to implementing mandated staffing plans rather than allowing nurses control over issues related to their professional practice. Because of the commonalities related to the topic of staffing, it would be helpful if all nurses supported the right to define the appropriate work environment in which RNs could practice safely and effectively. The Institute of Medicine (2004) completed a study entitled *Keeping Patients Safe: Transforming the Work Environment of Nurses*. The results of the study have led to significant recommendations that, if implemented, would begin to address the chronic shortage of sufficient RN staff without resorting to mandatory regulations from the legislatures.

Staffing requirements are already mandated by various agencies. For example, Medicare, state health department licensing requirements, and The Joint Commission (TJC) each publish staffing standards that define the need to have sufficient, competent staff for safe and quality care. All organizations that address staffing indicate that the nurse must demonstrate competencies for the processes that are needed to ensure the safety of the patients. The ANA has launched a campaign for safe staffing: Safe Staffing Saves Lives. The ANA encourages nurses to establish safe staffing plans through legislation (Trossman, 2008). Please refer to Chapters 17 and 25 for further discussion regarding staffing issues.

Objection to an Assignment. Professional duty implies an obligation to not accept an assignment for which one is not competent to complete. RNs cannot abandon their assigned patients but are obligated to inform their supervisor of any limitations they have in completing that assignment. To not inform and not complete the assignment or to not inform and attempt to complete the assignment risks untoward patient outcomes and resultant disciplinary action up to and including some potential action taken by the Board of Nursing.

The right and means for a nurse to register objection to a work assignment are considered essential elements in a union contract that incorporates the values of a profession as the basis of the contract agreement. This same process must be provided to nurses not represented by a union since nurses are obligated to only provide care, which they are competent to provide. Also, this is one way that issues can be brought to the attention of those in a decision making capacity. Nurses are encouraged to submit reports indicating an objection to the assignment when the assignment is not appropriate. The report should follow the process defined in the contract or facility policy. These same problems should also initiate constructive follow-through by management or staff-management committees to improve the situations described in the reports. Inaction could serve as a basis for a grievance or negotiated change in a union contract or an incident or change in policy in a nonunion environment.

Concept of Shared Governance. Many facilities are implementing a variety of governance models called *shared governance, self-governance, participative decision-making,* or *decentralization of management.* Each of these models describe a system in which nurses have a defined degree of organizational autonomy as it relates to control over practice (Hinshaw, 2002). The concept of shared governance can be a concern to unions representing nurses for purposes of collective bargaining. It is important to ensure that staff nurses who participate in shared governance are not ultimately seen to be performing management functions.

Shared-governance models do not hide the fact that their purpose is to involve nurses in decision making related to control of their practice while the organization maintains the authority over the traditional management decisions. Although this does not violate the principles of participation in aspects of decision making, it can be considered a disadvantage to nurses employed by institutions if shared-governance models are adopted in lieu of collective bargaining agreements and if it is believed there would be greater latitude in shared decision making in a union environment. However, as more facilities are moving toward Magnet certification in which shared governance is a major function, it is recognized that some facilities that are unionized are also embracing the concepts of Magnet as a recognition of the professional aspect of bargaining and representing the profession of nursing.

Clinical or Career Ladder. The clinical ladder, or career ladder, has a place in both traditional and nontraditional styles of collective bargaining (Drenkard & Swartout, 2005). The clinical ladder was designed to provide recognition of a registered nurse who chooses to remain clinically oriented. The idea to reward the clinical nurse with pay and status along a specific track or ladder is the result of the contributions of a nurse researcher, Dr. Patricia Benner. Her descriptions of growth and development of nursing knowledge and practice provided the basis for a ladder model that can be used to identify and reward the nurse along the steps from novice to expert (Benner, 2009). Force 14 of the Forces of Magnetism, required for a facility to achieve Magnet certification, discusses the use of clinical ladders as a part of the professional development program for RNs (HCPro, 2006). Continued professional growth is an essential element identified in Magnet facilities.

Negotiations. Nurse negotiators represent a diverse population of constituents since nurses in a facility have varied educational backgrounds and represent the multiple practice specialties available to nursing. This variety leads to differences in practice needs, which must be addressed by the nursing negotiating team.

Professional goals and practice needs are appropriate topics for contract negotiations. Since personnel directors, hospital administrators, and hospital lawyers may have difficulty relating to these discussions, the nurse negotiating team has to be able to provide sufficient information to help prepare these individuals to understand the inclusion of professional goals and practice needs into the collective bargaining process and as entries into the agreed-upon contract. The resolution of disagreements about professional issues necessitates there be time for a thoughtful process by those who are appropriately prepared to reach agreements through the negotiating process. Perhaps the complex issues, such as recruitment, retention, staffing, and health and safety, are better addressed in the more collegial setting of the nontraditional model; however, many of these issues are paramount to the creation of a safe and effective work environment for nurses and need to be addressed in both types of negotiation (Institute of Medicine, 2004).

THE DEBATE OVER COLLECTIVE BARGAINING

Collective Bargaining: Perspectives of the Traditional Approach

Is There a Place for Collective Bargaining in Nursing? Should nurses use collective bargaining if they are members of a profession? Is nursing a profession or an occupation? These are questions nursing has debated since the late 1950s, and the discussion and debate continues today. Nursing often looks for assistance outside of the occupation/profession to help resolve issues, but these two questions can and should be resolved by nursing if there is the desire to be recognized as independent and in control of our practice.

A profession can be defined as a vocation that requires a long period of specialized educational, to prepare one for service to society (Blais et al, 2002). This specialized education is one that is generally a part of a baccalaureate program as is the minimum required for most professions. Because of their expertise and the value of their service, members of a profession are granted a measure of autonomy in their work. This autonomy permits practitioners to make independent judgments and decisions on the basis of a theoretical framework that is learned through study and practice. While there may still be some who do not agree with the need for baccalaureate education to be designated as a profession, consideration needs to be given to the fact that not being designated as a profession continues to keep nurses from reaching the potential of their contributions to patients and the health care system. In each state, registered nursing is categorized as an occupation by the respective labor boards and many decisions regarding the position of nursing in an organization are based on this definition as an occupation. For purposes of the discussion on traditional and nontraditional collective bargaining, the role of nursing will be addressed as that of a profession.

Conflict arises as nurse-employees advocate for a professional role in patient care when they are not classified as a profession by labor definitions and by the hiring facilities. The health care institutions hire nurses as members of an occupation who are essentially managed and led by the organization's formal leaders who often focus on productivity and savings. This is believed to be a factor leading nurses to consider unionization as the only way they can gain some control over their practice.

> "A myth widely subscribed to by hospital management is that big, powerful unions organize professional nurses. In fact, unions do not organize nurses; professional nurses organize themselves. They do this because administrators and nursing supervisors fail to recognize and address collective needs" (Stickler & Velghe, 1980, p 14). While this was written in 1980, it remains true today. One cannot organize a group that does not see this as a need.

Nursing has used collective action to its benefit, achieving professional goals while protecting and promoting public interest through lobbying efforts in the political arena. Many nurses support collective bargaining in the workplace as a way to control their practice by redistributing power within the health care organization.

> "The power bestowed upon the nursing profession should derive not from the hospital administrator's value of services provided by the practitioner" (Cleland, 1975, p 17).

Legal Precedents for State Nursing Associations as Collective Bargaining Agents. The legal precedent that determined that state nursing associations are qualified under labor law to be labor organizations is the 1979 Sierra Vista decision. The important consequence of this decision that affected nurses was that they were free to organize themselves and not be organized by existing unions (Kimmel, 2007). Many nursing leaders contend that these associations are not only proper and legal, but are the preferred representatives for nurses in this country for purposes of collective bargaining. Ada Jacox (1980) suggested that collective bargaining through the professional organization may be a way for nurses to achieve that collective professional responsibility that is a characteristic of a profession. It is felt by many that the state nursing association is the only safe ground that can be called a neutral turf on which nurses from all educational backgrounds can meet and discuss issues that are of a generic nature and of importance to all nurses, regardless of title.

Nurse Participation in Collective Bargaining. If the state nursing associations are logical bargaining agents for RNs, why are so few nurses joining associations and even fewer pursuing collective bargaining? Approximately 80% of all RNs belong to no association and have no professional or practice affiliation. It is important to recognize that this low membership rate is not unique to nursing but is the same for most disciplines and for society in general.

One of the problems with association memberships is that people tend to look at these associations and organizations for "what they can do for *me*"—for the work *I* do or the benefits *I* can receive. In reality, we need to look at these associations for what they can do for the profession and the population being served by the members of the profession/occupation. We then realize that the profession is only as strong as its members and the contributions they make to that occupation/profession. Perhaps looking at it in this way will encourage more to join and become members.

Collective bargaining for nurses occurs more frequently in states where there is significant union activity in other industries. The current labor climate is very volatile across the country. Unions are trying to organize new categories of workers, with special emphasis on the growing health care sector in states that have not traditionally been active in the labor movement. Some state nursing associations stopped providing collective bargaining services because of external pressures including challenges from competing unions, excessive resistance by employers, or state policies that make unionization difficult, such as right-to-work laws. In states with right-to-work laws, it is illegal to negotiate an agency shop requirement; membership and dues collection can never be mandatory, even if the workers are covered by a collective bargaining agreement. The cost of negotiating and maintaining a collective bargaining agreement in these states is often more than the income received for providing these services. Philosophical differences regarding the benefits and risks of a professional association as the bargaining agent have also led nurses in some states to abandon or avoid union activities.

There are 2.5 million working nurses, but only a few hundred thousand are organized for collective bargaining and only 20% of RNs belong to a professional organization. Fifty-nine percent of these registered nurses are employed by hospitals (Bureau of Labor Statistics, 2010-2011). How will collective professional goals be achieved if so many nurses depend on the time and finances of so few? Some believe that the profession's efforts to address workplace concerns from both the traditional and nontraditional perspectives will result in larger membership numbers in the near future. For now, there may be too few nurses involved in the nursing associations to make up the needed critical mass for the kinds of changes and support that need to take place. Perhaps learning that this is the case will motivate more RNs to join their professional organization to support the work that needs to be accomplished. The announcement of the implementation of the National Nurses United as the "RN Super Union" (National, 2010, p 1) may supplant the state nurses associations as the primary provider of collective bargaining services for registered nurses.

Where Does Collective Bargaining Begin?

Nurses in the private sector are guaranteed legal protection, as stated in the National Labor Relations Act, if they seek to be represented by a collective bargaining agent. Once a drive for such representation is under way and 30% of the employed RNs in an institution have signed cards signaling interest in representation, both the employer and the union are prohibited from engaging in any anti-labor action. Employers are prohibited from terminating the organizers for union activity and may not ignore the request for a vote for union representation. After the organizing campaign, a vote is taken; a majority made up of 50% plus one of those voting selects or rejects the collective bargaining agent.

Your employer may choose to bargain in good faith on matters concerning working conditions by recognizing the bargaining agent before the vote. This approach usually occurs only if management believes a large majority of potential voters support the foundation of a union. In other cases, your employer may appeal requests for representation to the NLRB. Before and during the appeal, other unions may intervene and try to win a majority of votes for representation.

As a part of this appeal process, arguments are made before the NLRB regarding why, by whom, or how the nurses are to be represented. For example, the hospital may raise the question of unit determination. The original policy interpretation of the labor law simultaneously limited the number of individual units an employer or industry would have to recognize, yet allowed for distinct groups of employees, like RNs, to have separate representation. Nurses historically have been represented in all-RN bargaining units, and most bargaining units throughout the country reflect that pattern.

What Can a Contract Do? Generally speaking, what can a union contract do in a hospital setting? In the article by Budd, Warino, and Patton (2004), it was stated that collective bargaining helped nurses gain some control over their practice which gave them "a voice in decisions that affect the patient care environment and their ability to deliver quality care" (p 2). The article also includes the statement indicating that unions protect nurses as they "demand that the standards of their profession be respected and enforced" (Gelinas & Bohlen, in Budd, et al, 2004, p 3). This respect and enforcement of standards has led to "a 5.7% lower risk-adjusted mortality for myocardial infarction patients in unionized hospitals" (Seago & Ash, in Budd, et al, 2004, p 3).

Wages. Wages and benefits are the foundation of a contract. Wages are the remuneration one receives for providing a service and reflect the value put on the work performed. In a 1990 article on the history of nursing's efforts to receive adequate compensation, Brider reaffirmed the need to continue efforts being made on behalf of achieving improvements in nursing salaries. The author correctly stated that "from its beginnings, the nursing profession has grappled with its own ambivalence which is how to reconcile the ideal of selfless service with the necessity of making a living" (Brider, 1990, p 77). The article confirmed the ambivalence of the nurses who recorded both their joy in productive careers and their disappointment with the way their work was valued. Nursing has certainly come a long way from the $8 to $12 monthly allowance in the early 1900s, but the challenge remains to bring nursing in line with comparable careers.

At the beginning of the 21st century, it is clear there is another shortage of nurses already in place. Like other occupations and professions, when the supply and demand favors the employee, wages are more critically evaluated. There is usually an adjustment of entry level wages (to address recruitment) and of wages paid to nurses who remain in practice (for retention). This current shortage of nurses seems to be less responsive to some of the traditional solutions such as wage adjustments. This clearly indicates that wages are not the only, or perhaps not even the primary, reason that individuals are not choosing nursing as a career or why many nurses are choosing to leave the field.

Another aspect of nurse compensation involves the challenge of addressing the negative effects of wage compression. This economic concept means that nurses who have been in practice for 10 and 12 years may make less money than recent graduates in their first nursing jobs! Unfortunately, it is not uncommon during times of shortages to see hiring or relocation bonuses to attract nurses into new positions. It would be preferable to see those dollars redistributed for the purposes of maintaining the base that is formed by the retention of experienced nurses in the facility.

Job Security versus Career Security. It is probably not news to any student enrolled in a nursing program that he or she has entered a field that is facing many challenges—both from within and outside nursing. The economic environment in the health care industry, coupled with rapid technological progress and a renewed interest in primary and preventive care has dramatically shifted a great deal of health care away from the hospital setting. The 2004 Division of Nursing Sample Survey (USDHHS, 2004) confirmed that nurses have practice opportunities across a diverse continuum, but it also validated that large numbers of nurses, over 59% of the 2.5 million working nurses, are still employed in hospital-based care.

Other changes include the introduction and implementation of managed care, managed care reform, shorter lengths of stay, new technologies and pharmaceuticals, limited resources, and a growing demand for all health services by the growing aging population. Each of these factors affects the world in which nursing care is delivered. These new paradigms have challenged nurses and their representatives to modify bargaining strategies and turn attention to issues of sustaining quality nursing care in the face of shortages, to overcome negative practices such as mandatory overtime, and to advocate for health and safety initiatives like safer needle devices and ergonomics.

Seniority Rights. Nurses who remain on staff at an institution accrue seniority, which is based on the length of time employed as a registered nurse at that facility. Seniority provides specific rights, spelled out in the bargaining agreement, to those who have the highest number of years of service. These rights derive from the idea that permanent employees should be viewed as assets to the organization and should therefore be rewarded for their service. In nurse employment contracts, there are provisions (seniority language) that give senior nurses the right to accrue more vacation time and to be given preference when requesting time off, a change in position, or relief from shift rotation requirements. In the event of a staff layoff, the rule that states "the last hired become the first fired" protects senior nurses. Seniority rules may be applied to the entire hospital registered nursing staff or may be confined to a unit. However, transfers and promotions must reward the most senior qualified nurse in the institution.

Resolution of Grievances. Methods to resolve grievances, which are sometimes explicitly spelled out in a contract, are an important element of any agreement. A grievance can arise when provisions in a contract are interpreted differently by management and an employee or employees. This difference often occurs when issues related to job security (a union priority), job performance, and discipline (a management priority) arise. *Grievance mechanisms* are used in an attempt to resolve the conflict with the parties involved. The employer, the employee, or the union may issue a grievance. Nurses who are covered by contracts should be represented at any meeting or hearing they believe may lead to disciplinary action being taken. Such representation can be provided by a co-worker, an elected nurse representative, or a member of the labor union's staff.

Arbitration. If the grievance mechanism does not lead to resolution of the issue, some contracts allow referral of the issue to arbitration. A knowledgeable—but neutral—arbitrator acceptable to both parties (union and hospital) will be asked to hear the facts in the case and issue a finding. In pre-agreed, binding arbitration, the parties must accept the decision of the arbitrator. For example, some contracts require that when management elects to discharge (suspend or terminate) a nurse, the case must be brought to arbitration. On the basis of the arbitrator's finding, the nurse may be reinstated, perhaps with back pay, remain suspended, or be terminated. If the contract states that the arbitrator's decision is final and binding, there is no further contractual or organizational avenue for either party to pursue.

Arbitration has also been used to resolve issues involving the integrity of the bargaining unit. Arbitrators have been asked to decide whether nurses remain eligible for bargaining unit coverage when jobs are changed and new practice models are implemented.

Mediation, arbitration, and fact-finding have all been used to resolve conflicts in union contracts. There is strong support for use of these methods, but hospital management personnel often resist using them. Nurses usually fare well when contract enforcement issues are submitted to an arbitrator and facts, not power or public relations, determine the outcome.

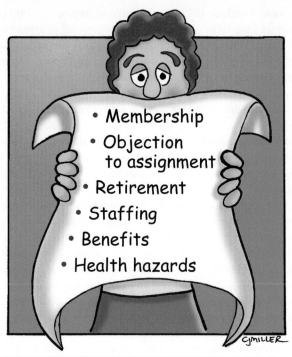

FIGURE 18-1
Effective elements of a sound contract.

What Are the Elements of a Sound Contract?

Membership. The inclusion of union security provisions is an essential element of a sound contract (Figure 18-1) and one of the defined goals of collective bargaining (union integrity). *Security provisions* include measures such as enforcement of membership requirements (collection of dues and access by the union staff to the members). A legal modification of the closed shop is the *agency shop*, in which new employees are required to join the union within a given period of time.

Retirement. The usual pension or retirement programs for nurses have been either the social security system or a hospital pension plan. Individual retirement accounts, which are transferable from hospital to hospital in case of job change, are becoming increasingly popular as defined pension plans are being eliminated by many employers. The method of addressing issues related to support at the time of retirement should be a topic of negotiations. The ANA has entered an agreement with a national company to provide a truly portable national plan, unrestricted by geographic location or employment site. Although this plan could be complicated by conflicting state laws governing pension plans, a precedent was set as long ago as 1976, when California nursing contracts mandated employer contributions to individual retirement accounts for each nurse with immediate vesting (eligibility for access to the fund) and complete portability for the participants (meaning that the nurse could take the established retirement account to another hospital and continue to add to this account either directly or roll it over into the new employers individual retirement account).

One of nursing's most attractive benefits has been a nurse's mobility, which is the opportunity to change jobs at will. A drawback of this mobility is the loss of long-term retirement funds. With financial cutbacks in the hospital industry, retirement plans are in danger of being targeted as givebacks in negotiating rights or benefits to be traded away in lieu of another issue or benefit that may be more pressing at the time. One of the major benefits of the individual retirement accounts is that they do belong to the employee and the employee's contributions to the plan plus the employer's contributions to the plan can be taken by with the employee when he or she leaves that employment, assuming all the defined rules of the plan are followed.

Health insurance coverage continues to be a key concern of employees and has been at the root of the majority of labor disputes in all industries in the last few years. It is not inconceivable that nurses may be asked to trade off long-term economic security (pensions) for short-term security (e.g., health benefits, wages). There is less chance this will occur if the organization has moved from the defined pension benefit. What is more likely to occur is that the employer will be asking to contribute fewer dollars to health insurance premiums and/or retirement accounts and asking employees to contribute an increased percentage of the cost of these benefits.

Other Benefit Issues. Most employees in the United States have been experiencing a dramatic reduction in their health insurance benefits packages. This trend is reflective of the crisis of the health care system and the escalating costs of health care. Nurses have not been immune to the reduction in health insurance benefits, and access to health insurance benefits will continue to be a major issue for nurses and all employees until substantial reform is accomplished. Other issues that have affected RNs as employees are family-leave policies, availability of daycare services, long-term disability insurance, and access to health insurance for retirees. These are the same issues that affect many workers in this country but may have a greater impact on employees such as nurses because of the 24-hour/7-day-a-week coverage that needs to be provided by them.

An issue of special concern to RNs involves the scheduling of work hours. Although more men have been joining the nursing occupation profession, nursing remains a 94% female occupation (USDHHS, 2004). That reality must be addressed by providing benefit packages that provide flexibility for women who assume multiple roles in today's society. Generally, it is women who provide ongoing care to both children and parents. The nurse in the family may be called upon to do this more than the spouse or the siblings. Nurses are asking nursing contract negotiators to secure leave policies that permit use of sick time for family needs and scheduling that is both flexible and allows part-time employment and work-sharing.

Staffing issues such as objection to an assignment, inadequate staffing, poorly prepared staff, mandatory overtime, nurse fatigue, and health hazards are all issues that can be addressed in a union contract; however, these are also issues of ongoing concern for all RNs, regardless of the type of bargaining situation in their respective states or organizations. These issues are discussed further in Chapter 25.

How Can Nurses Control Their Own Practice?

The essence of the professional nurse contract is control of practice. For example, nurse councils or professional performance committees provide the opportunity for nurses within the institution to meet regularly. These meetings are sanctioned by the contract. The elected staff nurse representatives may, for example, have specific objectives to:

- Improve the professional practice of nurses and nursing assistants.
- Recommend ways and means to improve patient care.
- Recommend ways and means to address care issues when a critical nurse staffing shortage exists.
- Identify and recommend the elimination of hazards in the workplace.
- Identify and recommend processes that work to ensure the safety of patients.

The importance and relevance of such professional practice committees were documented by a 1986 review of state nursing association contracts. When 381 agreements were analyzed, 424 references to professional practice committees were identified. This aspect of control continues to be a major aspect of most professional contracts.

Nurse Practice Committees. Nurse practice committees should have a formal relationship with nursing administration. Regularly scheduled meetings with nursing and hospital administrators can provide a forum for the discussion of professional issues in a safe atmosphere. Many potential conflicts over contract language can be prevented by discussion before contract talks begin or before grievances arise. Ideally, physicians should also be a part of these forums since they are an integral part of the care delivery system in a hospital and other settings. Joint-practice language has been proposed in some contracts to facilitate these discussions.

Since the recognition of Magnet hospitals by the American Nurses Credentialing Center (ANCC) began in 1994, approximately 6.3% of all health care organizations in the United States have achieved ANCC Magnet recognition status (ANCC, 2010). Approximately 20% of the facilities awarded the recognition have a collective bargaining agreement with the nurses. This helps to validate the fact that control of nursing practice by RN staff can be successfully achieved within the context of a collective bargaining agreement when both Magnet and collective bargaining have this as a common goal.

Strikes and Other Labor Disputes. What can nurses do in the face of a standoff during contract negotiations? The options that current RNs have are quite different from those before 1968, when nurses felt a greater sense of powerlessness. At that time, despite nurses' threats of "sickouts," walkouts, picketing, or mass resignations, the employer maintained an effective power base. Threats of group action attracted public attention, but nurses' threats had little effect on employers because nurses represented through the ANA had a no-strike policy. As negotiations became more difficult, it was apparent that nurses were in a weaker bargaining position because of the no-strike policy. The ANA responded to the state nursing associations, and in 1968, it reversed its 18-year-old no-strike policy. The National Nurses United union does not have a no-strike policy.

Strikes remain rare among nursing units, but as mentioned previously, when the efficacy of patient care and patient and staff safety are at risk, nurses may have to strike. Increased strikes were seen beginning in 2000 as facilities were imposing mandatory overtime to cover the staff shortages. Many nurses are uncomfortable with the idea of striking, believing that they are abandoning their patients. This image may conflict with the service ideal. It is important for nurses who contemplate striking to discuss plans for patient care with nurses who have previously conducted strikes so that they will be assured that plans to care for patients are adequate.

When an impasse is reached in hospital negotiations, national labor law requires nurses to issue a 10-day notice of their intent to strike. Every effort must be made to prevent a strike in the public's interest. Mediation is mandated by the NLRB, and a board of inquiry to examine the issue may be created before a work stoppage. The hospitals are supposed to use this time to reduce the patient census and to slow or halt elective admissions. In the meantime, the nurses' strike committee will develop schedules for coverage of emergency rooms, operating rooms, and intensive care areas. This coverage is to be used only in the case of real emergencies. Planning patient care coverage should reassure nurses troubled by the strike scenario. Nurses who agree to work in emergencies or at other facilities during a strike often donate their wages to funds set up for striking nurses.

Business and labor are both in search of more positive ways to work together to be able to avoid the possibility of a work stoppage. Strikes are not easy for either side—one side is not able to provide services, and the other side is not able to earn its usual income. In the middle, when health care is involved, is the patient who loses trust in both the facility and in the body of employees who choose to strike, requiring the patient to seek care elsewhere. National grants have been sponsored by the Department of Labor and the Federal Mediation and Conciliation Service to undertake alternatives to traditional collective bargaining. At least two Midwestern nursing organizations used win-win bargaining techniques and found them to be constructive methods of negotiation.

Collective Bargaining: Perspectives of the Nontraditional Approach

How to effectively address the concerns of the workplace advocacy, higher standards of practice, and economic security is not a new issue. These concerns have caused nurses in some areas of the country to organize and use unions and collective bargaining models. This section is designed to provide you with information and a rationale for a different approach to the position of the traditional collective bargaining. In the end, it will be up to you and your concept of the RN's role to grapple with this issue during your professional life.

Simultaneous Debates. Nursing today has acquired the majority of the generally recognized characteristics of a profession. One of these characteristics is a lengthy period of specialized education and practice preparation. The activities that are performed by professions are valued and recognized as important to society. In addition, a member of a profession has an acquired area of expertise that allows the person to make independent judgment, act with autonomy, and assume accountability. Nurses also have specialty organizations and are eligible in some areas to receive specialty credentialing.

Another aspect of professional nursing is its strongly written ethical code. It is the obligation of every licensed RN to follow the tenets of the 2001 ANA Code of Ethics for Nurses (see Chapter 19). The Code articulates the values, goals, and responsibilities of the professional practice of nursing. The provisions of the Code that outline our duties to care, advocate, and be faithful to those who entrust their health care to us are well integrated into the educational preparation of the RN. They are also widely recognized and respected by the public.

Collective Bargaining: The Debate That Continues. The debate over the appropriateness of collective bargaining continues. The combination of an explosion in knowledge and technology and an expanded population able to access health care quickly brought both public and private sector payers of health care to the inevitable quest to rein in the cost of health care. This gave birth and life to a growing collection of payment systems. We now have gatekeepers, specific practice protocols, contractual agreements between payers and providers, and provider and consumer incentives that govern the place, provider, type, and quantity of a patient's care.

These developments have affected everyday care in a growing number of settings. Nurses are challenged daily in practice environments that have, by necessity, taken on business models and processes to survive financially. The nurses who advocate for CAN feel that this business and financial environment is not conducive to the patient-focused model and ethical values that have been an inherent part of the professional education and practice preparation of nurses.

All too often, the intense clinical education of the RN practicing in today's health care has not prepared the individual to appreciate the financial and regulatory realities of a large industry. Perhaps even more discomforting is that as RNs enter this work environment, they may not see the magnitude of their potential for leadership and problem-solving within an environment that continues to evolve so quickly while also working hard to hold on to the traditional hierarchy of medicine.

The history of the position of nursing during the first half of the 20th century may, in part, explain our slow journey toward leadership and control of nursing practice. In the last half of the 20th century, some nurses organized and relied on collective bargaining units to speak for them. The debate about the fit of union membership and a profession is likely to continue for some time.

Traditional Collective Bargaining: Its Risks and Benefits. The goal of the traditional collective bargaining model is to win something that is controlled by another. There is an "us versus them" approach. The weapon is the power of numbers. Although a desired contract is achieved, long-lasting adversarial relationships may develop between the nurses and the employer (Budd et al, 2004).

With the soaring cost of health care, the changes in health care reimbursement, and the subsequent reining in of health care costs, where does that leave nursing in the collective bargaining process? Does this not further aggravate the already adversarial relationship of nurses and their employers? Traditional collective bargaining held promise and assisted the professional nurse's evolution toward economic stability. These were important gains. However, the full power and potency of nursing as an industry leader has not emerged through traditional collective bargaining efforts. This may explain the dissatisfaction of the nurses with traditional collective bargaining or may also be an indication that the other basic debates within the body of RNs need to be resolved before nurses take the place in the industry they feel is appropriate for them.

Can nursing effectively step away from the adversarial process of traditional collective bargaining into an effective leadership role? IBB may offer nurses a nonadversarial approach, but it will require nursing leaders to demonstrate an understanding of interests and outcomes that are important both to the nursing occupation/profession and to other members of the health care industry (Budd et al, 2004). As discussed earlier in this chapter, IBB is a nontraditional style of bargaining that attempts to problem-solve differences between the workforce and the employer—or the nurse and the hospital. Although this style of bargaining and mediation will not always eliminate the need for the more traditional and adversarial collective bargaining, this non-adversarial approach of negotiation may be closer to the basic beliefs underlying professional nursing as well as the nursing code of ethics.

In considering the IBB approach, it is important to recognize state associations that have made significant contributions to their local membership by offering IBB services to that membership. This has also resulted in contributions to the advancement of nontraditional, non-adversarial bargaining for the promotion of workplace advocacy on a national level (Box 18-3). Do these commitments sound familiar?

BOX 18-3   Eight Commitments to Workplace Advocacy

Workplace advocacy is a nurse-to-nurse strategy that can give RNs a meaningful voice in their workplace. As a result of Texas Nurses Association (TNA) workplace advocacy efforts in the past, Texas now has one of the strongest nursing practice acts in the country. The following are eight commitments to workplace advocacy. The Texas Nurses Association will:

Work to secure mechanism within health care systems that provide opportunities for registered nurses to affect institutional policies. Mechanisms include:
- Shared governance
- Participatory management models
- Magnet hospital identifications
- Statewide staffing regulations

Develop with stakeholders a conflict resolution process for nurse/nurse employers that addresses registered nurse concerns about patient care and delivery issues.
- Active participation with the Texas Hospital Association and the American Arbitration Association to develop a conflict resolution process that meets the needs of nurses in resolving patient care issues.

Provide legislative solutions to Texas registered nurses by reviewing issues of concern to nurses in employment settings and introducing appropriate legislation. Previous initiatives include:
- Whistle-Blower
- Safe Harbor Peer Review
- Support for Board of Nurse Examiners rules outlining strong nursing practice standards

Explore the development of a legal center for nurses that could provide legal support and decision-making advice as a last recourse to unresolved workplace issues. Its purpose would be to:
- Provide fast legal assistance
- Earmark precedent-setting cases that could impact case law and health care policy

Support the RN in practice with self-advocacy and patient advocacy information by providing products that increase knowledge about:
- Laws and regulations governing practice
- Use of applicable standards of nursing practice
- Conflict resolution techniques
- Statewide reporting mechanisms that allow the nurse to report concerns about health care institutions and professionals
- Professional behaviors, core values, and conduct that support effective negotiation

Promote to RNs those health care institutions in Texas that demonstrate outstanding nurse/employer relations.

Work with Texas schools of nursing to develop materials that incorporate self-advocacy and patient advocacy information into the nursing curriculum.

Advocate for the elimination of physician abuse of RNs with the physician community and employers by:
- Working with physician professional organizations to develop a campaign to end physician abuse of RNs
- Working with health care facilities to establish Zero Tolerance for physician abuse of RNs
- Developing model policies against physician abuse of nurses
- Encouraging nurse-to-nurse advocacy to stop abusive situations

Reprinted with permission from Texas Nursing Association, 2006, 7600 Burnet Rd, Ste 440, Austin, Texas 78757; tna@texasnurses.org.

FUTURE TRENDS

The public should be concerned about an inadequate supply of nurses. Based on that concern, along with terrorist attacks on America, there is increased interest by the press and policymakers to be sure nurses are prepared in adequate numbers and that their working environment supports quality nursing care. This attention is helping nurses achieve improvements in overall compensation and working conditions and must also lead to support for the preparation of sufficient numbers of nursing faculty and methods of financial support for the education of RNs.

The nursing community should take a step back and try to identify those factors that appear to keep nursing from becoming a profession of choice, which should result in eliminating the continuous cycle of shortage/staff reduction/shortage. One of the classic issues is that nursing is still not considered a profession by most definitions of a profession or by the labor bureaus, which classifies employee groups. Until the occupation/profession accepts the fact that we cannot just say we are a profession, without meeting the minimum criteria for this designation, we will continue to be classified as an occupation only.

The second issue that must be addressed by organized nursing is that which is defined by Buresh and Gordon (2000) when they discuss the silence of nursing. These authors completed extensive research to determine why nurses were rarely seen or heard in the various forms of media. They discovered that for the most part, the media cannot find nurses who are willing to talk, to be interviewed, or to write editorials stating opinions or positions. More importantly, when nurses were available to talk to the media, they "too often unintentionally project an incorrect picture of nursing by using a 'virtue' rather than a 'knowledge' script" (Buresh & Gordon, 2000, p 4). They also noted that nurses tend to downplay or devalue basic nursing bedside care, the heart of what we do, while focusing on the greater status of the advanced practitioner.

As with many things in life, there is a tendency to look outside of the problem to define a cause for the problem and look to others to find a solution. Nursing, as the largest group of health care providers and as the only group of providers entrusted to implement the majority of the medical plan of care, needs to look within to find how to most effectively communicate the vital role we take in the provision of health care.

> In survey after survey, the number-one reason nurses are unhappy with their nursing practice environment is their dissatisfaction with the care that they are able to give in that environment. Focusing on the creation of a safe work environment for nurses should address this area of dissatisfaction.

Nurses throughout the country have felt firsthand the effects of cost containment. Those effects have often been detrimental to the quality of care that RNs are charged to provide. From a professional practice perspective, mandatory overtime and short staffing are some of the factors contributing to the preponderance of medical errors documented in the Institute of Medicine report *To Err Is Human: Building a Safer Health System* (Institute of Medicine, 2000). The ANA was the initial voice in recognizing these as potential contributing factors and has led the way in encouraging research agendas that further quantify the number of work hours needed to provide safe care and further define how patient safety can be ensured. As with other major issues affecting the practice of RNs, the ANA and state nursing associations are in the lead in federal and state legislative efforts to address overtime and staffing in the context of safe patient care.

What lies ahead for collective bargaining and all forms of collective action for nurses must be viewed within the context of the overall changes occurring in the health care system and in the financing mechanisms for that system. As concerned nurses, we need to remain vigilant about our need to meet the basic obligation of licensure, which is to provide safe care to all patients. This issue of adequate access to health care services is one that will probably be with us for the rest of our professional lives. It is believed by many that one way to improve access to services is to deliver them in environments and by providers that have not traditionally been a part of our health care system. Each of these venues provides significant opportunities for RNs since the essence of our work is prevention of disease and adaptability to chronic disease processes that will enable our patients to remain as active as possible in their own environment.

CONCLUSION

Nursing has a unique contract with society to promote good health care and, as a natural outcome, promote the health and welfare of the nurse and the occupation/profession of nursing. The multipurpose nature of the professional nursing association will continue to work to preserve the future of nursing. This chapter cannot stand alone, nor can the nurses in the workplace stand alone, if they are to offset the forces that negate the contributions of nurses. Political action and lobbying, research, and education are necessary to further the cause of nursing and to meet the health care needs of the public we serve. As nurses work to transform aspects of the health system and to improve access to care, they will continue to depend on collective action and a collective voice through the structures and functions established within the ANA to advocate for optimal working conditions and standards of practice. Welcome to nursing! Join us in our efforts to unify our skills, knowledge, and voices as we ensure our vision is being met.

BIBLIOGRAPHY

American Nurses Credentialing Center (2010): *Magnet recognition program.* Retrieved from *www.nursecredentialing. org/ancc/magnet.*

Benner P: *Expertise in nursing practice,* ed 2, New York, 2009, Springer.

Blais K, et al.: *Professional nursing practice: concepts and perspectives,* ed 4, Upper Saddle River, NJ, 2002, Prentice-Hall.

Brider P: Professional status: the struggle for just compensation, *Am J Nurs* 90:77-80, 1990.

Brommer C, Buckingham G, Loeffler S (2003): *Cooperative bargaining styles at federal mediation and conciliation services: a movement toward choices.* Retrieved from *www.fmcs.gov/internet/ itemDetail.asp?categoryID=35&ite mID=15880.*

Budd K, Warino L, Patton M: Traditional and non-traditional collective bargaining: strategies to improve the patient care environment, *Online J Issues Nurs* 9(1), 2004.

Bureau of Labor Statistics (2010): *Occupational outlook handbook-2010-2011.* Retrieved from *www.bls.gov/oco/ ocos083.htm.*

Buresh B, Gordon S: *From silence to voice,* New York, 2006, Cornell University.

Center for American Nurses (2008): *Mission, vision, purpose, and values.* Retrieved from *www.can.affiniscape. com/displaycommon.cfm?an=1&subarti clenbr=2.*

Cleland V: Taft-Hartley amended: implications for nursing. The professional model, *Am J Nurs* 75:288-292, 1975.

Drenkard K, Swartwout E: Effectiveness of a clinical ladder program, *J Nursing Admin* 35:502-506, 2005.

HCPro: *Magnet status: a guide for the nursing staff,* Marblehead, Mass, 2006, HCPro.

Hinshaw A: Building magnetism into health organizations. In McClure ML, Hinshaw A, editors: *Magnet hospitals revisited: attraction and retention of professional nurses,* Washington, DC, 2002, American Nurses Publishing.

Institute of Medicine: To err is human: building a safer health system. In Kohn L, Corrigan J, editors: *IOM report*, Washington, DC, 2000, National Academy Press.

Institute of Medicine: Keeping patients safe: transforming the work environment of nurses. In Kohn L, Corrigan J, editors: *IOM report*, Washington, DC, 2004, National Academy Press.

Jacox A: Collective action: the basis for professionalism, *Supervisor Nurse* 11:22-24, 1980.

Kimmel N (2007): *Nurses and unions: changing times.* Retrieved from *http://EzineArticles.com/?expert= NancyKimmel.*

Meier E: Is unionization the answer for nurses and nursing? *Nurs Economic$* 18:36-37, 2000.

Michigan Nurse: New National Nurses United a Reality, *Michigan Nurse* 83(1):2-3, 2010.

National Nurses United (2010). Retrieved from *www.nationalnursesunited.org/ about/who-we-are.html.*

Nations New RN SuperUnion (2009). Retrieved from *www.prnewswire.com/ news-releases/nations-new-rn-superunion-names-executive-director-holds-first-public-rally-for-rn-rights-representation-78853232.html.*

Nursing World, March/April: 3, 2008.

Stickler KB, Velghe JC: Why nurses join unions, *Hosp Forum* 23:14-15, 1980.

Trossman S: ANA's Campaign to promote patient safety and quality health care, *Am Nurse* 40, 2008.

United American Nurse (UAN): 2008. UAN: Power of nurses. Retrieved from *www.uannurse.org/who/history.html.*

U.S. Department of Health and Human Services, Division of Nursing: *Sample survey*, Washington, DC, 2004, Bureau of Health Professionals, USDHHS.

Wendt A, O'Neill T: Report of findings from the 2005 RN practice analysis: linking the NCLEX-RN examination to practice, Chicago, 2006, National Council of State Boards of Nursing.

Williams K: Ethics and collective bargaining: calls to action, *Online J Issues Nurs,* 2004. Retrieved from *www.nursing world.org.*

Additional resources are available online at *http://evolve.elsevier.com/Zerwekh/nsgtoday/.*

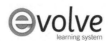

CHAPTER 19

Ethical Issues

Peter Melenovich, MS, RN, CCRN-CSC, CNE

People of Orphalese, you can muffle the drum, and you can loosen the strings of the lyre, but who shall command the skylark not to sing?
—KAHLIL GIBRAN, *The Prophet*

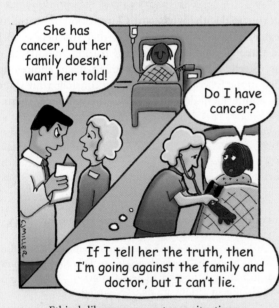

Ethical dilemmas are not easy situations.

After completing this chapter, you should be able to:

- Define terminology commonly used in discussions about ethical issues.

- Analyze personal values that influence approaches to ethical issues and decision making.

- Discuss the moral implications of the American Nurses Association and International Council of Nurses codes of ethics.

- Discuss the role of the nurse in ethical health care issues.

In developing the content for this chapter, a deliberate effort has been made to "simplify" the presentation of ethical issues and avoid complex philosophical debate. Many nurses shy away from formal ethical discussions because the terminology seems better suited to graduate school and a peer-reviewed journal. In reality, nurses deal with ethical issues every day in practice and need to have the tools to advocate effectively for patients, as well as themselves. The first step in equipping oneself for ethical debate is becoming

Thank you to Alice B. Pappas, PhD, RN, for her previous contributions to this chapter.

comfortable with the language and issues. Ethics refers to principles of right and wrong behaviors, beliefs, and values. Thompson et al (2007) add, "ethics is essentially concerned with our life as members of a community, and how we behave and function in society" (p 36).

Concern about ethical issues in health care has increased dramatically in the past three decades. This interest has soared for a variety of reasons, including advances in medical technology; social and legal changes involving abortion, euthanasia, patient rights, end-of-life care, reproductive technology; and growing concern about the allocation of scarce resources, including a shortage of nurses. Nurses have begun to speak out on these issues and have focused attention on the responsibilities and the possible conflicts that they experience as a result of their unique relationship with patients and their families and their role within the health care team.

UNDERSTANDING ETHICS

Let us begin by defining commonly used terms (Box 19-1).

What Are Your Values?

Your values represent ideas and beliefs that you hold with high regard. Clarification of your values is suggested as a strategy to develop greater insight into yourself and what you believe to be important. Values clarification involves a three-step process: choosing, prizing, and acting on your value choices in real-life situations (Steele, 1983). Opportunities to make choices and improve your decision making are included in the following pages. As you consider your values, you will, I hope, gain more understanding about the underlying motives that influence them. It

---

BOX 19-1	Definition of Terms

Advance directive: A written statement of a person's wishes about how he or she would like health care decisions to be made if he or she ever loses the ability to make such decisions independently.

Bioethics: Ethics concerning life.

Bioethical issues: Subjects that raise concerns of right and wrong in matters involving human life (e.g., euthanasia, abortion).

Durable power of attorney for health care: A document that allows a person to name someone else to make medical decisions for him or her if he or she is unable to do so. This spokesperson's authority begins only when the patient is incompetent to make those decisions.

Ethics: Rules or principles that determine which human actions are right or wrong.

Ethical dilemma:
(1) A situation involving competing rules or principles that appears to have no satisfactory solution.
(2) A choice between two or more equally undesirable alternatives.

Living will: A document that allows a person to state in advance that life-sustaining treatment is not to be administered if the person later is terminally ill and incompetent.

Moral or ethical principles: Fundamental values or assumptions about the way individuals should be treated and cared for. These include autonomy, beneficence, nonmaleficence, justice, fidelity, and veracity.

Moral reasoning: A process of considering and selecting approaches to resolve ethical issues.

Moral uncertainty: A situation that exists when the individual is unsure which moral principles or values apply in a given situation.

Values: Beliefs that are considered very important and frequently influence an individual's behavior.

is not intended as a "right" or "wrong" activity; rather, it is a discovery about the "what" and "why" of your actions. Do not be surprised if your peers or family hold different views on some topics. And remember, the values that are "correct" or "right" for you may not always be the "right" values for others, including patients and their families. Your values may also change over time as you face different life experiences.

Evaluate the critical thinking questions, write down your responses to them, and consider the possible reason or reasons for your choices. The critical thinking exercise (Critical Thinking Box 19-1), Listing Values, is suggested as a means of clarifying your values. Discuss your answers with peers and decide how comfortable you are in discussing and defending your values, especially if they differ from the values of your peers. Critical Thinking Box 19-2 involves reproductive issues and has been included here because of the proliferation of reproductive technology, including genetics, and the ongoing moral and political debate regarding abortion and the use of stem cells.

Moral/Ethical Principles

What Is the Best Decision, and How Will I Know? Despite different ideas regarding which moral or ethical principle is most important, ethicists agree that there are common principles or rules that should be taken into consideration when an ethical situation is being examined. As you read through each principle, consider instances in which you have acted on the principles or perhaps felt some conflict in trying to determine what was the best action to take (Figure 19-1).

Autonomy: A Patient's Right to Self-Determination Without Outside Control. Autonomy implies the freedom to make choices and decisions about one's own care without interference, even if those decisions are not in agreement with those of the health care team. This principle assumes rational thinking on the part of the individual and may be challenged when the individual infringes upon the rights of others.

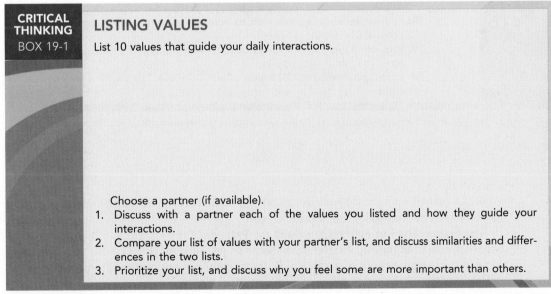

CRITICAL THINKING BOX 19-1

LISTING VALUES

List 10 values that guide your daily interactions.

Choose a partner (if available).
1. Discuss with a partner each of the values you listed and how they guide your interactions.
2. Compare your list of values with your partner's list, and discuss similarities and differences in the two lists.
3. Prioritize your list, and discuss why you feel some are more important than others.

From Steele S, Harmon V: *Values clarification in nursing*, ed 2, East Norwalk, Conn: Appleton-Century-Crofts, 1983, p 90; with permission.

CRITICAL THINKING
BOX 19-2

REPRODUCTIVE EXERCISE

Identify your degree of agreement or disagreement with the statements by placing the number that most closely indicates your value next to each statement.

1 = Strongly Disagree
2 = Disagree
3 = Ambivalent
4 = Agree
5 = Strongly Agree

_____1. Contraception is a responsibility of all women.
_____2. Some types of contraception are more valuable than other types.
_____3. Abortion as a form of contraception is completely unacceptable.
_____4. Abortion decisions are the responsibility of the pregnant woman and her physician.
_____5. The birth of a "test tube baby" is a valuable medical advance.
_____6. Genetic screening should be done frequently.
_____7. Genetic counseling should provide information so that patients can make informed choices about future reproductive decisions.
_____8. Amniocentesis should be required as part of prenatal care.
_____9. Genetic engineering should be advanced and promoted by federal funding.
_____10. Artificial insemination should be available to anyone who seeks it.
_____11. Sperm used in artificial insemination should come from all strata of society as do blood transfusions.
_____12. Fetal surgery should be done even when it places another fetus at risk (i.e., a twin).
_____13. Surrogate mothers play an important role in the future of families.
_____14. Fetuses who survive experimentation should be raised by society.
_____15. Women should be encouraged to participate in fetal research by carrying fetuses to desired dates and then giving the fetus to the scientist for research.
_____16. Contraception is reserved for women of legal age.
_____17. Adolescents should require a parent's signature for abortion.
_____18. Information about genetically transmitted diseases should be provided to all pregnant women.
_____19. Women at high risk for genetically transmitted diseases should be encouraged to have amniocentesis.
_____20. Infants born with severe defects should be allowed to die through a natural course.

From Steele S, Harmon V: *Values clarification in nursing*, ed 2, East Norwalk, Conn: Appleton-Century-Crofts, 1983, p 169; with permission.

Consider this:

What if a patient wants to do something that will cause harm to him or herself? Under what circumstances can the health care team intervene?

Beneficence: Duty to Actively Do Good for Patients. For example, you use this principle when deciding what nursing interventions should be provided for patients who are dying when some of those interventions may cause pain. In the course of prolonging life, harm sometimes occurs.

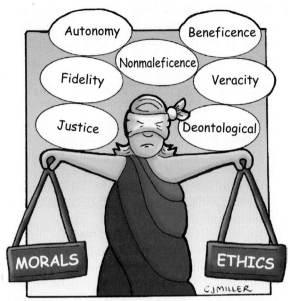

FIGURE 19-1

Moral/ethical principles.

Consider this:

Who decides what is good? Patient, family, nurse, or physician? How do you define good?

   Nonmaleficence: Duty to Prevent or Avoid Doing Harm, Whether Intentional or Unintentional. Is it harmful to accept an assignment to "float" to an unfamiliar area that requires the administration of unfamiliar medications?

Consider this:

Is it acceptable to refuse an assignment? When does an assignment become unsafe?

   Fidelity: The Duty to Be Faithful to Commitments. Fidelity involves keeping information confidential and maintaining privacy and trust (e.g., maintaining patient confidentiality regarding a positive HIV test or "blowing the whistle" about unscrupulous billing practices).

Consider this:

To whom do we owe our fidelity? Patient, family, physician, institution, or profession? Who has the right to access patient medical records? When should we "blow the whistle" about unsafe staffing patterns?

   Justice: The Duty to Treat All Patients Fairly, Without Regard to Age, Socioeconomic Status, or Other Variables. This principle involves the allocation of scarce and expensive health care resources. Should uninsured patients be allowed to use the emergency department (ED) for nonemergency care—the most expensive route for delivering this type of care? Who should be paying for their care?

Consider this:

What is fair, and who decides? Why are some patients labeled very important persons (VIPs)? Should they receive a different level of care? Why or why not? What kind of access to health care should illegal immigrants receive: preventive or more costly ED care?

Veracity: The Duty to Tell the Truth. The principle of veracity may become an issue when a patient who suspects that her diagnosis is cancer asks you "Nurse, do I have cancer?" Her family has requested that she not be told the truth because their culture believes bad news takes away all hope for the patient.

Consider this:

Is lying to a patient ever justified? If a patient finds out that you have lied, will that patient have any reason to trust you again?

Each of the aforementioned principles sounds so right; yet the "consider this" questions indicate that putting principles into practice is sometimes much easier said than done. Reality does not always offer textbook situations that allow flawless application of ethical principles. As Oscar Wilde, an Irish playwright, once said, "The truth is rarely pure, and never simple." You will encounter clinical situations that challenge the way in which you apply an ethical principle or that cause two or more principles to be in conflict, creating moral distress, which is often referred to as an ethical dilemma.

Which Principle or Rule Is Most Important? Current thinking on the part of ethicists favors autonomy and nonmaleficence as preeminent principles because they emphasize respect for the person and the avoidance of harm. However, there is no universal agreement, and many individuals rely on their spiritual beliefs as the cornerstone to ethical decision making.

Another possible approach to decision making is to consider the relative benefits and burdens of an ethical decision for the patient. If patients are capable of rational decision making, they may choose a different treatment approach than the care team. This fact is sometimes difficult for health care team members to accept, especially if it involves a decision to stop treatment. If patients are not capable of autonomous decision making, substituted judgment (decision making) by their designated family is then used. Problems frequently arise when family members disagree regarding a treatment choice or quality-of-life issues, as evidenced by the Terry Schiavo case in Florida (2003), when the husband's wishes to discontinue life support for his wife were granted after a prolonged court case that included attempted government intervention.

Traditional and contemporary models of ethical reasoning offer worldviews from which ethical principles, spiritual values, and the concepts of benefits and burdens can be derived, interpreted, and comparatively emphasized. Nevertheless, models of ethical reasoning are not without their critics, including nurses, who feel that abstract ideas about right and wrong are not helpful or "practical" at the bedside.

In recent years, nursing ethicists have advanced a new approach to ethical issues emphasizing an ethic of caring as the moral foundation of nursing. Nurses have been encouraged to consider all ethical issues from the central issue of caring. Because caring implies concern for preserving humanity and dignity and promoting well-being, the awareness of rules and principles alone does not adequately address the ethical issues that nurses confront, such as suffering or powerlessness. Research regarding the application of caring to ethical issues is underway, but a practical model for applying this ethic of caring to clinical situations does not yet exist. Currently, the most care-centered approach to ethical dilemmas is to consider the relative "benefits versus burdens" that any proposed solution offers to the patient. Health team members need to try to consider benefits and burdens from the patient's perspective versus their own values on life, death, and the vast degrees of illness between the two. It is a difficult task to undertake.

So How Do I Make an Ethical Decision? A number of approaches to ethical decision making are possible. The following is a brief overview of the three most commonly applied models of ethical reasoning. The first two types are considered normative because they have clearly defined parameters, or norms, to influence decision making. The third type is a combination of the other two models.

Deontological. Derived from Judeo-Christian origins, the deontological normative approach is duty-focused and centered on rules from which all action is derived. The rules represent beliefs about intrinsic good that are moral absolutes revealed by God. This approach reasons that all persons are worthy of respect and thus should be treated the same.

All life is worthy of respect.

As a result of the rules and duties that the deontological approach outlines, the individual may feel that he or she has clear direction about how to act in all situations. Right or wrong is determined on the basis of one's duty or obligation to act, not on the consequences of one's actions. Therefore abortion and euthanasia are never acceptable actions because they violate the duty to respect the sanctity of all life, and lying is never acceptable because it violates the duty to tell the truth. The emphasis on absolute rules with this approach is sometimes seen as rigid and inflexible, but its strength is in its unbending approach to many issues, emphasizing intent of actions.

Teleological. Derived from humanistic origins, the teleological approach is outcome-focused and places emphasis on results. *Good* is defined in utilitarian terms: That which is useful is good. Human reason is the basis for authority in all situations, not absolutes from God. Morality is established by majority rule, and the results of actions determine the rules. Because results become the intrinsic good, the individual's actions are always based on the probable outcome.

That which causes a good outcome is a good action.

Simplistically, this view is sometimes interpreted as "the end justifies the means." Abortion may be acceptable because it results in fewer unwanted babies. Euthanasia is an acceptable choice by some patients because it results in decreased suffering. Giving preference for a heart transplant to a foreign national who can pay cash and donate money for a transplant program is acceptable because this will create a greater good for others. Using this approach, the rights of some individuals may be sacrificed for the majority.

Situational. Derived from humanistic and Judeo-Christian influences and most commonly credited to Joseph Fletcher (1966), an Episcopalian theologian, the situational view holds that there are no prescribed rules, norms, or majority-focused results that must be followed. Each situation creates its own set of rules and principles that should be considered in that particular set of circumstances. Emphasizing the uniqueness of the situation and respect for the person in that situation, Fletcher appeals to love as the only norm. Critics of this approach argue that this can lead to a "slippery slope" of moral decline.

Decisions made in one situation cannot be generalized to another situation.

Chemically restraining a disruptive patient who has Alzheimer's disease provides a calmer atmosphere for other patients in a long-term care facility. This approach is used after all other efforts to calm the patient have failed. "Pulling the plug" on a terminally ill patient who does not want any more extraordinary care is an act of compassion. Withholding or withdrawing treatment is ethically correct from the individual patient's perspective if the burden of treatment outweighs the benefit of merely extending life. Defining *burden* has to be approached from the patient's perspective, not from others who may feel burdened by the patient's need for care. Viewing a situation from the perspective of benefit versus burden can assist patients and families to make difficult decisions on the basis of the patient's clear or intended wishes discussed over a period of time. Nurses and other health care providers need to be patient advocates, speaking out for those who are disadvantaged and cannot speak for themselves.

Table 19-1 compares the relative advantages and disadvantages of each approach. Remember that there is no perfect world view. If there were, debate would stop, and the need for continued ethical deliberation would cease. The ethical models presented here are not intended to be all-inclusive or exhaustive in depth. Rather, they should whet your appetite for further content. Many journals and texts are devoted to clinical ethics, and you are encouraged to see how ethicists apply these and other models to issues that affect your area of practice. Surveys of nurses indicate an ongoing interest and expressed need for ethical discussion and support in practice.

TABLE 19-1 Three Approaches to Ethical Decision Making: Comparison of Advantages and Disadvantages

ETHICAL APPROACH	ADVANTAGES	DISADVANTAGES
Deontological	Clear direction for action. All individuals are treated the same. Does not consider possible negative consequences of action.	Perceived as rigid. Does not consider possible negative consequences of actions.
Teleological	Interest of the majority is protected. Results are evaluated for their good, and actions may be modified.	Rights of individual may be overlooked or denied. What is a good result? Who determines good? Morality may be arbitrary.
Situational	This approach mirrors the way most individuals actually approach day-to-day decision making. Merits of each situation are considered. Individual has more control/autonomy to make decisions in his or her own best interest.	What is good? Who decides? Morality is possibly arbitrary. Lack of rules of generalizability limits criticism of possible abuse.

Nurses experience ethical distress along with physicians and other team members, but the 24/7 experience of nursing is unique from the perspective of patient continuity and opportunities for advocacy. Nurses increasingly serve on hospital ethics committees and are encouraged to contribute their perspective to ethical debates.

How Do I Determine Who Owns the Problem? The decision to choose a particular model of ethical reasoning is personal (see Table 19-1) and based on your own values. Familiarize yourself with various models to decrease your own moral uncertainty and gain some understanding of the values of others. The following guidelines are suggested as a means of analyzing ethical issues that will confront you in nursing practice. You will not be a pivotal decision maker in all situations, but these guidelines can assist you in making up your own mind and helping patients to voice their wishes and ask questions.

First, Determine the Facts of the Situation. Make sure you collect enough data to give yourself an accurate picture of the issue at hand. When the facts of a situation become known, you may or may not be dealing with an ethical issue. As an ICU nurse, you believe that the wishes of patients regarding extraordinary care are being disregarded. In other words, resuscitation is performed despite expressed patient wishes to the contrary. You need to

- Determine whether discussion about extraordinary care is taking place among patients, their families, and attending physicians.
- Clarify the institution's policy regarding cardiopulmonary resuscitation (CPR) and do-not-resuscitate (DNR) orders.
- Determine what input the families have had in the decisions (i.e., whether the families are aware of the patient's wishes).
- Explore the use of advance directive documentation at your institution, and determine whether patients are familiar with the use and possible limitations of living wills.
- Share your concerns with attending physicians to obtain their views of the situation. Discuss the situation with your clinical manager to clarify any misconceptions regarding policy and actual practice.

Second, Identify the Ethical Issues of the Situation. In the ICU scenario, if competent patients have expressed their wishes about resuscitation, this should be reflected in the chart. If a living will has been executed and is recognized as valid within your state, its presence in the chart lends considerable weight to the decision. The patient should be encouraged to discuss his or her decision with family to decrease the chances for disagreement if and when the patient can no longer "speak" for himself or herself. If immediate family members disagree with the living will, the physician may be reluctant to honor it, at least in part because of concern regarding possible liability. If a living will is executed without prior or subsequent discussion with the attending physician, there may be reluctance to honor the will because the physician was not informed of the patient's decision. The physician may feel that the patient did not make an informed decision. However, a durable power of attorney for health care (DPAHC), combined with a living will and completed before the patient's present state of incapacitation, would stand as clear and convincing evidence of the patient's wishes, preventing such a problem. The example of extraordinary care in the ICU illustrates the existence of values and principles in conflict. When the care team, family, and patient have different views of the situation, the patient is likely to be burdened with less than the best outcome, unless differences are resolved. The nurse can facilitate communication between the family and patient in resolving differences among all those involved.

Patient: Values autonomy, including the right to decide when intervention should stop.

Family: May value the patient's life at all cost and be unwilling to "let go" when a chance exists to prolong life regardless of life quality.

Physician: May feel that the patient has a fair chance to survive and that the living will was executed without the patient being "fully informed." The duty to care or cure may outweigh the physician's belief in the exercise of patient autonomy and fidelity.

Nurse: Values patient autonomy and the need to remain faithful to the patient's wishes. Concern for the needs of the family, in addition to respect for the physician-patient relationship, may cause some conflict.

Institution: Examination of institutional policy may reveal a conflict between stated policy (e.g., honoring living wills) and actual practice (e.g., code all patients unless written physician orders indicate otherwise).

In this situation, the ethical components of this second step involve autonomy and fidelity versus beneficence.

Third, Consider Possible Courses of Action and Their Related Outcomes. Having collected data and attempted discussion on the issue with all involved parties, you are faced with the following three options:

1. Advocate for the patient with physicians and the family by facilitating communication.
2. Encourage the patient and family to share feelings with each other regarding desires for care.
3. Encourage the family, patient, and attending physicians to discuss the situation more openly.

If the advocacy role does not bring about some change in behavior, consider the possible input and assistance of an interdisciplinary ethics committee (IEC). In the past two decades, such committees have evolved in response to the growing number of ethical issues faced in clinical practice. Most hospitals now have an IEC, which is typically composed of physicians, clergy, social workers, lawyers, and increasingly, nurses. Any health team member can access the committee with the assurance of receiving at least a helpful, listening ear. If necessary, the committee will convene to review a clinical case and will offer an unbiased opinion of the situation. Committee members may be helpful in clarifying issues or offering moral support; they may also be persuasive in suggesting that involved parties (i.e., family, physician, patient, and nurse) consider a suggested course of action. The authority of an IEC is usually limited, because the majority of IECs are developed with the understanding that the advice and opinions offered are not binding to the individual. However, it can serve as a potent form of moral authority and influence if used.

Taking the initiative to express your values and principles is not necessarily easy. As a recent graduate, it may seem safer to "swallow hard," remain quiet, and invest your energies in other aspects of your role. You may risk ridicule, criticism, and disagreement when you speak out or have questions on an ethical issue, especially if your view is different or unpopular. However, you risk something far more important if you do not speak out and ask questions for clarification. Silence diminishes your own autonomy as a person and as a professional. Depending on the situation, it may raise eyebrows, but it is important to make your concerns known because some values may be imposed on the patient or you in the clinical setting and those values may not be morally correct. You may not agree with these values or feel that they are in the best interest of the patient. Unresolved moral distress is also cited as a cause of job resignation (Pendy, 2007). Find your voice, ask questions, and speak up so you can more effectively control your practice.

Fourth, After a Course of Action Has Been Taken, Evaluate the Outcome. In the ICU scenario, did improved communication occur among patients, families, and physicians? Were your efforts to advocate met with resistance or a rebuff? What could you try differently the next time? What values or principles were considered most important by the decision makers? What kind of assistance did you receive from the IEC? What role did nursing play in this situation, and was it appropriate?

What Other Resources Are Available to Help Resolve Ethical Dilemmas? Professional resources are also available to provide direction about ethical issues and behavior. The first of these is the American Nurses Association (ANA) *Code of Ethics for Nurses* (2001b) (see Box 19-1). The code is a statement to society that outlines the values, concerns, and goals of the profession. It should be compatible with the individual nurse's personal values and goals. The code provides direction for ethical decisions and behavior by repeatedly emphasizing the obligations and responsibilities that the nurse-patient relationship entails.

The provisions of the *Code of Ethics* allude to the ethical principles mentioned earlier in this chapter and certainly imply that fidelity to the patient is foremost. A copy of the code with interpretive statements is available from the ANA. If you did not purchase a copy as a reference for school, consider buying it for your own use in practice. A copy of the code should be accessible within your place of employment.

Critics of the *Code of Ethics for Nurses* cite its lack of legal enforceability. This is a valid criticism because the code is not a legal document like licensure laws. However, it is a moral statement of accountability and can add weight to decisions involving legal censure. Many practicing nurses claim ignorance of the *Code of Ethics for Nurses* or believe that it is a document for students only. However, the *Code of Ethics* is for all nurses and was developed by nurses. In 2001, the American Nurses Association published a *Bill of Rights for Registered Nurses*, a first ever document of "rights" in contrast to the traditional focus on responsibilities. Box 19-2 lists the

---

| BOX 19-2 | American Nurses Association Bill of Rights for Registered Nurses |

Nurses have the right to practice in a manner that fulfills their obligations to society and to those who receive nursing care.

Nurses have the right to practice in an environment that allows them to act in accordance with professional's standards and legally authorized scopes of practice.

Nurses have the right to a work environment that supports and facilitates ethical practice, in accordance with the Code of Ethics for Nurses and its interpretative statements.

Nurses have the right to freely and openly advocate for themselves and their patients, without fear of retribution.

Nurses have the right to fair compensation for their work consistent with their knowledge, experience and professional responsibilities.

Nurses have the right to a work environment that is safe for themselves and their patients

Nurses have the right to negotiate the conditions of their employment, either as individuals or collectively, in all practice settings.

From www.Nursingworld.org/MainMenuCategories/ThePracticeofProfessionalNursing/workplace/RightsofNurses/BillofRights.aspx.

seven rights. Awareness of these rights may provide nurses with a sense of comfort in voicing their advocacy for patients as well as for themselves. Take the opportunity to become familiar with its contents (ANA, 2001a). Box 19-3 presents the *International Council of Nurses Code for Nurses*. The international code is valuable because it points out issues of universal importance to all nurses.

In 1973, the American Hospital Association published a *Patient's Bill of Rights*. Now revised (Box 19-4) and called The Patient Care Partnership, this document reflects acknowledgment of patients' rights to participate in their health care and was developed as a response to consumer criticism of paternalistic provider care. The statements detail the patient's rights with corresponding provider responsibilities. Read over each statement and consider whether they seem reasonable. When first developed, many of the statements were considered radical. This document reflects the increasing emphasis on patient autonomy in health care and defines the limits of provider influence and control. Earlier beliefs that the hospital and physician know best (paternalism) have been challenged and modified. This document is likely to be further refined as joint responsibilities between patients and health care providers grows.

Consider the settings in which you have had clinical experiences and decide how well these rights have been acknowledged and supported. In your future practice keep these rights in mind. Observing them is not only the "right thing to do," it is enforceable by law.

As a response to the rapidly growing home health care area of community nursing, the National Association for Home Care established a *Home Care Bill of Rights* for patients and families to inform them of the ethical conduct they can expect from home care agencies and their employees when they are in the home (National Association for Home Care & Hospice, n.d.). This document is widely used and addresses the rights of the patient and provider to be treated with dignity and respect; the right of the patient to actively participate in decision making; privacy of information; financial information regarding payment procedures from insurance, Medicare, and Medicaid; quality of care; and the patient's responsibility to follow the plan of care and notify the home health nurse of changes in his or her condition. Surprising as it may seem, there are instances of nurses who have lost their license as a result of unethical behavior toward patients in their homes. These abuses include financial and sexual exploitation—major violations of professional boundaries.

Home care nurses often face difficult ethical dilemmas about the delivery of care to patients. For example, a patient will require or desire more care or visits than Medicare or private insurance will pay for. All home care agencies have policies written to guide them through the decision-making process when they can no longer receive reimbursement for a patient's care. Often it is the responsibility of the home care nurse to find another community agency that can meet the patient's needs at a cost the patient can afford.

An additional document that you should be familiar with is the *Nuremberg Code* (Box 19-5). This code grew out of the blatant abuses perpetrated by Nazi war criminals during World War II in the name of science. Experiments were conducted by health care professionals without patient consent and resulted in horrific mutilations, disability, and death. The *Nuremberg Code* identifies the need for voluntary informed consent when medical experiments are conducted on human beings. It delineates the limits and restrictions that researchers must recognize and respect. Because of the preponderance of research in many clinical settings, nurses have a responsibility to understand the concept of voluntary informed consent and support the patient's rights throughout the research process. After reading this code, you should have increased awareness

BOX 19-3   International Council of Nurses Code for Nurses

ETHICAL CONCEPTS APPLIED TO NURSING

- The fundamental responsibility of the nurse is fourfold: to promote health, to prevent illness, to restore health, and to alleviate suffering.
- The need for nursing is universal. Inherent in nursing is respect for life, dignity, and rights of man. It is unrestricted by considerations of nationality, race, creed, color, age, sex, politics, or social status.
- Nurses render health services to the individual, the family, and the community and coordinate their services with those of related groups.

NURSES AND PEOPLE

- The nurse's prime responsibility is to those people who require nursing care.
- The nurse, in providing care, promotes an environment in which the values, customs, and spiritual beliefs of the individual are respected.
- The nurse holds in confidence personal information and uses judgment in sharing this information.

NURSES AND PRACTICE

- The nurse carries personal responsibility for nursing practice and for maintaining competence by continual learning.
- The nurse maintains the highest standards of nursing care possible within the reality of a specific situation.
- The nurse uses judgment in relation to individual competence when accepting and delegating responsibilities.
- The nurse, when acting in a professional capacity, should at all times maintain standards of personal conduct which reflect credit upon the profession.

NURSES AND SOCIETY

- The nurse shares with other citizens the responsibility for initiating and supporting action to meet the health and social needs of the public.

NURSES AND COWORKERS

- The nurse sustains a cooperative relationship with coworkers in nursing and other fields.
- The nurse takes appropriate action to safeguard the individual when his care is endangered by a coworker or any other person.

NURSES AND THE PROFESSION

- The nurse plays the major role in determining and implementing desirable standards of nursing practice and nursing education.
- The nurse is active in developing a core of professional knowledge.
- The nurse, acting through the professional organization, participates in establishing and maintaining equitable social and economic working conditions in nursing.

From International Council of Nurses: *ICN Code for Nurses: ethical concepts applied to nursing,* Geneva: Inprimeres Populaires, 1973; with permission.

BOX 19-4	The Patient Care Partnership: Understanding Expectations, Rights, and Responsibilities

Our goal is for you and your family to have the same care and attention we would want for our families and ourselves. The sections explain some of the basics about how you can expect to be treated during your hospital stay. They also cover what we will need from you to care for you better. If you have questions at any time, please ask them. Unasked or unanswered questions can add to the stress of being in the hospital.

WHAT TO EXPECT DURING YOUR HOSPITAL STAY

- High-quality hospital care. Our first priority is to provide you the care you need, when you need it, with skill, compassion, and respect. Tell your caregivers if you have concerns about your care or if you have pain. You have the right to know the identity of doctors, nurses, and others involved in your care.
- A clean and safe environment. We use special policies and procedures to avoid mistakes in your care and keep you free from abuse or neglect. If anything unexpected and significant happens during your hospital stay, you will be told what happened and any resulting changes in your care will be discussed with you.
- Involvement in your care. Please tell your caregivers if you need more information about treatment choices. When decision making takes place, it should include:
  - *Discussing your medical condition and information about medically appropriate treatment.* To make informed decisions with your doctor, you need to understand:
    The benefits and risks of each treatment and whether the treatment is experimental or part of a research study.
    What you can reasonably expect from your treatment and any long-term effects it might have on your quality of life.
    What you and your family will need to do after you leave the hospital.
    The financial consequences of using uncovered services or out-of-network providers.
  - *Discussing your treatment plan.* When you enter the hospital, you sign a general consent to treatment. In some cases, such as surgery or experimental treatment, you may be asked to confirm in writing that you understand what is planned and agree to it.
  - *Getting information from you.* Your caregivers need complete and correct information about your health and coverage so that they can make good decisions about your care. That includes:
    Past illnesses, surgeries, or hospital stays; past allergic reactions; any medicines or dietary supplements (e.g., vitamins, herbs) that you are taking; and any network or admission requirements under your health plan.
  - *Understanding your health care goals and values.* Make sure your doctor, your family, and your care team know your wishes.
  - *Understanding who should make decisions when you cannot.* If you have signed a health care power of attorney stating who should speak for you if you become unable to make health care decisions for yourself, or a living will or advance directive that states your wishes about end-of-life care, give copies to your doctor, your family, and your care team.
- Protection of your privacy. State and federal laws and hospital operating policies protect the privacy of your medical information. You will receive a Notice of Privacy Practices that describes the ways that we use, disclose, and safeguard patient information and that explains how you can obtain a copy of information from our records about your care.
- Preparing you and your family for when you leave the hospital. The success of your treatment often depends on your efforts to follow medication, diet, and therapy plans. You can expect us to help you identify sources of follow-up care and to let you know if our hospital has a financial interest in any referrals. You can also expect to receive information and, when possible, training about the self-care you will need when you go home.

BOX 19-4 The Patient Care Partnership: Understanding Expectations, Rights, and Responsibilities—cont'd

- Help with your bill and filing insurance claims. Our staff will file claims for you with health care insurers or other programs, such as Medicare and Medicaid. If you have questions about your bill, contact our business office. If you need help understanding your insurance coverage or health plan, start with your insurance company or health benefits manager. If you do not have health coverage, we will try to help you and your family find financial help or make other arrangements.

This is an abridged text. Full text is available at *www.aha.org*. Reprinted with permission of the American Hospital Association, copyright 2003. All rights reserved.

BOX 19-5 The Nuremberg Code

The great weight of the evidence before us is to the effect that certain types of medical experiments on human beings, when kept within reasonably well-defined bounds, conform to the ethics of the medical profession generally. The protagonists of the practice of human experimentation justify their views on the basis that such experiments yield results for the good of society that are unprocurable by other methods or means of study. All agree, however, that certain basic principles must be observed in order to satisfy moral, ethical, and legal concepts:

1. The voluntary consent of the human subject is absolutely essential. This means that the person involved should have legal capacity to give consent; should be so situated as to be able to exercise free power of choice, without the intervention of any element of force, fraud, deceit, duress, overreaching, or other ulterior form of constraint or coercion; and should have sufficient knowledge and comprehension of the elements of the subject matter involved as to enable him to make an understanding and enlightened decision. This latter element requires that before the acceptance of an affirmative decision by the experimental subject there should be made known to him the nature, duration, and purpose of the experiment; the method and means by which it is to be conducted; all inconveniences and hazards reasonably to be expected; and the effects upon his health or person which may possibly come from his participation in the experiment.

   The duty and responsibility for ascertaining the quality of the consent rests upon each individual who initiates, directs, or engages in the experiment. It is a personal duty and responsibility that may not be delegated to another with impunity.
2. The experiment should be such as to yield fruitful results for the good of society, unprocurable by other methods or means of study, and not random and unnecessary in nature.
3. The experiment should be so designed and based on results of animal experimentation and a knowledge of the natural history of the disease or other problem under study that the anticipated results will justify the performance of the experiment.
4. The experiment should be so conducted as to avoid all unnecessary physical and mental suffering and injury.
5. No experiment should be so conducted where there is an a priori reason to believe that death or disabling injury will occur; except, perhaps, in those experiments where the experimental physicians also serve as subjects.
6. The degree of risk to be taken should never exceed that determined by the humanitarian importance of the problem to be solved by the experiment.
7. Proper preparations should be made and adequate facilities provided to protect the experimental subject against even remote possibilities of injury, disability, or death.
8. The experiment should be conducted only by scientifically qualified persons. The highest degree of skill and care should be required through all stages of the experiments of those who conduct or engage in the experiment.

Reprinted from *Trials of war criminals before the Nuremberg Military Tribunals under Control Council Law* No. 18, vol. 2, Washington, DC: U.S. Government Printing Office, 1949, p 181.

of the patient's right to autonomy and the health care provider's responsibility to be faithful to that right.

Controversial Ethical Issues Confronting Nursing

Situations that raise ethical issues affect all areas of nursing practice. The following is a sampling of issues that consistently cause controversy.

Abortion. The debate over this issue has raged in the United States since the 1973 *Roe v. Wade* Supreme Court decision. The resolution of this case struck down laws against abortion but left the possibility of introducing restrictions under some conditions. Efforts toward that end continue today with mixed results for both "pro-choice" and "pro-life" factions. Increasing efforts are focused on the need for parental notification/consent. The right to reproductive choice and access continues to be debated and the argument affects nursing practice in both acute care and community settings.

Historical references to abortion can be found as far back as 4500 BC (Rosen, 1967). It has been practiced in many societies as a means of population control and terminating unwanted pregnancies; yet sanctions against abortion are found in both ancient biblical and legal texts. It is interesting to note that the ancient sanctions against abortion generally related to fines payable to the husband if the pregnant woman was harmed. This form of sanction derived from the concept of woman and fetus as male property. Greek philosophers, including Aristotle and Plato, made a distinction between an unformed fetus and a formed fetus. A fine was levied for aborting an unformed fetus, whereas the aborting of a formed fetus required "a life for a life." The number of gestational weeks that determine whether a fetus was formed was not stated, although the time of human "ensoulment" was understood: Aristotle believed that a male fetus was imbued with a soul at 40 days gestation *(quickening)* versus 90 days for a female (Feldman, 1968). The subject of ensoulment became part of the ongoing debate regarding the time when the developing fetus becomes human. In other words,

> When does life begin?

Judeo-Christian theologians generally came to identify the beginning of life at conception or the time of implantation. However, even within this tradition, the Jewish Talmud and Roman law stated that life begins at birth because the first breath represents the infusion of life. These varied views continue to the present.

Social customs and private behavior regarding abortion have frequently differed from theological teaching. The first legal sanctions against abortion in the United States began in the late 19th century. Before that time, first-trimester abortions were not uncommon and, in fact, were advertised, supporting the idea that abortion before quickening was acceptable.

The ethical debate about abortion today is a continuing struggle to answer the question of when life begins and to determine an answer to the following questions:

- Does the fetus have rights?
- Do the rights of the fetus (for life) take precedence over the right of the mother to control her reproductive functions?
- When is abortion morally justified?

- Should minors have the right to abortion without parental consent or awareness?
- Should fetal stem cells be used for research, helping to end the suffering of patients with chronic disorders such as Parkinson's disease?

The struggle to answer these questions has polarized individuals into pro-life or pro-choice camps. Yet opinion polls on the subject have found very few people to be against abortion in all circumstances or to favor abortion as a mandatory solution for some pregnancies. Most Americans express views somewhere between these extremes, and the legal battle to maintain or restrict abortion access continues. The controversy has escalated into violence in some areas of the country, with abortion clinics and personnel subjected to attack; some abortion providers have been killed. This violence has resulted in the decreased availability of abortion services in many areas. In recent years, some pharmacists have refused to fill prescriptions for birth control pills and the "morning after" pill, claiming that this violates their moral beliefs, an exacerbation of the pro-life/pro-choice debate.

The Roman Catholic Church has been the religious group most frequently identified with the pro-life movement, but there are other groups—religious and otherwise—that support a ban on abortion. Pro-life proponents generally condone abortion only to save the life of the mother. These antiabortion groups are often criticized by pro-choice as extremist, anti-woman, and repressive.

The pro-choice movement is vocal in championing the woman's right to choose and promoting the safety of legalized abortion. They cite the tragedy of past "back-alley" abortions and compare restrictions on abortion to infringements on the civil liberties of women. Within the pro-choice movement are many individuals who favor restrictions on abortions after the first trimester and oppose the use of abortion as a means of birth control. Pro-life proponents often view pro-choice supporters as anti-family extremists who do not represent the views of the majority of Americans.

How Does the Abortion Issue Affect Nursing? Nurses are involved both as individuals and professionals. Following are some general guidelines to consider.

Consider what your values and beliefs are in relation to abortion and how you can best apply these values to your work and possible political action.

If you choose to work in a setting in which abortions are performed, review Provision 1 of the ANA's *Code of Ethics for Nurses*: "The nurse, in all professional relationships, practices with compassion and respect for the inherent dignity, worth and uniqueness of every individual, unrestricted by considerations of social or economic status, personal attributes, or the nature of the health problems" (ANA, 2001b).

This statement outlines your responsibility to care for all patients. If you do not agree with an institution's policy or procedure regarding abortion, the patient still merits your care. If that care (e.g., assisting with abortions) violates your principles, you should consider changing your job or developing an agreement with your employer regarding your job responsibilities. If you cannot provide the care that the patient requires, make arrangements for someone else to do so.

You do not have to sacrifice your own values and principles, but you are barred by the ANA *Code of Ethics* from abandoning patients or forcing your values on them. Such abandonment would also constitute legal abandonment, and you would be subject to legal action.

Some hospitals have developed conscience clauses that provide protection to the hospital and nurses against participation in abortions. Find out if your institution has such a clause.

Consider your response and possible conflict in the following situations:

- You are a labor and delivery nurse working on a unit that performs second-trimester saline abortions in a nearby area. You are not a part of the staff for the abortion area, but today, because of short-staffing, you are asked to care for a 16-year-old who is undergoing the procedure.
- You work in a family-planning clinic that serves low-income women. Because of escalating violence against abortion providers, the nearest abortion clinic is 100 miles away. You are restricted from giving information regarding abortion services because of federal guidelines.
- A 41-year-old mother of five has expressed interest in terminating her pregnancy of 6 weeks' gestation. She confides that her husband would beat her if he knew she was pregnant and contemplating abortion.
- You are teaching a class on sexuality and contraception to a group of high school sophomores. Two of the girls state that they have just had abortions. In response to your information regarding available methods of contraception, one of the girls states, "I'm not interested in birth control. If I get pregnant again, I'll just get an abortion. It's a lot easier."
- You have a history of infertility and work in the neonatal ICU. You are presently caring for a 24-week-old baby born to a mother who admits to taking "crack" as a means of inducing labor and "getting rid of the baby." The mother has just arrived in the unit and wants to visit the baby.

These sample scenarios are meant to illustrate the conflicts that personal values, institutional settings, and patients may create for the recent graduate. In your responses, consider how you might lobby or participate in the political process to change or support existing policies regarding abortion and access to such services.

Euthanasia. *Euthanasia* is commonly referred to as "mercy killing." It is a Greek word that means "good death" and implies painless actions to end the life of someone suffering from an incurable or terminal disease. Euthanasia has been closely tied to a "right-to-die" argument, which has gained a good deal of attention in the past decade. Euthanasia is classified as *active, passive,* or *voluntary. Active euthanasia* involves the administration of a lethal drug or another measure to end life and alleviate suffering. Regardless of the motivation and beliefs of the individuals involved, active euthanasia is legally wrong and can result in criminal charges of murder if carried out. In recent years, incidents of active euthanasia have become periodic news events as spouses or parents have used measures to end the suffering of their mates or children from, for example, advanced Alzheimer's disease or persistent vegetative state. *Passive euthanasia* involves the withdrawal of extraordinary means of life support (e.g., ventilator, feeding tube). *Voluntary euthanasia* involves situations when the dying individual expresses his or her desires regarding the management and time of death to a sympathetic physician who then provides the means for the patient to obtain a lethal dose of medication.

Today, advanced technology routinely keeps alive patients who would never have survived a few short years ago. Concerns regarding prolonging life and suffering for those individuals have resulted in a movement to have right-to-die statutes and living wills accepted. In those states that have such statutes and recognize living wills, termination of treatment in such cases has become easier. Right-to-die statutes free health care personnel from possible liability for honoring a person's wishes that life not be unduly prolonged (Rudy, 1985).

Another legal document, the durable power of attorney for health care (DPAHC), helps ensure that a living will is carried out. The DPAHC identifies the individual who will carry out the patient's wishes in the event that he or she is incapacitated and also informs health care providers about the specific wishes of the patient regarding life-support measures.

A major impact on the availability of living wills and the DPAHC (which are referred to as advance medical directives) resulted from the introduction of the Patient Self-Determination Act in December 1991. Advance directives are federally mandated for all institutions receiving Medicare or Medicaid funds. On admission, all competent adults must be offered information about advance directives. This means that all adults are told about the purpose and availability of living wills *(treatment directive)* and DPAHCs *(appointment directive)*. They are then offered assistance with completing these documents if desired. After 15 years of having advance directive information available to patients, the impact of this document on decision making is varied. It certainly has influenced the communication that many patients have with their families, physicians, and other health care providers regarding their wishes at the timing of signing, but patients often change their minds when their health care status changes, frequently opting for the prolongation of life. A problem has surfaced regarding the timing of information to patients regarding advance directives. If patients first hear about advance directives on admission to an acute care setting, anxiety regarding their admission and the separate concept of advance directives may seriously affect informed decision making at that time. Advance directives should ideally be discussed *before* serious illness occurs, and at the very least in a noncrisis environment to encourage non-pressured decision making. Cultural, religious, and racial issues regarding DPAHC have also surfaced and need to be researched to determine the best approaches for providing this information within a culturally diverse society. Patients and families need reassurance that declining extraordinary care does not mean the abandonment of caring and palliative care when needed. Both patients and families need to be reassured that palliative comfort care will never stop, even when aggressive curative efforts are withdrawn.

Decisions to withdraw or withhold nutrition and hydration from patients are complex and the subject of ongoing debate by ethicists, health care personnel, and the legal system. In response to the issues of hydration and nutrition, the Ethics Committee of the ANA developed guidelines in 1988 and revised them in 1992. These guidelines state that there are instances when withholding or withdrawing nutrition and hydration are morally permissible. Although intended only as a guideline, this document provides direction for nurses who face such issues. Its wording has been both praised for its clarity and criticized for possible ambiguity. The primary exception to the withdrawal of hydration and nutrition is when harm from these measures can be demonstrated. This document is available from the ANA.

Futile Care and Physician-Assisted Suicide. Futile care (futility) and physician-assisted suicide (PAS) are two ethical and human rights issues that have drawn a great deal of attention and debate. In a survey conducted by the ANA's Center for Ethics and Human Rights in June 1994, respondents were asked to identify 10 of the most frequently occurring ethical issues. Approximately 55% identified "end-of-life decision" as one of the top four issues, and 37% identified "providing futile care" as an important priority issue facing nursing (Scanlon, 1994). These issues continue to be at the forefront for clinicians almost 15 years later (Robichaux & Clark, 2006).

What Is Futility? *Medical futility* refers to the use of medical intervention (beyond comfort care) without realistic hope of benefit to the patient. *Benefit* is defined as improvement of outcome. A concrete example of futility would be the continuation of ICU care for a patient in a persistent vegetative state who would, on discharge from the hospital, return to a nursing home incapable of interacting with the environment. The futility debate concerns the very nature of the definition of *benefit*, in addition to who defines it. The economic pressure to control health care costs is also causing a focus on ways to eliminate "unnecessary" intervention.

On paper, futility can be defined, but its application to diverse clinical situations remains a challenge. The debate involves multiple parties whose interests and values are not always compatible. For example, patients and families have argued both for the right to refuse care that they believe is futile and the right to receive all possible care in the face of a medical opinion of futility. This argument raises two related questions:

1. Do patients or families have the right to demand and receive treatment that health care providers believe to be futile?
2. Do physicians have the right to refuse to provide treatments that they believe to be futile, despite patient or family desire to initiate or continue such treatment?

Ethics committees have struggled to agree on a working definition of futility to provide support for clinicians and patients and families who are faced with difficult decisions regarding care. Many institutions have developed guidelines for the withdrawal of treatment (except for comfort care). These guidelines emphasize the importance of clear, ongoing communication among all health care team members and with the patient and family. Accurate, compassionate discussion is essential to convey a unified approach to the realities and limitations of possible medical care. The guidelines should never be used as a threat or to imply abandonment of care. They are, as their name implies, guidelines. Lack of agreement among the patient, the family, and the health care team is likely to delay or prevent withdrawal of treatment, primarily because of the fear of liability, even in cases of brain death. Supporting the patient or family decision may be difficult because of personal values and professional opinions. It is crucial to clarify where professional loyalties should lie and to keep the discussion patient-centered.

Pressures to eliminate unnecessary costs also influence the futility debate. Insurers, clinicians, and health care institutions increasingly question medical expenditures that produce futile outcomes and prolong the inevitability of impending death. Insurance reimbursement is likely to further limit and deny payment for treatment judged to be of no benefit to the patient. A possible risk is that beneficial treatment may be eliminated or denied solely because of economic concern in cases having an uncertain outcome. Nurses need to keep informed on institutional guidelines regarding medical futility and communicate clearly with patients, families, and physicians regarding expected goals and likely outcomes of care. The patient's welfare—and not economic concerns—should be the primary driving force for withdrawal of treatment. Studies continue to show that nurses experience moral distress when inappropriate treatments are used to prolong the dying process. Speaking out on behalf of the patient is an essential advocacy role even if the final decision regarding care differs from what the nurse believes is appropriate. Passivity in such situations only increases frustration and a sense of professional resignation (Robichaux & Clark, 2006).

Physician-Assisted Suicide (PAS). PAS has gained national attention because of Dr. Jack Kevorkian's persistent efforts to publicize and bring legitimacy to a formerly taboo topic. Kevorkian assisted or attended in the deaths of more than 130 terminally and chronically ill patients (Hyde, 1999). His work caused the state of Michigan to pass legislation barring PAS. Proponents of PAS managed to put the issue on the ballot in three Western states since 1991. In 1994, Oregon approved PAS legislation. It was immediately challenged in the Oregon court by right-to-life advocates but the Death with Dignity Act finally went into effect October 27, 1997. Between 1998 and 2006, 292 people in Oregon have died as a result of prescriptions for lethal medications. Approximately 85,000 other Oregonians with similar conditions died during this time frame pointing out the relatively small number of people and clinicians who chose to use approved lethal injections (State of Oregon, 2006). In 2008, voters in the state of Washington approved a measure, which legalized PAS making it the second state to legalize PAS. The law took effect in early 2009. For right-to-life advocates even one of these deaths is too many and a step down the path of state approved murder. Quality-of-life advocates support PAS as an example of personal autonomy and control. The debate continues.

PAS has been debated for years, and opinions on both sides among physicians and the public are very strong. The American Medical Association opposes PAS because it violates the most basic ethical principle: "First, do no harm." Physicians have traditionally taken care of the living patient, and support for PAS threatens to destroy this fundamental relationship. Many individual physicians have, however, changed their minds in recent years because of their work with terminally ill patients. More than a few of these clinicians have come to believe that the only option for the relief of some patients' intractable pain and suffering is death.

Although the legalization of PAS continues to be debated in the courts, the practice goes on—generally in private without headlines. Both critics and supporters of PAS state that the secrecy goes on because of the fear of arrest for homicide. There have been some court rulings supporting the right to PAS by terminally ill patients on the basis of the 14th Amendment's guarantee of personal liberty. These decisions have been assailed by the right-to-life groups as an anti-life philosophy, which dishonors the intrinsic value of life.

PAS affects nursing practice because a decision to perform PAS may involve the nurse. The term *PAS* implies that the physician is the active agent, but a lethal dose may be ordered by the physician for the nurse to administer. Nurses need to be aware of the legal and ethical implications of such an order. The administration of a lethal dose for the explicit purpose of ending a patient's life is an illegal act that can be prosecuted as homicide. From an ethical point of view, many would consider this the ultimate act of mercy; yet it is an illegal act in the United States, except in Oregon and Washington state. Clinicians, ethicists, the public, and the courts continue to struggle with how best to respect the life and wishes of terminally ill patients without "doing harm." Nurses need to remain aware of their nurse practice acts and the *Code of Ethics for Nurses* as they balance patient needs with their conscience and value systems.

Ethicists generally agree that although the prolongation of life by extraordinary means is not always indicated, clarifying the circumstances when such care may be stopped (withdrawn) or possibly never begun (withheld) frequently creates controversy, particularly when the quality of life (coma, persistent vegetative state) is likely to be questionable.

Opponents of the right-to-die movement believe that it represents the erosion of the value of human life and may encourage a movement toward the acceptance of suicide as part of a "culture of death." They caution that the lives of the weak and disabled may come to be devalued as society concentrates on the pursuit of "quality life." If passive euthanasia achieves societal acceptance, who will speak out in favor of protecting incompetent or dependent individuals who are not living society's view of a quality life? The well-publicized Schiavo controversy demonstrates the political polarization that this topic can cause (Nagourney, 2005).

Proponents of the right-to-die movement believe that it provides a more natural course of living and dying to the individual and family by avoiding the artificial prolongation of life through technology. The availability of technology to prolong life often raises the question "We can, but should we?"

Surveys of medical and nursing school curricula in the United States continue to reveal minimal content on end-of-life care issues. Schools continue to focus curricula more on the curative approach to illness and disease, neglecting to address the palliative, comfort-directed needs of individuals who require care in the last months and days of their lives. This fact, combined with the aging of our population, points out the need for improvement in educating both current clinicians and students in health care institutions on ethical issues surrounding end-of-life care. A growing number of proactive clinicians and educators concerned with the quality of care provided to dying patients and their families have created an educational movement called *End-of-Life Care*. The specific program targeted for nursing is called *End-of-Life Nursing Education Consortium Project*, targeting nursing faculty and nursing leadership in many specialty organizations. This consortium project has educated hundreds of nurses in the past few years, slowly influencing a change in both education and clinical practice. Studies of patients facing end-of-life issues indicate that pain and symptom management, communication with one's physician, preparation for death, and the opportunity to achieve a sense of life completion are the most consistently important issues (Steinhauser et al, 2000). It will be interesting to see the impact of these efforts on patient care over the next decade. Perhaps we will be better prepared to accept the reality that everyone does die. As nurses, we are challenged to make this last event of life a better experience for all. The growing popularity of the palliative care movement in the United States is a significant paradigm change, acknowledging the value and complexity of supportive, noncurative care for many conditions. Supporting the broader picture of palliative interventions that may continue for months or years will increase our understanding of the needs of patients who do not have a cure awaiting them but who want to embrace the time they have left with our support.

Consider your response and possible conflict in the following critical thinking situations:

A 22-year-old quadriplegic repeatedly asks you to disconnect him from the ventilator. His family rarely visits, and he believes that he has nothing to live for.

The spouse of a patient with advanced Alzheimer's disease states that he can no longer watch his wife of 43 years suffer. "She would not have wanted to live this way." His wife is being treated for dehydration, malnutrition, and a urinary tract infection. She is confused and is frequently sedated to manage her combativeness. The use of a feeding tube is being contemplated because of her refusal to eat.

The attending physician for a patient with terminal AIDS refuses to order increasing doses of pain medication because of her concern that it may cause a repeat episode of respiratory depression. The patient's pain is unrelieved, and he begs you for medication. "Please help me. I know I'm dying."

A patient on long-term dialysis wants to discontinue treatment citing the side effects of dialysis and her medications. She feels that the quality of her life has disappeared. Her life partner died a year ago, and she sees no reason to continue suffering. She has been on the transplant list for 6 years. She has indicated that her last appointment will be in 1 month, and she would like to know what kind of supportive care will be available.

For each of these scenarios, consider what your reaction would be and the possible resources you would use to resolve the conflicts.

What Are the Ethical Issues Regarding Transplantation? There are almost 110,000 people on transplant lists in the United States today, and the majority of these individuals will die without a transplant because of the shortage of available organs (United Network for Organ Sharing, 2010). On what basis should someone receive an organ? Should severity of illness serve as the primary criteria, or what other factors should be taken into consideration? Should economic status be used as a contributing factor in the process? How are donors solicited? What are the religious and cultural issues that influence someone's decision to be considered as a potential donor? Should the government intervene to enlarge the donor pool by making a decision that victims of accidents imply donor consent if their driver's license does not have a statement specifically refusing donation? What protections need to be put into place to prevent coercion for organ donation, a reality in many countries where organs are paid for or where condemned prisoners are sources for donation?

All of the above questions offer a window into the complexity of issues surrounding organ transplantation. The technology exists with ever-increasing precision, but there is a tremendous scarcity of organs. On what basis do we as a society attempt to create a process of organ access that is just and equitable? Who decides?

What Is the Ethical Issue Regarding the Use of Fetal Tissue? Fetal tissue from elective abortions has been identified as potentially beneficial in the treatment of Parkinson's disease and other degenerative disorders because of its unique embryonic qualities. Proponents argue that it is available tissue that can be put to some beneficial use in patients who at present do not have any other hope of significant improvement or cure. They further argue that the availability of fetal tissue from elective abortions is a separate issue from the later use of the tissue for stem cell research. The abortion would have occurred regardless. Later use of the stem cell derives some good from the discarded tissue.

Critics who assail the use of fetal tissue for stem cell research as a further erosion of respect for the unborn were successful in spurring a federal ban on the use of fetal tissue for research in the United States during the 1980s. They believe that the limited research that has already occurred regarding fetal tissue has created the mentality that pregnancy can be used as a means of providing parts and tissues for others. This ban was removed in early 1993 after President Clinton took office, and in 2001, use of stem cells received narrowly defined approval by the Bush administration for genetic research. Individual states also have the authority to pass laws to permit human embryonic cell research using state funding. This state right has not been overridden by any congressional ban (NIH, 2007). Access any electronic news source or a print newspaper and you are likely to see at least one article related to the continuing debate regarding the ethics of stem cell research. As the largest group of health care providers, nurses need to be informed regarding the issues. Consider your own viewpoint and how it can affect your nursing care. Does the good (beneficence) achieved from the use of fetal tissue for patients with Parkinson's disease outweigh the harm inflicted by viewing a fetus as a source of parts?

What Are the Ethical Issues Regarding In Vitro Fertilization? This procedure involves the fertilization of a mother's ovum with the father's sperm in a glass laboratory dish followed by implantation of the embryo in the mother's uterus. Since the birth of the first successful in vitro fertilization baby in 1978, the procedure has gained popularity as a last-chance method for some infertile couples to have a child. The availability of the technique has created a new subspecialty practice in obstetrics and raised ethical issues for consideration. Opponents of the procedure argue that it is an unnatural act and removes the biological act of procreation from the intimacy of marriage. The cost of the procedure is also a source of criticism, calling into question whether it should be covered by insurance and whether the procedure should be available to all couples, regardless of ability to pay. Many couples are now lobbying to select the sex of their baby, choosing the desired embryo for implantation and destroying the undesired embryos. If technology can be made to meet our desires for a "designer baby," does that make it a morally correct course of action?

Questions concerning informed consent for the procedure merit attention as well. Many infertility clinics offer this service but have not been upfront about their success rates or qualifications. Standardized methods of reporting this information have just recently been established. To be ethical, all such clinics should define success the same way; for example, success equals pregnancy or success equals live birth. The two definitions are very different. Information about the qualifications of the staff should be available to patients, and the subspecialty should lobby for standards of practice that are enforceable and available to the public. Possible side effects from the drugs used to induce hyperovulation and from anesthesia or surgical injury during the laparoscopy should be explained.

Should anyone who desires the in vitro procedure have access, or should the procedure be limited to those in a heterosexual marriage? Most clinics have limited their services to heterosexual couples to avoid adverse publicity, but this policy is starting to change as single and lesbian women seek out avenues of becoming biological parents. Most important, to whom does the embryo belong and what are the embryo's rights? There have been court cases involving marital disputes regarding the custody of frozen embryos. What are the rights of the embryos in such instances? Can a parent choose to destroy the embryos over the objection of the estranged spouse, or should one parent be able to obtain custody of the embryos when his or her spouse wants them to be thawed out and destroyed? What responsibility does the staff have for maintaining parental ownership of the embryos?

What Are Genetics and Genomics? The study of genetics and genomics has led to the increased ability of health care professionals to assist patients in improving health outcomes and treatments of disease processes. Genetic research has led to an 'improved understanding of the genetic contribution to the disease, the development of targeted drug therapy (pharmacogenomics) ... and new and better ways to treat diseases such as gene therapy" (Greco & Salveson, 2009, p 558).

"Genetics is a term that refers to the study of genes and their role in inheritance—the way certain traits or conditions are passed down from one generation to another."
"Genomics is a relatively new term that describes the study of all of a person's genes including interactions of those genes with each other and the person's environment." (Lea, 2009, p 2)

But, what is the role of nursing in this emerging area? Nurses will provide education to patients about genetic and genomic testing, research, and treatment. As research-based improvements in the recognition of familial disease traits are identified and emerging disease treatments are discovered, nurses will play an increasingly important role in the study and application of genetic findings and the role of genetics and genomics in the health of the patients they serve. The role of genetics and genomics will undoubtedly play a significant role in current and future patient care. Nurses of all levels have the opportunity to engage in this opportunity and provide needed education, support, and treatment based in the most current research, even though ethical challenges may arise as the result of this emerging research and treatment.

How Should the Ability to Prenatally Diagnose Genetic Defects Be Used? Genetic disorders such as Tay-Sachs disease, cystic fibrosis, Huntington's chorea, and retinoblastoma can be diagnosed early in pregnancy. As this technology advances, how should it be used? Should screening remain voluntary, or as some have suggested, should it be mandatory to detect fetal disorders that could be aborted or possibly treated? Should the results of such genetic screening be made available to insurance companies? Critics argue that this information could be used as a means of coercion for couples regarding reproductive decisions if future insurance coverage is then limited. As this technology advances, safeguards need to be applied to prevent invasion of privacy and any societal movement toward eugenics. As the human genome project allows us to become capable of knowing our genetic code and possibilities for disease, it raises the question of who should have access to that information. And for what reason(s)? If a family with a known genetic disorder chooses to have more children with that disorder, is it the obligation of society to pay for their care? Is there any reason for insurance or the government to become involved with genetic counseling, or is this a private family affair?

Allocation of Scarce Resources. When the subject of scarce resource allocation is mentioned, justice is the core issue. What is fair and equal treatment when health care financing decisions are made? Who should make such decisions and on what basis? Critics argue that health care is not a scarce resource in this country but that the *access* to such care is scarce for many. They believe that this scarcity of access could be eliminated if our priorities in governmental spending were altered. Managed care put a temporary brake on runaway costs in the 1990s, but that brake failed in the past few years. Nearly 50+ million individuals living in the United States are without health insurance or a reasonable means of accessing anything but stopgap emergency care (U.S. Census Bureau, 2009). The solution to this issue remains unclear and highly politicized. In the meantime, managed care of one form or another is influencing a larger and larger share of the insured population, raising related issues of restricted access to specialized care and loss of patient and physician autonomy.

Allocation also raises a number of questions. For example, do all individuals merit the same care? If your answer is an immediate "yes," would you change your mind if the patient were indigent, with no chance of paying the bill? If you still say "yes," should this same indigent patient receive a liver transplantation as readily as someone who has insurance or cash to pay for it? Should taxpayers be responsible for the medical bills for organ transplants, cardiac bypass surgery, or joint replacements for incarcerated felons? These and other questions continue to be asked by individuals, government, and ethicists, in addition to health care providers. Perhaps at the core of this subject is a more fundamental question: Is health care a right or a privilege that comes with the ability to pay? If access to health care is a right that should be provided to all citizens, are we as a society prepared to pay the bill? And is there a level of health care that is essential for all, beyond which financing becomes a private matter?

The type of care that is provided and supported is another aspect of the debate. For example, should health promotion and prevention be emphasized as much as or more than illness-oriented and rehabilitative care? It is widely acknowledged that each dollar spent on preventive care (e.g., prenatal care) saves three or more dollars in later intervention (e.g., neonatal ICU); yet our national and state health care expenditures (Medicare and Medicaid) are traditionally weighted in favor of an illness model for reimbursement. Managed care is an effort to control health care costs, but it is increasingly criticized as prioritizing the financial bottom line over the quality of care.

What Are Some of the Possible Solutions Being Debated? In recent years, some individuals have proposed the idea of health care rationing for the elderly, specifically as it relates to the use of expensive technology that often prolongs the last few weeks of life and suffering (Lamm, 1986). Proponents of health care rationing argue that high-tech "11th-hour expenditures" are unwanted by many older adults and consume disproportionate amounts of health care resources. Proponents of rationing stress the need to acknowledge the finite resources of society. As our society continues to age, younger workers will increasingly be asked to pay the costs for Medicare, Medicaid, and social security. Disparities between generations will increasingly become part of the conversation regarding health care financing.

Many believe that more vulnerable groups, such as uninsured children, should be given a more equitable portion of health care services (e.g., well-baby clinics, universal health insurance for children). Others argue that health care is already being rationed and that we should recognize this fact and articulate our priorities. Few would disagree that our present health care financing is in need of a comprehensive overhaul before we experience a chaotic breakdown.

The state of Oregon has gone one step further, imposing guidelines on the type of care that its Medicaid funds will cover. Deciding that preventive care affects a majority of its citizens, Oregon made funding for such measures as immunizations and prenatal care a priority, whereas extraordinary care that benefits only a few individuals, such as a bone marrow transplantation is not covered (Rooks, 1990). This utilitarian approach, emphasizing the greatest good for the greatest number, is not without its critics, but it is an effort to provide direction for health care priorities. Oregon's plan was initially vetoed by the federal government and has undergone some revision, still emphasizing preventive care and treatment for disorders that affect a majority of citizens. Other states are now looking at the Oregon model as they plan health care reform. Another state to watch is Massachusetts, universal coverage was implemented in 2007 (Belluck, 2007).

Health Care Rationing. You may have already experienced situations of health care rationing or limited access. As a nurse you may, on one hand, feel powerless and frustrated when patients do not receive care because they cannot afford it or, on the other hand, feel angry because indigent patients are placing heavy burdens on both private and public facilities. Consider your values and professional responsibilities as you think through this issue. As an individual and a nurse, you need to take a stand regarding health resource allocation and support efforts to improve access, while determining in your mind what type of health care you believe to be ethically justifiable.

CONCLUSION

As medical technology advances, ethical issues and concerns will play an ever-increasing role in your nursing practice. The general public, health care professions, religious traditions, increasing cultural diversity, and the legal system will all have influence in the attempts to resolve the ethical issues affecting health care in the 21st century. Keeping an open mind in these controversial dilemmas is difficult, but it is hoped you will examine your personal values and continue to make decisions that are based on the welfare of your patients.

BIBLIOGRAPHY

American Nurses Association (2001a): *Nurses' Bill of Rights.* Retrieved from *www.nursingworld.org/MainMenu Categories/ThePracticeofProfessional Nursing/workplace/RightsofNurses/ BillofRights.aspx.*

American Nurses Association: *Code of ethics for nurses,* Kansas City, Mo, 2001b, ANA.

Belluck P: Massachusetts universal care plan faces hurdles, *New York Times,* July 1, 2007. Retrieved from *www.nytimes. com/200707/01/health/policy/01.insure. htm.*

Feldman DM: *Marital relations, birth control and abortion in Jewish law,* New York, 1968, Schocker.

Fletcher JF: *Situation ethics,* Philadelphia, 1966, Westminster.

Greco K, Salveson C: Identifying genetics and genomics nursing competencies common among published recommendations, *J Nursing Educ* 48:557-565, 2009.

Hyde J (1999): *Prosecutors drop assisted suicide charge against Kevorkian.* Retrieved from *www.detnews.com/ 1999/metro/9903/13/031301.htm.*

Lamm RD: Rationing of health care: the inevitable meets the unthinkable, *Nurs Pract* 11:57, 61-64, 1986.

Lea DH: Basic genetics and genomics: a primer for nurses, *OJIN: the Online Journal of Issues in Nursing* 2(14):1-11, 2009. Retrieved from *www.nursing world.org.*

Nagourney A: 44 million with no health insurance and more to come, *New York Times* A:14, March 23, 2005.

National Association for Home Care & Hospice (n.d.): *What are my rights as a patient?* Retrieved from *www.nahc.org/ consumer/rights.html.*

National Institutes of Health (2007): *Stem cell information.* Retrieved from *www. stemcells.nih.gov/info/faqs.asp.*

Pendy PS: Moral distress: recognizing it to retain nurses, *Nurs Econ* Jul-Aug (4): 217-221, 2007.

Robichaux CM, Clark AP: Practice of expert critical care nurses in situations of prognostic conflict at the end of life, *Am J Crit Care* 15:480-491, 2006.

Rooks JP: Let's admit we ration health care—then set priorities, *Am J Nurs* 90:38-43, 1990.

Rosen H, editor: *Abortion in America,* Boston, 1967, Beacon Press.

Rudy EB: The living will: are you informed? *Focus Crit Care* 12:51, 1985.

Scanlon C: Ethics survey looks at nurses' experiences, *Am Nurse* 26:22, 1994.

State of Oregon (2006): *Characteristics of 292 DWDA patients who died during 1998-2006 after ingesting a lethal dose of medication compared with 85,755 Oregonians dying from the same underlying diseases.* Retrieved from *www. egov.oregon.gov/DHS/ph/pas/docs/ yr9-tbl-2.pdf.*

Steele SM: *Values clarification in nursing,* ed 2, East Norwalk, Conn, 1983, Appleton & Lange.

Steinhauser KE, et al: Factors considered important at the end of life by patients, family, physicians, and other health care providers, *JAMA* 284:2476-2482, 2000.

Thompson IE, et al. *Nursing ethics,* ed 5, St. Louis, MO, 2007, Churchill Livingstone, Elsevier.

United Network for Organ Sharing (2010): *Data.* Retrieved from *www.unos.org.*

U.S. Census Bureau (2009): *Income, poverty, and health insurance coverage in the United States.* Retrieved from *www. census.gov/newsroom/releases/archives/ income_wealth/cb10-144.html.*

Additional resources are available online at *http://evolve.elsevier.com/Zerwekh/nsgtoday/.*

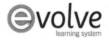

CHAPTER 20

Legal Issues

Judy Irvin, RN, JD

> *The law is good, if a man use it lawfully.*
> —THE FIRST EPISTLE OF PAUL THE APOSTLE TO TIMOTHY 1:8

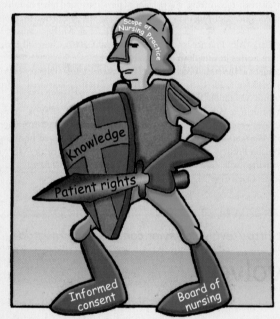

Knowledge regarding legal aspects is the best defense a nurse can have.

After completing this chapter, you should be able to:

- Discuss various sources and types of law.

- Relate the Nurse Practice Act to the governance of your profession.

- Understand the functions of a state board of nursing.

- Describe your responsibilities for obtaining and maintaining your license.

- Be able to identify the elements of nursing malpractice and how they are proved in a malpractice claim.

- Incorporate an understanding of legal risks into your nursing practice and recognize how to minimize these.

- Identify legal issues involved in the medical record and your documentation, including the use of electronic medical records.

- Take an active role in improving the quality of health care as required by legal standards.

- Participate as a professional when dealing with nurses who are impaired or functioning dangerously in the work setting.

- Discuss the concerns surrounding at least two controversial legal issues in nursing practice.

*W*hen you graduate and become a registered nurse, you will also be achieving a new status under the law. An example of this change is that after meeting certain criteria, you will have a license to practice nursing. This license sets certain standards that you must follow as a nurse in the state in which you are both licensed and practice. Should you not live up to these standards, your state can take away your ability to practice as a nurse. If your actions are not what a reasonable nurse with the same knowledge and education would do, and this causes someone to be injured, you can be sued for malpractice. Of course, a person can always be sued if his or her behavior is negligent (unreasonable) and someone gets harmed. However, when you are working as a professional, the expectations for your behavior are higher than simply being a reasonable person. You are expected to perform as a reasonable professional nurse. People react to these changes in legal status differently. Some nurses see the law as a big monster that is unpredictable, very frightening, and out to do harm to them. Other nurses find the law to be quite interesting and attempt to learn all they can about how it may affect their practice. These nurses often find the law to be a very helpful tool to ensure safe practices. I hope that this chapter is a start in your becoming a legally educated nurse. Remember, though, that the law is always changing, and as a nurse it is your responsibility to keep up with the changes taking place in the state in which you practice.

Before beginning a discussion of legal aspects in nursing, there is some practical advice that you can use in any situation in which you wonder whether what you are doing or proposing to do is legal. It is called the "Mother Rule." When such a question about the legality of an action comes to you, ask yourself if you would feel comfortable telling your mother about what you are doing or propose to do. If your answer to this question is "no," then it probably is not advisable. Why?

If you are uncomfortable with what you are doing, it may involve lying in some manner, which is involved in a claim for **fraud** or **defamation.** Perhaps you are doing something outside your scope of practice or something that is unsafe for the patient and could cause injury. These types of actions are involved in **malpractice. Invasion of privacy** and **breach of confidentiality** are claims that involve gossip or talking about patients unnecessarily.

In addition to the aforementioned, mothers are on juries. As jurors, they are instructed about laws, but they often make their decisions based on what they think is "right" or "wrong." In every lawsuit, jurors are faced with evidence for both sides. In some respects, this forces them to simply make a human decision regarding the events. If you can feel comfortable when telling your mother (a jury) about what happened—truthfully and without hiding anything—then it is likely that you can do the same confidently with a jury. It is also likely that you will be believed and found to have acted reasonably. In simplified terms, that is all you need to do. Now let us address the more formal aspects of this thing called "law."

SOURCES OF LAW

Where Does "The Law" Come From?

People will often tell you that you cannot do something because it is "illegal." Or, they will make a statement that the law is this or that. Some nurses, who are afraid of laws, will simply believe what they are told. Other nurses will ask, "What law?" This is an important question because there is often much misinformation regarding the law floating around institutions where nurses work.

The most common type of law affecting nurses is **"statutory law"** or **"statutes"** or **"laws."** These are the documented rules for living in your state (state laws) or in the United States (federal laws) that are passed by state legislatures and by Congress. Statutes cover the rules for our relationships with one another and can be viewed as the ethics of our society written down. The section on definitions is one of the most important parts of a statute. There you can find what the authors of the statute mean when they use a certain word. We all use words differently, but when reading laws, a more precise understanding is necessary. (Box 20-1 lists definitions of common legal terms.)

Nurse practice acts are examples of state statutory laws and can be easily found online, in a public library, or obtained from the state board of nursing. It would first be important to see how a "registered nurse" is defined in your state to see whether there is a clue there about what nurses can or cannot do. Usually, however, these laws are quite general and might not answer specific questions—for instance, whether or not registered nurses in your state can administer intravenous (IV) conscious sedation.

■ CASE STUDY 1

You are working in a hospital where a very well-known actor is admitted with a diagnosis of pneumocystic pneumonia. You know that this is usually associated with AIDS. During the patient's stay, you are asked by a physician to give an IV drug to sedate this patient while the physician does a procedure. The patient becomes oversedated, has a respiratory arrest, and dies. You are so upset about this that you call your best friend, who is also a nurse, to talk about the incident. You mention the actor's name and the fact that he had AIDS. Your friend says that it was "illegal" for you to be giving what he calls "IV conscious sedation" and you are in deep trouble. Where might you be able to search to determine whether this is true? What type of legal trouble might you have?

The next type of law is constitutional law. This type of law refers to the rights, privileges, and responsibilities that were stated in, or have been inferred from, the U.S. Constitution, including the Bill of Rights. States may not pass laws or institute rules that conflict with constitutionally granted rights or rules because the Constitution is the highest law of our country. Freedom of speech and religion are such rights. The right to privacy is an example of a right inferred from the Constitution (Critical Thinking Box 20-1).

The third type of law to consider is **administrative law.** This body of law is made by administrative agencies that have been granted the authority to pass rules and regulations and render opinions, which usually explain in more detail the state statutes on a particular subject. Examples of this type of law are the rules and regulations passed by boards of nursing to control nursing practice in each state. This might well be a source for finding out specifically about nurses giving

CRITICAL THINKING BOX 20-1   In Case Study 1, can you identify where a constitutional law might have been broken?

BOX 20-1   Common Legal Terms

Advance directive: A document made by a competent individual to establish desired health care for the future or to give someone else the right to make health care decisions if the individual becomes incompetent; examples include living wills and medical powers of attorney.

Defamation: A civil wrong in which an individual's reputation in the community, including the professional community, has been damaged.

Defendant: The person who is being accused of wrongdoing. The person then must defend himself or herself against the charges. In a malpractice claim, the nurse or other health care provider.

Deposition: Out-of-court oral testimony given under oath before a court reporter. The purpose is to enable attorneys to ask and have answered questions related to a case. The deposition process may involve expert witnesses, fact witness, defendants, or plaintiffs. It may be used to impeach (find inconsistencies or untruths) testimony in trials.

Diversion program: A program for treatment and rehabilitation of substance abusers. Such programs may be used by boards of nursing for encouraging treatment but are independent of such boards.

Expert witness: A person who has specific knowledge, skills, and experience regarding a specific area and whose testimony will be allowed in court to prove the standard of care.

Good Samaritan law: A law that provides civil immunity to professionals who stop and render care in an emergency. Care rendered cannot be done so in a grossly negligent manner.

Interrogatory: A process of discovering the facts regarding a case through a set of written questions exchanged through the attorneys representing the parties involved in the case.

Jurisdiction: The court's authority to accept and decide cases. May be based on location or subject matter of the case.

Malpractice: Improper performance of professional duties; a failure to meet the standards of care that results in harm to another person.

Negligence: Failure to act as an ordinary prudent person when such failure results in harm to another.

Plaintiff: The person who files the lawsuit and is seeking damages for a perceived wrongdoing. In medical malpractice, the patient, and/or the patient's family.

Reasonable care: The level of care or skill that is customarily rendered by a competent health care worker of similar education and experience in providing services to an individual in the community or state in which the person is practicing.

Standard of care: A set of guidelines based on various types of evidence as to what is reasonable and prudent behavior for a health care professional.

Statutes of limitations: Laws that set time limits for when a case may be filed. Differ from state to state.

Telemedicine: Using telecommunication technology, usually interactive, to provide medical information and services.

Torts: Civil (not criminal) wrongs committed by one person against another person or property. Includes the legal principle of assault and battery.

Whistleblower: Individual "on the inside" who reports incorrect or illegal activities to an agency with authority to monitor or control those activities.

Whistleblower statute: Law that protects a whistleblower from retaliation. Usually involves specific criteria about how whistle was blown.

IV conscious sedation in your state. There may also be an "advisory opinion" given by the state board of nursing on this topic. Your state board of pharmacy may also have other regulations that describe their rules for administering medications and who may do this.

Another type of law is **common law,** which includes decisions made by judges in court cases or is established by rules of custom and tradition. **Case law** is composed of the decisions rendered in court cases by appeal courts. Often, nurses will hear about something happening in a court case and think that there must be a document somewhere talking about that case. This is not necessarily true, because not all cases reach the level of an appeal court, where a record of the court's opinion and reasoning is recorded. Cases are usually appealed to higher courts because there is an issue of statutory law involved. Many cases do not have such issues and are therefore not appealed or recorded.

Once there is a recorded court opinion, the result is the legal principle of *stare decisis,* which means that if an issue has been decided, all other cases concerning the same issue should be decided the same way. Another word for this is **precedent.** Although you may hear of a case in which a nurse was found negligent in administering IV conscious sedation, there may not be case law on this issue to set a legal precedent in your state. Each state has its own case law. Each state's body of case law differs because it is based on the decisions of individual judges, who often do not resolve issues in the same way as judges in another state and who base their decisions on differing state statutes.

COURT ACTIONS BASED ON LEGAL PRINCIPLES

There are two major classifications of legal actions that can occur as a result of either deliberate or unintentional violations of legal rules or statutes. In the first category are **criminal actions.** These occur when you have done something that is considered harmful to society as a whole. The trials will involve a prosecuting attorney, who represents the interests of the state or the United States (the public), and a defense attorney, who represents the interests of the person accused of a crime (defendant). These actions can usually be identified by their title, which will read "*State v. [the name of the defendant]*" or "*U.S. v. Smith [the name of the defendant].*" Examples include murder, theft, drug violations, and some violations of the Nursing Practice Acts, such as misuse of narcotics. Serious crimes that can cause the perpetrator to be imprisoned are called **felonies.** Less serious crimes resulting in fines are **misdemeanors.** The victim, if there is one, may or may not be involved in a decision to prosecute a case and is considered only a witness in the criminal trial. Laws differ in states as to victim rights and/or if the person or the state will receive any of the money from fines. In Case Study 1, your actions would not likely result in a criminal action. Recently, however, there have been instances in which a nurse was thought to have recklessly caused a patient's death, and a case was brought in criminal court for negligent homicide. The issues involved in such criminal actions will be discussed later in this chapter.

In the second category of legal claims are **civil actions.** These actions concern private interests and rights between the individuals involved in the cases. Private attorneys handle these claims, and the remedy is usually some type of compensation that attempts to restore injured parties to their earlier positions. Examples of civil actions include malpractice, negligence, and informed consent issues. The victim (patient) or victim's family (patient's family) brings the lawsuit as the **plaintiff** against the **defendant,** who may be the individual (nurse) or company (hospital) that is believed to have caused harm. In the situation presented, you might be sued for malpractice by the actor's spouse if it is felt that you acted below a standard of care and caused the actor's death.

Sometimes an event can have both criminal and civil consequences. When that happens, two trials are held with different goals. The amount of evidence required to support a guilty verdict is different for each type of trial. The criminal case requires that the evidence show that the defendant was guilty beyond a shadow of a doubt. The civil case requires only that the evidence show that the defendant was more likely guilty than not guilty. This is what makes it possible for someone such as O. J. Simpson to be found "not guilty" in a criminal trial but "guilty" or negligent in a civil trial.

LEGAL CONTROL OVER NURSING PRACTICE

Having a license to practice nursing brings you into close contact with laws and government agencies. The nurse practice act is the statute governing nurses in your state. The board of nursing is the agency designated to apply the laws to individuals.

There are nurses who do not understand their responsibilities in relationship to their licensing board. Do not become one of these. State boards act under the police power granted each state from the federal government to protect the safety of its residents. Persons serving on such boards take this responsibility seriously. They expect that you will also.

■ CASE STUDY 2

After your incident with the actor, you decide to leave the state. You have to answer detailed questions on your licensure application for the new state about any previous malpractice claims. You had heard something about a claim being filed against your former hospital but had left shortly after that. Now you have received a notice from the state board of nursing of your previous residence inquiring about the incident with the actor and asking for a response within 2 weeks. The letter has taken a long time to be forwarded to you, and the 2-week deadline has passed. What should you do?

What Are the Legal Aspects of Licensure?

Receiving a license to practice nursing is a privilege, not a right. Even the successful completion of an educational program in nursing and/or passing the National Council Licensure Examination for Registered Nurses (NCLEX-RN) does not guarantee that a license will be granted. A license is granted by a state after a candidate has successfully met *all* the requirements in that particular state. Examples of these requirements may include high school education, successful completion of a nursing education program, application to the appropriate national and state agencies, fee payment, not being a felon (i.e., .not having a criminal record), and passing the national examination for the appropriate level of licensure (NCLEX-RN or PN). Because the license is intended to guarantee public safety, the level of expertise necessary to pass the test is the minimum level needed to provide safe care. The state also continues to monitor your practice and to investigate complaints regarding this practice.

When you move to a new state, you need to make certain decisions with regard to your license. You may want to continue being licensed in the state of past residence. It is important to keep your past state board informed of your current residence so that you receive important documents in a timely fashion that can affect your future ability to practice. You also need to be informed of licensure and practice requirements of a new state of residence before you begin to practice there.

Each state's practice act may be different from any other state's act. In the past, this has posed many hurdles for nurses who traveled or had practices across state lines. States have attempted to resolve these issues by developing a licensure model that will allow participating states to recognize licensure of another state. This works in the same manner as driver's licenses—your state driver's license is recognized in other states, but when driving in another state, you must adhere to *that* state's driving laws. As of June, 2010, according to the National Council of State Boards of Nursing (NCSBN), 24 states had passed laws to accept the Nurse Licensure Compact, or the Mutual Recognition Model (NCSBN, 2010). You can practice in those states if your home state is part of the model.

If you travel to another state or cross state lines in the normal course of your practice, either to care for a specific patient or to perform other nursing services in another state, you need to check with the board of nursing in the states in which you are performing nursing care to determine their rules about practice within their borders. An example of this would be telephone triage or telemedicine programs with patients outside of your state. You can obtain copies of a state practice act from the board of nursing or licensing agency for nurses in that state. (See Appendix A on the Evolve website.)

Some practice acts regulate nursing by controlling who may use the titles "registered nurse" and "licensed practical nurse" or "licensed vocational nurse." Others regulate by controlling the scope of practice and determining the specific activities for each level of nursing—that is, who can perform what functions. In most states, the nurse practice act does the following:

- Describes how to obtain licensure and enter practice within that state.
- Describes how and when to renew your license.
- Defines the educational requirements for entry into practice.
- Provides definitions and scope of practice for each level of nursing practice.
- Describes the process by which individual members of the board of nursing are selected and the categories of membership.
- Identifies situations that are grounds for discipline or circumstances in which a nursing license can be revoked or suspended.
- Identifies the process for disciplinary actions, including diversionary techniques.
- Outlines the appeal steps if the nurse feels the disciplinary actions taken by the board of nursing are not fair or valid.

Some practice acts are very specific and detailed; others simply grant the board authority to declare the rules and regulations (administrative law) and to establish the details. To understand the scope of practice within a specific state in which you are practicing or wish to practice, you must obtain a copy of the state's nurse practice act that includes the law, rules, and regulations that the board or administrative agency has established in that state.

Because you have gone to a great deal of expense and effort to obtain your nursing license, you should guard it carefully. Never ignore or take lightly any document received from your state board of nursing. Even if you think you have received a notice in error, contact the board of nursing immediately (Box 20-2).

The power of the board to discipline is the power that can have an adverse effect on the nurse's ability to practice. It is important that each nurse carefully review the power of the board within the state of their practice. Several levels of disciplinary actions can occur based on the severity

BOX 20-2	Protect Your License

- Do not let anyone else borrow it.
- Do not let anyone copy it unless you write "copy" across it. In some states it is illegal to copy your license.
- If you lose it, report it immediately and take the necessary steps to obtain a duplicate.
- Be sure that the Board of Nursing knows whenever you change your address, whether you move across the street or across the nation.
- Practice nursing according to the scope and standards of practice in your state.
- Know your state law so you will not do anything that could cause you to be disciplined by the removal of your license.
- Meet all renewal requirements on time.

of the problem. Boards of nursing have the authority to censure, to suspend, to revoke, or to deny licensure. Each of these actions can be temporary or permanent. It would be prudent to consult an attorney who is versed in health care law if you should receive notice of any possible action against your license. Such a person can be your advocate and explain your rights and how best to deal with the state board. Seeking legal advice is an investment to protect your investment. Some institutions assist nurse employees in these instances, and some nurse insurance policies will also defend nurses in these "administrative actions."

What About the Impaired Nurse?

Impaired nurses are nurses who are unable to function effectively because of some type of substance abuse (i.e., alcohol, prescription drugs, illegal drugs). The American Nurses Association (ANA) has recently estimated that 6% to 8% of nurses abuse drugs or alcohol at a level sufficient to impair their professional judgment (Dunn, 2005). One of the most common reasons for state board action against nurses involves the taking of hospital medications for personal use (Brent, 2001). Boards of nursing are increasingly concerned about this issue, because it has significant impact on rendering safe, effective patient care (NCSBN, 2001). Some states discipline nurses who know about but fail to report an impaired colleague. Allowing an impaired nurse to practice not only puts the nurse and her patients at risk but also negatively impacts the facility's reputation and the nursing profession as a whole. It is important that you know what the reporting requirements are for your state board of nursing and your facility.

Do not ever assume that you or your colleagues are immune from impairment. High stress and easy access to drugs seem to contribute to this common problem for health care providers. A slippery slope occurs when a nurse first takes any medication, even an aspirin, that does not belong to him or her. It is best to see that first wrong as a prelude to many future wrongs and to never do it. If you do find yourself in trouble with drugs or alcohol, it is far better to voluntarily report this to your state board of nursing rather than to be caught or to harm other persons. Most boards react more favorably to the nurse who seeks assistance than to one who is reported by law enforcement agencies or a hospital as required by law. At least 37 states have taken a rehabilitative approach to this problem rather than a punitive one, recognizing how important it is to return an abstinent nurse to the work force (Dunn, 2005).

These states have programs set up to allow nurses to meet specific behavioral criteria, such as blood or urine testing, ordered evaluations, and attendance at rehabilitation programs, either while disciplinary action is being taken or instead of bringing formal proceedings. The primary concern is to assist the impaired nurse back to full and appropriate nursing practice. If a nurse is involved in a voluntary rehabilitation program through a contract with a state board and backslides or has additional problems, the board may bring formal action against the nurse that will negatively affect licensure for the rest of his or her life and can also involve criminal sanctions.

Who Knows About the Disciplinary Actions Against Nurses?

When an action is taken by a state board against a nurse, states have differing methods of reporting such action to health care providers and others to protect the public. **NURSYS** is a comprehensive electronic information system that includes the collection and warehousing of nurse licensing information and disciplinary actions. Previously called NIS and ELVIS, as it underwent different stages of development, the term "NURSYS" is a derivative of "nurse" and "system." NURSYS contains data on a nurse's personal information (identity, residence), license information, education information, disciplinary action information, verification and fee tracking requests, and historical information (any changes to the aforementioned data). NURSYS is the information system that supports the mutual recognition of nurses' licenses. In 2003, NURSYS announced that it would be available to the public for nursing license verification. Nurses can also access the system to provide nursing license verification for a fee of $30 (NCSBN, 2010).

Another national storehouse of information is The National Practitioner Data Bank (NPDB), which was part of a federal law under Medicare called The Healthcare Quality Improvement Act. Although initially set up to identify physicians who had committed malpractice and/or who had licensure problems across state lines, it now extends to many licensed individuals, including nurses. Information related to malpractice payments made on behalf of a nurse and licensing actions are required to be made by professional insurance companies, federal and state agencies, and health care institutions. Individual states may restrict information that may be accessed through the National Practitioner Data Bank (NPDB, 2006).

TORTS

Civil, as opposed to criminal, actions are also called *torts*. Remember that civil actions occur when a plaintiff files a lawsuit to receive compensation for damages he or she suffered as a result of a perceived wrong. The economic reason for filing the suit should never be forgotten. This is important to keep in mind should you or a colleague become involved in a tort action. Try not to interpret everything in terms of a personal insult and/or an intentional desire to cause you personal and professional harm. This is not a criminal action, and the terms "guilty" or "innocent" are not appropriate, nor are words such as "killed" that can sometimes be heard in the gossip mill or read in the media.

There are two categories of tort actions. Unintentional torts are those that usually involve an inadvertent, unreasonable act that causes harm to someone. We might call these acts "incidents" or "accidents." Intentional torts are those acts done deliberately by a defendant. Although sometimes occurring in the heat of a moment, they are not considered accidental in nature.

NURSING MALPRACTICE

The most common unintentional tort action brought against nurses is a malpractice claim.

According to the NPDB 2006 report, 24,736 nurses and nursing-related practitioners had a report made against them between the years 1990 to 2006. There have been 6208 cases over the history of the NPDB in which malpractice payments were made on behalf of a specifically named nurse. This does not include the number of claims naming only a facility, yet involving nursing actions. Because malpractice can potentially affect every nurse, it is important to explore what this means.

■ CASE STUDY 3
You are a nurse working in a hospital. The physician tells you that you need to give an injection of Vistaril (hydroxyzine pamoate). You make sure that the order is documented in the medical record. The medication comes up from the pharmacy, and you check it against the physician's order and find it to be correct. You walk into the patient's room and use at least two patient identifiers to make sure it is the right patient. You give the injection in the patient's right dorsogluteal muscle and document this in the medical record.

The patient leaves the hospital. A year later, you are told that a lawsuit has been filed against the hospital by the patient. It seems the patient is claiming that the injection you gave him caused sciatic nerve damage and his whole leg is numb (Critical Thinking Box 20-2).

Legal Commentary

Many times nurses worry about being sued for something when, in the eyes of the law, no malpractice has occurred. Not all poor outcomes are malpractice. A nurse also may legitimately make an error in judgment. Therefore, it is important for a nurse to know the basic elements that must be proved before malpractice can occur. Then the nurse can evaluate incidents realistically.

Basic Elements of Malpractice

What are the basic elements of malpractice?
1. You must have a duty. In other words there must be a professional nurse-patient relationship.
2. You must have breached that duty. In other words you must have fallen below the standard of care for a nurse.
3. Your breach of duty must have been a foreseeable cause of the injury.
4. Damages or injury must have occurred.

CRITICAL THINKING BOX 20-2   Who may have malpractice liability in this situation and why? You? The physician? The hospital? What defenses may be available to you?

These four elements need to be present in each malpractice case. The job of the patient's (plaintiff's) attorney is to prove to a jury that each element has occurred. Your attorney, on the other hand, defends you by proving that all or even just one element did not happen. This is not always a black-and-white process, which can be frustrating and confusing. Still, it is important for the nurse to evaluate events in light of these elements and to know how they are proved in court.

Do You Have a Professional Duty? To make a claim of malpractice against a nurse, the plaintiff must establish that there is a nurse-patient relationship, or in legal terms, that you had a professional duty to a patient. A duty is implied if you are employed by and render services at a health care institution such as a hospital or nursing home. This would also be true if you work as a registered nurse for a home health agency in the home, or in a school, or in a physician's office.

In the case studies, you are working as a nurse in a hospital, and the nurse-patient relationship is implied. Therefore the first element can easily be proved. What if you are giving medical advice in your home informally as a friend, relative, or neighbor? In this setting, it is not implied that you are acting as a nurse, and proving that you owed your friend a duty as a professional might be difficult. There is no payment, or institution, or formal contract. Therefore, although nurses are continually warned about being sued in this situation, it is unlikely that a plaintiff's attorney would easily prevail on the element of duty for such casual comments to others outside your employment.

What if you stop at an accident to assist someone who is injured? Because most states want to encourage medical professionals to help people at accidents without fear of a lawsuit, Good Samaritan statutes have been passed. These laws give immunity from malpractice to those professionals who attempt to give assistance at the scene of an accident. In essence, you do not have any professional duty to stop, although you may feel an ethical duty to do so. If you do, know that in most—if not all—states you cannot be sued for malpractice for what you might or might not do. That is, you do not have a professional standard of care to adhere to unless you are a professional at the scene as part of your employment. All persons, of course, are expected not to leave a victim in a position that is more dangerous than when found. Once you stop to help the injured person, stay with him or her until you are given clearance by emergency responders.

Sometimes nurses volunteer to give nursing assistance at sports events or other activities in which it is foreseen that professional services may be needed. In thinking about this, you may see that such a situation is not quite as clear as other situations. If you are at a first aid station and/or wear a badge indicating you are a nurse, then you have the appearance of a professional and people may rely on that when seeking advice or assistance.

It is important to know your status under such circumstances in your state. You should know whether you have immunity and whether you are covered by malpractice insurance.

What Is the Professional Duty Owed? Once it is established that you owe a duty to the person, the question becomes, "What is that duty?" How does a plaintiff's attorney establish what the duty might be? The duty owed by a nurse is different from that owed by a physician or nursing assistant. The duty of a nurse will be to act as a reasonable nurse under the same or similar circumstances. The duty or standard of care for the physician will be to act as a reasonable physician. You can see that the two will be different. Of course, the most interesting question in any malpractice case will be, "How will my attorney prove that I acted as a reasonable nurse?" The following will be considered when attempting to establish through evidence what the standard of care for the nurse might be.

What About the Nurse Practice Act? Perhaps the most important guideline for nurses will be the nurse practice act in the state in which you are practicing. Most acts describe in fairly general terms what a nurse may do. Prohibitions, or things that are considered unprofessional conduct, are usually more specific. A violation of such a license prohibition means that you have fallen below a standard of care set by the state for nurses. It also may mean that you risk an action against your license. If you do not know what these prohibitions are, you are putting yourself in jeopardy. As stated previously and applied here to the standard of care, it is important that you obtain a copy of the nurse practice act for the state(s) in which you are or will be licensed to practice, and be sure to stay current with your licensing standards. For instance, Texas now requires that all applicants for licensure pass a nursing jurisprudence examination, which is based on the Texas Nursing Practice Act and the Texas Board of Nursing Rules and Regulations (Texas BON, 2010).

What Is an Expert Witness? The most common way to establish the duty owed by a nurse is by the testimony of a registered nurse usually, but not always, with training and background similar to yours. This expert witness will then testify regarding what a reasonable nurse in the same or similar circumstances would be expected to do—and that you did not do it. If a plaintiff's attorney cannot find an expert nurse to testify that you did not act reasonably, then in most instances the case cannot go forward. In general, a patient cannot simply claim professional malpractice without having a professional witness to prove this.

In the same manner, if the plaintiff has an expert witness to prove you fell below the standard of care, you will need an expert witness to testify that you did not. Some nurses enjoy being expert witnesses either for the defense of a nurse or as part of the plaintiff's claim against a nurse. Either role requires both integrity and professionalism to be effective and believed by a jury (Di Luigi, 2004).

There is a type of malpractice case in which an expert is not required. This type of claim is called *res ipsa loquitur*, or "the thing speaks for itself." This claim is very difficult to prove, because the patient must have enough evidence to show that: (1) the injury would ordinarily not occur unless someone were negligent; (2) the instrumentality causing the injury was within the exclusive control of the defendant; and (3) the incident was not owing to any voluntary action on the part of the plaintiff. If a patient can prove that all of these exist, the burden then shifts to the defendant nurse to prove that malpractice did not take place. Incidents such as operating on the wrong body part or leaving a surgical sponge in a patient fall into this category of claims.

What Are Established Policies and Procedures? Policies and procedures established by the institution in which you work are the most crucial pieces of evidence for establishing a standard of care. Most good attorneys representing plaintiffs will request a set of hospital policies as soon as a lawsuit is filed. For instance, in Case Studies 1 and 3, a lawyer might ask for the hospital's policies on documentation and administration of medications. If you did not follow that policy, then you fell below a standard of care set by your institution.

You can see why you need to know and read the policies within your health care facility or corporation. These policies should also be a resource when you have questions about how to do certain procedures or what your rights are in a certain situation. Policies are the laws under which you must live. It is also important for you as a professional to participate in making or changing policies so that they accurately reflect what nurses are doing in your institution. In addition, the policies set standards for giving quality and consistent patient care. If you have followed a policy, it can also be used proactively to prove that you followed the standard of care set by your institution.

What About Accreditation and Facility Licensing Standards? Most health care facilities and other health care organizations such as health maintenance organizations (HMOs) must go through a process whereby they become licensed and/or accredited. The Joint Commission (TJC) and the National Committee of Quality Assurance (NCQA) are two such organizations that set standards for health care organizations. These standards can often be used as evidence of the standard of care for nurses working in such facilities. For instance, The Joint Commission has issued National Patient Safety Goals (NPSG) for 2010 that include standards to improve safe identification of patients and their medications, prevent infections using proven guidelines and improve communication among care providers (TJC, 2010). A state facility-licensing requirement would be that the facility develop policies and procedures to optimize patient safety when administering medications. Should a malpractice claim involving medications occur, the patient's attorney will require proof that these requirements have been followed.

What About Textbooks and Journals? Articles, textbooks, or portions of such publications may be used as evidence of the standard of care for nurses to follow. For instance, if a nursing journal has published a recent article on correct administration of intramuscular injections, that may be used to demonstrate what you should have done.

What Are Professional Standards for Organizations? Professional organizations such as the American Nurses Association (ANA) or the Association of Perioperative Registered Nurses (APRN) may publish certain standards or practice guidelines. These may also be used as evidence for what a reasonable nurse should do under certain circumstances.

In summary, there are many different types of evidence used by plaintiff attorneys to demonstrate an expected standard of care. The nurse needs to remember that these same documents can be used to demonstrate that you did follow the standard of care. Let us see how.

Applying the Standard of Care to the Case Study. In Case Study 3, the plaintiff will have to find a nurse who will testify to the correct method of giving intramuscular injections. If you did not give the injection in such a manner, then the jury can infer that you did not act reasonably. However, if the correct method is to give the injection intramuscularly in the right dorsogluteal site and you have documented that you did this, an expert's testimony will not help prove anything. Also, if you can show that you followed hospital policies in the administration of the medication, again, there will be no proof of falling below a standard of care.

What if the patient attempts to claim a case using the theory of *res ipsa loquitur*? Again, the patient's lawyer must prove that the claimed injury could not have happened unless there was negligence. As demonstrated earlier, you would be able to prove through your documentation that you were not negligent. In addition, your attorney would also demonstrate your lack of liability through the third element of malpractice. Do you remember what that is?

Was There a Breach of Professional Duty? Not only must a plaintiff prove what the standard of care is in a given situation, the plaintiff must prove that you did not meet the standard of care. Other legal terms used regarding this needed element might be that you "fell below the standard of care" or you "breached the duty owed the patient." In other words, the plaintiff must demonstrate through the evidence listed earlier that you did not act as a reasonable and prudent nurse under the circumstances. Please remember that even if you did not act reasonably, there are other elements that must be proved to have a malpractice claim.

Did the Breach of Duty Cause the Injury? Causation is an element often overlooked by the nurse; yet this is often the most strongly argued by attorneys. Did the difficult birth cause the child to have cerebral palsy or did a genetic birth defect cause the baby to have a difficult delivery? Was the injury caused by the auto accident or by the medical care? Did the patient have the physical problem before the medical care or after? Was the injury caused subsequently by the patient's lack of compliance with the treatment plan, or did the patient subsequently injure herself after the medical care was rendered?

The causation requirement must be proved by the plaintiff's attorney, and as you can imagine, this may not be easy. Certain well-documented observations will make such proof impossible.

1. Clearly document the patient's physical and mental condition upon admittance to and discharge from your health care facility or unit. Both of these observations can be used to demonstrate that either the patient had the symptom when she came and/or did not have the symptom when leaving. Therefore whatever happened during her stay in your unit or facility did not cause the problem.

2. After any incident, such as a patient fall, the patient's physical and mental condition must be documented. This will help demonstrate that subsequent complaints cannot be attached or caused by the incident.

3. Document clearly any actions of a patient that demonstrate noncompliance with medical directives. When a patient states or clearly demonstrates that he is not taking medications as ordered or is not following a prescribed physical therapy regimen, this can cause therapeutic failure, rather than the treatment itself. A documented "no show" at an outpatient clinic can dispel later claims that you ignored a patient's complaints and so caused the injury.

4. Document clearly when a patient complains and does not complain. If, in Case Study 3, it is documented that the patient has been up and walking after the injection and has no complaints, it will be very difficult to prove that the injection caused the problem.

5. Be very careful when documenting what a patient states as opposed to what you think may have happened. If a patient states that an injection caused a problem, it is best to document "Patient states, 'My leg has felt numb since I received an injection in the hospital,'" rather than document "Hospital injection caused patient's leg to be numb." The latter documentation may inadvertently be condemning a health care provider who has done nothing wrong.

6. Document the patient's own admissions. "I knew I shouldn't have gotten out of bed so soon" can be helpful if a patient falls and then later tries to blame the nursing staff. "My wife tried to remove the stitches, but she could not get that deep one" can raise doubt regarding what caused the incision to become infected. Infection is very rarely considered to be malpractice unless it can be proved to have been caused by negligence such as not using good aseptic technique.

7. Document discharge instructions clearly. In today's managed care environment, many acutely ill patients are sent home to care for themselves. If they and/or their families have not been given clear instructions—not only about their care but also about symptoms to watch for that may need immediate medical attention—they may attempt to blame health care professionals for what occurs at home. A clear, documented discharge plan is imperative after any procedure

that can have adverse outcomes, not only to prevent law suits, but to promote good patient care. A warning to a patient to call a specific number if adverse symptoms occur can save a life *and* prevent a lawsuit. Emergency departments have long understood the importance of such instructions, and the age of specialized computer software programs makes them easily accessible to everyone.

8. Document allergies. Recording a patient's allergies or lack thereof is another way of preventing a malpractice claim. Neither nurses nor physicians cause patients to have allergies. They do have a duty to not give medications to patient when previous experience has demonstrated that the medication has caused an allergic reaction. "No known allergies" can completely eliminate a claim involving an allergic reaction.

Applying "Causation" to Case Study 3

Returning to Case Study 3, the patient will have to prove that your injection caused the numbness in his leg. There are many intervening factors that could have caused this numbness. You do not have to prove anything because you, as a defendant, do not have the "burden of proof." The plaintiff may have a very difficult time, especially if there are no documented complaints by the patient of problems at the time of the injection or shortly thereafter.

Just remember that a patient's claim that you or another provider caused some particular injury or problem should not automatically be assumed to be true. Although you do not have to argue the point with the patient, you also do not have to agree. Injuries have many causes and many stories behind them:

- Document the facts.
- Document what you see and do.
- Your role is to render nursing services, not to judge or give your opinion.
- Leave the determination of fault to the courts.
- Your actions and truthful documentation will be your best defense.

Did the Patient Suffer Damages or Injury? The last element that must be proved is that your breach of duty caused injury to the patient. This last element of malpractice can also be overlooked when the nurse becomes embroiled in the fact that a mistake has been made. For instance, in many cases of medication error, the patient is not permanently harmed, because a single dose of most medications will not cause a permanent change. This does not mean that medication errors should be taken lightly or that some medications cannot cause death with a single mistake. They can. It only means that it is very unlikely that a malpractice claim will be brought for a medication error that does not cause injury.

Damages can be viewed as the sum of money a court or jury awards as compensation for a tort action. **General damages** are those given for intangibles such as pain and suffering, disfigurement, interference with ordinary enjoyment of life, and loss of consortium (marital services) that are inherent in the injury itself (Guido, 2006). **Special damages** are the patient's out-of-pocket expenses such as medical care, lost wages, and rehabilitation costs. **Punitive damages** are those damages that seek to punish those whose conduct goes beyond normal malpractice. Claims in which this might occur are rare, but they involve issues such as changed medical records, lies being told to patients, or intentional misconduct while under the influence of alcohol or drugs. Such punitive awards can add millions of dollars to an otherwise low-damage claim. Some states have limited the amount for specific types of damages that a plaintiff can receive (Critical Thinking Box 20-3).

Does your state limit the amount of damages a plaintiff can receive?

For a malpractice plaintiff's attorney to take a claim to trial, it may cost that person more than $100,000, and this does not include the attorney's time. Malpractice claims take much expertise and are time-intensive (Larson, 2005). Because malpractice claims are brought on a contingency fee basis, the attorney will get paid only if he or she wins the claim. In this situation the damages must be greater than the costs to make the claim worthwhile. When worrying about an incident and whether a suit will result, it is helpful to understand what factors make claims worthwhile:

1. In the majority of claims, the most important factor involved with damages is **the age of the patient.** The younger the patient with a permanent injury, the longer will be the time of suffering, the costs of future medical care, the loss of wages or income, and the emotional loss to the family. Therefore to assess damages, the first question an attorney asks is the age and status of an individual. An 83-year-old widower who has a numb leg will not have a large claim for damages. He will not lose wages. He does not have to support a family. It is likely that he has other illnesses or physical problems that might contribute to difficulty with ambulating. His life expectancy is not great. On the other hand, a 30-year-old single mother with three dependent children who has made her living as a waitress might well have costly damages if a numb leg hinders her ability to walk and provide for her family. However, in recent years, claims by nursing home patients have become more common because of statutes involving abuse of "vulnerable adults." These statutes can give plaintiffs triple damages and other monetary awards, including the right to "punitive damages," thus making these claims very attractive to attorneys.

2. **The nature of the injury** is also a consideration in evaluating damages. Is the injury permanent? Is it one for which a jury will have great sympathy, as when there is a huge disfiguring facial scar? Is it one that demonstrates a blatant mistake such as surgery performed on the wrong limb?

3. Does the claim involve any act of **malicious misconduct** or an **intentional cover up?** Such acts inflame juries and can cause them to award punitive damages.

Again, the principles of good documentation can make the damages of a claim not worth pursuing. It is particularly important that there is accurate evidence of damages at the time the injury occurred. Any time there is an incident involving a patient, such as a fall, an immediate and thorough examination can greatly assist in substantiating the patient's condition and thus affect the awarding of damages. The examination and findings need to be accurately documented. Subsequent examinations and evaluations should be completed. Documentation of the patient's complaints, or lack of complaints, at the time of an incident can prove extremely beneficial. A simple "No complaints" or "Denies pain" could refute a patient's later claim that "I was terribly injured by the fall."

Sometimes when a clear mistake has been made that falls below the standard of care and has caused an injury, your attorney will admit negligence. This is often a relief to the nurse who does not wish to try to defend a mistake and/or not tell the truth. The case is then brought solely on the amount of damages. Often the patient's perception of the injury is greatly augmented. Usually, the patient will have to go through what is called an independent medical examination (IME) to substantiate injury.

Damages Applied to the Case Study. In Case Study 3, numbness of a limb may be difficult to prove. Nerve conduction studies may be performed in an independent medical examination to demonstrate that the injection could not have caused the neurological injury of which the patient complains. Numbness also does not mean lack of function and would not usually prevent any activity of daily living. Again, the age and status of the claimant would play an important role, as would your documentation of the patient's lack of complaints and ability to ambulate.

Who Might Have Liability (Responsibility) in a Claim?

■ CASE STUDY 4

You are a nurse working on a surgical unit in a hospital. One evening you are asked to float to pediatrics. The only experience you have had with children was when you were a student. A physician asks you to give digoxin to an infant and writes an order for 2 mL. This seems like a lot of medication to you, so you ask the head nurse on the unit about the dose. The head nurse assumes you are speaking about an oral dose of the medication and states that this is normal. You give the medication by injection and shortly thereafter the child's heart stops beating and he is coded. When you attempt to use an Ambu bag, it is not on the crash cart. The child eventually recovers; however, 21 years later, you receive notice that a young man is suing you for giving him the wrong dose of digoxin when he was an infant.

Personal Liability. There is often confusion about who can be held accountable for your actions as a nurse. You may hear things such as, "Don't worry, I'll take responsibility for this." Understand that in the eyes of the law, each individual is accountable for their own actions. There is no defense called "She made me do it." Even if you are not personally named in a lawsuit, you will be asked to give evidence regarding your involvement and will have to be able to defend your actions under oath. "I was just following orders" does not explain why you as a professional made a medication error. You are held to a professional standard of care to know about the medications you are administering, including the correct dose. In Case Study 4, you may be named and would most likely have liability.

Physician and Other Independent Practitioner Liability. For many years, physicians were seen as the "Captain of the Ship" and thus ultimately responsible for everything that happened to the patient. This doctrine is no longer true. Unfortunately, some physicians still mislead nurses by ordering them to do things and then assuring them that they will assume any risk involved. Although nurses do have a duty to follow physician's orders under most circumstances, this is never true if the nurse believes or has reason to believe that the order is unsafe for the patient or not within the nurse's scope of practice. In Case Study 1, receiving an order to give IV conscious sedation does not relieve the nurse of a duty to determine whether this is within his or her scope of practice. If not, the order must be refused. In Case Study 4, if the nurse did not know the correct dose of IV digoxin, there was a duty to look up the correct dose. It is also true that if the physician's order is wrong or done in a negligent manner such as in the case study, it does not relieve the physician from having liability in addition to the nurse.

In instances when a nurse is hired directly by a physician to work in an office practice, the physician, as the employer, can be held vicariously liable on a theory of ***respondeat superior.*** This is a Latin term meaning that "the master is responsible for acts of the servant," translated in modern terms to "the employer is responsible for the acts of the employee." The physician, then, rather than the nurse, may be named in the lawsuit. Remember, though, that you will still have to answer for your actions.

Another issue is what the nurse should accept as delegated or ordered by other independent health care practitioners, such as nurse practitioners (NPs), and physician assistants (PAs). States may have different rules about who can give orders to the RN.

The general rule is that the RN can accept orders from other licensed health care providers who are working within their scope of practice. To be sure about your state, contact the board of nursing. When accepting delegated duties, remember that you should only accept duties you are competent to carry out and that are within your scope of practice.

Supervisory Liability. Questions often arise regarding the nurse's responsibility for acts of those working under him or her. The standard of care for a supervisor is to act as a reasonable supervisor under the same or similar circumstances. A supervisor can be expected to ensure the following:

- The task was properly assigned to a worker competent to safely perform it.
- Adequate supervision was provided to the worker if needed.
- The nurse provided appropriate follow-up and evaluation of the delegated task.

As in Case Study 3, a supervisor could be expected to more closely supervise a float nurse or a recent graduate than someone who is an experienced nurse on a pediatric unit. It is also incumbent upon a person being supervised to ask for assistance if they are faced with a problem for which they lack the necessary skills to resolve. In Case Study 4, this was done, but the nurse administering the medication and the supervisor miscommunicated regarding the method or route of administration. How common do you think this is?

Delegation of nursing duties to unlicensed health care workers presents supervisory nurses with some special risks. Changes in health care delivery systems and financing are resulting in some unfamiliar categories of unlicensed caregivers with a wide variety of skills and expertise. Some boards of nursing have informed their licensees that each nurse remains personally liable for any task delegated to an unlicensed worker on the theory that the delegated task is considered the nurse's responsibility, rather than within the scope of practice of the unlicensed worker. Other boards of nursing have stated that they will apply to delegation the traditional standards for supervising any health care worker as described earlier.

Certain nursing responsibilities, such as nursing diagnosis, assessment, teaching, and some portions of planning, evaluation, and documentation should not be delegated to unlicensed staff. Contact the board of nursing in your state to better understand your responsibilities in the delegation of nursing duties.

Institutional Liability. As in the aforementioned case involving physician liability, health care institutions such as hospitals are usually sued under a theory of *respondeat superior* for the actions of their employees. Of course, an institution cannot do or not do any act that can cause a lawsuit except through its employees or agents. That is why almost all health care institutions carry insurance to cover the acts and omissions of their employees. Otherwise, a corporation could go bankrupt if sued. For the most part, institutions, not individual nurses, are named defendants in a lawsuit, but again this does not relieve the nurse from having to formally answer to the court for his or her own actions or inaction. An institution's policies or lack thereof is also a common claim in a lawsuit. For instance, there can be a claim in Case Study 4 that the institution should have had a policy on floating nurses to other units in the hospital and that such persons should never be given the responsibility of transcribing physician's orders. Additionally, in this case, there may be institutional liability through the pharmacy. If the pharmacy filled the wrong medication dose and there are systems in place to check dosages, the pharmacist and/or technician may also be brought into the claim through the institution. There are certainly more systems in place in most hospitals to prevent medication errors than ever before. When they all fail, many persons can be involved in the liability.

Student Liability. Nursing students have responsibility for their own actions and can be held liable (Guido, 2006). Again, the adage that "students practice under their instructor's license" is not true. As a student, you may have an instructor supervising you closely in the early stages of your education, but at the end of your program, it is likely that you will have less supervision. Student nurses at all times will be held to the standard of an RN for the tasks they perform (Guido, 2006). It is therefore important that students never accept assignments beyond their preparation and that they communicate frequently with their instructors for assistance and guidance.

Instructors are responsible for reasonable and prudent clinical supervision, a standard that may be higher than other worker supervision because of the student's lack of experience. An instructor could be held liable for inadequate supervision in determining that a student was competent to perform a skill, which she indeed was not (Shinn, 2001).

> It is important to know your status under such circumstances in your state, and/or if you have immunity and/or are covered by malpractice insurance.

Instructors and preceptors need to remember that the level of expertise of individual students may vary, and the standard used to evaluate the student's performance usually requires more supervision than some more experienced workers may need.

What Defenses Might Be Available in Malpractice Claims?

If the plaintiff in a malpractice claim does not prove each of the elements previously discussed, the defense can ask for a dismissal of the claim by making various motions (formal requests) to the court. There are several other issues that may have an effect on the outcome of a malpractice claim.

A **statute of limitations** is a law that sets a time period after an event during which a lawsuit must be filed. States have different statutes and case law surrounding this time limit. Usually, the limit is measured from the time of the event or incident, last date of treatment, or the time the event was discovered (or should have been discovered). For minors, some states allow the time to be counted from the time they reach majority (usually 18 years old), unless a suit has already been brought on their behalf by parents or others. Therefore, in Case Study 4, a suit could be brought 2 or 3 years after a person turns 18 years (majority) for an injury occurring as an infant. Other states do not permit this delay. Lack of mental competence will also delay the time requirements in some states.

Failure to file the lawsuit within the statute of limitations time results in the loss of the right to sue. This can be considered a defense, because filing after the date allows the defendants to have the case dismissed. It is important to know, however, that in most states, the statute starts running when the patient knows of the injury. If there is any type of cover-up regarding an incident, the statute will not run.

Proving that the patient assumed the risk of harm or that the patient contributed to the harm by his or her actions provides another type of defense. **Assumption of the risk** defense states that plaintiffs are partially responsible for consequences if they understood the risks involved when they proceeded with the action (Guido, 2006). An example would be a mentally competent patient who has been warned to use a call light but instead crawls out of bed and thus injures herself.

Contributory negligence is an older doctrine that was at one time an "all or nothing" rule. Plaintiffs who had any part in the adverse outcome were barred from compensation. Today, most jurisdictions use a comparative negligence theory and reduce the money award by the injured party's responsibility for the ultimate harm done (Guido, 2006). One case found that a patient could be negligent and thus be at least partially responsible by (1) refusing to follow advice or instructions; (2) causing a delay in treatment or not returning for follow-up; (3) furnishing false, misleading, or incomplete information to a health care provider; or (4) causing the injury that results in the need for medical care (*Harvey v. Mid-Coast Hospital,* 1999).

What Evidence Can Help Me in a Lawsuit?

The Medical Record. An estimated one in four malpractice cases are decided on the basis of what is in the medical record (Sullivan, 2004). In many instances, you can become a nurse hero or be in deep trouble based on the accuracy and timeliness of your documentation in the medical record. One of the most important tools for all providers in a malpractice claim is the medical record. This is the first piece of evidence asked for by the attorney for the plaintiff. The nurses' notes are often the first part of the record to be examined. Their integrity, accuracy, and completeness will make a claim defensible or indefensible. Good documentation, therefore, is one of the best defensive actions a nurse can take. By recording the care administered, the specific time it was administered, the patient's response, and the overall status of the patient's condition, the nurse can demonstrate that the standard of care was met (Figure 20-1).

Your defense attorney will use the medical record extensively and will make a timeline of events that surrounded the incident. The most effective defense is to "put on a play" for a jury regarding what occurred to demonstrate all that was done for the patient. A good educational exercise is to take any patient's chart and see whether you can present a play regarding what happened to that patient during your care.

Some nurses have advocated the maintaining of personal notes regarding the circumstances of a particular incident. The rationale for this is so they can carefully review the notes; it will also assist them to more clearly recall the situation should they be required to do so. However, these notes are also discoverable by the plaintiff's side and may be damaging to your case. Personal notes are frequently written on an emotional level. In most states what you write, unless to your attorney or under a peer-review privilege, will have to be produced. Personal documentation about what others did or did not do or what you think they did wrong or should have done will almost certainly come back to haunt you. Documentation regarding an incident should be

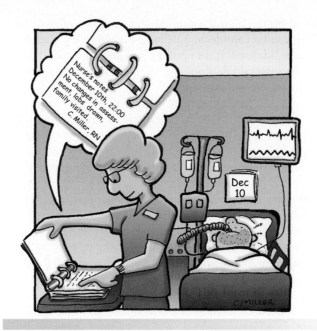

FIGURE 20-1

It is critical that the nurse's notes reflect the current condition of the patient.

thoroughly and factually done in the medical record and not in personal records or a diary (Figure 20-2).

There is an adage that states, "If it is not documented, it wasn't done." In reality, it is simply difficult to prove something was done if there is no documentation and the plaintiff claims it was not done. It is then a "he said/she said" type of argument. A more accurate statement might be "If it is documented, it was done." Once it is documented at the time of the event, there is a strong presumption that the documentation is accurate and whatever a patient says to the contrary is simply self-serving. That is why it is so important to document extensively, accurately, and very factually in the medical record (Box 20-3). This is especially true when there is an adverse event.

Forms often provide a difficult problem for defense attorneys when they are not completed. A blank space on the form or a box that is not checked when it appears that the space or box was to indicate the performance of a needed therapy can be very detrimental to the nurse involved.

> Do not have forms in the record if they are not routinely completed in a correct manner.

Most institutions are in the process of implementing the electronic medical record (EMR) or electronic health record (EHR). The federal government is encouraging all health care agencies to make the transition to an EHR by 2014. The conversion to an EHR will significantly improve the accessibility, quality, and efficiency of health care (NLN, 2008). The cardinal rules of

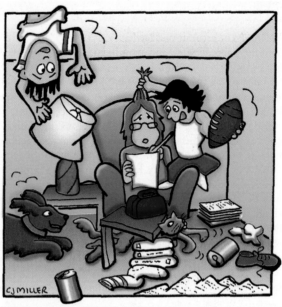

FIGURE 20-2

Charting in the home setting can be challenging.

documentation still apply, but additional safeguards will have to be considered. This is especially true when some of the health records are paper and some electronic. Both records will have to be accessed, coordinated, and made complete to manage and safeguard the patient. It is believed that the EHR will promote more accurate and safe record keeping. For instance, the problem of illegible handwriting will be eliminated. Additionally, certain programs have automatic safeguards to catch errors. It is therefore tempting to think that EHRs will solve all problems (Sullivan, 2004). Of course, this is not true as long as there are humans entering information. No jury will appreciate blame being placed on a computer glitch. NLN has issued a position paper that calls for nursing programs to prepare nursing graduates with up-to-date knowledge in the critical areas of computer literacy, information literacy, and informatics (NLN, 2008). Education and problem solving to ensure safe EHRs and effective computer documentation systems must continue as always.

How Can I Avoid a Malpractice Claim?

There are certain situations that involve a high risk for a lawsuit against nurses. These situations most often relate to patient safety, improper treatment, problems with monitoring, medication errors, and failing to follow proper procedures and policies.

Medication Errors. A study by the Institute of Medicine (IOM) in 2006 reported that medication errors harmed 1.5 million people every year. The additional medical cost of treating drug related injuries in the hospital was at least 3.5 billion per year. The study did not indicate whether the source of the error was nurses, physicians, and/or pharmacists. The reporting

---

BOX 20-3   Guidelines for Defensive Charting

- All entries should be accurate and factual.
- Make corrections appropriately and according to agency or hospital policies. Do not ever obliterate or destroy any information that is or has been in the chart.
- If there is information that should have been charted and was not, the nurse should make a "late entry," noting the time the charting actually occurred and the specific time the charting reflects. Example: "10/13/03, 10:00 late entry, charting to reflect that on 10/13/03 …"
- All identified patient problems, nursing actions taken, and patient responses should be noted. Do not describe a patient problem without including the nursing actions taken and the patient response.
- It is often as important to document why you did not do something that you would routinely do, as why you did do something. For instance, "Pt. refused to ambulate because of …"
- Be as objective as possible in charting. Rather than charting "The patient tolerated the procedure well," chart the specific parameters checked to determine that conclusion. Example: "Ambulated, tolerated well" would be more effective if charted "Ambulated complete length of hall, no shortness of breath noted, pulse rate at 98, respirations at 22."
- Each page of the chart should contain the current date and time. Frequently, chart forms are stamped ahead of time. Each time you enter information on a new page, make sure it reflects the current time of charting.
- Each page of the chart should include the full name and professional designation of every person making an entry on that page.
- Follow through with who saw the patient and what measures were initiated. Particularly note when the physician visited; if you had to call a physician for a problem, record the physician's response, the nursing actions, and the patient's response. If orders were received, be sure they are signed according to policy. This is especially important if you had to make several calls to the physician.
- Make sure your notes are legible and clearly reflect the information you intended. It is a good idea to read over your nurses' notes from the previous day to see whether they still make sense and accurately portray the status of the patient. If the notes do not make sense to you the next day, imagine how difficult it would be to decipher the information at a later date.
- Pertinent notes from other providers should also be reviewed. The medical record is for communication. A jury will never understand if team members are not coordinating efforts and thought.

---

committee found that medication errors are common at every stage, from the writing of the prescription, to the filling of the prescription, to the administration of a drug and the monitoring of the patient's response (IOM, 2006). Claims involving medication errors are augmented when the nurse fails to record the medication administration properly, fails to recognize side effects or contraindications, or fails to know a patient's allergies. Any initiative that improves patient safety also lowers the chance of someone being sued. At the same time, it sets a standard on which the standard of care may rest and thus becomes important for every nurse to know and follow.

The nurse's ability to listen to a patient or family member who notices that a medication is new, or recheck when anything such as color or amount seems unusual, may prevent a serious error. Many nurses feel rushed by the amount of work they are expected to accomplish and do not want to take extra time for anything. Making this check a priority will prove to be time well spent. Dealing with an error and the consequences to the patient will be longer and more painful.

BOX 20-4 Tips for Being at Your Best When Administering Medications

- Be very careful if you have been interrupted during a task. This is very common in nursing. Many accidents happen because nurses did not remember what they had been doing or where they were in a task. Shift change is also a common time for mistakes.
- If you are fatigued, you are more likely to make mistakes. Follow all the steps thoroughly when you are tired. This is one of the reasons that double or long shifts may not be wise.
- Listen to your patients. Often they will tell you if what you are planning to do is different or unusual. Being able to take the time to do a second check may save you and your patient trouble.
- Never do a procedure you do not know how to do at the appropriate standard of performance. It is better to be embarrassed by admitting you need help or supervision than to risk hurting someone.
- Never be afraid to admit you made a mistake. Corrective action may stop or at least reduce harm.
- Keep current and up to date in your practice knowledge base. An article in a professional journal may keep a lawsuit away.
- Do not rush when you are extra busy. Set priorities on what must be done, and do it carefully.

Although many medication errors do not cause permanent or serious damage to patients, there are certain medications that can. TJC standards require each institution to identify high-risk medications used in the institution and to initiate safety procedures for managing these medications. Medications, such as chemotherapy, should be stored separately, ordered on a special form to verify dosages, and attached to protocols that help ensure safe administration by qualified staff with specialized training. In TJC's NPSGs for 2010, there are specific guidelines for safety in administering anticoagulants and in communicating without interruptions to other health care providers on the patient's status, hands-off report, and when receiving telephone and verbal orders (TJC, 2010).

Whenever a medication error occurs, the source of the error and the system failure should be carefully investigated. Most institutions are now attempting to ensure that punitive measures are not attached to medication errors. This is to facilitate reports to be made and systems involving the team of ordering practitioner, dispensing pharmacy, and administering nurse to have checks and balances to prevent any team member from causing harm to a patient (Kohn et al, 2000) (Box 20-4). TJC also requires that health care organizations have a plan for responding to adverse drug events and medication errors (e.g., send reports to the Medication Error Reporting Program operated cooperatively by U.S. Pharmacopeia [USP] and the Institute for Safe Medication Practices) (IOM, 2006).

Provide a Safe Environment. Patient safety is being more and more recognized as a duty of health care institutions. Providing a safe environment and preventing falls are included in TJC's 2010 NPSGs (TJC, 2010). Ensuring patient safety has many aspects. Nurses sometimes do not recognize the multiple roles that they must play in this area. They are responsible for knowing how equipment should work and not using it if it is not functioning correctly; removing obvious hazards such as chemicals, which might be mistaken for medications; and making the environment free of hazards such as inappropriately placed furniture or equipment and spills on the floor. An additional preventive measure is knowing how to document correctly if an incident occurs, so that there cannot be a doubt regarding the facts of what happened and all you did to protect the patient.

CRITICAL THINKING BOX 20-4   What fall protocols have you observed in your clinical settings? How are they the same, and how are they different? How are fall protocols in acute care hospital settings different from long-term care settings?

Patient Falls. TJC has specific safety goals that are directed toward preventing harm to patients resulting from falls (TJC, 2010). These may include falls out of bed, slips and falls from slipping on something spilled on the floor, or falls due to inadequate nurse supervision of the patient. Falls, particularly repeated falls, are a major source of both physical and psychological injury to older patients (Tideliksaar, 1998).

Much time and effort has been spent in an attempt to change patient care so that falls do not occur. Proposals coming out of such efforts range from total lack of restraints (Walker, 1992), to environmental modifications (Tideliksaar, 1998), to decreasing the number of certain types of medications (Haumschild et al, 2003). It is important to keep up with the latest information in order not to be caught without defenses in a malpractice claim (Critical Thinking Box 20-4).

Nurses are best able to defend themselves in these cases when their institution has a policy regarding protecting vulnerable patients against falls, sometimes called a "fall protocol." These policies establish levels of risk in patients, such as age, confusion, sedation, and steps the nurse must take to protect the patient, such as side rails, soft restraints, or bed position. If the nurse follows such a protocol, it is difficult for a plaintiff to prove that the nurse fell below a standard of care. In developing such protocols, however, it is important to know the laws in your state, Federal CMS guidelines, and TJC standards regarding restraints. Unnecessary and unsafe restraining of patients has become the focus of public and private attention, and restraint injuries can also be the basis of legal action (Medscape Medical News, 2000).

Documentation is extremely important when a patient falls. The following should be considered:

- Document factually how the fall was discovered, where the patient was found, and the facts surrounding the fall. An example is to document that the patient was found beside the bed, with the side rails up and the bed in the low position.
- Document the nursing assessment data, any obvious injuries, and nursing actions to maintain patient safety.
- Document what the patient says in regard to the fall. A statement such as "I know you told me to put on the call light, but you all seemed so busy that I didn't want to bother you," can be of great benefit to the nurse. Of course, a patient's statement "I put on the call light, but nobody came" can have the opposite effect.
- Document whom you notified, such as the physician or the family.
- Document what was done for the patient, such as an examination, radiographs, orientation to surroundings, monitoring after the incident, restraints, and assistance with further ambulation.
- Document your adherence to any policies of the hospital regarding vulnerable patients or those at risk for falls.

In *Shaw v. Plantation Management*, a nurse found a patient on the floor with a puddle of liquid next to him. The patient stated that the liquid was urine from another patient and that this caused him to fall. The nurse assessed the patient and got him the medical attention that he needed. The patient later died after surgery for a broken hip. The nurse did not know what the liquid was, and she did not know whether or not the patient had actually urinated after he fell. The nurse only charted what she had actually seen and what she did. Her clear documentation later prevented the patient's family from being able to prove that the incident was caused by any negligence on behalf of the facility (*Shaw v. Plantation Management*, 2009).

Equipment Failure. Today many nurses feel that they spend more time nursing equipment than patients. This can be true. What some nurses do not understand is that there is a certain standard of care connected with equipment. It must be used as directed by the manufacturer, and the nurse has a duty to know what that is and to follow such directions. There is also a duty to make sure that the equipment is properly maintained and that records are kept of this maintenance. The equipment needs to be working properly and should not be used when a known defective condition exists. Additionally, the device must be available for use. For instance, in Case Study 4, the fact that the Ambu bag was not available can be viewed as a liability for either the nurse responsible for checking crash carts, or the institution for not seeing that the carts are checked.

When there is a failure of a device or piece of equipment and a patient is injured, the focus should of course initially be on helping the patient. After that, it is extremely important that the device (e.g., catheter, pump, instrument) be sequestered and a clear record of its handling (chain of custody) be maintained. In a lawsuit, the nurse will need to prove that equipment failure, rather than human error, caused the injury. Part of that proof will rest in the piece of equipment itself. Therefore one of the most important aspects of the defense will be to not lose or let go of the equipment or device before it is thoroughly evaluated by a neutral party after an incident. Often the manufacturer will ask for the equipment, but their interests might be adverse to yours to prove user error rather than equipment failure. Information regarding the failure can be given, but never let the device or equipment out of the custody of the institution. In addition, the nurse should adhere to any institutional policies regarding incidents involving equipment failure.

Nurses may also have a duty to be sure their institution complies with the Safe Medical Device Act of 1990. This federal law requires that all medical device-related adverse incidents be reported to manufacturers and in the case of death, to the U.S. Food and Drug Administration (FDA), within 10 days. The purpose of this act is to protect the public from devices that may be defective (Guido, 2006).

■ CASE STUDY 5

A 67-year-old woman with chronic obstructive pulmonary disease is having increasingly difficult respirations, increased cyanosis, and increased anxiety. She tells you she just cannot breathe. You have done all the measures for which you currently have orders, without her getting relief. It is 2 AM. You call the physician. She orders Valium 10 mg intramuscularly now. Even as a recent graduate, you know that Valium is contraindicated in a patient with this respiratory status. You call your supervisor, who tells you that Dr. Jones is a good physician and must know what she is doing. What should you do?

Failure to Adequately Assess, Monitor, and Obtain Assistance. Most often, the nurse should not delegate to another the responsibility of assessing and evaluating patient care and progress. If some portions of this duty are done by others (e.g., another RN, LPN/LVN, unlicensed personnel), the nurse primarily responsible for the care of the patient must still be aware of the findings and confirm them when they indicate a change in patient condition or progress. Documentation of the changes and events surrounding the changes is critical. The 2010 NPSGs from TJC specifically address improving the effectiveness of communication between caregivers when reporting changes in a patient's condition. Effective communication includes clear documentation of critical events.

In Case Study 5, there may also be liability for failure to challenge an inappropriate order. These areas are uncomfortable for many experienced nurses, not just for the recent graduate. Frequently, these situations involve challenging a physician or other health care professional. They require that the nurse have current and accurate information. They also require the difficult balance between assertiveness and diplomacy.

> It is not enough to identify problems. The nurse must identify the problems and contact the physician or other individuals to get appropriate care and follow up the chain of command as deemed necessary.

Of most help in situations such as Case Study 5 is a policy that clearly delineates the chain of command for the institution. With a policy in place, the nurse can be clear about who must be notified about a potentially problematic order, and it can be documented appropriately. It is important that the nurse be protected from any retaliation in such instances by the institution that stands to lose if the patient's safety is not put first.

Accurate documentation of the nursing assessment and of frequent monitoring will be required to prove what you have done. Flow charts and forms can be timesaving devices in this area. Electronic communications now make such time-consuming documentation more readily available. This documentation is especially important in the critical care setting and in the obstetric suite. The attachment of accurate times to such monitoring activities will be your best defense tool in many malpractice claims.

Failure to Adequately Communicate. Perhaps the most important role of everyone on the health care team is to adequately communicate. The patient's total care rests on this communication, whether it is verbal or written in the medical record.

> The most frequent claim against nurses in this area is the failure to communicate changes in the patient's condition to a professional with a need to know.

This is especially true in acute care settings during the night hours, as in Case Study 5. Communication is not always welcomed in the middle of the night and is impaired because it is not face to face and because the receiver may not be fully awake and alert. TJC now requires a verification "read back" of all verbal and telephone orders (not limited to medication orders) by the person taking the order and the use of a standardized set of abbreviations, acronyms, and symbols throughout the organization. Thorough documentation of the communication will protect the nurse, but it should not be done defensively or thought of as a substitute for proper care.

Communication with certain hearing- and speech-impaired patients and with ethnically and culturally diverse patients will often provide a challenge to good nursing care. The Americans with Disabilities Act is a federal statute that has requirements for institutions rendering health care to have certain translators available for key health care interactions. The failure to do so may put the institution at risk for fines and penalties (*Freydel v. New York Hospital,* 2000).

Failure to Report. States have many statutes that require health care providers to report certain incidences or occurrences. If the provider fails to report as required and a person is injured, there can be negligence per se, and no expert testimony will be needed to prove a case. In addition, both institutional and professional licensure can be affected. It is important that nurses be aware of the reporting statutes in the state in which they are practicing. In some states, it is not only a duty, but also the law to report certain incidences. The following are examples of such statutes involving a duty to report.

- A duty to report other health care professionals whose behaviors are unprofessional and/or could cause harm to the public. This includes drug and alcohol abuse.
- A duty to report evidence of child or adult or elder abuse and neglect, including any acts of a sexual nature against vulnerable (i.e., anesthetized) patients.
- A duty to report certain communicable diseases.
- A duty to report certain deaths under suspicious circumstances, including deaths during surgery.
- A duty to report certain types of injuries that are or could be caused by violence.
- A duty to report evidence of Medicare fraud.
- Emergency Medical Treatment and Labor Act (EMTALA) violations.

The nurse needs to know what areas must be reported, who should report, how the report should be accomplished, and to whom a report should be made. Institutional policies and nurse practice acts on these topics are invaluable. In *State v. Brown,* criminal charges were brought against an emergency room nurse who failed to report suspected child abuse to a physician or agency when a 2-year-old boy was brought in with suspicious bruises. The trial court dismissed the charges on the grounds that the Missouri statute was unconstitutionally vague as to the term "reasonable cause to suspect"; however, the Missouri Supreme Court later reversed that decision, reinstating criminal charges against the nurse (*State v. Brown,* 2004).

Many nurses are afraid to report their employers, other professionals, or other agencies because of the possibility of retaliatory action against them. Most mandatory reporting statutes give immunity to those who report in good faith. Some states have specific "whistleblower statutes" that not only protect nurses from retaliatory action but also may reward them. The content of these statutes differs from state to state, so the nurse must find out whether one exists in his or her state of practice and learn what protection is provided. A federal statute, the False Claims Act, provides protection under certain situations for reporting Medicare fraud. Additionally, federal compliance standards require that institutions maintain a mechanism to report unlawful activities such as a "hotline" where problems can be reported anonymously. In response to such reports, institutions must demonstrate that they responded appropriately and disciplined all individuals engaged in the illegal activities (Critical Thinking Box 20-5) (Green, 2000).

CRITICAL THINKING BOX 20-5   Which states have "whistleblower" protection?

INTENTIONAL TORTS

Intentional torts are civil claims that are closely related to criminal acts in that they involve intent to do the wrong. Instead of seeking to put the defendant in jail, however, these claims attempt to right the wrong by compensating the plaintiff. These lawsuits are less common than malpractice claims, but the following can be brought against a nurse.

Assault and battery are the legal terms that are applied to nonconsensual threat of touch (assault) or the actual touching (battery). Of course, in health care, there is a lot of touching. Permission to do this touching is usually implied when the patient seeks medical care. Sometimes, however, a patient refuses to have certain procedures done or has certain procedures done without giving an informed consent. The Louisiana Supreme Court awarded $25,000 to a patient's family in a lawsuit wherein the nurses had ignored the patient's refusal of a Foley catheter. The patient was ultimately injured in the process of removing the catheter, and the Court determined that the nurses had committed battery by performing an invasive procedure against his wishes (*Robertson v. Provident House*, 1991). Also, a patient may wish to leave an institution "against medical advice" (AMA). If nurses use physical restraint or touching to keep this patient from leaving, these actions can lead to a civil claim of assault and battery.

False imprisonment means making someone wrongfully feel that he or she cannot leave a place. It is often associated with assault and battery claims. This can happen in a health care setting through the use of physical or chemical restraints or the threat of physical or emotional harm if a patient leaves an institution. Threats such as "If you don't stay in your bed, I'll have to sedate you" constitute false imprisonment. This tort might also involve telling a patient that he or she may not leave the emergency department until the bill is paid. Another example is using restraints or threatening to use them on competent patients to make them do what you want them to do against their wishes. Unless you are very clearly protecting the safety of others, you may not restrain a competent adult (Critical Thinking Box 20-6) (Guido, 2006).

Even in a psychiatric case in which someone is thought to be a danger to self or others, there are many very specific state and federal laws to follow. The challenge, of course, is preventing the patient from committing suicide while also maintaining the patient's rights to liberty. This is not an easy balance, and very specific policies are needed to give legal guidance for those in the many difficult situations of the emergency department and psychiatric nursing. There are also many restrictions on the appropriate use of both hard and soft restraints and elevated scrutiny on their use in long-term care facilities (Tideliksaar, 1998). Claims of elder abuse have been filed for the misuse of restraints. You must be aware of the policies in your agency and state statutory requirements.

Defamation (libel and slander) refers to causing damage to someone else's reputation. If the means of transmitting the damaging information is written, it is called **libel;** if it is oral or spoken, it is called **slander.** The damaging information must be communicated to a third person. The actions likely to result in a defamation charge are situations in which inaccurate information

CRITICAL THINKING BOX 20-6   In what situations would it be acceptable to restrain a patient?

from the medical record is reported, such as in Case Study 1, or speaking negatively about your coworkers (supervisors, doctors, other nurses).

Two defenses to defamation accusations are *truth* and *privilege*. If the statement is true, it is not actionable under this doctrine. However, it is often difficult to define truth, because it may be a matter of perspective. It is better to avoid that issue by not making negative statements about other people unnecessarily. An example of privilege would be required good-faith reporting to child protective services of possible child abuse or statements made during a peer review process. If statements made during these processes are made without maliciousness, state statutes often protect the reporter from any civil liability for defamation.

Recovery in defamation claims usually requires that the plaintiff submit proof of being injured—for instance, loss of money or job. Some categories, such as fitness to practice one's profession, do not require such proof, as they are considered sufficiently damaging without it. Comments about the quality of a nurse's work or a physician's skills in diagnosing illness would fit in this category. You can avoid this claim by steering clear of gossip and/or writing negative documents about others in the heat of the moment and without adequate facts.

Invasion of Privacy and Breaches of Privilege and Confidentiality

A good general rule in relationship to torts involving the sharing of patient information is to always ask yourself, "Do I have the patient's consent to share this information, or is it necessary to the health care services for this patient?" If the answer to either is "no," then the information should not be communicated.

The public's attention has been recently focused on privacy because of new privacy regulations under an older federal law called the Health Insurance Portability and Accountability Act of 1996 (HIPAA). These specific privacy regulations became effective in April 2003 and include an elaborate system for ensuring privacy for individually identifiable health information. Information used to render treatment, payment, or health care operations does not require the patient's specific consent for its use. This includes processes such as quality assurance activities, legal activities, risk management, billing, and utilization review. However, the rules require that the disclosure be the "minimum necessary," and a clear understanding of what information can be shared under this exception is necessary (Annas, 2003). Notice must be given to the patient of how the information will be used. All nurses working in health care must be aware of this law and how their institutions specifically comply with it.

Another aspect of HIPAA has to do with electronic information and security measures necessary to make sure that protected patient information is not accessed by those without a right or need to know. These rules came into effect in April 2005. Each institution must have data security policies and technologies in place based on their own "risk assessment." Many institutions will now require that any health information transmitted under open networks, such as the Internet, telephones, and wireless communication networks, be encrypted (coded).

Many states have physician-patient privilege laws that protect communications between caregivers and their patients. This enables information to pass freely between physician and patient without concern that it will be shared with those who do not need to know it. This includes law enforcement. The privilege usually extends to information about a patient in the medical record or obtained in the course of providing care. Most states extend physician-patient privilege to nurses and sometimes to other health care givers as well. This privilege belongs to the patient, not the health care giver, which means that only the patient can decide to give it up.

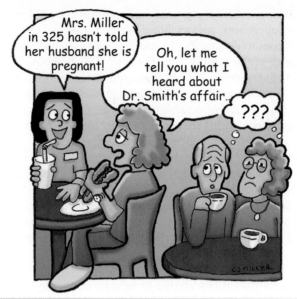

FIGURE 20-3
Maintaining confidentiality is both an ethical and a legal consideration in nursing.

As a professional it is important to observe **confidentiality** when talking about patients at home and at work (Figure 20-3). Nurses must be very careful to keep information about the patient or from the patient to themselves and to share it only with health care workers who must know the information to plan or give proper care. This is often difficult to do, as seen in Case Study 1.

EHRs and national clearing houses for health information present significant confidentiality issues. Such technologies offer many advantages, including easier and broader access to needed information and more legible documentation. These same advantages also present concerns because it is more difficult to ensure confidentiality. Many hospitals and agencies already have policies and procedures in place, such as access codes, limited screen time, and computers placed in locations that promote privacy. The nurse is still responsible for the protection of confidentiality when computers, faxes, e-mail, or other rapid communication techniques are used.

A similar cause of action is for **invasion of privacy.** This cause of action can apply to several behaviors, such as photographing a procedure and showing it without the patient's consent, going through a patient's belongings without consent, or talking about a patient's private life publicly.

Miscellaneous Intentional Torts and Other Civil Rights Claims Involved with Employment

The aforementioned torts and others can be relevant to nurses in regard to their employment. These intentional torts can be brought personally against the nurse and are not usually covered by any insurance. **Tortious interference with contract** is a claim that someone maliciously interfered with a person's contractual (often employment) rights. This can occur, for instance, if a nurse attempts to get another nurse fired through giving false or misleading facts to a supervisor. **Intentional infliction of emotional distress** is described by its name and can also be attached to malicious acts in the employment setting. These and certain civil rights claims such as **sexual harassment** and **discrimination** are both rights and potential liabilities for every person in the work force. Although beyond the scope of this text, policies and information regarding these issues demand further investigation by each health care employee to ensure that their rights and the rights of others are not violated.

What Is a Defense to Intentional Torts?

Informed Consent. Consent is usually a complete defense to all of the aforementioned intentional torts. You cannot have a claim for assault and battery if the patient has given consent for the procedure. Likewise, there can be no invasion of privacy if the patient has given consent to share confidential information with someone else, such as his or her lawyer.

There is much confusion about informed consent in that many people believe that it must be a piece of paper with "Informed Consent" written on it. This is not true.

Informed consent in the health care setting is a process whereby a patient is informed of:
1. The nature of the proposed care, treatment, services, medications, interventions, or procedures;
2. The potential benefits, risks, or side effects, including potential problems related to recuperation;
3. The likelihood of achieving care, treatment, and service goals;
4. Reasonable alternatives and their respective risks and benefits including the alternative of refusing all interventions (TJC, 2008a).

After being thus informed, the patient then gives consent for the procedure to be done. The piece of paper is simply evidence that the informed consent process has taken place.

The nurse's role in the consent process is often confusing. Remember that it is ultimately the responsibility of the person doing the procedure to provide the basic explanation of its risks, benefits, and alternatives. In regard to most procedures and operations, this means the physician. However, in some settings, the nurse is part of an educational process involving videos, booklets, handouts, and other aids to the patient's understanding.

As nurses perform more invasive procedures, the process of informing the patient of what is to occur is the nurse's.

For surgeries and other physician-performed procedures, nurses may be asked "to get the consent." Be clear about what this means. In essence, it means to witness the patient's voluntary signature on a form that should be filled out by the person performing the procedure. That is all. However, as a witness to a signature, documentation of the patient's level of understanding, or the patient's refusal to receive information, or reluctance to have the procedure done, is critical to the witnessing role.

Consent forms must be signed when a patient is considered able or competent to make informed decisions and before the procedure is done. This means that the form must be signed before the administration of preprocedure medications, which often contain narcotics or other mind-altering drugs. Nurses are sometimes asked to obtain a patient's signature consenting to a procedure that has not yet been explained. The nurse is told that the physician will explain the procedure when the patient arrives to the procedure area and that for convenience it is better to have all forms signed prior to sending the patient. As an advocate for the patient and in order to protect your license, never obtain a patient's consent to a procedure that has not been fully explained to him or her.

The patient is the only person who may give consent if he or she is competent. Competency (also called "capacity") is defined differently from state to state, and the nurse should be aware of how it is defined in his or her state of practice. Competency is presumed, and therefore any claim of incompetence would have to be proved. Some situations may require special consideration. An example would be a patient suffering from "sundowning" syndrome who shows no signs of cognitive impairment during the day but is quite confused and/or agitated throughout the night. Although the patient may verbalize understanding of an upcoming procedure and you believe that he is currently competent to sign a consent form, his competency could possibly be brought into question in a malpractice case if the record reflects periods of confusion.

Advance Directives. It is important to allow patients to direct the course of their care and treatment whenever possible; however, they must be protected from making harmful decisions when their cognitive status is unclear or fluctuates. States differ with regard to how consent can be given if the patient is incompetent or lacks capacity to make medical decisions. Advance directives such as a medical power of attorney or a living will may give information about the patient's wishes. These documents allow individuals to prepare for possible incompetence in advance by formalizing their wishes about their further health care decisions in writing. The living will is used to allow a competent adult to direct what he or she wishes in regard to health care upon becoming incompetent. This may include that the person does not want any unusual medical procedures or lifesaving equipment used to prolong life.

Often used in conjunction with the living will is the "durable" or "medical" power of attorney. This document allows the competent adult to appoint a specific person to authorize care if he or she becomes incompetent. The durable power of attorney does not usually become effective until a person loses competency. This document may be used in conjunction with or without a living will (see Chapter 19 for more information on advance directives). Congress has passed the Patient Self-Determination Act of 1990 requiring hospitals to inform their patients of the availability of advance directives. State law defines the required wording for these documents and any other formalities necessary in their preparation. Because patients must be educated on these laws and documents, so should nurses. If not, you could be caught in violation of law at a crucial moment of life and death.

If a family challenges a living will or a medical power of attorney, a nurse will need to go through the administrative chain of command. A general rule is for nurses to follow the advance directives unless or until there is a court order to do otherwise. This means that families need to obtain legal services and go to court to overturn or challenge these documents. All persons, no matter what their age, should complete advance directives. The Terri Schiavo case is a sad demonstration of the difficulties faced by families when there are no documented advance directives and family members differ in beliefs about what should or should not be done. Questions then arise as to whether acts or omissions of health care providers prolong life or prolong the dying process. Judges are certainly not the preferred ultimate decision makers.

When a patient does not have an advance directive and is incompetent, there are also state laws that give guidance regarding who can act as a *surrogate decision maker*. Parents must usually sign for minor children. Spouses or immediate family members may sign for unconscious adults. In other instances, if no one is available or designated, a court can appoint someone for the purpose of medical decisions in a very short time. Informed consent is not required if the procedure is necessary to save a life and is done during an emergency. A special consent under stricter standards applies to research studies, and often surrogates may not be able to make such decisions (Truog, 2002).

Competent patients may always decline to give consent for a procedure, even if doing so may have serious consequences for their health status. This legal standard respects the fundamental liberty interest in personal autonomy protected by American jurisprudence (Moore, 1999). In certain instances, pregnant women may not be permitted to refuse a treatment if doing so will result in serious harm to the fetus. Such a case should be referred to risk management and resolved before the procedure is done. Consent may be withdrawn at any time before the procedure.

Documentation of informed refusal should be accurate, complete, and in accordance with the policies and procedures for your facility. It should include the results of a mental status assessment to show that the patient was neurologically and psychologically capable of refusing treatment. Clearly document what information was provided to the patient, quoting the patient's reason(s) for refusing treatment, any questions he or she may have, and your responses (Smith, 2004).

CRIMINAL ACTIONS

Nurses who violate specific criminal statutes (such as those having to do with illegal drug use, negligent homicide, and assault and battery) risk criminal prosecution. Conviction of certain types of crimes must be reported to the state board of nursing and will usually result in a review of licensure status. You must be aware of the rules in the state in which you practice.

What Criminal Acts Pose a Risk to the Nurse?

Theft and Misappropriation of Property
- Protect patient's property by thoroughly documenting and locking up all valuables upon admission to the facility.
- Keep all items and property owned by the facility at the facility. This includes tape, bandages, and pens to name a few.

Sometimes, nurses fail to adequately protect a patient's property and thus open themselves up to claims of theft. Many patients bring valuables to health care facilities or think that they do. Clear notice to the patients before admittance to leave valuables at home is helpful. A thorough and documented list of property upon admission is imperative to prevent such claims, as is the locking up of valuables. When dentures and other property have not been adequately stored or monitored, the nurse may be held responsible.

Another aspect of this problem is theft from the employer. Because of the extensive and costly nature of this problem, many employers have developed elaborate systems to try to discourage theft. With an ever-increasing focus on lowering health care costs, those related to employee theft will not be tolerated. Occasionally, nurses accidentally leave the job with tape, bandages, or other supplies in their pockets. These should be returned. Better yet, establishing a routine of checking your pockets before leaving for home will help reduce this risk. No employer's property should ever be intentionally taken by a nurse.

Nursing Practice Violations. Scope-of-practice violations that result in the death of a patient may be the result of nurses doing tasks or procedures that have not been accepted by the state board of nursing as within the appropriate scope for nurses or doing actions that have been approved for advanced practice nurses only. In some states these violations and other possible violations of the nurse practice act are misdemeanors, but in other states they may be felonies.

In rare cases, charges of murder or negligent homicide may be filed against the nurse (Kowalski & Horner, 1998). In November 2000, the State of Hawaii convicted an individual of manslaughter in the death of a nursing home patient for permitting the progression of decubitus ulcers without seeking appropriate medical help (Di Maio & Di Maio, 2002). In November 2006, the Wisconsin State Attorney General's Office charged nurse Julie Thao with "neglect of a patient causing great bodily harm" when she accidentally connected an epidural infusion bag instead of penicillin to an IV, resulting in the death of a 16-year-old mother during childbirth. The felony charge was later reduced to two misdemeanors through a plea bargain, and the nurse's license was suspended for two years (Weier, 2007).

This fairly new trend should be of concern to all nurses because mistakes will always occur in medicine. To err is human. According to Kohn and colleagues (2000), "It may be part of human nature to err, but it is also part of human nature to create solutions, find better alternatives, and meet the challenges ahead (p. 15). If fear of criminal prosecution and prison are added to these personal responses, how can we believe thoughtful, caring people will continue in the profession? As Curtin (1997) asks, "What conceivable social good will be achieved by putting these nurses in jail?" (Kowalski & Horner, 1998, p 127).

Violations of the Food and Drugs Act. Participating in any activity with illegal drugs or the misappropriation or improper use of legal drugs may result in criminal action against the nurse. Conviction for a crime in this area will almost always result in action against a nurse's license. As described earlier, there is a high incidence of substance abuse in the medical profession, so nurses need to be aware of the risks and avoid them. Writing prescriptions for drugs without the authority to do so is a criminal activity. Obtaining drugs illegally for friends and/or family needs, even if they seem legitimate, will still have criminal consequences.

RISK MANAGEMENT AND QUALITY IMPROVEMENT

How Do I Protect Myself and My Patient From All These Risks?

The safety of patients often involves many different formalized processes in institutions. One involves quality and goes by many names such as "quality assurance" (QA), "continuous quality management" (CQM), or "continuous quality improvement" (CQI). In relationship to nursing practices, *peer review* is the process of using nurses to evaluate the quality of nursing care. This means that you, as a professional nurse, will be continuously involved in evaluating the care that you and other nurses provide. In the past, this was only done through retroactive review of care using techniques such as nursing audits to evaluate care already given. The current focus is on looking for ways to do better all the time. Examples of activities that may be involved in this process include the following:

- Evaluation of what nurses are doing for patients
- Policy and procedure development
- Staff preparation, competency, and skill documentation
- Continuing education and certification
- Employee evaluations
- Ongoing monitoring, such as infection control and risk management systems

TJC requires that peer review be driven by the following: (1) the organization's delineation of circumstances that require review; (2) the designation of who will participate in the process; (3) the time frame of the review; (4) the timely reporting of the results (TJC, 2008b).

Risk management is a process that becomes involved when incidents or untoward events occur that may pose a financial risk or risk of lawsuit to the institution. This department, through a risk manager, will often take the first step, which is to gather evidence surrounding the event in "anticipation of litigation." Such evidence will include interviews with those involved and physical evidence such as relevant documents. If you are being interviewed, understand that a truthful accounting is the most important aspect of this process and will best serve the institution and yourself.

Risk management will then often evaluate how to prevent a reoccurrence by changing systems that have broken down to allow an adverse occurrence. This might mean setting a new standard that can then be evaluated and ensured through a quality assurance process.

One tool used by risk management is the **incident report.** Incident reports generate many legal concerns as in most states they must be produced in a lawsuit and can be used as evidence against individuals and the institution (Guido, 2006). Therefore extreme caution should be used when completing an incident report, and only the person directly involved should objectively document the facts. Conclusions, opinions, defensiveness, and judgment or blame of others have absolutely no place in this document or process. In addition, the form should never be used for punitive reasons, since this will almost certainly increase the possibility that it will not be filled out honestly if at all (Kohn et al, 2000).

Although you would not mention that you filled out an incident report in the medical record, the same objective, factual documentation of an incident should be made in the medical record by the person involved in the incident. Lack of documentation in the face of a known occurrence will always be considered a cover-up and thus will be extremely detrimental to any subsequent legal action. Never speculate about who or what caused an incident, because this may inadvertently give the plaintiff "causation" proof, which may not be true.

An example of risk management and quality assurance working together would be the following. A fire breaks out in the operating room, and a patient is burned. Immediately after this event, a risk manager might be notified through a telephone call and then later an incident report. The risk manager would come immediately to the scene and collect all items and/or equipment involved in the fire (evidence) to determine the cause of the fire. He or she would also interview those who saw the fire (witnesses) to determine facts involved. The risk manager may also take specific actions to assist the patient and/or family, in addition to giving advice to those involved regarding documentation of the event and/or communications. Sometimes financial settlements are made very early to avoid the costly process of a lawsuit. Risk management might also identify ways to prevent another occurrence, such as removal of all alcohol-based skin preparations from the operating room. This standard may then be periodically evaluated by the quality assurance department to ensure the continued safety of a patient.

Risk managers usually work very closely with insurance companies that cover institutions and their employees for all types of financial risk, including malpractice and general liability. The defense and prevention of many claims start with good risk management. Yet such efforts must also be made by every individual on the health care team who identifies a risk to patient safety and does something constructive to correct it. Several simple risk management actions by nurses can often prevent a lawsuit. These include the following:

- Approaching angry patients with an apology and an offer to help (Gutheil et al, 1984). Moving toward the patient who has experienced an unexpected outcome rather than away is always the best policy. Isolation and a feeling of abandonment in the face of an untoward event can only augment the feeling that a wrong was done.
- Sharing uncertainties and bringing patient's expectations down to a realistic level during the informed consent process can also prevent claims based on disappointment that an outcome is not perfect (Gutheil et al, 1984).
- Refusing to participate in hospital gossip, to joust in the medical record, or to judge others on the medical team will contribute to an atmosphere of teamwork and compassion, rather than competition, blame, and retaliation. The latter can ultimately contribute to unsafe patient care. An inadvertent negative remark to patients and families about a physician, the pharmacy, the laboratory, or other nurses is very frequently the genesis of a lawsuit. Such remarks are often based on limited knowledge and personal bias. Making such remarks could cause you to end up as a witness in a malpractice claim against your peers and/or other medical team members. This is seldom a desirable position for anyone.

Malpractice Insurance

One of the more controversial topics for nurses involves the need for nurses to purchase individual malpractice insurance policies. There is often misinformation about what these individual policies will do or cover, and there is little substantiation for what most authors say. Part of the problem is that lawyers, rather than insurance professionals, talk about what the policies mean. In addition, sometimes insurance companies use scare tactics to induce nurses to purchase their products.

As the nurse's role continues to expand, so does the amount of liability exposure in a medical malpractice claim. According to the U.S. Department of Health and Human Services 2003 Annual Report on Malpractice, a nurse can expect at least 1.11 malpractice reports against her during her career. This means that careful consideration should be given to a decision as to whether or not to carry an individual malpractice insurance policy. An informed nurse should at least know what questions to ask.

What About Individual Malpractice Insurance?

Some individual nurse policies claim that you can prevent settlement of a claim if you wish to do so (have a consent clause). However, a close reading of the policy might demonstrate that should the case then be lost at trial or settled for more than the insurance company wished to offer, the company has the right to collect that difference and the cost of defense from you. Therefore the consent you have a right to withhold has very little meaning.

The fact that registered nursing insurance costs have not changed much since introduced on the market, although all other malpractice insurance costs have risen drastically, is an indication of its lack of use. The cost for a nurse to purchase an individual malpractice policy is based on the area of nursing and the state of practice. Check your professional journals and your professional associations for insurance companies that offer malpractice insurance for nurses.

What Is Institutional Coverage?

Almost all health care corporations or institutions carry very large insurance policies that specifically cover acts or omissions of their employed nurses. This includes cases in which only the institution is named under the previously described *respondeat superior* doctrine or when an individual nurse employee is named. Most individual personal nursing malpractice policies are secondary to this policy. This means they cannot be used in any manner if the institutional policy is used to cover the claim. It is not correct to assume that you can have your personal attorney present to represent your personal interests in addition to the institutional attorney. Even if you could, having two attorneys will often divide the defense and augment the claim.

A representation that the institutional attorney will only look out for the institution's interests and not yours is questionable in that attorneys ethically must represent both your interests and those of the institution. In addition, the institution's interests are rarely, if ever, adverse to yours. Both of you wish to settle claims that have liability and defend claims when there is no liability.

The claim that an institution will insure you but then turn around and sue you is belied by the fact that one cannot find statistics to verify this common claim. Institutions spend millions of dollars on insurance to specifically cover the acts of nurses. In addition, if institutions sued the nurses working for them, they would not keep many nurses.

It is true that if an employee commits a criminal act that by its nature is outside the scope of their employment, such as forced sexual intimacies with a patient, an institution may not defend the employee or cover costs. In this regard, however, criminal acts are not insurable under laws in most states and therefore are not covered by any policy (Simpson, 1998).

What Should I Ask About Institutional Coverage?

There are certain things that a prudent nurse concerned about coverage should do. All nurses should request and have a right to a document that gives them the following information regarding their employer's insurance coverage for them:

- The name of the institution's insurance carrier, the limits of the policy, and the rating of the insurance company (Best Rating A+++ is the highest).
- Whether they are covered for all acts occurring within the scope of their employment and during the time they are employed.
- The acts for which they do not have coverage.
- Whether the hospital will cover them if they need to appear before the state board of nursing in relationship to a malpractice claim. If not, an individual insurance policy that clearly does may be valuable.
- How the nurse is covered by the institutional employer. This is particularly important if the nurse is an independent practitioner and/or in an extended practice role.

What Happens When I Go to Court?

Sometimes, despite all your efforts, you find yourself in litigation as a defendant. Know that very few claims go to trial. Therefore you do not need to picture yourself in a setting from "Law and Order" with a prosecutor tearing you apart. In reality, 95% of personal injury lawsuits are either dismissed or settled out of court, usually after an investigatory process called "discovery" (Fish et al, 1990). This involves written questions about situations surrounding a case called **interrogatories,** as well as a recorded oral questioning process called a **deposition.**

Depositions are oral statements given under oath and are extremely important in any malpractice claim. They are used to evaluate the merits of the case, the credibility of the witnesses, and the strength of the defendants. Cases are won or lost in this process; thus with the help of your attorney, you must be very well prepared. If you have not been offered the chance to meet with your attorney long before your deposition, request the time to do so. This is your right and an ethical obligation of the attorney. Being prepared ahead of time can have a significant effect on your performance under stress. Many attorneys will role-play situations with you so that you can get the feel of the process. Helpful books, videos, and other aids are available. Ask your attorney, or check with your hospital risk management department, in addition to public libraries and websites (Box 20-5).

Depositions occur in a less formal setting than the courtroom. Attorneys for both sides will be present, but this is not the time to tell your story. The attorney questioning you will be either the attorney for the plaintiff or for the other defendants, whose interests may be adversarial to yours. Your attorney can object to certain questions, but on the whole you will have to answer them anyway because in the deposition there is no judge to rule on the objections.

Remember, in a deposition you are there to answer questions in a truthful manner, but not to teach or inform.

BOX 20-5	Tips for Testifying in a Deposition

1. You need to look and act like a professional. That means that you must be prepared. Know the case and review your documented record ahead of time.
2. Be clear, accurate, and very concise. It is often said that if you say more than seven words, it is too much. If you do not know an answer, say so—do not guess.
3. Never give opinions unless asked for them. Stick to the facts!
4. Speak slowly and in a well-modulated tone of voice. Do not allow yourself to be rattled by the opposing attorney.
5. If you do not remember a question or do not understand it, ask for it to be repeated or clarified. Many attorneys use long, multipart questions to confuse you. Do not get caught in this trap.
6. If you have made a statement and later realize it is not correct, do not be afraid to say so, rather than to skirt issues or contradict yourself.
7. Do not allow yourself to be goaded into an angry or emotional response. You can always ask for a break during a deposition to collect yourself and your thoughts.
8. Avoid the use of "always" and "never" and vague comments like "maybe," "I think," or "possibly."
9. Do not answer more than is asked for by the question. This helps maintain focus and clarity. The attorney wants to catch you in contradictory statements. The shorter your statements, the less likely that is to happen.

A lawsuit is a very disconcerting and disheartening process to everyone involved. Your ability to realize this and not feel alone in the process is extremely important. Often institutions mandate that persons involved in litigation receive counseling to help them resolve the anger and depression that almost inevitably occurs. Be sure to use resources available to you, including your lawyer. Your risk management team also is often a good resource and can usually answer questions or help resolve problems you might be having in relationship to the case. Remember that the old adage of "this too will pass" is true.

CONTROVERSIAL LEGAL ISSUES AFFECTING NURSING

Because developments and advances in medical and nursing care occur constantly, many areas of practice do not have firm rules to follow when making decisions. Changes in health care delivery and society's values have sparked controversy about a variety of issues.

Health Care Costs and Payment Issues

One example is third-party reimbursement, or the right of an individual nurse, usually a nurse practitioner, to be paid directly by insurance companies for care given. Medicare has passed rules that allow nurse practitioners to bill independently under their own provider number. This is a very important step in the field of independent practice for nurses, because many health care insurers follow the lead of Medicare in billing issues.

In relationship to the right to bill, all nurses need to understand billing and reimbursement rules so that they cannot be accused of participating in fraudulent billing schemes. For instance, although a bill can be generated for certain follow-up care performed by nurses in the outpatient clinic as services rendered "incident to" what the physician does, there are strict requirements of physician involvement that nurses must understand. Nurse practitioners need to be careful that their services are not also being illegally billed for by physicians with whom they collaborate.

The seven most frequent areas where nurses can inadvertently become involved in fraud and abuse claims are the following:
1. Questionable accuracy and monitoring of physician visit coding
2. Improper use of diagnosis codes
3. Failure to provide patient care or providing patient care that is sloppy
4. Anesthesia services
5. Unneeded critical or acute care services
6. Billing for physician assistant services
7. Improper billing of nursing or physician services (Nelson, 2005)

To avoid these areas, it is important to know about and understand your institution's compliance plan and to report suspected abuses through the required "hotline" or directly to nursing administration (Green, 2000).

From another perspective, the high cost of health care is also driving the proliferation of health care workers with less training and education than nurses, who can be hired for less money. Often these unlicensed workers have no laws circumscribing their practice and are doing tasks that have traditionally been done by RNs or LPN/LVNs, such as administering medications and giving injections. This is an important issue for nurses, especially when asked to supervise such workers and/or compete for positions in the health care market.

Controversial legislative changes have been made in an attempt to address some of these problems. In response to concerns of whether or not increased acuity of patients, increased caregiver workload, and declining levels of training among patient-care personnel have threatened the quality of patient care, California passed Assembly Bill 394. This bill set a minimum nurse-patient ratio in acute care general, special, and psychiatric hospitals (Lang et al, 2004). A year after it went into effect, nurses were battling Governor Arnold Schwarzenegger to keep what they fought so hard to obtain—an RN-to-patient ratio of 6 to 1 in 2004 and 5 to 1 in 2005. The controversy seems to stem from the difficulty of maintaining ratios "at all times" and in finding enough nurses to fulfill the ratios.

Related topics involve practice models and case management. Practice models involve attempts by institutions to answer what types and ratios of health care providers should constitute a patient-care team. Case management looks at how patient care teams can best derive better outcomes and continuity for patients while effectively managing the variable costs of care delivery. Decisions on these matters by institutions become policies and thus the "laws" under which you must deliver patient care.

Your knowledge of the issues, participation in the processes, and support for legislation and policies that are favorable for your profession and for patient care will be important when your state and/or institution decides such issues. Professional behavior includes concern with and participation in the direction health care, and particularly nursing care, will take in the future.

Health Care Delivery Issues

Changes made in the types of systems used to deliver health care and in the techniques used by the systems have created many concerns for nurses. Hospitals and other expensive acute care settings are giving way to outpatient clinics and same-day surgery centers. This means that people are being sent home while still acutely ill to take care of themselves or to be cared for by relatives without the benefit of hospital nursing services. This makes the nurse's role in discharge planning and patient education an extremely important one to prevent deterioration of certain health or surgical conditions in the home. In addition, it means that home health care nurses are routinely organizing care that used to be rendered only in hospitals. For example, respirators in the home are not unusual. With this change, however, come more independent responsibilities for nurses. Responsibility can translate into liability.

Telephone nursing triage and telemedical nursing care present new and unusual legal concerns because of the difficulties of providing accurate long-distance care and the independent nature of these tasks. Although these nurses bring nursing care to many areas that have not had access to this care in the past, selecting appropriately prepared individuals to provide the care and educating them to function effectively when they cannot see the patient are challenging tasks.

HMOs and other forms of prepaid health care have helped reduce the rapidly growing costs of health care through a process called **utilization review.** Nurses hired to do this review are often asked to make judgments regarding whether or not a patient should be discharged. Early discharge of patients and limits on insurance reimbursements for certain allowable medications, equipment, and external services have sometimes caused ethical and legal problems for health care professionals (Deloughery, 1998).

Past laws protecting the HMOs from malpractice claims when patients were harmed because of flawed utilization review practices are now being challenged. There is a growing public concern that managed care organizations are making large profits while patients covered under their programs are not receiving adequate care. Both Congress and state legislatures are attempting to pass statutes to curb this practice (Kongstvedt, 2001).

The many changes occurring in the workplace often create levels of confusion and frustration, which make it more difficult to focus on the quality of the care being given on a day-to-day basis. These issues are examples of how legal issues interweave with all the other events in your professional life. Nurses must remain involved in these matters to stay aware of how their legal responsibilities are influenced by them.

Issues About Life-and-Death Decisions

Controversial ethical issues surrounding life and death also, of course, present controversial legal issues. Scientific research and new technologies can blur the line between life and death. As a nurse, you can often find yourself in the center of such controversies, so you need to be very aware of what your state's laws are on at least the following subjects.

Abortions. Where can abortions be performed? Who can perform them? When can an abortion be performed? Under what conditions? Under what, if any, conditions can teenagers obtain an abortion without parental consent?

Fetal Rights. If a fetus is born alive, what rights does it have? What rights do the parents have? What rights do health care workers have? What are the laws surrounding fetal death and/or the cessation of life-preserving treatments?

Human Experimentation or Research. What can be done legally with the products of conception? What types of consent are necessary to enroll a patient in research studies? What types of boards and oversight must be involved to approve and monitor human research studies?

Patient Rights. What rights do patients have in your state in relationship to medical records, medical information, giving consent, participating in their care, suing providers, dictating issues surrounding their death, donating organs, being protected from abuse, receiving emergency treatment, being protected from the practice of unlicensed providers, transplantation of organs, accessibility of the disabled to health care, privacy, and confidentiality?

CONCLUSION

As time goes on, laws will be changing and new areas will arise that nursing will have to address. Continuing education, critical thinking, and an open mind will help you to learn about and deal with the legal issues that will touch your professional life daily. Get involved whenever possible with safety, quality, and risk management processes in your institutions. Be someone who has an educated opinion about conflicts inherent in medicine and nursing. Take the opportunity to visit the hearings conducted by your state's board of nursing and by the state legislature. By becoming involved with the legal and disciplinary process, you will be much more aware of how you can protect yourself and your patients and influence the direction of health care issues. By concluding this chapter, it is hoped that you also feel more confident when faced with "the law."

BIBLIOGRAPHY

Annas GJ: HIPAA regulations—a new era of medical-record privacy? *N Engl J Med* 348:486-1490, 2003.

Brent N: *Nurses and the law*, ed 2, New York, 2001, Saunders.

Curtin LL: When negligence becomes homicide, *Nurs Manage* 28:7-8, 1997.

Deloughery G: *Issues and trends in nursing*, St. Louis, 1998, Mosby.

Di Luigi K: What it takes to be an expert witness, *RN* 67:65-66, 2004.

Di Maio VJ, Di Maio TG: Homicide by decubitus ulcers, *Am J Forensic Med Pathol* 23:1-4, 2002.

Dunn D: Substance abuse among nurses: defining the issue, *AORN J*, October 2005. Retrieved from *www.findarticles.com/p/articles*.

Fish RM, Ehrhardt ME, Fish B: *Malpractice: managing your defense*, Montvale, NJ, 1990, Medical Economics Books.

Freydel v. New York Hospital, No. 97 Civ 7926 (SHS), Jan 4, 2000.

Harvey v. Mid-coast Hospital, 36 F., Supp. 2d 32, D. Maine, 1999.

Green E: Creating an effective corporate compliance program, *Drug Benefit Trends* 12:37-38, 2000.

Guido G: *Legal and ethical issues in nursing*, ed 4, Upper Saddle River, NJ, 2006, Prentice Hall.

Gutheil TG, Bursztajn H, Brodsky A: Malpractice prevention through the sharing of uncertainty: informed consent and the therapeutic alliance, *N Engl J Med* 311:49-51, 1984.

Haumschild M, et al: Clinical and economic outcomes of a fall-focused pharmaceutical intervention program, *Am J Health-Syst Phar* 60:1029-1032, 2003.

Institute of Medicine (2006): *News medication errors injure 1.5 million people and cost billions of dollars annually*. Retrieved from *www.nationalacademies.org/onpinews/newsitem.aspx?RecordID=11623*.

Kohn LT, Corrigan JM, Donaldson MS: *To err is human: building a safer health system*, Washington, DC, 2000, National Academy Press.

Kongstvedt PR: *Essentials of managed health care*, ed 4, Rockville, Md, 2001, Aspen.

Kowalski K, Horner MD: A legal nightmare. Denver nurses indicted, *MCN Am J Maternal Child Nurs* 23:125-129, 1998.

Lang TA, et al: Nurse-patient ratios: a systematic review on the effects of nurse staffing on patient, nurse, employee and hospital outcomes, *JONA* 34:326-327, 2004.

Larson A (2005): *Medical malpractice law and litigation*. Retrieved from *www.expertlaw.com/library/malpractice/malpractice.html*.

Medscape Medical News (2000): *Joint Commission releases revised restraints standards for behavioral healthcare*. Retrieved from *www.doctor.medscape.com/viewarticle/411832*.

Moore R: A guide to the assessment and care of the patient whose medical decision-making capacity is in question, *Medscape Gen Med* 1, 1999.

National Council of State Boards of Nursing: *Chemical dependency handbook for nurse managers—a guide for managing chemically dependent employees*, Chicago, 2001, NCSBN.

National Council of State Boards of Nursing: NCSBN introduces online public access to NURSYS (letter), February 12, 2003.

National Council of State Boards of Nursing (2010): *Participating states in the NLC, 2010 Nurse Licensure Compact*. Retrieved from *www.ncsbn.org/nlc*.

National League for Nursing: (2008) *Workforce to practice in 21st-century, technology-rich health care environment*, New York. Retrieved from *www.nln.org/aboutnln/PositionStatements/informatics_052808.pdf*.

National Practitioner Data Bank (2006): *Fact sheet on the National Practitioner Data Bank*. Retrieved from *www.npdb-hipdb.hrsa.gov/pubs/stats/2006_NPDB_Annual_Report.pdf*.

Nelson R: Staffing in California one year later, *AJN* 105:25-26, 2005.

Robertson v. Providence House, 576 So. 2d 992 (La. 1991).

St. Anthony's Hospital v. Whitfield, 946 SW2d 174 (Tex App 1997).

Shaw v. Plantation Management, 2009 WL 838680 (La. App., March 27, 2009) cited in Patient's Fall: Solid Nursing Documentation Afterward, Negligence Lawsuit Dismissed. *Legal Eagle Eye Newsletter* 17(5), 2009. Retrieved from *http://nursinglaw.com*.

Shinn LJ: Yes, you can be sued, *ANA continuing education. The nursing risk management series. An overview of risk management*. Retrieved from *www.nursingworld.org/mods/archive/mod310/cerm101.htm*.

Simpson KR: Should nurses purchase their own professional liability insurance? *Am J Maternal Child Nurs*, 23:122-123, 1998.

Smith LS: Documenting refusal of treatment, *Nursing* 34:79, 2004.

State v. Brown, No. SC85582 (Mo. Aug. 03, 2004).

Sullivan GH: Does your charting measure up? *RN* 17:61-65, 2004.

Texas Board of Nursing (2008): *Eligibility and disciplinary sanctions for nurses with substance abuse, misuse, substance dependency, or other substance use disorder*, Austin, Texas, 2008, Texas Board of Nursing. Retrieved from *www.bon.state.tx.us/practice/pdfs/chemical.pdf*.

Texas Board of Nursing (2010): *Examination information*. Retrieved from *www.bon.state.tx.us/olv/examination.html*.

The Joint Commission (2010): *2010 national patient safety goals*. Retrieved from *www.jointcommission.org/PatientSafety/NationalPatientSafety Goals*.

The Joint Commission (2008a): *Ethics, rights, and responsibilities*. Retrieved from *www.jointcommission.org/NR/*

rdonlyres/940FBF10-AB6A-410C-B396-53FEEB11E58C/0/LTC2008RIChapter.pdf.

The Joint Commission: *Comprehensive accreditation manual for hospitals: the official handbook*, Oakbrook Terrace, Ill, 2008b, TJC.

Tideliksaar R: *Falls in older patients: prevention and management*, Baltimore, 1998, Health Profession Press.

Truog R: *Inadequacies in use of informed consent may limit potential for research in intensive care*, 15th Annual Congress of European Society of Intensive Care Medicine, Sept 19-Oct 2, 2002, Barcelona, Spain.

Walker RS: *Falls and serious injuries before, during and after a nursing home became restraint free (thesis)*, Tucson, Ariz, 1992, University of Arizona.

Weier A: St. Mary's nurse case spurs proposal to halt health care worker prosecution, *The Capital Times*, Madison, WI, Jan. 26, 2007.

Additional resources are available online at *http://evolve.elsevier.com/Zerwekh/nsgtoday/*.

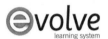

CHAPTER 21

Cultural and Spiritual Awareness

Tim J. Bristol, PhD, RN, CNE

十人十色
[10 People, 10 Colors]
—JAPANESE PROVERB

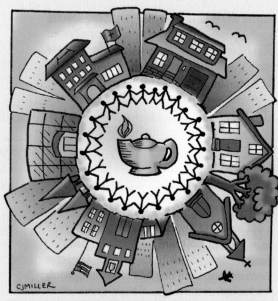

Our communities need culturally competent nursing care.

After completing this chapter, you should be able to:

- Define cultural competence.

- List practice issues related to cultural competence.

- Identify challenges in defining spirituality.

- Determine cultural and spiritual beliefs of patients in the health care setting.

- Assess spiritual needs of patients in the health care setting.

Thanks to the previous author of this chapter—Valerie Eschiti, PhD, RN, CHTP, AHN-BC.

CULTURE AND SPIRITUALITY

What Is Meant by Cultural Competence?

In today's global society, cultural competence is necessary for excellence in nursing care. People can travel like never before. Nurses are connecting to patients through the Internet. Medical "tourism" is now a reality. These factors demonstrate the need for nurses to understand cultural and spiritual differences in themselves and others.

The American Nurses Association (ANA) asserts that the necessity of the nurse being sensitive to individual needs in the *Code of Ethics:* "The need for health care is universal, transcending all individual differences. The nurse establishes relationships and delivers nursing services with respect for human needs and values, and without prejudice. An individual's lifestyle, values system, and religious beliefs should be considered in planning health care with and for each patient" (ANA, 2005).

Dr. Margaret Leininger, considered a top authority on culture care diversity, proposes that cultural understanding would allow for peaceful relations among people groups (Leininger, 2007). This philosophy was considered so important by some, that Dr. Leininger was nominated for the Nobel Peace Prize. Cultural competence is essential for nurses.

But what exactly is cultural competence? It is defined as "developing an awareness of one's own existence, sensations, thoughts, and environment without letting it have an undue influence on those from other backgrounds; demonstrating knowledge and understanding of the patient's culture; accepting and respecting cultural differences; adapting care to be congruent with the patient's culture" (Purnell & Paulanka, 2008, p 6).

> The culturally competent nurse has enhanced ability to provide quality care, which fosters better patient understanding of the plan of care.

"Inattention to cultural competence in patient care leads, at best, to sub-optimal patient outcomes and, at worst, to active harm," says Carla Serlin, PhD, RN, director of ANA's Ethnic/Racial Minority Fellowship Programs. "When we fail to address issues of difference such as language, ethnicity and race, our patients will have lower levels of compliance with care instructions and longer hospital stays" (as cited in Stewart, 1998, p 1).

A mnemonic, CULTURE, developed by Zerwekh and Claborn (2006) can be helpful for nurses to assess and improve their level of cultural competence (Box 21-1). In addition, nurses need to use effective cultural interviewing questions, which are best if left semistructured and open-ended. Spector (2000) has identified nine suggestions for enhancing communication when gathering cultural data (Box 21-2).

What Practice Issues Are Related to Cultural Competence?

Barriers to Cultural Competence. Two categories of barriers to cultural competence exist: provider barriers and systems barriers (Mazanec & Tyler, 2003). Provider barriers are those such as a nurse may have, including lack of information about a culture's customs regarding end-of-life care. Systems barriers are those that exist in an agency, because the agency's structure and policies are not designed to support cultural diversity (Mazanec & Tyler, 2003).

BOX 21-1 CULTURE—A Nursing Approach

Consider your own cultural biases and how this affects your nursing care.
Understand the need to recognize cultural implications in planning and implementing nursing care.
Learn how to utilize cultural assessment tools.
Treat patients with dignity and respect.
Use sensitivity in providing culturally competent care.
Recognize opportunities to provide specific cultural-based nursing care.
Evaluate own previous encounters with patients from other cultures and backgrounds.

Zerwekh J, Claborn J: *CULTURE: a mnemonic for assessing and improving cultural competence*, Ingram, Tex: Nursing Education Consultants, Inc, 2006.

BOX 21-2 Nine Suggestions for Gathering Cultural Data

1. Determine the patient's level of fluency in English and arrange for an interpreter if needed.
2. Ask how the patient prefers to be addressed.
3. Allow the patient to choose seating for comfortable personal space and eye contact.
4. Avoid body language that may be offensive or misunderstood.
5. Speak directly to the patient, whether an interpreter is present or not.
6. Choose a speech rate and style that promotes understanding and demonstrates respect for the patient.
7. Avoid slang, technical jargon, and complex sentences.
8. Use open-ended questions or questions phrased in several ways to obtain information.
9. Determine whether the patient's reading ability before using written materials in the teaching process.

Spector RE: *Cultural diversity in health and illness*, ed 5, Upper Saddle River, NJ: Prentice-Hall Health, 2000, as cited in Ignatavicius D, Workman L: *Medical-surgical nursing: critical thinking for collaborative care*, St. Louis: Elsevier, 2008.

For instance, an American Indian family may wish to spend the night in the intensive care unit room with a critically ill family member. However, the room does not have a cot on which to sleep, and the waiting room is not large enough to accommodate all the family and extended family members who are present to support the patient. The community in which the hospital is located has a large American Indian population. The nurse, as an advocate for patients and their families, can intervene through activities such as joining a hospital committee focused on hospital redesign. The nurse can point out the need for space for family members to stay the night near their loved ones. In this way the nurse supports the needs of the cultural diversity in her community.

Many organizations are involved in improving cultural competency in the health care industry. One governmental organization (Office of Minority Health) provides extensive continuing education for health care professionals (AHRQ, 2009). Through a web resource *(www.thinkculturalhealth.org)* and other offerings, they assist providers in delivering respectful, understandable, and effective care to patients of all ethnicities. Education like this is crucial because of the increasing diversity of the American population.

Health and Health Care Disparities. One of the goals of *Healthy People 2020* is to eliminate health disparities (*Healthy People 2020*, 2010). Health disparities are inequalities in disease morbidity and mortality in segments of the population. These disparities may be due to differences in race or ethnicity. They are believed to be the result of the interaction among genetic variations, environmental factors, and health behaviors. For instance, the infant death rate among blacks is more than double that of whites. American Indians and Alaska Natives have an infant death rate almost double that for whites. Also, their rate of diabetes is more than twice that for whites. Hispanics are almost twice as likely to die of diabetes than are non-Hispanic whites. New cases of hepatitis and tuberculosis also are higher in Asians and Pacific Islanders than in whites (*Healthy People 2010*, 2000).

OFFICE OF MINORITY HEALTH AND DISASTER PREPAREDNESS
OMH is a part of the Department of Health and Human Services. In 2009, OMH launched an initiative to help first-responders better manage disaster and crises in diverse populations. Some of the issues addressed include:
- Using interpreters
- Using bilingual materials
- Managing cultural variation
- Implementing culturally based standards

Visit *www.thinkculturalhealth.org.*

Inequalities in income and education are at the root of many health disparities. In general, those populations who have the worst health status are those that have the highest poverty rates and the least education. Low income and low education levels are associated with differences in rates of illness and death, including heart disease, diabetes, obesity, and low birth weight. Higher incomes allow better access to medical care, enable people to afford better housing and live in safer neighborhoods, and increase the opportunity to engage in health-promoting behaviors. Recent initiatives are even focusing on increasing the minority representation amongst workers in the health care industry (*Healthy People 2020*, 2010).

According to the Institute of Medicine (IOM) report *Unequal Treatment*, conscious and unconscious bias from health care professionals affects quality of care and hence leads to health disparities (Smedley et al, 2003; White-Means et al, 2009). Some of the causes of health care disparities include provider variables and patient variables. Provider variables are provider/patient relationships, lack of minority providers, as well as provider bias and discrimination. Studies have clearly demonstrated that providers will often make different plans for different patients when the only difference is culture or skin tone. Patient variables are mistrust of the health care system and refusal of treatment (Baldwin, 2003). Often this mistrust comes from barriers in communication.

Nurses can carry *Rapid Rescue Spanish* on their smart phone for translation assistance. *www.skyscape.com/estore/productdetail.aspx?productid=2023.*

Can you think of ways to decrease disparities in health and health care in your community? What projects could you do as a nursing student to make a positive impact? Could you devise a project as part of a class assignment or a Student Nurses Association activity?

The solutions to challenges of health and health care disparities are complex and still being discovered (Critical Thinking Box 21-1). Some solutions are increasing the diversity of health care providers; ensuring that all people have access to affordable, basic health care; promoting wellness and a healthy lifestyle; strengthening provider/patient relationships; increasing cultural competency of health care providers; and conducting research to determine why certain diseases affect minorities so greatly and to discover effective intervention strategies (Baldwin, 2003).

Culturally Diverse Work Force. In order to meet the health care needs of an increasingly diverse society, it would be beneficial to have such diversity represented in the nursing profession. Unfortunately, the diversity of the nursing workforce does not mirror that of the U.S. population (AACN, 2009). For instance, in 2007 the U.S. Census Bureau reported that 34% of the American population was from a minority background. However, in 2004 the *National Sample Survey of Registered Nurses* showed that minorities accounted for 10.7% of registered nurses. It is also important to have minority faculty to mentor nursing students. In 2008, 10.7% of nursing faculty listed a minority for their ethnicity.

The American Hospital Association (2002) recommends that exposure to health careers begin early in the education of minority populations, as well as males, in order to reach out to those who are currently underrepresented in nursing and who will account for an increasing share of the labor pool. The AHA states, "Improving diversity will not only help solve the workforce crisis, but also enhance the cultural competencies of hospitals, making them more responsive to their communities' health care needs" (p 47). See Evidence-Based Practice Box 21-1 for information about culturally diverse nurse-patient interactions.

What Is the Meaning of Spirituality?

One of the challenges for the nurse in providing spiritual care to patients is that there is not yet a clear definition of spirituality (MacLaren, 2004). Many people confuse religion with spirituality, when in fact, they can be separate entities. Pesut et al (2008) contend that current trends in health care tend to define religion as a set of institutionalized beliefs and rituals, whereas spirituality can be defined "as an individualized journey characterized by experiential descriptors such as meaning, purpose, transcendence, connectedness and energy" (p 2804).

McSherry (2006) presents several components of spirituality with relevance to nursing, which is a helpful framework for understanding the concept (Box 21-3). At times, a spiritual advisor or chaplain may be called upon for a patient's or family's spiritual needs. But there are times these spiritual needs may be met most appropriately by the nurse (Bokinskie & Evanson, 2009).

A definition of spiritual nursing care is "an intuitive, interpersonal, altruistic, and integrative expression that is contingent upon the nurse's awareness of the transcendent dimension of life but that reflects the patient's reality" (Sawatzky & Pesut, 2005, p 23). Spiritual distress is an approved nursing diagnosis (Carpenito-Moyet, 2007). Examples of spiritual nursing

BOX 21-1   EVIDENCE-BASED PRACTICE

Cultural Diversity

PRACTICE ISSUE

With the increasing diversity of patients, relationships between nurses and patients may become strained if there is lack of cultural awareness between them. It is vital to maintain positive nurse-patient interactions, in order for patients to achieve the highest level of health and well-being.

IMPLICATIONS FOR NURSING PRACTICE

Three themes emerged from this study—shared tension, perceived differences, and held awareness.
- *Shared tension* was reported in nurse-patient relationships, notably involving racial and gender differences between nurse and patient and surrounding the issue of family visitors.
- There were *perceived differences* between nurses and patients in regard to culture and beliefs; there was a focus on perceived differences rather than similarities.
- Patients and nurses *held awareness* (or were being attentive) regarding language, as well as the need for information. There were not always interpreters available when needed, which created potential for misunderstanding.
- The level of involvement between nurses and patients remained task-oriented, in a detached manner, rather than a level of reciprocity and connectedness.

Considering This Information:

How might you improve relationships with your culturally diverse patient?

Reference for the Evidence

Cioffi J: Culturally diverse patient-nurse interactions on acute care wards, *Int J Nurs Pract* 12:319-325, 2006.

BOX 21-3   Components of Spirituality

- Spirituality is a universal concept relevant to all individuals.
- The uniqueness of the individual is paramount.
- Formal religious affiliation is not a prerequisite for spirituality.
- An individual may become more spiritually aware during a time of need.

From McSherry W: *Making sense of spirituality in nursing practice: an integrative approach*, Edinburgh, 2006, Churchill Livingstone, p 48.

interventions include prayer, presence, scripture reading, peaceful environment, meditation, music, pastoral care, inspiring hope, active listening, validation of patients' thoughts and feelings, values clarification, sensitive responses to patient beliefs, and developing a trusting relationship (Callister et al, 2004).

Free services are online for your patients to listen to religious works such as the Bible. This is useful for the patient that is too ill to read or for family members who would like to offer this to their loved one. *www.biblegateway.com/resources/audio.*

CULTURAL AND SPIRITUAL ASSESSMENT

What Are Cultural and Spiritual Beliefs About Illness and Cures?

Patients will have different responses to illness based on their cultural and spiritual beliefs. It is vital for the nurse to be aware of the variety of responses that may be encountered (Box 21-4).

> The nurse needs to be careful, however, not to stereotype a patient based on his or her cultural or spiritual background.

People of many cultures may use complementary, alternative, or integrative modalities that can affect their health status (Box 21-5). Complementary and alternative medicines are often grouped together using the acronym of CAM. The National Center for Complementary and Alternative Medicine (NCCAM, 2010) defines CAM as "a group of diverse medical and health care systems, practices, and products that are not presently considered to be part of conventional medicine." Because the public is increasingly using CAM in the United States (Barnes et al, 2002; Eisenberg et al, 1998), it is vital that the nurse have a basic understanding of various therapies,

---

BOX 21-4	Cultural and Spiritual Beliefs Affecting Nursing Care

AFRICAN-AMERICAN

Extended family has large influence on patient.
Older family members are honored and respected, and their authority is unquestioned.
Oldest male is decision maker and spokesman.
Strong emphasis on avoiding conflict and direct confrontation.
Respect authority and do not disagree with health care recommendations—but, they may not follow recommendations.

CHINESE

Chinese patients will not discuss symptoms of mental illness or depression because they believe this behavior reflects on family; therefore, it may produce shame and guilt. As a result, there may be psychosomatic symptoms.
Use herbalists, spiritual healers, and physicians for care.

JAPANESE

Believe physical contact with blood, skin diseases, and corpses will cause illness.
They also believe improper care of the body, including poor diet and lack of sleep, cause illness.
They believe in healers, herbalists, and physicians for healing, and energy can be restored with acupuncture and acupressure. Their high regard for the status of physicians decreases the likelihood that they will question their care.
They use group decision making for health concerns.
Disability is a source of family shame. Mental illness is taboo.
Pain is not expressed as it is considered a virtue to bear pain.
Addiction is a strong taboo.

BOX 21-4 Cultural and Spiritual Beliefs Affecting Nursing Care—cont'd

HINDU AND MUSLIM

Indians and Pakistanis do not acknowledge a diagnosis of severe emotional illness or mental retardation because it reduces the chance of other family members getting married.

Medical beliefs are a blend of modern and traditional practice.

VIETNAMESE

Vietnamese are slow to trust authority figures due to their refugee experiences. They accept mental health counseling and interventions particularly when they have established trust with the health care worker.

Very patriarchal society.

Although home remedies are tried first, they are compliant with Western health care treatment, once sought.

HISPANIC/LATINO

Older family members are consulted on issues involving health and illness.

Patriarchal family—men make decisions for family.

Illness is viewed as God's will or divine punishment resulting from sinful behavior.

Prefer to use home remedies and consult folk healers known as curanderos or curanderas rather than traditional Western health care providers.

Many believe in the hot and cold theory of disease, although they may differ about what constitutes hot or cold.

ASIAN/PACIFIC ISLANDER

Family- and church-oriented.

Extensive family bonds.

Key family member is consulted for important health-related decisions.

Illness is a punishment from God for wrongdoing or is due to voodoo, spirits, or demons.

Illness is prevented through good diet, herbs, rest, cleanliness, and laxatives to clean the system.

Wear copper and silver bracelets to prevent illness.

Some distrust health care providers, especially due to an under representation of African-American health care providers.

AMERICAN INDIAN

Oriented to the present.

Value cooperation, family, and spiritual beliefs.

Strong ties to family and tribe.

Believe state of health exists when patient lives in total harmony with nature.

Illness is viewed as an imbalance between the person and natural or supernatural forces.

May use medicine man or medicine woman instead of or in conjunction with seeking Western health care.

Illness is prevented through rituals and prayer.

Some mistrust health care providers, due to historical conflicts in the United States, lack of culturally competent care, and underrepresentation of American Indians as health care providers.

Adapted from Smith SF, Duell DJ, Martin BC: *Clinical nursing skills: basic to advanced skills*, ed 6, Upper Saddle River, NJ: Pearson-Prentice Hall, 2004, p 111.

BOX 21-5	Definitions of Terms

Complementary therapies: those that are used in conjunction with mainstream treatments.
Alternative therapies: those that are used instead of mainstream medical therapies.
Integrative therapies: those for which there is some scientific basis for usage.

From National Center for Complementary and Alternative Medicine (2010): *What is complementary and alternative medicine?* Retrieved from *www.nccam.nih.gov/health/whatiscam/*.

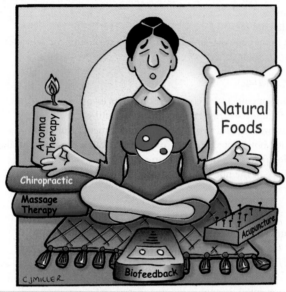

FIGURE 21-1

Complementary health care therapy is on the rise.

as well as their benefits and risks. For instance, a patient with diabetes may be ingesting ginger for general health or to address a concern (e.g., nausea). However, the nurse needs to know that ginger may decrease blood glucose levels (Al-Amin et al, 2006). It is possible that ginger ingestion by the patient could influence the dosage of an oral antidiabetic agent needed by the patient (Figure 21-1). The nurse will also need to consider that ginger could increase bleeding times if the patient is taking an anticoagulant (Kee et al, 2009).

The American Holistic Nurses Association (AHNA) says that holistic nursing is defined as "all nursing practice that has healing the whole person as its goal" (AHNA, 2008). Holistic nursing is an attitude, a philosophy and a way of being; it is not just something a person or a nurse does. Vital components of a holistic nursing assessment are identification of cultural and spiritual practices (AHNA, 2008). Nurses need to be aware of all aspects of a patient's life as there are many factors that must be considered for providing adequate care (Migrant Clinicians Network, 2009). Having access to a comprehensive assessment tool will assist in identifying important transcultural variations for each patient (Figure 21-2).

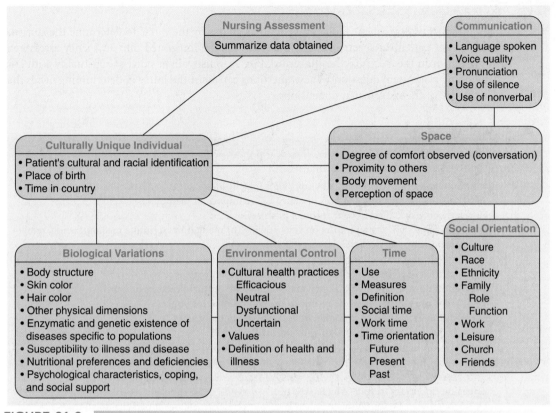

FIGURE 21-2
Giger and Davidhizar's Transcultural Assessment Model. *(From Giger JN, Davidhizar RE:* Transcultural nursing: assessment & intervention, *ed 5, St. Louis: Elsevier, 2008.)*

CRITICAL THINKING BOX 21-2

How much knowledge do you have regarding various CAM therapies, such as acupuncture, reiki, herbal medicine, and aromatherapy? Use the NCCAM website *www.nccam.nih.gov/health/bytreatment.htm#r* to enhance your knowledge base. Identify possible referral sources for integrative therapies in your community. You never know when a patient may ask you for information and/or referral regarding integrative therapies.

The Joint Commission (TJC; formerly JCAHO) acknowledges a patient's right to care that respects their cultural and spiritual values: "JCAHO recommends that health care organizations (1) acknowledge patients' rights to spiritual care and (2) provide for these needs through pastoral care and a diversity of services that may be offered by certified, ordained, or lay individuals" (LaPierre, 2003, p 219). It is imperative that the nurse perform a spiritual assessment to assess the patient's individual needs (Critical Thinking Box 21-2).

How Do You Assess Spiritual Need?

Specific spiritual assessment tools can be used as guides by the nurse to determine the spiritual needs of her patients. Aspects of these tools may also be integrated into an agency assessment document or in the electronic health record. Box 21-6 lists dimensions of spirituality with corresponding assessment questions. These questions can assist the nurse in determining needs that exist in any of the six spiritual dimensions.

BOX 21-6   Dimensions of Spirituality with Corresponding Assessment Questions

SPIRIT-ENHANCING PRACTICES OR RITUALS

How do you express your spirituality (or philosophy of life)?
What spiritual or religious practices or activities are important to you?
How has being sick affected your spiritual practices?
How does being sick have an impact on your praying (or meditation, scripture reading, fasting, receiving sacraments, service attendance, etc.)?
How and for what do you pray?
What spiritual or religious books or symbols are helpful to you?
What effect do you expect your illness to have on your spiritual practices or beliefs?
What kinds of readings, artwork, or music are inspirational for you?
How do Holy Scriptures (e.g., Koran, Bible) help you in daily life?
How can I as a nurse help you with your spiritual practice?
How do your religious practices help you to grow spiritually?

EXPERIENCE OF GOD OR TRANSCENDENCE

Is religion important to you? Why or why not?
Does God/Higher Power/Ultimate Other/The Transcendence, etc. seem personal to you?
Do you feel close now?
How does God or a deity function in your personal life?
How is God working in your life?
How would you describe your God and what you worship?
What is your picture of God?
What do you feel you mean to God?
Are there any barriers between you and God? Is there anything you think God could not forgive you?
How do you make sense of feeling angry with God?
How does God respond when you pray?
Do you feel a source of love from God or any spiritual being? Where is God in all this?
What kind of relationship do you have with the leader of your spiritual community (e.g., priest, rabbi, guru)?
In what ways does your spiritual community help you when times are bad?
What kinds of confusion or doubt do you have about your religious beliefs?
Are you having difficulty carrying out your religious duties?

SENSE OF MEANING

What gives most meaning to your life? What is the most important thing in your life?
When you are sick, do you have feelings that you are being punished or that it is God's will for you to be sick?

| BOX 21-6 | Dimensions of Spirituality with Corresponding Assessment Questions—cont'd |

What are your thoughts about or explanations for suffering? Are these beliefs helpful?

What do you see as the cosmic plan/God's plan or purpose for your life?

Have you been able to answer any of the "why" questions that often accompany illness?

What, if any, have been the good outcomes from having this difficult time in life?

What, if anything, motivates you to get well?

GIVING AND RECEIVING LOVE, OR CONNECTEDNESS TO SELF (DEGREE OF SELF-AWARENESS) AND OTHERS

What do you do to show love for yourself?

What are some of the most loving things that people have done for you?

What are the loving things that you do for others?

How do others help you now? How easy is it to accept their help?

For what do you hope? How do you experience hope?

How have you experienced forgiveness during your life/illness (Forgiveness toward self, toward or from others and God)?

SOURCES OF HOPE AND STRENGTH

What helps you to cope now?

What (or who) is your source of hope? Of strength? How do they help?

To whom do you turn when you need help? Are they available?

What helps you most when you feel afraid or need special help?

How can I help you maintain your spiritual strength during this illness?

To what degree do you trust your future to God?

What brings you joy and peace in your life?

What do you believe in?

What do you do to make yourself feel alive and full of spirit?

LINKAGE BETWEEN SPIRITUALITY AND HEALTH

How does your spirituality affect your experience of being sick?

How has your current situation/illness influenced your faith?

How has being sick affected your sense of who you are (or how has being sick affected you spiritually)?

What has bothered you most about being sick (or in what is happening to you now)?

What do you do to heal your spirit?

Has being sick (or your current situation) made any difference in your feelings about God or your faith experience (or in what you believe)?

Is there anything especially frightening or meaningful to you now?

Do you ever wish for more faith to help you with your illness?

Has being ill ever made you feel angry, guilty, bitter, or resentful?

How involved in a spiritual/religious community/organization (e.g., church, temple, covenant group) are you? (As a visitor? Member? Leader?)

From Taylor EJ: *Spiritual care: nursing theory, research, and practice*, Upper Saddle River, NJ: Pearson-Prentice Hall, 2002, pp 121-124.

CRITICAL THINKING BOX 21-3	If your patient asked you to pray with him, would you feel comfortable? If not, what other resources could you call upon to meet the spiritual needs of this patient?

CONCLUSION

As you enter the world of nursing, you will come into contact with patients from various cultures, and they will have many different spiritual beliefs (Critical Thinking Box 21-3). As nurses, we must be able to address these issues as they relate to health care. Nurses need to become more "culturally competent" to better understand the health care needs of our vast, multicultural patient population. It will not be enough to recognize and accept these cultural implications; we must plan nursing and health care that will achieve the most positive patient results. With the melting pot of cultures in the patient population, nurses must begin to implement a more holistic approach to providing health care. The place to begin is with each individual nurse, who must begin with an assessment of his or her own value system and become more culturally competent. "Cultural humility and a desire to better understand your patients are essential" (Migrant Clinicians Network, 2009).

In clinical settings, spiritual assessment tools can help the nurse gain a deeper understanding of the patient from a holistic perspective. However, these tools are merely guides, not multipurpose checklists that can be completed all at once during an initial assessment period.

BIBLIOGRAPHY

Agency for Healthcare Research and Quality (2009): *National healthcare disparities report 2008.* Retrieved from *www.ahrq.gov/qual/nhdr08/nhdr08.pdf.*

Al-Amin ZM, et al: Anti-diabetic and hypolipidaemic properties of ginger (*Zingiber officinale*) in streptozotocin-induced diabetic rats, *Br J Nutr* 96:660-666, 2006.

American Association of Colleges of Nursing (2009): *Fact sheet: enhancing diversity in the nursing workforce.* Retrieved from *www.aacn.nche.edu/Media/pdf/diversityFS.pdf.*

American Holistic Nurses Association (2008): *What is holistic nursing?* Retrieved from *www.ahna.org/AboutUs/WhatisHolisticNursing/tabid/1165/Default.aspx.*

American Hospital Association (2002): *In our hands: how hospital leaders can build a thriving workforce. Broaden the base.* Retrieved from *www.aha.org/aha/content/2001/pdf/Ioh06Chap3.pdf.*

American Nurses Association: *Code of ethics for nurses with interpretive statements,* Kansas City, Mo, 2005, ANA. Retrieved from *www.nursingworld.org/ethics/code.*

Baldwin DM: *Disparities in health care: focusing efforts to eliminate unequal burdens,* Washington, DC, 2003, American Nurses Association. Retrieved from *www.nursingworld.org/mods/mod560/cebrdnfull.htm.*

Barnes P, et al: CDC Advance Data Report #343. Complementary and alternative medicine use among adults: United States, 2002, May 27, 2004. Retrieved from *www.nccam.nih.gov/news/report.pdf.*

Bokinskie JC, Evanson TA: The stranger among us: ministering health to migrants, *J Christian Nurs* 26:202-209, 2009.

Callister LC, et al: Threading spirituality through nursing education, *Hol Nurs Practice* 18:160-166, 2004.

Carpenito-Moyet LJ: *Handbook of nursing diagnosis,* Philadelphia, Lippincott, 2007, Williams & Wilkins.

Eisenberg DM, et al: Trends in alternative medicine use in the United States: 1990-1997, *JAMA* 280:1569-1575, 1998.

Healthy People 2010: understanding and improving health, Washington, DC, 2000, U.S. Department of Health and Human Services. Retrieved from *www.healthypeople.gov/Document/html/uih/uih_2.htm#goals.*

Healthy People 2020: Proposed objectives, Washington, DC, 2010, U.S. Department of Health and Human Services. Retrieved from *http://www.healthypeople.gov/hp2020/Objectives/TopicAreas.aspx.*

Kee JL, Hayes ER, McCuistion LE: *Pharmacology: a nursing process approach,* ed 6, St. Louis, MO, 2009, Saunders Elsevier.

LaPierre LL: JCAHO safeguards spiritual care, *Holistic Nurs Pract* 17:219, 2003.

Leininger M: Theoretical questions and concerns: response from the theory of culture care diversity and universality perspective, *Nurs Sci Q* 20:9-15, 2007.

MacLaren J: A kaleidoscope of understandings: spiritual nursing in a multifaith society, *J Adv Nurs* 45:457-462, 2004.

Mazanec P, Tyler MK: Cultural considerations in end-of-life care: how ethnicity, age, and spirituality affect decisions when death is imminent, *Am J Nurs* 103:50-58, 2003.

McSherry W: *Making sense of spirituality in nursing practice: an integrative approach*, Edinburgh, 2006, Churchill Livingstone.

Migrant Clinicians Network-cultural competency, Chico, CA, 2009, Author. Retrieved from *www.migrantclinician. org/clinical_topics/cultural-competency. html*.

National Center for Complementary and Alternative Medicine (2010): *What is complementary and alternative medicine?* Retrieved from *http://nccam. nih.gov/health/whatiscam/*.

Pesut B, et al: Conceptualizing spirituality and religion for healthcare, *J Clin Nurs* 17(21):2803-2810, 2008.

Purnell LD, Paulanka BJ: *Transcultural healthcare: a culturally competent approach*, ed 3, Philadelphia, 2008, FA Davis.

Sawatzky R, Pesut B: Attributes of spiritual care in nursing practice, *J Holistic Nurs* 23:19-33, 2005.

Smedley BD, Stith AY, Nelson AR: *Unequal treatment: confronting racial and ethnic disparities in health care, Institute of Medicine report*, Washington, DC, 2003, National Academy Press.

Stewart M: Nurses need to strengthen cultural competence for next century to ensure quality patient care, Washington, DC, January-February, 1998, *Nursing World*. Retrieved from *www. nursingworld.org/MainMenu Categories/ANAMarketplace/ANA Periodicals/TAN/1998/TANJan Feb98FeaturesCulturalCompetence. aspx*.

White-Means S, Dong Z, Hufstader M, Brown LT: Cultural competency, race, and skin tone bias among pharmacy, nursing, and medical students, *Med Care Res Rev* 66:436-455, 2009.

Additional resources are available online at *http://evolve.elsevier.com/Zerwekh/nsgtoday/*.

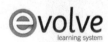

CHAPTER 22

Quality Patient Care

Theresa M. Pape, PhD, RN, CNOR

Reality is merely an illusion, albeit a very persistent one.
—ALBERT EINSTEIN

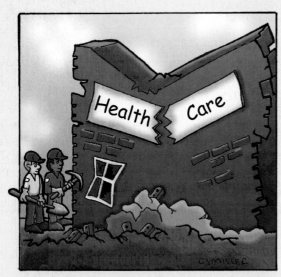

By working together in our quality circles, we can fix our broken health care system

After completing this chapter, you should be able to:

• Define quality standards in health care management.

• Describe the history and evolution of quality in health care.

• Define and discuss core measures.

• Identify the role of regulatory agencies in health care quality.

• Discuss the use of key indicators to measure performance.

• Describe your role in quality and performance improvement.

• Identify tools and processes for continuous quality improvement.

• Identify the role of regulatory standards and agencies.

• Incorporate successful process improvement strategies.

• Consider the value and requirements of quality credentialing.

 ou may wonder why nurses need to know about quality issues to provide patient care. All nurses know to give high-quality care, right? Of course they do—at least in an ideal world—but soon many new graduates find out that not all nurses do the right thing all the time for the patient and the health care environment. That is why we have

480

quality improvement departments within health care settings. Someone must monitor quality care compliance.

Look at almost any news show or sensational tabloid and you will find health care errors featured. Today more than ever, these stories seem to have become the focus of news stories. Who or what makes this happen?

Issues that are on the forefront of news will take precedence over those that are routine or commonplace. Recently, medical errors have become of primary concern. Quality departments have the job of helping nurses and healthcare team members avoid errors by implementing various prevention methods. They also ask for the help of nurses in mobilizing process improvement teams that work to identify risk areas and develop prevention plans. Quality care can be likened to fire prevention instead of fire fighting. Illegible handwriting continues to be a contributing factor to errors and has led to regulations about what medical abbreviations are appropriate. (See Table 11-1, The Joint Commission Official "Do Not Use" List of Abbreviations.)

In the 1980s, the topic of human immunodeficiency virus (HIV) and hepatitis B virus caused increased use of gloves to prevent transmission of infection. The increased need for more gloves led to a need to produce them quickly, which resulted in the introduction of foreign supplies of latex gloves. More latex allergies surfaced. In the 1990s, more emphasis was placed on using needleless systems to prevent needlestick injuries, resulting in legislation. In the 2000s, there has been concern and controversy regarding the nursing shortage and access to health care. In the 2010s, increasing demands will continue to be placed on nurses and health care providers to provide high-quality care with less money and fewer resources. Each decade brings new topics that need to be addressed with quality initiatives, demonstrating how history and events shape the quality paradigm.

STANDARDS OF QUALITY HEALTH CARE MANAGEMENT

Several agencies have established standards that guide quality in health care. Some of these include the American Nurses Association (ANA) Standards of Nursing Care, accrediting group standards such as those of The Joint Commission (TJC), which accredits health care organizations. The Agency for Healthcare Research and Quality (AHRQ) has established clinical practice treatment guidelines. These guidelines are designed to improve patient outcomes and reduce costs. Each health care facility also sets its own standards of practice.

TJC publishes a sentinel event alert monthly. A *sentinel event* is an unexpected occurrence involving death or loss of limb or function. Such events are called "sentinel" because they sound a warning of the need for immediate investigation and response (Figure 22-1) (TJC, 2010b).

A pessimist sees the difficulty in every opportunity; an optimist sees the opportunity in every difficulty.
—SIR WINSTON CHURCHILL

What Is Root Cause Analysis?

When errors occur, the primary cause needs to be determined so that a solution can be found. *Root cause analysis* (RCA) is a process designed for use in investigating and categorizing the root causes of events that occur. In the health care setting, there are many factors that can contribute to the cause of errors. Rather than placing blame on any one person or thing, RCA, when conducted appropriately, can identify all factors leading up to the error. Often an RCA is conducted by a hospital's risk management department, and the results are presented to the *quality improvement* (QI) department for follow-up action. The role of the QI department is to become proactive at finding ways of preventing similar incidences from occurring.

Imagine an occurrence during which a nurse administers the wrong dose of a medication instead of the correct dose. The typical investigation would probably conclude that the nurse was at fault. However, if the analysis stops here, the reasons for the mistake may not be fully understood, and we may never discover what to do to prevent it from occurring again.

In the case of the nurse who gave the wrong medication dose, we are likely to make recommendations such as reprimanding the nurse, re-educating the nurse, and reminding all other nurses to be alert when giving the same medication. However, this does little to resolve the real problem. That is because medication administration involves a complex set of steps in order to get the correct medication to the correct patient in a timely manner. Many things contribute to medication errors as nurses encounter problems within the system, work-design problems, or human and environmental factors. This means that there may be problems getting medications to the nursing unit, or there may be problems with the labels.

Common causes of medication errors include wrong-dose errors, lack of drug knowledge, rule violations, slips, memory lapses, inadequate monitoring, misuse of infusion pumps,

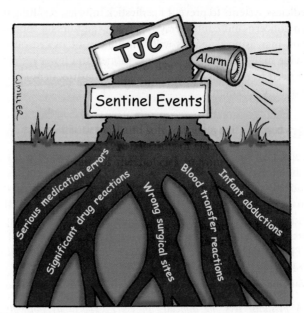

FIGURE 22-1

Root causes of sentinel events.

faulty-dose checking and failure to identify the correct drug, medication stocking problems, and using the wrong technique. System failures include lack of easy access to drug information, look-alike packaging, sound-alike drug names, transcription errors, lack of patient information, poor communication, distractions, interruptions, and excess workloads (Pape, 2003). The environment plays a part through the many distractions the nurse must attend to.

The environment and behavior are as much a part of the system as they are the processes within the organization. Nurses are often interrupted as they prepare medications for their patients. Sometimes the lighting is bad or there is a great deal of noise and confusion that can distract a nurse. Technology can be helpful and is an integral part of the system components, but it cannot solve the human factor issues. Therefore, each aspect of medication errors should be considered when evaluating a cause-and-effect relationship of medication errors (Pape, 2006).

A root cause factor chart should be generated to find the real origin of the error. Figure 22-2 depicts a simplified version of the root cause analysis performed as an example. As the

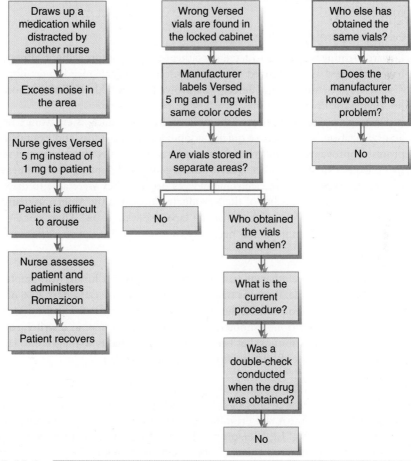

FIGURE 22-2

Root cause factor chart.

investigation proceeded, it became evident that the nurse was not entirely at fault because of a look-alike vial. In addition, distractions and hurriedness also contributed to the error.

HISTORY AND EVOLUTION OF QUALITY IN HEALTH CARE

The advent of quality in health care began when hospitals found the need to look outside their own expertise for error prevention strategies. The year is not as important as the fact that health care organizations found a need to borrow from other industries that were successful at managing risk. Manufacturing industries began focusing on error prevention in the early 1920s, whereas the evolution of improved quality techniques in health care was not adopted until the 1960s and is still evolving.

Historically, the focus of quality improvement was in controlling processes by inspection so that errors were prevented. Later, the emphasis changed from inspection to proactive approaches to error prevention. Included with prevention are monitoring processes to keep errors under control.

Who Is Edward Deming?

Edward Deming is often considered the father of quality improvement, although quality concepts have developed and improved over several decades. What once began simply as a method for discovering how to prevent defects has evolved into highly skilled methods for tracking and improving quality today.

Deming's teachings embraced the philosophy that quality is everyone's responsibility within an organization. The Japanese quickly adopted Deming's ideas and extended the application of process improvement from manufacturing to administrative functions and service industries so that the quality concept affected the whole organization. Japanese companies started taking over product markets on small electronic devices because they were able to drive down their costs, while improving the quality of their products. Subsequently, American manufacturers began to use the same quality techniques that the Japanese were using. That is one reason why we have better cars today than just a few decades ago.

Who Is Joseph M. Juran?

Another valuable forefather of quality initiatives is Joseph Juran, who emphasized the meaning of the Pareto principle. It means that 80% of problems are caused by 20% of sources, people, or things. Therefore if you can fix the 20%, you can fix almost the entire system. From his entry-level job as a factory troubleshooter, Juran developed a career as a writer, educator, and consultant. His major contribution has been in the field of quality management. His work marked the beginning of the idea of *total quality management* (TQM).

Who Is Phillip Crosby?

Phillip Crosby published 14 books about quality management and has also been credited with paving the way for the quality revolution in the United States and Europe. He is considered the father of *"zero defects."* He often proposed simplifying things so that everyone could understand. (Where was he when your Nursing Fundamentals textbooks were written?) He also believed in the importance of communicating quality efforts and their results to the entire organization.

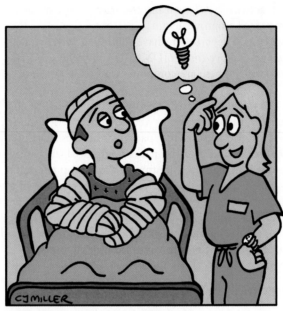

FIGURE 22-3

Bedside nurses often have great ideas!

Afterward, ideas such as "lean" manufacturing, "just-in-time" product delivery, and *"Six Sigma"* methods crossed over into health care.

Recently, there has been a real change in how we view quality improvement within health care settings. What once was considered only work for the QI department is now brought to the front-line workers, who can best affect the outcomes. By front-line workers, we mean the nurses at the bedside and other workers in direct patient care areas, who know the problems that need to be changed. An ongoing commitment to improvement strategies supports an atmosphere of teamwork. The focus is on the process, rather than blaming the people doing the work according to what they have been taught (Figure 22-3).

Still, the regulation of health care is conducted at the national level by regulatory governmental bodies. These governmental agencies are responsible for approving many of the licenses for educational institutions that educate personnel. Institutional accreditation is also conducted by these government agencies. That is why knowledge of what these regulatory agencies do is important. TJC is the primary agency used for hospital accreditation. Their role has not changed, just the name (from JCAHO to The Joint Commission [TJC]).

The mere mention of a visit by TJC can strike fear in the minds of nurses and hospital administrators. This is because hospitals must meet certain quality standards to pass TJC's inspections to maintain accreditation.

In the 1990s, TJC first began to mandate the use of *continuous quality improvement* (CQI) and recommended that organizations adopt a quality improvement model for all process improvement activities. TJC typically endorses the use of the *plan-do-study-act* cycle (PDSA) as one tool for process improvement.

Some hospital QI departments have combined newer strategies with PDSA, including *define-measure-analyze-improve-control* (DMAIC) and *rapid cycle changes* (RCCs), which further incorporate a team focus. These are components of CQI, but more discussion of these methods will come later.

TJC has also mandated specific quality outcome measures for all hospitals. Outcome measures mean looking for real patient results to determine whether the organization's goals were achieved. They want to know if the care that patients receive is meeting standards or is improving. Some of these measures include those for patients admitted with a diagnosis of acute myocardial infarction, congestive heart failure, community-acquired pneumonia, surgical-infection prophylaxis, pregnancy-related conditions, deep vein thrombosis, and whether specific best practices were implemented within the health care setting. . These measures are those that the public consumer considers important for choosing one hospital over another. However, discussion of the specific techniques for measuring these institutional indicators is beyond the scope of this text. Instead, we will focus on general CQI outcomes for nursing units.

JUST WHAT IS THE JOINT COMMISSION?

TJC is the major accrediting body for health care institutions that are Medicare and Medicaid funded. The Center for Medicare and Medicaid Services (CMS) is a part of the U.S. Department of Health and Human Services. Both organizations set the standards for safe practice and evaluate compliance. Having TJC accreditation symbolizes the organization's commitment to quality. This means that nearly all hospitals must be TJC-accredited in order to stay in business.

In the past, TJC standards have directly addressed patient safety in many areas. Beginning on July 1, 2001, additions to these standards required hospitals to develop a systematic approach to error reduction and to design patient care processes with safety in mind. For CQI initiatives, TJC recommends using things like flow charts, Pareto charts, run charts or line graphs, control charts, and histograms to depict data. We call these "tools" or "instruments," because they help depict the measurements and track the problems and improvements. Once the data have been collected, these tools help visualize results of performance improvement understood by most nurses. Other valuable tools are discussed later.

What Are Patient Safety Goals?

A primary driving force for CQI activities is TJC National Patient Safety Goals (NPSG). In 2001, TJC began instituting annual patient safety goals intended to improve the quality of health care. The goals for 2010 are summarized in Table 22-1 (TJC, 2010a).

The first NPSGs were approved by TJC's Board of Commissioners in July 2002. TJC established these goals to help accredited organizations address specific areas of concern regarding patient safety. Each goal includes no more than two brief, evidence-based recommendations. Evidence-based means the goals are based on real world research and/or expert opinions. Each year, the goals and associated recommendations are re-evaluated; some may be continued, whereas others will be replaced because of emerging new priorities. New goals and recommendations are announced in July and become effective on January 1 of the following year (TJC, 2010a; for more information on the NPSGs for specific organizations, one can access TJCs website).

TABLE 22-1 The Joint Commission 2010 Proposed Hospital National Patient Safety Goals

Goal 1: Improve the accuracy of patient identification
Goal 2: Improve the effectiveness of communication among caregivers
Goal 3: Improve the safety of using medications
Goal 4: Improve the safety of using infusion pumps
Goal 7: Reduce the risk of health care-associated infections—hand hygiene, report infections that are sentinel events
Goal 8: Accurately and completely reconcile medications across the continuum of care
Goal 9: Reduce the risk of patient harm resulting from falls
Goal 13: Encourage the active involvement of patients and families in the patient's care as a patient safety strategy
Goal 14: Prevent health care-associated pressure ulcers
Goal 15: The organization identifies safety risks inherent in the patient population
Goal 16: Improve recognition and response to changes in patient's conditions

UNIVERSAL PROTOCOL—THE ORGANIZATION MEETS THE EXPECTATIONS OF THE UNIVERSAL PROTOCOL

For more information on the National Patient Safety Goals, visit the Joint Commission website: *www.jointcommission.org/PatientSafety/NationalPatientSafetyGoals/*

UNIVERSAL PROTOCOL FOR ELIMINATING WRONG SITE, WRONG PROCEDURE, WRONG PERSON SURGERY

Preoperative Verification Process

The Joint Commission believes that delegation of site marking to another individual is acceptable in limited situations as long as the individual is familiar with the patient and involved in the procedure.

Performance for UP.01.02.01

Identify those procedures that require marking of the incision or insertion site. At a minimum, sites are marked when there is **C** more than one possible location for the procedure and when performing the procedure in a different location would negatively affect quality or safety.

NOTE: *For spinal procedures, in addition to preoperative skin marking of the general spinal region, special intraoperative imaging techniques may be used for locating and marking the exact vertebral level.*

Mark the procedure site before the procedure is performed and, if possible, with the patient involved. The procedure site is marked by a licensed independent practitioner who is ultimately accountable for the procedure and will be present when the procedure is performed. In limited circumstances, the licensed independent practitioner may delegate site marking to an individual who is permitted by the organization to participate in the procedure and has the following qualifications:
- An individual in a medical residency program who is being supervised by the licensed independent practitioner performing the procedure; who is familiar with the patient; and who will be present when the procedure is performed
- A licensed individual who performs duties requiring a collaborative agreement or supervisory agreement with the licensed independent practitioner performing the procedure (that is, an advanced practice registered nurse [APRN] or physician assistant [PA]); who is familiar with the patient; and who will be present when the procedure is performed.

Continued

TABLE 22-1 The Joint Commission 2010 Proposed Hospital National Patient Safety Goals—cont'd

The method of marking the site and the type of mark is unambiguous and is used consistently throughout the hospital.

NOTE: *The mark is made at or near the procedure site and is sufficiently permanent to be visible after skin preparation and draping. Adhesive markers are not the sole means of marking the site.*

A written, alternative process is in place for patients who refuse site marking or when it is technically or anatomically impossible or impractical to mark the site (for example, mucosal surfaces or perineum).

NOTE: *Examples of other situations that involve alternative processes include:*
- Minimal access procedures treating a lateralized internal organ, whether percutaneous or through a natural orifice
- Interventional procedure cases for which the catheter/instrument insertion site is not predetermined (for example, cardiac catheterization, pacemaker insertion)
- Teeth
- Premature infants, for whom the mark may cause a permanent tattoo

Performance for UP.01.03.01

A time-out is performed before the procedure.

The purpose of the time-out is to conduct a final assessment that the correct patient, site, and procedure are identified. This requirement focuses on those minimum features of the time-out. Some believe that it is important to conduct the time-out before anesthesia for several reasons, including involvement of the patient. A hospital may conduct the time-out before anesthesia or may add another time-out at that time. During a timeout, activities are suspended to the extent possible so that team members can focus on active confirmation of the patient, site, and procedure.

A designated member of the team initiates the time-out and it includes active communication among all relevant members of the procedure team.

The procedure is not started until all questions or concerns are resolved. The time-out is most effective when it is conducted consistently across the hospital.

Elements of Performance for UP

Conduct a time-out immediately before starting the invasive procedure or making the incision.

The time-out has the following characteristics:
- It is standardized, as defined by the hospital.
- It is initiated by a designated member of the team.
- It involves the immediate members of the procedure team, including the individual performing the procedure, the anesthesia providers, the circulating nurse, the operating room technician, and other active participants who will be participating in the procedure from the beginning.

When two or more procedures are being performed on the same patient, and the person performing the procedure changes, perform a time-out before each procedure is initiated.

During the time-out, the team members agree, at a minimum, on the following:
- Correct patient identity
- The correct site
- The procedure to be done

Document the completion of the time-out.

NOTE: *The hospital determines the amount and type of documentation.*

MONITORING QUALITY OF HEALTH CARE

It is important for nurses to know how to design and conduct simple quality improvement projects to improve processes on their nursing units. Nurses need to know the basics of collecting and analyzing data, and what to do with the results. They must be able to teach other nurses about performance improvement as well.

What Is Quality Improvement?

Quality improvement (QI) refers to the process or activities that are used to measure, monitor, evaluate, and control services, so that we can provide some measure of confidence to health care consumers. It includes reports that must be generated to track progress. Incidence reports are sometimes referred to as QI reports or variance reports. These help guide the hospital risk management (RM) department and QI department to make system improvements (Box 22-1).

How Do We Monitor Quality?

As stated earlier, someone must monitor quality care compliance; otherwise, people tend to go back to their old ways of doing things. The QI department is typically the department that receives data, analyzes trends, and recommends actions to facilitate improvement in the organization. However, there should also be a Continuous Quality Improvement (CQI) Council as a primary decision-making nursing team, as well as *quality circles* (QCs) that function along service lines, collaborating to improve care for a group of patient types.

Examples of service lines include surgical units, medical units, neurological units, rehabilitation units, and outpatient units. These teams review specific problems or indicators each month to determine whether quality care is being delivered. The idea is to keep patients safe by encouraging nurses to practice according to established standards.

Each service line sets out an annual quality plan for the next year, based on recent problem areas or hot topics. Because it is impossible to track everything that nurses consider important to quality care, QCs use various methods to prioritize or target their reviews. They establish unit-specific *quality indicators* for tracking problems on the nursing unit using measurable questions that provide data for trending improvements.

What Is an Indicator and a Metric?

A *quality indicator* is an item of concern that has come about because of a nursing practice problem. It is often a risk management problem as well. For example, a QC team may have identified a problem with urethral catheters being secured properly. This seems to be a recurrent issue. Perhaps several patients had urethral catheters that were inadvertently pulled out. After some investigation and collecting baseline data, the problem was identified as having to do with not properly securing the catheters. Thus the team will collect data for a specific time period and track the nurses' practices. They would count the number of urethral catheters not secured correctly and divide that by the total number of urethral catheters during a specific time frame to get the rate. The metric is the actual rate of urethral catheters that are secured properly (Table 22-2). The correct practice would be clarified with all nurses according to an established policy. Later, when most of the nurses were securing urethral catheters correctly, there may not be a need to monitor this particular practice any longer. Basically, the indicator is the problem, and the metric is the measurement of that problem.

BOX 22-1	Common Quality Terms

Audit: A formal periodic check on quality measures to verify correctness of actions.

DMAIC: A Six Sigma process for improving existing processes that fall below institutional goals or national norms. DMAIC stands for *define, measure, analyze, improve, control.*

Outcome or core measures: Measures that the public consumer considers important for choosing one hospital over another.

Quality indicators: Data that indicate whether high-quality care is being maintained. Items of concern that have come about due to a nursing practice problem (i.e., Foley catheter securing).

Quality assurance: Activities that are used to monitor, evaluate, and control services providing some measure of quality to consumers.

Key indicators: Selected data based on TJC mandates or on specific problem areas that may reveal the need for more extensive data collection or remedial action to resolve an identified problem (i.e., fall rates, medication error rates).

Key performance indicators (KPI): Reflect the things that the team wants to change. These are a part of the DMAIC and RCC process. Typical KPIs are time, costs, distance, numbers of incidents, or items.

Metric: A measurement to determine the rate of compliance or noncompliance with an indicator.

Monitor: Similar to auditing; checking or verifying that an established practice has been retained.

Operational definitions: A statement detailing the thing or event using specific identifiable and measurable wording with written inclusion and exclusion criteria.

Pareto principle: 80% of the problems are caused by 20% of sources, people, or things. If you can fix the 20%, you can fix the system.

Patient safety goals: Annual goals established by TJC that highlight problematic areas in health care and describe evidence and expert-based solutions to these problems. Goals are derived primarily from informal recommendations made in TJC's safety newsletter, *Sentinel Event Alert.*

Plan-do-study-act (PDSA): Contained within an RCC for planning, doing, studying, and carrying out actions intended to drive and maintain change.

Performance improvement: A plan and documentation method that demonstrates what procedures have been and will be implemented for changes in the quality of services based on previous data collection.

Total quality management (TQM): A management style where the goal is producing quality services for the customer and where the customer defines what *quality* means.

Rapid cycle changes (RCC): A strategy for process improvement as a part of DMAIC where changes are tried for very short time frames (3 to 7 days).

Six Sigma: A measurement standard in product variation that began in the 1920s when Walter Shewhart showed that three sigma from the mean is the point where a process requires correction. No fewer than 3.4 errors per million opportunities.

Stakeholders: Key people who will be affected by change and who can either positively or negatively influence the improvement.

A unit-based QI nurse is usually assigned the responsibility to audit charts or verify a procedure by direct observation to determine compliance with a specific nursing practice. The results are compiled and sent to the QI department. After nurses are re-educated about the correct practice, the same indicator is tracked for several months to see whether there has been an improvement. This is done until noncompliance reaches pre-established criteria (e.g., below 5%) and/or compliance is 95%.

TABLE 22-2 Indicator and Metric Descriptors

Indicator	Metric Descriptors
Admission documentation	Metric 1—Rate of patient's identified learning needs not documented within 24 hours of admission. Metric 2—Rate of skin assessment (Braden scale) not documented within 24 hours of admission. Metric 3—Rate of patient's identified spiritual needs not documented within 24 hours of admission.
Foley securing	Metric 1—Rate of Foley catheters not secured in place according to the procedure described in Potter and Perry.
IV tube labeling	Metric 1—Rate of continuous flow IV tubing that has not been labeled with the date and time it is due to be changed. Metric 2—Rate of intermittent flow tubing (IVPB) has not been labeled with the date and time it is due to be changed.
Skin care	Metric 1—Rate of high-risk patients, as defined by the Braden scale (<17), who have pressure ulcers within 2 to 4 days of admission. Metric 2—Rate of those patients with pressure ulcers that are: Stage 1 Stage 2 Stage 3 Stage 4 Eschar
TORAV/VORAV Telephone or verbal orders	Metric 1—Rate of telephoned physician's orders that did not contain read back verification by using "TORAV" *(telephone order read back and verified)* documentation with signature of person taking the order on the first two charts of each odd-numbered day.

Indicators are sometimes selected based on a risk issue. For example, there may have been a patient who suffered an injury because a catheter was not secured to her thigh correctly. The critical thinking exercise (Critical Thinking Box 22-1) can help you discover another example of how important chart auditing can be.

Some examples of metrics are in Table 22-2. Metric descriptors contain more detailed information about what is to be measured and not measured. For example, if nurses were measuring the rate of IV tubing labeled according to policy, they would further define what type of IV tubing. Further exploration would be to determine whether data should include only primary IV lines or both primary and piggyback lines. Most likely, it would include both, but it is always best to be specific about what is to be counted. TJC surveyors typically look at these details.

Most important, metrics and key indicators are developed after baseline data have been collected and careful consideration has been given to how things really are. They are not simply based on hearsay or what someone *thinks* the problems are. The QI nurse does not tell anyone what indicator is being measured until baseline data are collected. In this way, the true patterns of clinical practice can be discovered. Otherwise, the results will not be as accurate.

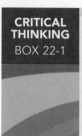

CRITICAL THINKING BOX 22-1

An audit review committee composed of the quality coordinator, three nurses, two case managers, a physical therapist, and a pharmacist, was charged with the task of reviewing the care of the patients having a total hip replacement. The patients' care did not seem to conform to the expected length of stay (LOS) as established by Medicare DRG reimbursement charts. As committee members reviewed the chart and discussed the care of all 20 patients, they noted that Mr. Garcia had been ready for discharge at 10:00 AM on Tuesday, but the case manager for that nursing unit was not able to place him in a rehabilitation unit until 48 hours later. Many of the other 19 charts depicted this same scenario. As a result, the hospital was not reimbursed for the entire LOS, at a loss of approximately $4000 per incident.

1. Who is responsible for the error?
2. What do you think should be done in this situation?
3. What steps can be taken (if any) to prevent the situation in the future?

The results are analyzed on a monthly or quarterly basis by the QI department, tracked, and trended with graphic displays and written committee reports. Based on the results, over time, new processes may need to be developed or more education done. The QI department develops the final reports for several major hospital committees, for the Chief Nursing Officer, and for other Councils. Such reports are usually reviewed at each TJC visit. Thus we see that the contributions of the bedside nurse and the unit QI nurse are quite valuable in TJC survey process. TJC often commends hospitals based on their QI efforts.

What Are Core Measures?

TJC mandates that organizations continuously track certain core measures in order to monitor quality care. Some of these include advance directives, autopsy rates, leaving against medical advice (AMA) and elopement rates, blood-product use rates, blood-transfusion reaction rates, code blue rates, conscious-sedation complication rates, fall rates, medication error rates, mortality rates, pain management effectiveness, restraint use, perinatal care, rates of deep vein thrombosis, and surgical-site infection rates. Simply put, these remain a part of TJC accreditation standards. Core measures are selected based on TJC problem areas that tend to reoccur. These may reveal the need for more extensive data collection or remedial action to resolve an identified problem. Regardless of whether there is improvement, TJC core measures must be continually tracked.

What Is Performance Improvement?

Performance improvement (PI) is practically synonymous with quality improvement (QI), and the terms are used interchangeably. PI is a plan and documentation method that demonstrates what the standard procedures will be for nurses and others within the hospital. It includes changes that have been implemented based on previous data collection. PI is similar to the nursing process (assess, diagnose, plan, implement, and evaluate). Often QI nurses are called on to conduct small data collection processes and provide reports. Critical Thinking Box 22-2 provides a sample scenario for you to try out these skills.

Once the RM and QI departments assess performance within the hospital system regarding the patient care services rendered, a diagnosis of sorts is made that demonstrates where the

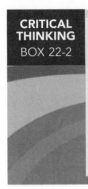

METRICS AND INDICATORS

Your nursing unit has experienced a problem with the IV tubing not being labeled to show when it needs to be changed. You are the QI (quality improvement) nurse who must collect data for a process improvement project. The nurse manager has asked you to determine baseline data for a month and report your findings to her.
1. How would you go about doing this?
2. What would be your indicators?
3. What would be the metrics?
4. Pretend you have some results after a month. How will you report the information to the manager?

majority of problems lie. We often use the Pareto principle by looking for the 20% of sources that caused 80% of the problems. Planning involves fixing the 20% that contributed to the problem. Implementation occurs as new strategies are put into place to resolve the problems or errors. Evaluation takes place as data are collected over a period of time, demonstrating compliance or noncompliance with the new technique. If noncompliant, in-service education may be conducted to emphasize the problem areas, and the measurement process continues.

The United States Pharmacopeia (USP) has played a major role in collecting and trending medication error rates related to patient deaths. This organization has existed since 1820, in order to promote quality standards for the use of medications. In 1991, the USP began more intense investigation on prevention of medication errors. This organization has been instrumental in focusing on problems with both the product and the system where medications are prescribed, dispensed, administered, and used. Many hospitals establish medication policies and quality initiatives based on USP standards (United States Pharmacopeia, 2010a).

One important quality initiative started by the USP is that of the ongoing MEDMARX study, in which hospitals can enter their medication error data in an effort to help other hospitals understand why errors occur. MEDMARX reports help hospital QI departments and nurses avoid future similar errors (USP, 2010b).

What Are the Barriers to Quality Improvement?

One of the primary barriers to implementing effective QI programs is cost. The cost of providing high-quality services within the health care organization has increased greatly over the past few decades. This is due to decreased payments from health insurance companies, including Medicare and Medicaid, as well as to the increased costs of doing business. Health care organizations continue to look for ways to cut expenses by reducing the high cost of supplies or by reducing staff. However, with the continuing shortage of qualified registered nurses, reducing the number of nurses is neither advisable nor acceptable, especially when we think about the errors that can occur as a result. Nevertheless, improving quality can help offset many of the internal costs of care. When quality is high, liability costs are typically low and vice versa. Liability risks are often reduced as quality initiatives prevent problems from happening. Soon, the organization begins to reap the rewards of "fire prevention" rather than constant "fire fighting." Once the hospital organization realizes that the cost of a lawsuit for each death or disability related to medication error far outweighs the cost of nurses, then quality becomes critical.

Other barriers to QI are nurses' loyalty to old practices and failure to recognize that changes are needed. Hospital administrators often oppose change of any kind, because they may value traditional practices, have an authoritative management style, or may not value innovators.

Nurses are often unaware or unwilling to change their practice from the way they have always done things. Many practicing nurses remain resistant to change because it seems threatening and because it requires effort, retraining, and restructuring of habits. However, if we always do things the same old way, we will always get the same results, which might not be good.

Many nurses have learned about how evidence-based practice (EBP) can help them in evaluating current practice. By looking into research studies about hospital issues and using EBP, nurses can make process changes that are tested in practice. This new knowledge provides the confidence nurses need when telling patients, physicians, and other nurses why they used specific practices. In addition, it is important to remain a lifelong learner of new information, especially since there is always uncertainty in decision making.

WHAT ARE SOME OTHER PATIENT SAFETY AGENCIES?

The National Patient Safety Foundation (NPSF) is a nonprofit organization that for years has demonstrated a commitment to patient safety in health care by providing resources for both health care providers and consumers. Part of their mission is to promote understanding among caregivers and consumers. The NPSF holds an annual conference where patient safety knowledge is shared, and where patient safety research results are presented. The organization also funds research to improve safety and quality care (National Patient Safety Foundation, 2010).

The Institute for Healthcare Improvement (IHI) is another nonprofit organization that is highly involved in patient safety initiatives. Founded in 1991, the IHI works to advance quality improvements, and conducts seminars and conferences on patient safety topics. Their website has free open school courses in quality where anyone can take these mini courses. They are also involved in helping organizations implement patient safety ideas (Institute for Healthcare Improvement, 2010).

A new quality and safety educational site has been developed to help prepare future nurses who will be needed in their health care environment to improve patient safety. The organization has developed specific competencies, which are being pilot tested in various universities in the United States. The Quality and Safety Education for Nurses (QSEN) project is funded by The Robert Wood Johnson Foundation (RWJF). In addition, the Institute of Medicine (IOM) provided some of the competencies to be addressed. These include patient-centered care, teamwork and collaboration, evidence-based practice, quality improvement and informatics, and safety. Teaching strategies are provided on their website for faculty members. The development of such an initiative demonstrates how dedicated nursing faculty and nursing leaders are in the future of nursing education in terms of patient welfare (Quality and Safety Education for Nurses, 2010).

QUALITY IMPROVEMENT METHODS

There are several methods used with quality improvement. Whatever approach is used, the values of the institution will be evident in the quality plan. For example, if an organization places emphasis on worker injury prevention, their CQI program will include this idea. Leadership personnel must be genuinely committed to CQI, or it will not work. They must empower nurses and other employees to help plan and carry out the needed strategies for change. Data must be collected systematically—not sporadically or on a whim. Blaming previous personnel for making mistakes does nothing to improve things. The work involves examining systems issues with a proactive approach rather than always being reactive. This means anticipating risks and preventing them.

Many organizations use quality teams, working groups, or quality circles (QCs), to conduct much of the data collection and improvement techniques. These groups need to have a sense of collaboration and appreciation for the value and ideas each person brings to the table. They must be committed to being a part of the solution, not a part of the problem.

Some problems we typically encounter in hospitals are delays in room assignments, medication delivery, treatments or other care, and internal system delays (e.g., dietary, linen). All of these time delays ultimately cost us more. Yet efficient people may not even realize these time traps are occurring because they are so accustomed to developing "work arounds" to eliminate them (Pape, 2006). Working around something means getting around the problem instead of solving it. An example of a "work around" would be the habit of borrowing medications from another patient in the interest of saving time. This type of practice is dangerous and does nothing to solve the system problem. Perhaps the pharmacy technician missed placing the medication in the patient's drawer or put it in the wrong one. Other people simply ignore these time traps or delays in getting their work done. Instead, they just put in their 8 or 12 hours and go home, hoping perhaps tomorrow will be better. This is also not a productive way to solve problems on the nursing unit.

> Everyone wins when nurses join those who are willing to make things work well. Thus, it is critical to be knowledgeable about current CQI methods.

TOOLS AND PROCESSES FOR CONTINUOUS QUALITY IMPROVEMENT

Tools include forms, methods, and analytical techniques that assist in understanding a problem. Quality tools are more specific, because they include tools applied to solving organizational or unit-specific problems. This discussion does not include all the tools that can be used for CQI, but it provides an overview of the more up-to-date tools used today (Figure 22-4).

What Is Six Sigma?

Six Sigma (SS) quality improvements methods are the newest wave of change initiatives for CQI. As with any new wave before it (root cause analysis; pain as the fifth vital sign), TJC will most likely be inclined toward recommending SS methods in the future for accreditation purposes. If this is the case, CQI employees will need SS education to understand and use the information to benefit the institution.

SS is a measurement standard that began in the 1920s, when Walter Shewhart showed that three sigma from the mean is the point where errors start to occur. Shewhart was one of Edward Deming's teachers and is responsible for the PDSA cycle of process improvement. Credit for coining the term "Six Sigma" goes to Bill Smith of Motorola.

SS uses statistics to improve the efficiency of business processes. The primary goal of SS is to increase profits and reduce problems by improving standard operating procedures, reducing errors, and decreasing misuse of the system.

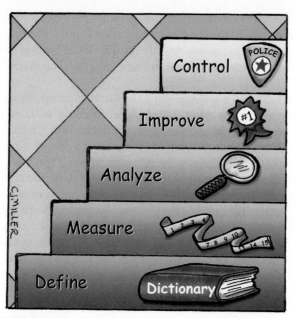

FIGURE 22-4

Stair steps to quality health care.

SS methodology is based on strategies that focus on CQI and reducing variation in practice through the application of DMAIC. In other words, once a protocol is found to be effective, everyone is trained to do it the same way. The SS DMAIC process (define, measure, analyze, improve, control) is used primarily for improving existing processes that do not meet institutional goals or national norms. DMAIC can save companies thousands of dollars per project. SS means having no more than 3.4 defects per million opportunities, or 99.99966% accuracy. The idea is to focus on the voice of the customer (VOC), whether internal or external, and to reduce risks associated with high-volume, high-risk, problem-prone areas of practice. Internal customers are nursing staff that we work with and personnel from other departments. External customers include patients and visitors. This means that even the bedside nurse has a voice as an internal customer of the system.

From the time DMAIC is adopted, nursing administrators must be supportive and trained in rapid cycle changes (RCC). They must provide both financial and human resources and allow sufficient time for project teams to work. Then they need to be supportive of the efforts put forth. The entire organization must be behind the effort and be enthusiastic about change. Nurses and other health care providers need to have education on the DMAIC and RCC processes, as well. If the organizational culture is too resistant to change, it will be difficult. Often a cultural change is needed before the process will be successful. Every organization tends to have a certain culture by which it operates. When an organization is dealing with DMAIC, the culture should be one that rewards innovative ideas and is not resistant to change.

When referring to *data-driven methods,* we mean looking at real results that have been measured using numbers (calculations). The bottom line is that we know that we are not perfect, but we can strive to perform up to this 99.99966% goal.

> Let's put this goal into perspective. If you take a million blood pressure readings, there should be no fewer than 3.4 that were incorrect.

Another important point is that most processes function more effectively if they are kept within a certain range of error. The intent is to control peaks and valleys in performance (those things that are way off target). In this instance, a flat line is a good thing, as long as it is near the 100% mark of compliance.

The DMAIC process (Table 22-3) provides more reliability and validity than other QI models and has become a national trend in QI strategies. Many companies will only do business with those who are using DMAIC.

Recent use of the DMAIC model was found useful in improving medication administration and reducing medication errors for one hospital. Rapid cycle testing was used as part of DMAIC for this process improvement project. As a result, a medication administration checklist improved focus and standardized practice. Signs with the words "Do Not Disturb During Medication Administration" reminded other people of the process. The protocol checklists and signs remained as reminders to reduce distractions and were simple, inexpensive tools to keep patients safe. Nurses also liked them because they could get their work done quicker (Pape et al, 2005).

In another QI project, an operating room team improved patient outcomes from postoperative hypothermia by using the DMAIC model. Because of the DMAIC team approach and the use of real data, patients' temperatures showed improvement in the postanesthesia care unit (PACU) because they warmed patients in the preoperative holding area before surgery (Bitner et al, 2007). (See Evidence-Based Practice Box 22-1.)

HOW DO WE USE DMAIC?

The DMAIC flow diagram (Figure 22-5) provides an overview of the DMAIC process. The framework shows how the process flows from start to finish and on to the next project. However, depending on the project, the steps may not always follow the path directed by the arrows. Depending on the situation, teams may need to change direction at times.

TABLE 22-3 DMAIC	
DMAIC is pronounced *DUH-MAY-ICK* and includes:	
DEFINE	Define the issue, possible causes, and goals.
MEASURE	Measure the existing system with metrics.
ANALYZE	Analyze the gap between existing and goal.
IMPROVE	Improve the system with creative strategies.
CONTROL	Control and sustain the improvement.

Prevention of Postoperative Hypothermia

PRACTICE ISSUE

Postoperative hypothermia (PH) is often a complication for patients undergoing surgery. Not only is the operating room a very cold environment, but patients are dehydrated and their skin is exposed, not to mention the strain on body systems that tends to cool the body. In addition, hypothermia during all phases of surgery increases the risk of postoperative infections and other complications.

IMPLICATIONS FOR NURSING PRACTICE

- Patients often experienced high levels of postoperative hypothermia (PH).
- Older adults are more at risk for PH and increased lengths of stay in the PACU.
- The DMAIC model provided a method to include staff members in the improvement process.
- With the creation of an easy-to-use tool, the team successfully improved core temperatures in postoperative patients.
- The implementation of preoperative forced air-warming blankets created a practice change for nurses, anesthesia care providers, and surgeons and eventually became a standard practice.
- Regardless of the initial financial strain of purchasing more equipment, the ultimate savings in patient complications would offset the funds.

Considering This Information:

What can you do to improve outcomes for surgical patients?

Reference for the Evidence

Bitner, J, et al: A team approach to the prevention of unplanned postoperative hypothermia, *AORN J* 85:921-929, 2007.

Sometimes the process may need to stop at the measure phase and go back to the design phase to develop formats for measuring. For example, the team may want to do some brainstorming or conduct RCCs to develop the best data collection form before moving on. Other times the form that was developed did not work and the team might make a different one to use for data collection. Now we see that the plan-do-study-act (PDSA) cycle also fits well with DMAIC (Figure 22-6).

PDSA is used to plan and conduct rapid cycle changes (RCC). However, there is no "one size fits all" for organizations using DMAIC. Nevertheless, the organization needs to standardize the DMAIC process somewhat so that everyone understands his or her roles and functions during each step.

As indicated, the PDSA cycle is contained with the RCC. Thus each project will be done slightly differently. The main focus is to keep on track with the goal in mind and to use real data, not guesswork or gossip, to direct decisions. As they say, if you do not measure it, you cannot fix it.

The Define Phase

In the define phase, a charter is developed as a written document of the work the team will accomplish. The charter is an agreement among the team members as to what they see as the problem and where they want to go. First, they identify the business case, main goals, team leaders, and team responsibilities or roles. The business case is a statement about why it is important to consider resolving the problem in terms of cost, injury, or standards.

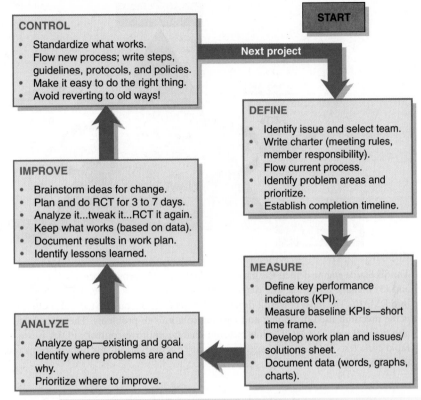

CONTROL
- Standardize what works.
- Flow new process; write steps, guidelines, protocols, and policies.
- Make it easy to do the right thing.
- Avoid reverting to old ways!

START

Next project

DEFINE
- Identify issue and select team.
- Write charter (meeting rules, member responsibility).
- Flow current process.
- Identify problem areas and prioritize.
- Establish completion timeline.

IMPROVE
- Brainstorm ideas for change.
- Plan and do RCT for 3 to 7 days.
- Analyze it...tweak it...RCT it again.
- Keep what works (based on data).
- Document results in work plan.
- Identify lessons learned.

MEASURE
- Define key performance indicators (KPI).
- Measure baseline KPIs—short time frame.
- Develop work plan and issues/solutions sheet.
- Document data (words, graphs, charts).

ANALYZE
- Analyze gap—existing and goal.
- Identify where problems are and why.
- Prioritize where to improve.

FIGURE 22-5

This flow diagram provides an overview of the define-measure-analyze-improve-control (DMAIC) process. The framework depicts the flow from the starting point of Define through Control to the next project. However, depending on the project, the process may not always follow the path directed by the arrows. Depending on the situation, teams may need to change direction at times.

When team members are chosen, it is important to include only those who want to be a part of the solution, and not a part of the problem. This is no place for "whiners" or complainers. Then set team rules (attendance, absence, how decisions are made). During meetings, ask that only one conversation go on at a time (no sidebars). Determine what the limits are on resources (financial, personal, time) and plan to discuss those.

Allow brainstorming during meetings. **Brainstorming** is a process by which a group of people think, talk about, and list many solutions to the problem. Some ideas may sound crazy at first, but group members should not make fun of them. The oddest ideas can often be changed into very useful ones. Although this may cause some delays in meeting goals, it is a valuable part of the process. That is how great innovative ideas start. During meetings, identify who the stakeholders are and how they will be affected. Stakeholders are key people who will be affected by change and those who can either influence or derail the improvement. Consider how to sell ideas to the stakeholders. Also, identify support resources and people. Who will provide the money and/or support the recommended changes?

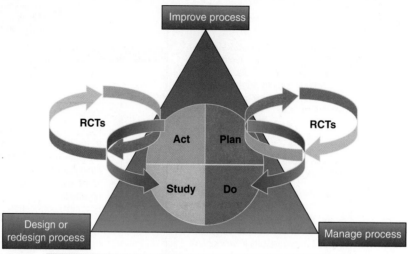

FIGURE 22-6

The Six Sigma engine depicts the parts of DMAIC to (1) improve processes, (2) design or redesign processes, and (3) manage processes. The diagram here, designed by Dr. Pape, depicts how the PDSA and RCCs tie into DMAIC. The most powerful difference between Six Sigma's DMAIC and other improvement methods is the precision used in finding and keeping solutions to problems. The plan-do-study-act (PDSA) cycle also fits well with DMAIC (define-measure-analyze-improve-control). PDSA is used to plan and conduct rapid cycle tests (RCCs) of change. There is no "one size fits all" for organizations using DMAIC to move toward Six Sigma.

Next, write the problem statement and goal statement. The problem statement will be similar to the business case. Write down the cost of doing nothing different (fire fighting) versus the cost of improving. These costs can be in dollar amounts or lost time, injury, errors, or dissatisfaction, for example. Set the goal in terms of how much saving is planned—10%? 25%? By what date?

Example: Problem statement—The number of patients waiting to be seen by an MD in the emergency department (ED) is excessive, and patients are dissatisfied. Controls are needed so that there are a limited number of minutes between bed placement and MD arrival to bedside. Patients need to be cared for efficiently so that they can get through the system in a timely manner, thus making room for more patients who are waiting in the waiting room. The hospital needs to contain costs and improve patient satisfaction.

Example: Goal Statement = There will be a 25% decrease in amount of time patients must wait in the ED after being placed in a bed.

In the example, the team would "flow out" or make a diagram of the processes (Figure 22-7) that take place within the problem or the unit. When flow diagramming, use large sheets of paper or write on a dry erase board. If a board is used, someone should still take notes and record the flow process on paper so that it can be kept as a record. Flow the current, "as is" process. At this point, the team needs to know how things are actually happening, not how they are supposed to happen.

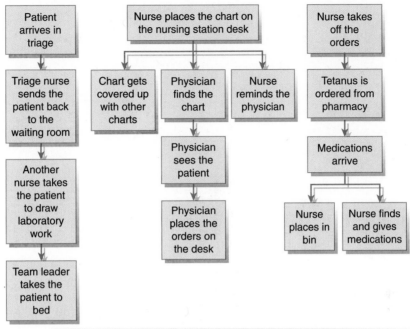

FIGURE 22-7

This is a process flow example. There are inputs, processes, and outputs in a typical flow diagram.

Ask lots of questions, such as why things happen at each step. Identify problem areas for improvements. Think "outside the box" and slay "sacred cows!" This means being willing to be innovative and objective in thinking of possible solutions.

At the start of each team meeting, review the agenda or plan for the meeting. Ask for any additions to the agenda, listen to each person's past assignment results, and review the overall progress individuals have made. It is important to allow time for discussion and brainstorming. At the end of the meeting, review what lessons have been learned and set assignments for the next meeting.

Develop the work plan (Table 22-4). This is usually done with an Excel spreadsheet used for tracking plans. The issues/solutions sheet, also done with an Excel spreadsheet, keeps the team focused and is used to track brainstorming sessions. Both the issues/solutions sheet (Table 22-5) and the workplan keep the team progressing on track. Figure 22-8 provides another flow process example with a medication delivery process diagrammed step by step as a group.

The Measure Phase

Everyone within the team needs to agree on what is to be measured. These are called *key performance indicators* (KPI). KPIs should reflect the things that the team sees as problem areas. Typical KPIs are time, costs, distance, numbers of incidents, or items. It is best to use whole numbers (with decimals) and measurable facts. Never use what someone *thinks* is a problem. Measure the problem first. It is also important to identify who will be responsible for data collection, retrieval, and analysis. Ultimately, if the team fails to document everything, things will fall apart quickly.

TABLE 22-4 Emergency Center Rapid Cycle Changes

RCC #	DATE	RCC INITIATIVE	WORKPLAN	RESPONSIBLE PERSONS	DATA COLLECTION PROCESS	SUMMARY RESULTS	KPI MOST AFFECTED	% IMPROVED
1	7/1/09	MD Awareness: Time in Bed	Use a special table called the "deck" to place the charts for the MDs. The RN Team Leader is to place the time patient placed in a bed on the triage note so MD aware.	Team Leader (TL) and/or Patient Care Coordinator (PCC or Charge Nurse)	We collected pre-RCC data via First Net (bed-tracking software) for July 1-3 on 278 patients and compared it with RCC data for July 4-6 on 268 patients (for time from bed placement to seen by MD). The times were 121 minutes vs. 110 minutes.	This RCC is considered successful. Implement immediately. At first, nurses that received ambulance patients placed chart on "deck" and did not place the time initially.	Bed Placement to MD Exam	10%
2	7/10/09	Chart on Deck	Implement chart placement on bedside table (deck) with log book. Record time when placed on "deck" and when chart is picked up.	PA, MD	Manual tracking; pre-RCC: Mon, Tues, Wed; post-RCC: Thurs, Fri, Sat. Data revealed an average turnaround time for MD to receive charts of 2.5 hours.	RCC was successful. The MD saw the patient after charts placed on deck an average of 60 minutes instead of 2.5 hours = a 40% improvement.	Bed Placement to MD Exam	40%

3	7/16/09	"Deck" Officer	Creation of a "Deck" Officer concept to enhance MD awareness initiative. A PA is assigned to monitor the "deck" and assign patients to MD/PAs if patient's chart not picked up within 15 minutes of bed placement.	Medical Director, PAs	First Net (tracking system): pre-RCC days without Deck Officer. RCC data: Days with Deck Officer by secretary July 24-26 Pre RCC = 61 minutes, RCC; after 26 minutes	RCC overall was successful. Barriers include not always having the extra person to act as Deck Officer. On days when the Deck Officer used, most patients were seen in <30 minutes.	Bed Placement to MD Exam 42%

TABLE 22-5 Brainstorming Results: Hospital Solutions Issues Sheet

Date	Persons	Issue	Detail	Proposed Solution	Responsible
6/1/09	MDs	MD to see patient	Average time from patient arrival to bed placement is 3 hours. Delays in time for MDs to see patients still remain problematic. A new RCC is being developed for this.	When patients are placed in a bed, a copy of the triage note is placed on the "deck." "Deck" is a term used for the location of charts on patients pending MD evaluation. The MD cannot determine how long the patient has been in a bed based on a chart that only has a triage time.	TL, charge nurse
6/3/09	EC staff nurses	Chart on deck	Some of the nurses failed to put the time on the note as directed. Nurses that receive ambulance patients place their note on "deck" and did not place the time initially. The Team Leader (TL) had to go back and remind them for a couple of days.	The TL had to go back and remind them for a couple of days. Most patients brought from waiting area by TL were done correctly.	TL, charge nurse
6/6/09	EC staff	Chart on deck	Still having problems getting charts in hands of MDs so that they will see patients quicker.	Discussion about the possibility of assigning an MD or PA to be the Deck Officer to more closely monitor charts.	MD, PA
7/10/09	EC	EC patient flow	Arrival to bed for admitted patients is an average of 235 minutes.	Focus on having TL aggressively look for possible EC discharges and move patients to the dismissal area.	TL, charge nurse

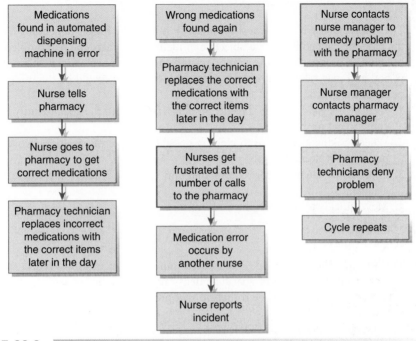

FIGURE 22-8

This is a process flow example. There are inputs, processes, and outputs in a typical flow diagram.

Identify what specifically will be measured to determine improvements and what will not be measured. Operational definitions for the KPIs detail the thing or event using specific wording with written inclusion and exclusion criteria. These are similar to metric descriptors discussed earlier. They define in detail what is to be measured. These definitions tell the team what is not going to be measured. This helps get everyone in agreement on what is identifiable and measurable.

For example: KPI #1 = The number of near-miss medication incidences on the nursing unit due to wrong medications found in the automated dispensing machine. We are including only those kept in the automated dispensing machine and excluding any kept in other areas.

Begin by measuring baseline numbers. That is, start with what exists currently before any changes are made. In other words, do not meddle with things until you know how bad the problem is. Do not tell anyone what is being investigated. Otherwise, you will not see any true changes when you do RCCs. Baseline measures can be retrospective if data have already been collected, or you can go forward for a couple of weeks to find out what the real data show. Find out what the actual losses are in time, errors, or dollars.

1. Get all the facts about the numbers of errors first. Record them in the work plan.
2. Measure and track the issue over a defined period of time based on what would be a realistic time frame to obtain a sample of what is occurring. This may need to be done for 2 to 4 weeks or longer.
3. Document data in words, graphs, pie charts, and bar charts.

The Analyze Phase

The analyze phase is usually a short phase, but it can be longer depending on the issue. Analyze the baseline data collected. Be objective in identifying where the real problems exist. These may be indicated by peaks in the graphs related to the number of incidences over a 2- to 4-week period and may relate to problems with processes. What could be the underlying causes of the peaks in the graph?

1. Identify the *gaps* between the current performance and the goal. Identify how far you need to come to get to the goal.
2. When looking at the data to identify possible sources of variation, avoid blaming people or past ways of doing things.
3. Look at the current process flow diagram again and determine where to begin making a change.
4. Move quickly to the next phase to improve.

The Improve Phase

The improve phase is a good place to determine whether measures reflect the true problems. The problem statement and goal statement may need to be revised based on the findings. The data collected may have shown that no real problem exists or that the problem involves other issues.

Now use the PDSA cycle (Table 22-6) to plan and implement some RCCs. The idea is to think of creative ways to improve things. Brainstorm ideas for the RCCs that you might try based on a problem process step within the flow diagram and the baseline metrics.

Brainstorming is the process where all team members spontaneously contribute and gather ideas without excluding any idea given. It is usually performed rapidly with all ideas considered and recorded. Be clear about what the target is and play off of each other's suggestions.

The group may consider using a fair voting method or writing out RCC ideas. Otherwise, whoever talks the loudest gets heard. Sometimes some great ideas come from those quiet people, who may be more comfortable writing their ideas. The collective ideas can then be reviewed by the group leader and then presented to the group.

1. Ask yourself: Can a step in the process be eliminated? Simplifying steps and deleting steps in a process can often eliminate big defects.
2. Could you try a new method?
3. Next, conduct the RCC using the PDSA cycle (see Table 22-6) for 3 to 7 days. Include staff education before starting the RCC so that everyone understands what is expected.
4. Conduct the RCC and study the results. Document everything in the workplan.
5. Analyze the data with percentage calculations for improvements over baseline for last week.
6. Document all brainstorming sessions in the issues/solutions sheet.

Use data to determine whether there were improvements or a lack of improvement. What percentage of improvement was there this week compared with last week? Compared with the baseline measure? How many minutes difference is there? Make decisions based on fact, not assumptions. Small improvements still mean improvement and help determine whether you are on the right track or not.

Small changes may need to be made in the process that was tried … so tweak it … and test it again with a change in the RCC over 3 to 7 days. Compare percentages again (against baseline or the previous week) and determine whether there was any improvement.

TABLE 22-6 The PDSA Cycle Within the RCC

PLAN	1. State the goal of the RCC cycle. Make predictions about what will be expected to happen. Who will be responsible, at what time, and place? When will it occur? Where will it take place first?
	2. What are we trying to accomplish?
	3. How will we know when we get there? Roughly, how far do we expect to come (percentage, minutes)? Use only data that are reflective of the KPIs. For example, you would not measure the time it takes to do something if you are looking at the number of incidences.
	4. What change can we feasibly make that will result in improvement? Be realistic about what can be changed.
	5. How long should it take? How many days should you run the RCC to see a result. Keep it as short as possible … 7-10 days.
Use the workplan and issues/solutions sheet to document, track, and analyze the data during and after RCCs. The workplan is very important to project successes in keeping track of each RCC and results.	
DO	First, carry out the RCC on one or two nursing units for 3-7 days. If it needs tweaking, make a small change and RCC again for 3-7 days or longer, depending on the issue. Then move to another nursing unit.
STUDY	Compare the resulting data to your predictions, to baseline, and contrast it to previous time frames. For example: What was the improvement in time compared with last week?
ACT	Act on what was discovered after the initial RCC. What are the new changes the team can make based on results? What might be the next cycle? Go on to do another RCC to improve the process further.

Market the solutions to the people whose cooperation is needed. If front-line people have been involved at the outset, this part is easier. Prepare for possible objections to the implementation of the change and plan to overcome them.

The Control Phase

Now you are ready to establish controls to keep things going in the right direction. Controlling and sustaining the improvement is not easy and requires the development, documentation, and implementation of an ongoing monitoring plan.

1. Standardize the steps in the new process and detail new flow diagrams. Write standard operating procedures, protocols, steps, guidelines, or policies so that it will be easier for people to do the right thing and harder for them to do the wrong thing.

2. Educate everyone about the new practice. Distribute the information in a systematic manner so that everyone in the organization has an equal chance of being informed. Educate new employees in correct procedures and be an example for them to follow.

3. Keep people informed of any changes.
4. Prevent reversion back to old ways or breaks in the "critical links" in the process by developing a process to monitor that changes have stuck and gains are sustained. Keep the process on the new course and maintain the new practices you worked so hard to develop. Backsliding can occur easily since people tend to return to old habits. Change is difficult for some people who are used to tradition or who have been absent from the job for a time.
5. Continue to measure KPIs on a routine basis to see whether solutions are still working. If slipping occurs, reinforce the new change or do more RCCs.

Box 22-2 provides a simplified example of DMAIC used successfully in one emergency center. Many of the important details have been left out for space. However, the basic process can be seen. Now see what you can do with the DMAIC process on a small scale using the scenario in Critical Thinking Box 22-3.

Practice improves results with time, and it can be a lot of fun.

HEALTH CARE PROVIDER CREDENTIALING FOR QUALITY IMPROVEMENT

Some larger health care organizations require that an individual obtain a certification in health care quality within a certain period of time of the hire date. Persons can become a *Certified Professional in Healthcare Quality* (CPHQ) after taking a certification test to determine one's knowledge of quality management, quality improvement, case/care/disease/utilization management, and risk management at all employment levels and in all health care settings.

Although there is no longer a minimum education requirement, those who test should have worked in quality management for a minimum of 2 years and review testing requirements before investing money into taking the examination. Approximately 75% of those who apply to test actually achieve certification.

CONCLUSION

Quality is about fire prevention, not fire fighting, and accountability for one's actions is critical in nursing. We must provide quality care that is cost-effective and meets the health needs of our patients. We do not have the luxury of giving a patient all the time we would like, or to use any equipment and supplies we want. That is why it is important to find solutions that save time and money. Nurses must be accountable to both the quality of care and the economics of providing that care. In quality improvement, the organization must first consider the voice of the customer, whether internal or external. The "squeaky wheel" issues are sometimes where organizations start. However, action should be taken first on those matters that are associated with high-volume, high-risk, problem-prone practices, and where errors frequently occur. Proven methods for quality improvement should be emphasized in all health care settings.

DMAIC is one of those, and it should be taught as a standard process so that everyone in the organization understands the roles and functions during each step. PDSA is used to plan and conduct RCCs. Certainly each organization must evaluate using DMAIC to move toward Six Sigma. The future of quality and patient safety is promising, as more and more health care providers and organizations get on the "band wagon" for safety changes.

BOX 22-2   Example of DMAIC in the Emergency Center

Problem statement: Emergency department patients are not seen by an MD in a timely manner.

DEFINE

The team *Defined* the cause of the problem as having to do with where the charts are placed.
Goal—Get the charts to the MDs sooner.
Business case—Cost of doing nothing different = Unhappy patients, possible patient complications, lack of bed space, and bottlenecks in throughput.

MEASURE

Key performance indicator (KPI) #1 = Time between patient bed placement and being seen by MD.
The team *Measured* the actual average baseline data (KPI #1) over a period of 2 weeks. Baseline = 90 minutes (15 min).
Target = Patients should be seen within 30 minutes of bed placement (a 50% improvement) within a month.

ANALYZE

The team *Analyzed* the gap between existing situation and goal of 30 minutes (gap is 60 min). The gap also depended on which MD was on duty.
Can something be done about which MD was on duty? Not really.
The team brainstormed for other ideas. Can something be done about where charts are placed? Yes.

IMPROVE

The team *Improved* by doing RCCs.
KPI #1 = Time of patient bed placement to seen by MD.
RCC #1: For the next 5 days, the team members involved placed charts in a separate bin and measured KPI #1.
Result = The MD saw patients on time 34% of the time. So they tweaked the plan and did more RCCs.
RCC #2: For the next 5 days they placed charts on separate bedside table (the deck) and set up a log book of times that charts were placed and picked up.
Still measured KPI #1 = Time of patient bed placement to seen by MD and added another KPI.
KPI #2 = Time between charts placed on deck and picked up from deck.
Result = MD saw patients on time 20% of the time.
The team again brainstormed, tweaked the plan, and did more RCCs.
Next 5 days, one MD was assigned as deck officer to oversee the process.
Result = MD saw patients on time 99% of the time within 30 minutes.

CONTROL

The team *Controlled* and sustained the improvement by establishing a standard practice.
They wrote a protocol and announced the new practice:
The protocol was to always have charts placed on deck and to assign a deck officer to monitor timeliness of chart retrieval.
The Department Director monitored effectiveness of the protocol and watched for slippage into old ways.

CRITICAL THINKING
BOX 22-3

A retrospective review of several charts revealed that documentation for 40% of PRN medications was lacking a prior assessment of pain. About 50% of the charts did not have documentation that the pain was evaluated according to policy within 30 to 45 minutes after the PRN medication was given. You have been asked to lead a team to resolve the problems that occurred mostly on your nursing unit.

1. What standard of practice has been violated?
2. How would you go about conducting your problem resolution using the DMAIC approach for process improvement?
3. Who would you include on your team?
4. Who will develop the workplan and issues solutions sheet?
5. When will meetings be held? What are the ground rules?
6. What is the business case?
7. What are the goals and targets?
8. What are the KPIs?
9. What RCC can be done?
10. Imagine that you have some excellent RCC results. What will you do to control the improvement?

Change is inevitable! It is the one thing you can always count on. Things will never be the same as they once were. So if you want to prevent other people from making changes for you, you have to get involved in the process. Rather than resist change, embrace it and make it yours! He who fails to invent change is at the mercy of those who will!

BIBLIOGRAPHY

Bitner J, et al: A team approach to the prevention of unplanned postoperative hypothermia, *AORN J* 85:921-929, 2007.

Institute for Healthcare Improvement (2010:) Retrieved from *www.ihi.org.*

National Patient Safety Foundation (2010): Retrieved from *www.npsf.org.*

Pape TM: Applying airline safety practices to medication administration, *MEDSURG Nurs: J Adult Health April* 12:77-94, 2003.

Pape TM (2006): Workaround error, *AHRQ WebM&M.* Retrieved from *www.webmm.ahrq.gov/case.aspx?caseID=118.*

Pape TM (2010): ATRANE: A Timely Resource for Advancing the Nursing Environment. Retrieved from *www.atrane.org.*

Pape TM, et al: Innovative approaches to reducing nurses' distractions during medication administration, *J Cont Educ Nurs* 36:33-39, 2005.

Quality and Safety Education for Nurses (2010): Quality and Safety Education for Nurses (QSEN). Retrieved from *www.qsen.org.*

TJC (2010a): Sentinel event alert. Retrieved from *www.jointcommission.org/SentinelEvents/SentinelEvent Alert/.*

TJC (2010b): The 2010 National Patient Safety Goals PowerPoint Presentation. Retrieved from *www.jointcommission.org/PatientSafety/NationalPatientSafety Goals.*

TJC (2007, November 12). The joint commission news conference to discuss progress and healthcare quality facing American hospitals on November 12, 2007 at 11:45 a.m. central time. TJC.

United States Pharmacopeia (2010a): About the United States Pharmacopeia. Retrieved from *www.usp.org.*

United States Pharmacopeia (2010b): MEDMARX® data reports. Retrieved from *www.usp.org.*

Additional resources are available online at *http://evolve.elsevier.com/Zerwekh/nsgtoday/.*

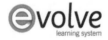

CHAPTER 23

Nursing Informatics

JoAnn Zerwekh, MSN, EdD, RN, and Cheryl D. Parker, MSN, PhD, RN

> *If we cannot name it [nursing practice], we cannot control it, finance it, research it, teach it, or put it into public policy.*
> —Norma M. Lang, PhD, RN, FAAN, FRCN

> *When computers (people) are networked, their power multiplies geometrically. Not only can people share all that information inside their machines but they can reach out and instantly tap the power of other machines (people), essentially making the entire network their computer.*
> —Scott McNeely

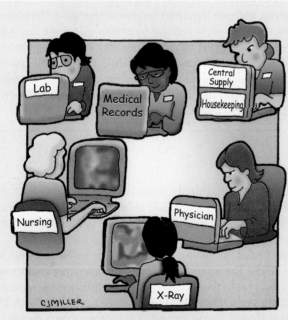

Nursing informatics—a specialty practice of nursing.

After completing this chapter, you should be able to:

- Define nursing informatics.

- Discuss the necessity of using recognized taxonomies and standardized nursing languages in nursing documentation.

- Discuss trends associated with the computerized electronic record, e-health, mobile devices.

- Describe what a nurse specializing in nursing informatics might do.

- Review the steps in evaluating the validity of a website.

- Discuss future trends in nursing informatics.

omputer technology is pervasive today. Everywhere we turn technology is in evidence. The neighborhood grocery store has automated scanners and checkout lines. Your bank has automated tellers, check scanners, wire transfers, and online services. The local library has automated catalogs, interlibrary lending, and books online. From our homes and smartphones, we can access the world through the Internet, researching any question, sending e-mail, and purchasing just about anything via an Internet connection. A litany of computerized marvels could fill volumes.

The explosion of new technology during the past 30 years that makes all this possible is truly phenomenal. What is even more incredible, and perhaps a bit frightening to some, is that this seems to be just the beginning. The time has come when the thoughts, communications, creations, manuscripts, learning material, and financial assets of the civilized world will exist primarily in electronic form. If the lights went out, civilization as we know it would cease to exist as most of modern society depends on the electrical and information infrastructure.

Health care is not immune. Some of the most complex automated systems and certainly some of the most complex requirements for these systems can be found in the health care environment. Systems to serve the diverse needs of the health care industry—from the administration and financial departments to the many clinical disciplines—need to be implemented and integrated across the continuum of care of modern health care organizations. As a result, the demand for health care professionals who are knowledgeable in the application of this technology is growing rapidly.

Even with technology all around us, we as users do not always feel comfortable with it. Technology is sometimes confusing, intimidating, and—in large part because it changes so rapidly—downright bewildering to some. Even so, there are some relative constants that make the field less confusing and easier to manage. One of the biggest challenges we face is how to properly harness and apply the available technology. The good news is that while the technology will continue to change and become more robust, the fundamentals of nursing care do not. The goal of this chapter is to explore how nursing and health care are embracing, harnessing, and using technology to increase the quality of patient care in all health care settings.

NURSING INFORMATICS

What Is Nursing Informatics?

In 1994, the American Nurses Association (ANA) recognized the field of nursing informatics. In 2008, the ANA updated the definition of nursing informatics (NI) as "a specialty that integrates nursing science, computer science, and information science to manage and communicate data, information, knowledge, *and wisdom* in nursing practice" (ANA, 2008, p 1).

The ANA further identified two distinct roles in nursing informatics: the informatics nurse (IN) and the informatics nurse specialist (INS). The informatics nurse has experience in nursing informatics but does not have an advanced degree in the specialty. The informatics nurse specialist has graduate level education in informatics or a related field (ANA, 2008). Nurses in both IN and INS roles "support consumers, patients, clinical nurses, and other providers in their decision-making in all roles and settings. This support is accomplished through the use of information structures, information processes, and information technology" (ANA, 2008, p 1).

With the advent of both specialty and integrated clinical information systems (CIS), the longitudinal electronic health record (EHR) has become the ultimate goal of health care organizations and is now supported by federal mandate. The EHR will reflect a record of patients' health care throughout their life. Although this realization of 100% integration of all patient data in one longitudinal electronic record is becoming more available, few organizations have actually reached this goal. There are still outstanding issues of what to do with outside information that comes into your facility, that is, old systems not able to interface with new ones, corrupt data from old systems, and not enough resources to enter all the data from old charts. Although solutions are being developed to solve some of these problems, it will take time to reach the ultimate goal.

Information is power. The extensive clinical background of the IN/INS is invaluable to the success of the implementation of the software applications. Nurses have a unique understanding of workflow, the hospital and clinical environment, and the specific procedures that are necessary for effective health care information infrastructure. Moreover, the IN/INS is critical to the translation of standard information into practical models that can be applied to improve the health care work environment (Delany, 2004).

But not all nurses in IN/INS roles work on implementation of the EHR. Some work for health care product vendors in both the hardware and software areas. They help to inform the next generation of existing products, and they work with engineers/design teams to create new products, always bringing the patient care viewpoint and the needs of the end user to the design process. Others work for consulting firms and specialize in workflow improvement using technology while still others work for government and educational institutions. The variety is seemingly endless.

The 2009 Healthcare Information Management Systems Society (HIMSS) Informatics Nurse Impact Survey asked organizational leaders to provide input on the roles and impact of informatics nurses in their organizations. Organizations responding included hospital or health systems (75%), vendor or consulting firms (11%), and other organizations such as home health, ambulatory care facilities, and academic or government facilities. Nearly all respondents noted that informatics nurses play a significant role in user education. Informatics nurses are also widely involved in system implementation, user support, workflow analysis, and gaining buy-in from end users. A primary success indicator for the informatics nurse was making sure that information technology did no harm to the patient (HIMSS, 2009).

So, how does one become an expert in this unique field of nursing? What does a nurse specializing in nursing informatics do on a daily basis? And, how does informatics impact the work of a clinical nurse?

Experience and Education

Many nurses in informatics roles today do not have formal education beyond their nursing preparation. They were "recruited" by their employers to help build and implement an electronic medical record application. These nurses learned as they went. However, this is changing rapidly as many of these nurses are returning to graduate school to pursue a master's degree in nursing informatics or related discipline. Those informatics nurses who want to hold a leadership role in informatics will need graduate level preparation. A student in a nursing informatics master's program said that she thought she knew all about nursing informatics but she learned in graduate school that she only knew about it at her own organization level. Her graduate school education had broadened her perspectives and introduced her to new concepts and ways of thinking.

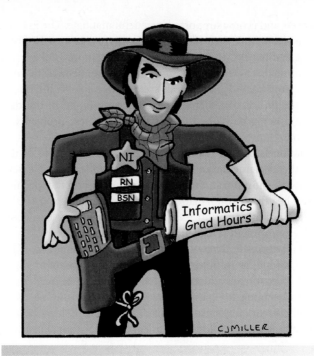

FIGURE 23-1

Nurses are finding technology can support many areas of nursing practice.

The Certification Process

In 1994, the American Nursing Credentialing Center (ANCC) *(www.nursecredentialing.org/default.aspx)* provided a method for nurses to become certified in this specialty. The baccalaureate degree is the minimum requirement to take the certification exam. The focus is to improve patient care with health care technology that encourages caregivers and physicians to make more accurate and timely decisions (Figure 23-1). Nurses can obtain RN-BC certification in informatics nursing through the ANCC.

Role of the IN/INS

The IN/INS must have a basic knowledge of how computers and networks work as well as systems analysis and design principles and information management. It is important for the IN/INS to converse with both the clinical staff and the technology staff regarding hardware, software, communications, data representation, and security (Figure 23-2). An IN/INS will become comfortable with software implementation, training, testing, presenting, and facilitating knowledge (Critical Thinking Box 23-1).

CRITICAL THINKING BOX 23-1	What has been your experience and exposure to the use of technology in the hospital? Your school? At home? Think of ways to become more familiar with the use of computers and other technology.

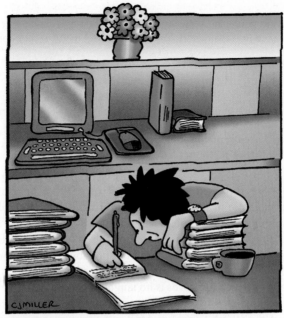

FIGURE 23-2
Even with technology all around us, we do not always feel comfortable with it.

PROFESSIONAL PRACTICE, TRENDS, AND ISSUES

What Are Regulatory and Accreditation Requirements?

Although there are many regulatory and governmental agencies instituting health care policy, the Health Insurance Portability and Accountability Act (HIPAA) and The Joint Commission (TJC) impact the daily work of every clinician and organization. The nurse must have a clear understanding of both HIPAA regulations and TJC requirements to be able to provide safe nursing care.

HIPAA. In 1996, the HIPAA was signed into law. The law defines standards that were developed to ensure that health care organizations collect the right data in a common format so that the data can be shared, as well as protect the privacy and security of patient data (Simpson, 2001). The major impact from this regulatory legislation is in these areas:

- Health information privacy law
- Data security standards
- Electronic transactions standards

Among many requirements, health care entities must adopt written privacy policies and procedures that define how they intend to abide by the highly complex regulations and protect individually identifiable health information. Each health care organization must ensure that all staff members who have access to patient information have an understanding of the consequences of noncompliance (Gale Group, 2001).

How has your clinical facility and/or school made changes to accommodate the Health Insurance Portability and Accountability Act (HIPAA) requirements?

Do you know your clinical facility's policies on cell phone/smartphone use in patient care areas? How about picture taking, Internet use, Internet access policy, information security access, and user-ID/password agreement?

In 1998, it was proposed that all health plans, health plan providers, and health care clearing-houses that maintain or transmit health information electronically be required to establish and maintain responsible and appropriate safeguards to ensure the integrity and confidentiality of the information. Although this seems logical, it is a very difficult and time-consuming task when using automated systems that did not previously meet these requirements (Critical Thinking Box 23-2).

Violation of HIPAA standards is no laughing matter. Violations of health information privacy can include termination of employment and even indictment and prison time. In 2010, a former researcher at the UCLA School of Medicine was sentenced to 4 months in federal prison for violations of the HIPAA privacy rule (Goedert, 2010, para 1).

HIPAA and the Use of Mobile Computing Devices. Knox and Smith (2007) encourage everyone to think about patient privacy and HIPAA compliance in the clinical area, especially with the growing use of laptops, tablet PCs, and cell/smartphones that take pictures and record videos (Critical Thinking Box 23-3).

You can violate an organization's HIPAA policies and not even realize it!

The influx of new mobile computing technology, such as tablet computers or smartphones, is creating new implications for protection of privacy and security. How to protect confidential information is something that we learn at the beginning of our nursing career; however, protecting that same information on a mobile device may not be so easily understood. The following is a list of some simple precautions that can be taken to help secure patient information that may be stored on a mobile device. These recommendations should be followed as standard practice.

- Keep careful physical control of the device at all times.
- Use data-encryption technology to protect the information.
- Use a password when turning on any computing device and a time-out to reactivate the password.
- Disable the infrared ports except when they are actually being used.
- Do not send infrared transmissions in public locations (Pancoast et al, 2003, p 611).

With the use of new technologies there is potential to improve patient safety and outcome, as well as reduce potential injury; however, at the same time there is an increased risk for exposing confidential patient information. A cautionary approach along with assuming the responsibility

CRITICAL THINKING BOX 23-4

Have you had the opportunity to be in clinical during a visit by The Joint Commission? If so, what did you observe? How was the staff prepared for the visit?

for safeguarding the confidentiality of information should be used when you download patient information into a mobile device.

The Joint Commission. TJC wrote the information management (IM) standards in the mid-1990s. The 10 standards outline the need for information management regulation (Clark, 2004). Since that time, information management has been woven throughout the various standards and the national patient safety goals.

TJC sends out a team of experts for a review of every health care organization that wishes to be certified. This team inspects and reviews a variety of areas within each organization. The IN/INS may be called upon to lead the effort for preparing for TJC visit and for maintaining ongoing compliance (Critical Thinking Box 23-4).

Ethics

Privacy and Confidentiality. Every health care organization has a responsibility to itself, to its patients, and to the community at large to have good control of its information systems. Because the internal workings of health care rely on accurate and timely data and information, personal data about employees and patients must be kept safe and confidential. A corporate security plan is important to an organization.

Maintaining confidentiality implies a trust of the individuals who handle that data and information. These health care workers ensure the privacy of this information and use it only for the purpose for which it was disclosed.

Security policies must be explicit and well defined. Confidentiality agreements should be reviewed and signed upon start of employment and yearly thereafter. Breaches of security, confidentiality, or privacy should be dealt with quickly, and the offender should be charged accordingly. Every lapse should be treated openly and made an example for others to note. The informatics nurse may be involved in the investigation process and the writing of the policies and procedures. As this is outlined in both TJC and HIPAA standards, all nurses must be aware of the importance of these topics to the health care organization.

Models and Theories

Nomenclature, Classification, and Taxonomy. The quote from Dr. Lang at the beginning of the chapter has never been truer. Traditionally, nurses documented care using personal preference, unit standards, or facility policy (Keenan, 1999). Standardized nursing languages, sometimes called nomenclatures offer a recognized, systematic classification and consistent method of describing nursing practice. Nomenclatures act as descriptors or labels; classifications are group or class entities; and taxonomy is the study of the classifications.

In 1995, the ANA approved the establishment of the Nursing Information and Data Set Evaluation Center (NIDSEC) to review, evaluate against defined criteria, and recognize information systems from developers and manufacturers who support documentation of nursing care within automated nursing information systems (NIS) or within computer-based patient record systems (CPR). They recognized the following 13 nursing practice classification systems (ANA, 2003).

- North American Nursing Diagnosis Association International (NANDA-I) Approved List of Diagnostic Labels
- Nursing Interventions Classification System (NIC)
- Nursing Outcomes Classification System (NOC)
- Nursing Management Minimum Data Set (NMMDS)
- Clinical Care Classification (CCC) [formerly Home Health Care Classification (HHCC)]
- Omaha System
- Patient Care Data Set (PCDS)
- Perioperative Nursing Dataset (PNDS)
- SNOMED CT
- Nursing Minimum Data Set (NMDS)
- International Classification for Nursing (ICNP)
- ABC codes
- Logical Observation Identifier Names & Codes (LOINC)

If the unique nomenclature of these classification systems is used consistently, gathered data elements can be captured, stored, and manipulated accurately in the electronic medical record. Without a common language, data cannot be aggregated into useful language (Simpson, 2000). The need for consistency causes problems for software vendors as they attempt to produce unique and robust software packages that still use the recognized labels and groupings of nursing practice elements. So what happens?

Currently, each software vendor uses a unique, possibly patented naming convention for their specific functionality and then must "explain and define" these names and labels in their literature or presentations by relating them back to recognized nursing practice or data elements. This causes confusion to the user community.

The ANA Committee for Nursing Practice Information Infrastructure requires that classifications or languages meet certain criteria, including:

- The language provides a clinical useful terminology and rationale for development.
- The language consists of clear and unambiguous terms.
- The developer provides evidence of reliability, validity, and utility.
- The language includes a unique identifier for each item.

Each of these classifications or languages has made a unique contribution to knowledge development in nursing. Learning about and working with standardized nursing languages will ensure nursing contributions are an integral part of any electronic medical record. Understanding those contributions through research and teaching will help to further define the scope of nursing practice. Until complete standardization occurs, nurses must be prepared to use different classification systems at different facilities or even with systems from different vendors within a single facility (Critical Thinking Box 23-5).

Theories. From the inception of nursing informatics during the 1990s, *general systems theory* has served as a conceptual framework. Systems theory consists of six elements:

CRITICAL THINKING
BOX 23-5

What has been your experience or exposure to these different standard nursing languages? What does your clinical agency use?

- Interdependent parts—elements of the system that interact for processing
- Input—any outside element or factor that is brought into the system
- Process—the activity within the system
- Output—any product that is produced from the processing activity
- Control—rules or procedures within the system
- Feedback—reusing output from the system as input back into the system for validation or correction

This theory organizes interdependent parts working together to produce a product that none used alone could produce. Nursing informatics uses this theoretical foundation for analysis and design, implementation and support, and testing and evaluation of automated systems. It is used as a basis for decision-making, education curriculum needs, and foundation for system and project management.

Health care is in a state of constant change. Sometimes it is planned, and sometimes it happens quite unexpectedly. The effects of change range from positive to negative, from minor to major, from predictable to unpredictable. With the advent of computers and new technology, nurses and caregivers are being invited to use this technology. An understanding of the *theory of change* offers a foundation and approach to assist nurses and caregivers in the inevitable change that will occur with the implementation of a clinical information system. Review Kurt Lewin's change theory in Chapter 10.

It is common for informatics nurses to be called upon to answer some of these questions. They act as role models for nursing and caregiver users, as they themselves have moved from a clinical background to being very comfortable in a technical environment.

CLINICAL INFORMATION SYSTEMS

Every day nurses encounter technology, and this technology is changing the ways that health care is delivered in the hospital, physician's office, or the patient's home. CISs have replaced pencil and paper charting. Florence Nightingale expressed a desire for medical records that were standardized, organized, and legible and these goals are equally valid today.

> In attempting to arrive at the truth, I have applied everywhere for information, but in scarcely an instance have I been able to obtain hospital records fit for any comparison.
> —Florence Nightingale (Notes on a Hospital, 1873)

A 2001 Institute of Medicine (IOM) report, *Crossing the Quality Chasm: A New Health System for the 21st Century*, identified the development and application of CISs as essential for health care to be able to leverage state-of-the-art technology to deliver the highest-quality, lowest-cost patient care.

What Is a Clinical Information System (CIS)?

According to Sittig and colleagues (2002), "A clinical information system is a collection of various information technology applications that provides a centralized repository of information related to patient care across distributed locations. This repository represents the patient's history of illnesses and interactions with providers by encoding knowledge capable of helping clinicians decide about the patient's condition, treatment options, and wellness activities. The repository also encodes the status of decisions, actions underway for those decisions, and relevant information that can help in performing those actions. The database could also hold other information about the patient, including genetic, environmental, and social contexts" (p 1). Essentially, the CIS uses the computer to provide and store information and data about a patient from departments that are patient-focused or department-focused.

What Is the Electronic Health Record (EHR)?

There is still some debate about whether an electronic health record (EHR) and an electronic medical record (EMR) are the same or different. The experts are moving in the direction that the two are different. HIMSS defines the EHR as:

the longitudinal electronic record of patient health information generated by one or more encounters in any care delivery setting. Included in this information are patient demographics, progress notes, problems, medications, vital signs, past medical history, immunizations, laboratory data and radiology reports. The EHR automates and streamlines the clinician's workflow. The EHR has the ability to generate a complete record of a clinical patient encounter—as well as supporting other care-related activities directly or indirectly via interface—including evidence-based decision support, quality management, and outcomes reporting. (HIMSS, 2010, para 1)

Figures 23-3 and 23-4 illustrate screenshots from a patient's EHR.

The EMR is comprised of data from multiple software applications used by a facility such as a hospital or provider officer to order, document, and store patient information just as a paper medical record did so in the past. The ability of the computer systems to combine data from various EMRs to form a more holistic view of a patient is one of the major benefits of electronic documentation.

For example, a patient is seen in a primary care provider (PCP) office for complaints of indigestion. The PCP completes a history and physical, does an ECG and basic lab studies. All data are in the computer at the office comprising one EMR for that patient. The patient is sent home with instructions. Later that evening, the patient feels worse and goes to the emergency department. Because it is after hours, the data in the patient's EMR at the PCP office is not available. A new EMR is begun. An EHR would be able to access data from both of these EMRs.

There is movement toward inclusion of data collected by the patient into the EHR. This is called the personal health record (PHR). These data could include family history, real-time blood glucose readings or exercise information sent directly from glucometer to the personal health record. Then, with permission of the patient, these data elements could be uploaded into the patient's PCP's EMR. Advantages of the EHR are listed in Box 23-1.

As mentioned in the IOM report Key Capabilities of an Electronic Health Record System (2003), a listing of essential features of the EHR (Box 23-2) must be addressed for our outdated health care system model to take advantage of the potential benefits of the "e-revolution." With an estimated 100 million Americans going to the Internet daily to obtain information, including health information, to make decisions, it is imperative to recognize the influence the Internet can have on making changes to improve patient self-management, patient satisfaction, and health outcomes (Forkner-Dunn, 2003). With federal initiatives pushing the adoption of EHRs

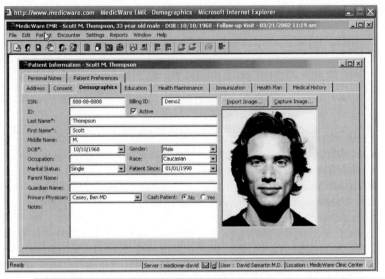

FIGURE 23-3

Patient information screen. *(Courtesy Medicware, Irwindale, Calif.)*

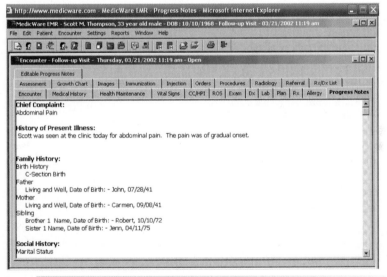

FIGURE 23-4

Patient encounter screen. *(Courtesy Medicware, Irwindale, Calif.)*

throughout all health care institutions by the year 2014, how nursing is practiced will be significantly changed. Nursing students need to know how to interact with informatics tools and systems to ensure safe and quality care. "In addition, there is a growing consumer movement wanting to interact with health care professionals through personal health records and various electronic communication devices" (NLN, 2008, p 1).

BOX 23-1   Advantages of Electronic Medical Records

- Simultaneous, remote access to patient from many locations
- Legibility of record—no handwriting
- Safer data—backup and disaster recovery system, so less prone to data loss
- Patient data confidentiality—authorized use can be restricted and monitored automatically
- Flexible data layout—can recall data in any order (chronically or in reverse chronological order)
- Integration with other information resources
- Incorporation of electronic data—can automatically capture physiological data from bedside monitors, laboratory analyzers, and imaging devices
- Continuous data processing—check and filter the data for errors, summarize and interpret data, and issue alerts and/or reminders
- Assisted search—can search free-text or structured data to find a specific data value or to determine whether a particular item has ever been recorded
- Greater range of data output modalities—data can be presented to users via computer-generated voice, two-way pagers, e-mail, and personal data assistants (PDA), smartphones
- Tailored paper output—data can be printed using a variety of fonts, colors, and sizes to help focus the clinician's attention on the most important data; images can be included to help see a more complete "picture" of the patient's condition
- Always up to date

BOX 23-2   Eight Core Functions of the Electronic Health Record

A committee of the Institute of Medicine of the National Academies has identified a set of eight core care delivery functions that electronic health records (EHR) systems should be capable of performing to promote greater safety, quality, and efficiency in health care delivery.

These eight core functions are:
- Health information and data
- Result management
- Order management
- Decision support
- Electronic communication and connectivity
- Patient support
- Administrative processes and reporting
- Reporting and population health

From Institute of Medicine (2003): Key capabilities of an electronic health record system, *Data Standards for Patient Safety*. Retrieved from *www.iom.edu/Reports/2003/Key-Capabilities-of-an-Electronic-Health-Record-System.aspx*.

Another IOM study, *Preventing Medication Errors* (2006), recommends greater use of information technologies in prescribing and dispensing medications, such as point-of-care reference information (handheld devices). Having detailed information about a medication at your fingertips addresses the issue of trying to keep up with all of the relevant information needed for the nurse to administer and the physician or health care provider to prescribe a medication safely (Figure 23-5). In addition, electronic prescriptions (e-prescriptions) can reduce many of the mistakes that occur with handwritten prescriptions. The e-prescription software guarantees that

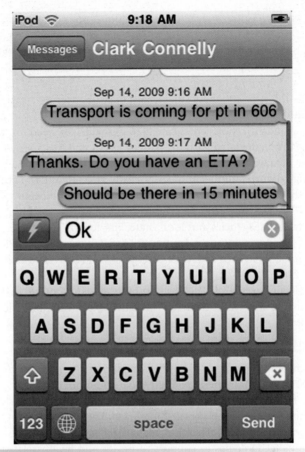

FIGURE 23-5

Smartphone communication application using text messaging. *(Courtesy Voalte, Sarasota, Fla.)*

all necessary information is filled out legibly. In addition, the software program correlates the patient's prescription with his or her medical history. This allows for automatic checking of drug allergies, drug-drug interactions, and overly high doses. According to *Preventing Medication Errors*, "In addition, once an e-prescription is in the system, it will follow the patient from the hospital to the doctor's office or from the nursing home to the pharmacy, avoiding many of the 'hand-off errors' common today. In light of all this, the committee recommends that by 2010 all prescribers and pharmacies will be using e-prescriptions" (IOM, 2006, p 3). Given that this book is being revised in early 2010, there is still a long way to go before this recommendation is achieved.

The American Hospital Association strongly supports the use of technology to protect and improve the quality of care in the hospital. Research data supports that the computerized physician order system (CPOE), computerized decision support systems, and bar-code medication administration (BCMA) and electronic medication administration record (eMAR) for medication administration can limit errors and improve care (AHA, 2006). In 2009, the *American*

Recovery and Reinvestment Act (ARRA) and the Centers for Medicare & Medicaid Services (CMS) released a proposed rule on Medicare and Medicaid payment incentives for "meaningful users" of EHRs by hospitals and physicians with financial incentives in the first few years and penalties thereafter. The AHA position on this proposed rule can be found at *www.aha.org/aha/content/2010/pdf/10-ib-def-meaning-use.pdf.*

Despite this new law, there still remain major barriers to the full integration health information technology. These barriers include:

- Lack of standardization across care areas—that is, the need for laboratory data and pharmacy systems to be integrated with the patient's EHR and the emergency department systems needs to share data with the inpatient systems.
- Funding—information technology is costly and often the major costs are borne by hospitals rather than shared by other providers, payers, and employers.
- Privacy laws—a single set of privacy laws is needed to simplify the task of communicating across facilities, agencies and local, state, and federal governments.
- Lack of a uniform approach (number) to match patients to their record—a single authentication number is needed to reduce safety risks and provide a uniform access to a patient's data (AHA, 2006).

Federal initiatives like ARRA are pushing the adoption of EHRs throughout all health care institutions by the year 2014, an initiative that will dramatically change how nursing is practiced.

What Is E-Health?

The all-encompassing term *e-health* is replacing the older term *telehealth*, and according to Mea (2001), "e-health presents itself as a common name for all such technological fields" (p 1)—e-health encompasses medical informatics and telemedicine and represents virtually everything related to computers and medicine. The World Health Organization (WHO) provides the following definition "eHealth is the cost-effective and secure use of information and communications technologies in support of health and health-related fields, including health-care services, health surveillance, health literature, and health education, knowledge and research" (WHO, 2005, p 121).

Although most "e-words" come from the commerce or business sector, the term is generally understood, despite its lack of precise definition, because of the dynamic environment of the Internet. E-health has come to characterize not only a technical development but also a state-of-mind, a way of thinking that focuses on improvement of health care via information and communication technology.

Eysenbach (2001) feels that it stands not only for "electronic" but implies a lot of other *e*'s, which he feels represent what e-health is all about (Box 23-3). He states that it should also be easy to use, entertaining, exciting, and most of all, in existence (Critical Thinking Box 23-6)!

TRENDS

When the first edition of this textbook came out more than 18 years ago, the section on computer technology was new and innovative. It was the cutting edge of technology that sent many nurse educators, students, and practicing nurses scrambling to make sense of how the computer might affect them. The explosion of knowledge and technology have visibly changed our mindset on

BOX 23-3 The 10 E's in "E-Health"

1. **Efficiency** leading to decreasing costs by avoiding duplicate or unnecessary diagnostic or therapeutic interventions, through enhanced communication possibilities between health care establishments, and through patient involvement.
2. **Enhancing quality of care** by allowing comparisons between different providers, involving consumers as additional power for quality assurance, and directing patient streams to the best quality providers.
3. **Evidence-based** intervention effectiveness and efficiency should not be assumed but proven by rigorous scientific evaluation.
4. **Empowerment** of consumers and patients by making the knowledge bases of medicine and personal electronic records accessible to consumers over the Internet, e-health opens new avenues for patient-centered medicine and enables evidence-based patient choice.
5. **Encouragement** of a new relationship between the patient and health professional, toward a true partnership, where decisions are made in a shared manner.
6. **Education** of physicians and health care providers through online sources (continuing education) and consumers (health education, tailored preventive information for consumers).
7. **Enabling** information exchange and communication in a standardized way between health care establishments.
8. **Extending** the scope of health care beyond its conventional boundaries.
9. **Ethics** e-health involves new forms of patient-physician interaction and poses new challenges and threats to ethical issues such as online professional practice, informed consent, privacy, and equity issues.
10. **Equity** to make health care more equitable is one of the promises of e-health, but at the same time there is a considerable threat that e-health may deepen the gap between the "haves" and "have-nots," deepening the "digital divide."

Adapted from Eysenbach G: What is e-health? *J Med Internet Res* 3(2), 2000. Retrieved from *www.jmir.org/2001/2/e20/*.

CRITICAL THINKING BOX 23-6

A June 2009 survey from the Pew Internet & American Life Project estimates that 61% of American adults surf the Web for health information. How have you (or your family) used the Internet for your own health or medical care?

the use of computer technology to the extent that computer literacy is integrated within nursing education. Being faced with devices, equipment, computer sensors, "smart" body parts, and EHRs that involve technological skills affects the way that nursing is practiced and delivered. In the *2010 NCLEX-RN Detailed Test Plan*, the subcategory of Information Technology is a content section under the category of Management of Patient Care, which is part of the patient need category of Safe and Effective Care Environment (Wendt et al, 2010) (Box 23-4).

As Forkner-Dunn (2003) so cleverly states, "time to byte the bullet ... the e-health train has not only left the station but is rapidly moving down the track carrying tens of millions of e-patients and many possibilities for transforming patient self-management, improving health outcomes, and enhancing [health provider] patient relationships" (p 8). Although there are numerous trend areas, using the Internet to communicate and to provide patient self-care, evaluating Internet resources, and using mobile computing devices are certainly in the forefront.

BOX 23-4 NCSBN Detailed Test Plan for NCLEX-RN® Examination

The following is an excerpt from the *2010 Detailed Test Plan for the NCLEX-RN®* about the content area of Information Technology on the NCLEX-RN exam:

- Receive and/or transcribe health care provider orders*
- Use information technology (e.g., computer, video, books) to enhance the care provided to a patient*
- Apply knowledge of facility regulations when accessing patient records
- Access data for patient through online databases and journals
- Enter computer documentation accurately, completely and in a timely manner
- Use emerging technology in managing patient health care (e.g., telehealth, electronic records)*

*Activity Statements used in the 2009 RN Practice Analysis.
Wendt A, Kenny L, Schultz L (2010): 2010 NCLEX-RN® Detailed Test Plan Candidate Version, *National Council State Board of Nursing*. Retrieved from *www.ncsbn.org/2010_NCLEX_RN_Detailed_Test_Plan_Candidate.pdf*.

USING THE INTERNET: THE NEXT GENERATION OF HEALTH CARE DELIVERY

Undoubtedly, the Internet has transformed our ability to locate health information and to connect via e-mail, social networking software (e.g., Facebook) or Web bulletin boards with other individuals who have similar interests. The federal government recognizes the importance of having access and quality information and has established a series of goals in the *Healthy People 2010* action plan. According to Forkner-Dunn (2003), Internet-based patient self-care is the "next generation of health care delivery" (p 1). Health information on the Internet can dramatically improve patients' abilities to manage their own health care conveniently. Of course, not all Web-based information is accurate, which raises concerns about the quality of information individuals are using and the impact this information has on the overall health of an individual.

> Internet users must still proceed with caution when seeking health care information online, because there is a plethora of incomplete and inaccurate information that can be dangerous.

As nurses, we need to better understand how consumers find health information on the Internet, how to evaluate the quality of information retrieved, and how to help our patients to critically evaluate and manage information (Greenberg et al, 2004).

A 2001 study by RAND for the California Healthcare Foundation showed that information on health websites is often incomplete or out of date and highly commercialized. This might be of little concern if consumers routinely consulted health care professionals about the information. However, the Pew Internet and American Life Project (Pew) found that 69% of consumers did not discuss the information they found online with a doctor or nurse, and considering that most health information on the Internet is written in a style that is above the 9th grade reading level, many individuals come away from the source of information confused, especially the underserved populations who need the information the most.

As tools and security functions are refined and advanced, components of the EHR that are being implemented or are being considered via the Internet include the following:

- Remote access to EHR from a health care provider's home or office
- Access to multiple clinical information systems in lieu of purchasing stand-alone electronic records systems
- Creation of a virtual EHR by bringing together information from multiple systems in a way that appears seamless to the end user
- Use of application service providers to provide access to the EHR
- Direct patient access to the official version of the patient's EHR

Imagine having access to your complete EHR no matter where you are in the world and being able to download portions of it to a CD-ROM or removable drive (thumb drive) for whatever you need to have as documentation.

A study by Ross and colleagues (2004) describes how care for patients with chronic diseases, such as congestive heart failure is affected by a patient-accessible online medical record. They describe how clinic operations using SPPARO (System Providing Access to Records Online) software that consisted of a Web-based electronic health record (EHR), an educational guide, and a messaging system enabled electronic communication among patient and staff. A noted trend of improved satisfaction with physician-patient communication was found among patients; improvement was also noted in how well patients felt their problems were understood and how well doctors explained information. In interviews, the physicians and nursing staff did not feel that providing SPPARO to their patients resulted in a perceptible change in their workload.

E-Mail

Practically everyone is familiar with e-mail. Your instructor may require you to complete assignments and submit your work via e-mail attachment instead of submitting a hard copy. You probably send e-mail to family and friends on a daily basis. Although more than 380 million Americans now use the Internet and e-mail daily (and many access health information), few doctors communicate with their patients through e-mail (Patt et al, 2003; Internet World Stats, 2008). Considering the popularity of e-mail and despite its potential for rapid, asynchronous, documentable communication to improve both the quality and efficiency of health services delivery, the use of e-mail communication has not been widely adopted by many physicians.

In Patt's (2003) study, physicians reported improved communication via e-mail with patients who have chronic diseases that require frequent, small changes in their treatment plans. In addition, physicians noted several other benefits, including continuity of communication with patients, especially patients who travel, ability to respond to nonurgent issues on their own time, avoidance of "phone tag" with patients, and improved efficiency. Drug-refill requests and educational information, including links to reputable Internet sources, were also cited as examples of effective use of e-mail with patients. Physicians anticipated problems with e-mail communication, such as reimbursement problems, technical problems of failing servers or lost e-mails, and medico-legal consequences of e-mail used for urgent issues, but these had not frequently been experienced, as reported in the study. With standards and guidelines for e-mail developed by the American Medical Informatics Association (1998), technically minded, electronically equipped health care consumers will continue to accelerate the demand for e-mail access to their health care providers (Englebardt and Nelson, 2002).

DATA ACCESS AT THE POINT OF CARE

Point-of-care documentation has surfaced as a need in health care due to the interruption in workflow created by electronic documentation. Thirty plus years ago, patient's flow sheet documentation was kept on a clipboard at the bedside. Nurse walked into room, collected vital data, wrote it on the flow sheet, and went on to next patient. While this was an excellent workflow for the clinical nurse, it made aggregating data across patient visits or patient aggregates a monumental task. Picture the emergency department (ED) nurse with an unconscious patient who is confronted with a stack of paper records that have been rolled to the ED in a wheelchair by a medical records person—trying to put together a concise, cohesive picture of the patient's history was next to impossible.

Enter electronic clinical documentation. It made it easier to review patient data from previous visits and to do research across patient populations, and it completely changed the workflow of the clinician at the bedside. We went from collecting data on multiple patients until we finally had time to sit down in front of a computer to enter the data into the patient's chart. We then attempted to regurgitate all the data we have either scribbled on a piece of paper or worse yet, tried to commit to memory. Even worst, we have had multiple person-to-person conversations, telephone calls, alerts, etc., between data gathering and documentation all of which interfere with being able to recall the details of patient care that was given in the previous hours.

Research has shown that point of care documentation reduces data latency and data errors (Gearing et al, 2006; Parker & Baldwin, 2008; Wager et al, 2010). A variety of point of care devices are now available to return documentation back to the point of care and help us handle the vast amount of data that we receive every day.

Workstations on Wheels

In order to free clinicians from computers at the nurses' station, computers were put on carts. This was one of the first steps in point of care electronic point of care documentation.

Smartphones

The last edition of this textbook focused attention on the use of PDAs in health care. Because of the convergence of technology, cell phones and PDAs have merged together to form a new product category, "smartphones" (Critical Thinking Box 23-7). The most popular smartphones in use during the writing of this edition are the Blackberry by RIM, the iPhone by Apple, HTC Evo 4G by Sprint, and the Palm Pre Plus and HTC Droid by Verizon. Smartphones can run applications that can monitor blood glucose levels, blood pressure, diet, and activity, as well as allowing users to check for drug interactions, calculate dosages, analyze lab results, schedule procedures, order prescriptions, and automate other clinical tasks, thus reducing the probability of errors and increasing patient safety (Abrahamsen, 2003) but they can also be used for multiple modes of communication as well.

> **CRITICAL THINKING**
> **BOX 23-7**
>
> Do you have a smartphone? If so, how do you use it? If not, do you anticipate purchasing one in the near future? Do you find nurses in the hospital or clinic setting using smartphones on a regular basis? What programs do they or you use?

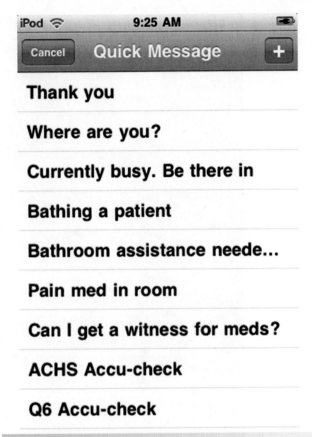

FIGURE 23-6

Smartphone Communication Application Text Messaging Templates. *(Courtesy Voalte, Sarasota, Fla.)*

Applications are now being developed to aid in managing the constant influx of information using multiple modes of communication such as text messaging, voice messages and calls, and alarms (Figures 23-6 and 23-7). However, due to their limited memory and scaled down operating systems, it is still impossible to access the entire scope of the patient's electronic record on a smartphone.

Tablet Computers

In 2007, the first tablet PC specifically designed for clinicians was introduced that was so different from anything that had previously been available that a new market category was created—the mobile clinical assistant (MCA). The MCA devices incorporated a camera, barcode scanner, and digitizer pen data entry in a fully functional Windows based slate tablet computer. One distinguishing feature of MCAs is that they are in a sealed device that is able to be disinfected. This class of computer has the ability to give the user access to the patient's entire electronic record rather than a scaled down version available using a smartphone. Combining MCA products with

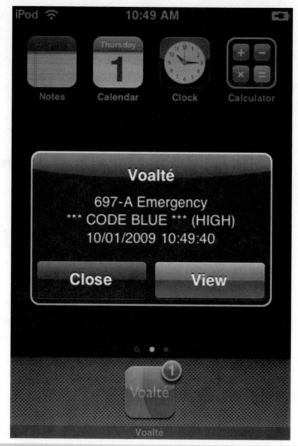

FIGURE 23-7

Smartphone communication application alarm. *(Courtesy Voalté, Sarasota, Fla.)*

workstations on wheels has resulted in a hybrid computing solution that is more flexible than either device alone. Figure 23-8 shows a nurse using an MCA product to document patient information.

EVALUATING INTERNET RESOURCES

What Do I Need to Know to Evaluate an Internet Resource?

McGonigle (2002) suggests a five-step plan to evaluate websites (Box 23-5).

> Remember that *anybody* can publish *anything* on the Web. Make sure you critically evaluate the source of the information.

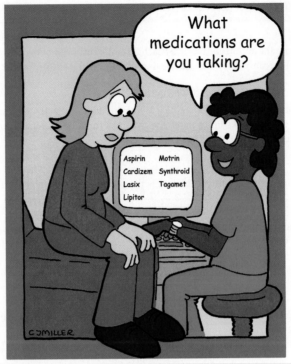

FIGURE 23-8

Nurse with tablet computer. *(Courtesy Motion Computing, Austin, Tex.)*

It is important to encourage patients to focus their Internet searching endeavors to well-known and reputable sites. For example, the U.S. Surgeon General's Family History Initiative is a great place to start with promoting the importance of a well-documented family health history. In addition to the Office of the Surgeon General, other U.S. Department of Health and Human Services (USDHHS) agencies involved in this project include the National Human Genome Research Institute (NHGRI), the Centers for Disease Control and Prevention (CDC), the Agency for Healthcare Research and Quality (AHRQ), and the Health Resources and Services Administration (HRSA). A downloadable, free tool, entitled "My Family Health Portrait," is available at *www.hhs.gov/familyhistory/download.html*. This tool helps patients organize their family trees and helps them identify common diseases that may run in their families. After completing the required information, the tool will create and print out a graphic representation of the patient's family generations and the health disorders that may have moved from one generation to the next. This is a powerful tool for predicting illnesses (USDHHS, 2004) and can be brought by the patient to a health care provider's appointment.

You can also limit your Internet search to specific domain sites by entering the search topic and then clicking on "Advanced search." At the bottom of the screen, a popup screen appears that reads: "search within a site or domain." You can type in the domain name such as .gov or .edu, and all of the articles that come up will be from a governmental agency or institution.

BOX 23-5	How to Evaluate Websites

STEP 1: AUTHORITY

Who is/are the author(s)? Describe each author's authority or expertise. Are professional qualifications listed? How can you contact the author(s)? Who is the site's sponsor? Is the site copyright protected?

STEP 2: TIMELINESS AND CONTINUITY

When were the site materials created? When did it become active on the Web? When was it last updated/revised? Are the links up to date? Are the links functional? When were data gathered? What version/edition is it?

STEP 3: PURPOSE

Who is the targeted audience? What is the purpose? Are the goals/aims/objectives clearly stated?

STEP 4: CONTENT: ACCURACY AND OBJECTIVITY

Does the information provided meet the purpose? Who is accountable for accuracy? Are the cited sources verifiable? What is the value of the content of this site related to your topical needs? How complete and accurate are the content information and links? Is the site biased? Does it contain advertisements?

STEP 5: STRUCTURE AND ACCESS

Does the site load quickly? Do multimedia, graphics, and art used on the page serve a purpose or are they just decorative or fun? Is there an element of creativity?

Is there appropriate interactivity? Is the navigation intuitive? Are there icons? Is this a secured site?

From McGonigle D: How to evaluate websites, OJIN 6(2), 2002. Retrieved from *http://eaa-knowledge.com/ojni/ni/602/web_site_evaluation.htm.*

The CARS Checklist. Acronyms are always helpful for remembering important key features. The CARS checklist (Credibility, Accuracy, Reasonableness, Support), developed by Harris in 1997 and updated in 2007, is designed for helping to evaluate a website. Although few sources will meet the majority of the criteria, the checklist will help in separating the high-quality information from the poor-quality information.

✓ Credibility—an authoritative source, includes author's credentials, evidence of quality control such as peer review.
✓ Accuracy—a source that is correct today (not yesterday); comprehensive
✓ Reasonableness—look at the information for fairness, objectivity, moderateness, consistency, and worldview.
✓ Support—a source that provides convincing evidence for the claims made; a source you can triangulate (find at least two other sources that support it)

Harris (2007) notes that you will also need a little "café" advice to live with the information you obtained from your Internet search.

▪ Challenge the information and demand accountability.
▪ Adapt and require more credibility and evidence for stronger claims—it is okay to be skeptical of the information.
▪ File new information in your mind rather than immediately believing or disbelieving it.
▪ Evaluate and reevaluate regularly. Recognize the dynamic, fluid nature of information.

NURSING INFORMATICS AND CLINICAL PRACTICE

Are you thinking—so why do I care about all this information related to nursing informatics? I will be taking care of patients not worrying about computers. Well, the truth be told, your practice will involve informatics on a daily basis. From electronic documentation, to using technology laden equipment such as smart IV pumps and beds, barcode medication administration and a variety of POC diagnostics equipment, to communication tools such as smartphone, and use of clinical decision support systems, technology will touch every part of your patient care (Evidence-Based Practice Box 23-1).

In addition, you may become part of the implementation team for a new software application as a super user. Super users are individuals who have been through additional training for a software application and who are responsible for helping others on your unit. You may be a subject matter expert (SME) at some point in your career and help design the data input screens of an application.

Basic computing and information literacy skills are rapidly becoming required for all nurses, whether working directly with patients in any environment, teaching or any of the other varied positions held by nurses today.

Informatics Competencies for the Practicing Nurse

Based on an extensive literature review, the TIGER Informatics Competency Collaborative (TICC) developed the *TIGER Nursing Informatics Competencies Model* that includes basic computer competencies, information literacy, and information management (Gugerty & Delaney, 2009). This is an outstanding self-assessment tool to determine if you have gaps in your skill set.

Basic Computer Competencies. There seems to be a lack of consensus of what skills are needed to demonstrate basic computer competence (Elder & Koehn, 2009). Rather than develop another set of skills, the TICC basic competencies recommendations are based on The European Computer Driving Licence [sic] (ECDL) Foundation's syllabus, which can be found at: *www.ecdl.org/programmes/index.jsp?p=102&n=2227.*

The basic skills include:

- Concepts of information and communication technology
- Using the computer and managing files
- Word processing
- Spreadsheets
- Using databases
- Presentation
- Web browsing and communication

Information Literacy. The second competency identified by the TIGER initiative is information literacy. The Association of College and Research Libraries (2010, para 1) defined information literacy as "the set of skills needed to find, retrieve, analyze, and use information." After a systematic literature review, Hart (2008) concluded that nurses in the United States are not prepared for evidence-based practice due to the lack of competency in information literacy skills. The TIGER recommendation is that all practicing nurses and graduating nursing students will have the ability to:

1. Determine the nature and extent of the information needed
2. Access needed information effectively and efficiently

BOX 23-1 **EVIDENCE-BASED PRACTICE**

Use of technology improves safety of medication administration

PRACTICE ISSUE

Approximately 1.5 million Americans are injured each year because of medication errors. Medication errors in the inpatient setting cost the health system well over $3.5 billion per year. Leape and colleagues broke medication errors into five phases: 39% of errors occurred during the prescribing phase, 12% during transcription, 11% during dispensing, and 38% during administration. It is the nurse at the patient's side who is the last link in the chain of medication administration. In a 300-bed community hospital, use of bar-code technology reduced medication errors by 80%. The Veteran's Administration in Eastern Kansas prevented 549,000 medication errors between 1995 and 2001. Most nurses have heard of the case of the newborn twins of actor Dennis Quaid and his wife Kimberly receiving 10,000 units of heparin instead of 10 units. While not all adverse drug events (ADEs) are preventable, those that are the result of a breakdown in the Five Rights of Medication Administration can be prevented by using bar-code technologies. But the technology only works when nurses use it. In a study by Koppel and colleagues (2008), nurses were found to use a work-around to using BCMA in more than 10% of the medications delivered.

NURSING IMPLICATIONS

- Don't use a work-around as a quick-fix solution to a bigger problem. If technology is hampering your work, tell your manager
- Don't try to save time by bypassing the BCMA process
- Many of the medication errors were made unknowingly by nurses—BMCA can help ensure that the Five Rights are followed every time

Considering This Information:

Have you used BCMA yet? Has anyone taught you a work-around? Why would you want to bypass a BCMA alert and when?

References for the Evidence

Coyle GA, Heinen M: Evolution of BCMA within the Department of Veterans Affairs. Bar Code Medication Administration, *Nursing Administration Q* 29:32-38, 2005.

Foote SO, Coleman JR: Success story. Medication administration: the implementation process of bar-coding for medication administration to enhance medication safety, *Nursing Economic$* 26:207-210, 2008.

Leape LL, Bates DW, Cullen DJ, et al: Systems analysis of adverse drug events, *JAMA* 274:35-43, 1995.

Institute of Medicine (IOM): Medication errors injure 1.5 million people and cost billions of dollars annually, 2006. Retrieved from *www.nationalacademies.org/onpinews/newsitem.aspx?RecordID=11623*.

Sakowski J, Newman JM, Dozier K: Severity of medication administration errors detected by a bar-code medication administration system, *AJHP: Official Journal of the American Society of Health-System Pharmacists* 65:1661-1666, 2008.

Koppel R, Wetterneck T, Telles JL, et al: Workarounds to barcode medication administration systems: their occurrences, causes, and threats to patient safety, *J Am Medical Informatics Assoc* 15:408-423, 2008.

3. Evaluate information and its sources critically and incorporates selected information into his or her knowledge base and value system
4. Individually or as a member of a group, use information effectively to accomplish a specific purpose
5. Evaluate outcomes of the use of information (Gugerty & Delaney, 2009, p 5)

CONCLUSION

Nursing informatics is a specialty grounded in the present while planning for the future. Informatics nurses face many challenges in their daily activities, because they are in a position to wear many hats and bear many responsibilities. Change is the only constant. The challenge will be for the INS to assume a leadership role in informatics, while the nurse educator and practicing nurse prepare to embrace the generalized applications of working within a computerized environment. No longer will it be sufficient to be able to turn on a computer and complete a simple task. A nurse will need to be able to use technology in all the forms found in health care organizations, access information, as well as evaluate the content of the information to provide to the patient population. Wishing will not make technology go away so savvy nurses will focus on the benefits technology brings to patient care, learn the skills they need, and embrace the future with all the changes it will bring.

BIBLIOGRAPHY

Abrahamsen C: Patient safety: take the informatics challenge, *Nurs Manage* 34:48-51, 2003.

American Hospital Association (2006): *Protecting and improving care for patients and communities health information technology.* Retrieved from *www.aha.org/aha/content/2006/pdf/Iss-Paper-Health-IT-06.pdf.*

American Nurses Association: *ANA scope and standards of nursing informatics practice*, Washington, DC, 2008, ANA.

American Nurses Association (2003): *Nursing Information and Data Set Evaluation Center (IN/INSDSEC).* Retrieved from *www.nursingworld.org/nidsec/.*

Association of College and Research Libraries (2010): *Introduction to information literacy.* Retrieved from *www.ala.org/ala/mgrps/divs/acrl/issues/infolit/overview/intro/index.cfm.*

Clark J: *Information management: the compliance guide to JCAHO standards*, ed 4, Danvers, MA, 2004, HCPro Inc.

DeGroote SL: The use of personal digital assistants in the health sciences: results of a survey, *JAMA* 92:341-349, 2004.

Delany C: IN/INSCTF activities: response to the President's Information Technology Advisory Committee, *CIN: Computers, Informatics, Nursing* 22:299, 302-305, 2004.

Englebardt SP, Nelson R: *Health care informatics: an interdisciplinary approach*, St Louis, 2002, Mosby.

Elder BL, Koehn ML: Assessment tool for nursing student computer competencies, *Nursing Education Perspectives* 30:148-152, 2009.

Eysenbach G: What is e-health? *J Med Internet Res* 3(2), 2001. Retrieved from *www.jmir.org/2001/2/e20/.*

Forkner-Dunn J: Internet-based patient self-care: the next generation of health care delivery, *J Med Internet Res* 5:e8, 2003. Retrieved from *www.pubmedcentral.nih.gov/articlerender.fcgi?artid=1550561.*

Gale Group: HIPAA privacy rule takes effect, *Healthcare Financial Manage* 55:9, 2001.

Gearing P, Olney CM, Davis K, et al: Enhancing patient safety through electronic medical record documentation of vital signs, *J Healthcare Information Management* 20:40-45, 2006.

Greenberg L, D'Andrea G, Lorence D: Setting the public agenda for online health search: a white paper and action agenda, *J Med Internet Res* 6(2), 2004. Retrieved from *www.jmir.org/2004/2/e18/.*

Goedert J (2010): Prison for HIPAA privacy violator, *Health Data Management.* Retrieved from *www.healthdatamanagement.com/news/hipaa_privacy-violation-conviction-breach-40202-1.html.*

Gugerty B, Delaney C (2009): *TIGER informatics competencies collaborative (TICC) final report.* Retrieved from *http://tigercompetencies.pbworks.com/f/TICC_Final.pdf.*

Harris R (2007): *Evaluating Internet research sources.* Retrieved from *www.virtualsalt.com/evalu8it.htm.*

Hart MD: Informatics competency and development within the US nursing population workforce: a systematic literature review, *CIN: Computers, Informatics, Nursing* 26:320-329, 2008.

HIMSS Nursing Informatics Awareness Task Force: An emerging giant nursing informatics, *Nurs Manage* 38:39-42, 2007.

HIMSS Informatics Nurse Impact Study (2009): *Final report.* Retrieved from *www.himss.org/content/files/HIMSS2009NursingInformaticsImpactSurveyFullResults.pdf.*

HIMSS (2010): *Electronic health record.* Retrieved from *www.himss.org/ASP/topics_ehr.asp.*

Institute of Medicine: Committee on Quality of Health Care in America. *Crossing the quality chasm: a new health system for the 21st century*, Washington, DC, 2001, National Academy Press.

Institute of Medicine (2003): Key capabilities of an electronic health record system. *Data standards for patient safety*. Retrieved from *www.providersedge.com/ehdocs/ehr_articles/Key_Capabilities_of_an_EHR_System.pdf*.

Institute of Medicine (2006): Preventing medication errors, *Report Brief*. Retrieved from *www.iom.edu/Object.File/Master/35/943/medication%20errors%20new.pdf*.

Internet World Stats (2008): *Internet world users by language*. Retrieved from *www.internetworldstats.com/stats7.htm*.

Keenan G: Use of standardized nursing language will make nursing visible, *Michigan Nurse* 72:12-13, 1999.

Knox C, Smith A: Handhelds and HIPAA, *Nurs Manage* 38(6):38-40, 2007.

McGonigle D: How to evaluate websites, *OJIN* 6(2), 2002. Retrieved from *http://eaa-knowledge.com/ojni/ni/602/web_site_evaluation.htm*.

McIntire S, Clark T: Essential steps in super user education for ambulatory clinic nurses, *Urologic Nursing* 29:337-342, 2009.

Mea VD: What is e-health (2): the death of telemedicine? *J Med Internet Res* 3:2001. Retrieved from *www.jmir.org/2001/2/e22/*.

National League for Nursing (2008): *Workforce to practice in 21st-century, technology-rich health care environment New York*. Retrieved from *www.nln.org/aboutnln/PositionStatements/informatics_052808.pdf*.

Pancoast PE, Patrick TB, Mitchell JA: Physician PDA use and the HIPAA privacy rule, *J Am Med Informatics Assoc* 10:611, 2003.

Parker CD, Baldwin K. Mobile device improves documentation workflow and nurse satisfaction, *CARING Newsletter* 23(2):14-18, 2008.

Patt MR, et al: Doctors who are using e-mail with their patients: a qualitative exploration, *J Med Internet Res* 5(2):2003. Retrieved from *www.jmir.org/2003/2/e9/*.

Pattillo RE, Brewer M, Smith CM: Tracking clinical use of personal digital assistant reference resources, *Nurse Educator* 32:39-42, 2007.

RAND Corporation: *Proceed with caution: a report on the quality of health information on the Internet*, San Francisco, Calif, 2001, Rand Corporation. Sponsored by the California Health Care Foundation. Retrieved from *www.chcf.org/documents/consumer/ProceedWithCautionCompleteStudy.pdf*.

Ross SE, et al: Providing a Web-based online medical record with electronic communication capabilities to patients with congestive heart failure: randomized trial, *J Med Internet Res* 6(2), 2004. Retrieved from *www.jmir.org/2004/2/e12/*.

Saba VK, McCormick KA: *Essentials of computers for nurses: informatics for the new millennium*, 3 ed, New York, 2001, McGraw-Hill.

Simpson R: A systems view of information technology, *Nurs Admin Q* 24:80, 2000.

Simpson R: Size up the big three, *Nurs Manage* 32:12, 2001.

Sittig DF (1999): Advantages of computer-based medical records, *The Informatics Rev*. Retrieved from *www.informatics-review.com/thoughts/advantages.html*.

Sittig DF, et al (2002): A clinical information system research landscape, *The Permanente J*. Retrieved from *http://xnet.kp.org/permanentejournal/spring02/landscape.html#*.

Smith CM, Patillo RE: PDAs in the nursing curriculum, *Nurse Educator* 31:101-102, 2006.

U.S. Department of Health and Human Services (2004): *U.S. Surgeon General's family history initiative*. Retrieved from *www.hhs.gov/familyhistory/*.

Wager KA, Schaffner MJ, Foulois B, et al: Comparison of the quality and timeliness of vital signs data during a multiphase EHR implementation. *Computers, Informatics, Nursing*, July-Aug:205-212, 2010.

Wendt A, Kenny L, Anderson J: *2010 NCLEX-RN detailed test plan*, Chicago, 2010, National Council of State Boards of Nursing.

Wilcox RA, La Tella RR: The personal digital assistant: a new medical instrument for the exchange of clinical information at the point of care, *Med J Aust* 174:659-662, 2001.

World Health Organization (WHO) (2005): *Resolutions and decisions*. Retrieved from *http://apps.who.int/gb/ebwha/pdf_files/WHA58/WHA58_28-en.pdf*.

Additional resources are available online at *http://evolve.elsevier.com/Zerwekh/nsgtoday/*.

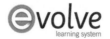

CHAPTER 24

Using Nursing Research in Practice

Mary Mackenburg-Mohn, RN, PhD, CNP

> *The new challenge is for nurses to use research methods that can clearly explicate the essential nature, meanings and components of nursing so that nurse clinicians can use this knowledge in a deliberate and meaningful way.*
> —MADELINE LEININGER

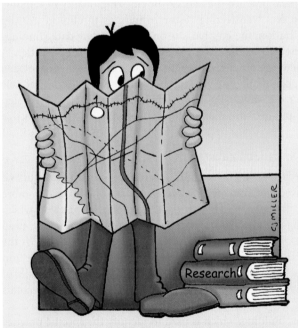

Nursing research is the road map to professional practice.

After completing this chapter, you should be able to:

- Identify the steps in the process of research utilization.

- Discuss the difference between conducting research and research utilization.

- Identify resources for evidence-based nursing practice.

- Identify the characteristics of your practice context.

- Describe ways in which nursing research can be used to guide your nursing practice.

- Describe the function of the National Institute of Nursing Research.

THE NEED FOR NURSING PRACTICE BASED ON RESEARCH

In the recent past, there has been a continuing increase in costs associated with the delivery and receipt of health care in the United States. At the same time, there has been more and more scrutiny of how those health care dollars are spent. The decision of which health care treatments receive funding from health care insurance is now based primarily on documentation of favorable patient outcomes. In addition, patients want to know that the dollars they spend on health care will help them to get well and feel better—they want to purchase something that works for them. As providers of today's health care, nurses must be able to demonstrate that the nursing care they provide is cost-effective and improves the health of patients.

Although in the past nursing care was largely based on traditional knowledge, given the current health care environment, today's nurses must base their practice on nursing care that has been documented as being beneficial to patients. Such practice is based on sound scientific research in which nursing care has been able to demonstrate cost-effective, predictable, and measurable practice outcomes. In this chapter, two methods of incorporating nursing research findings into nursing practice are discussed: *nursing research utilization* and *evidence-based practice.*

WHAT IS NURSING RESEARCH UTILIZATION?

The ability to transfer research into clinical practice is essential for ensuring quality in nursing. The process of research utilization involves transferring research findings to clinical nursing practice. In the process of research utilization, the emphasis is on using *existing* data (findings or evidence) from previous nursing research studies to evaluate a current nursing practice. A major component of the process is reviewing completed nursing research studies that have been published in the literature. In contrast, conducting new research involves the collection of *new* data to answer a specific clinical practice question. Nursing research utilization is a step-by-step process incorporating critical thinking and decision making to ensure that a change in practice has a sound basis in nursing science.

What Are the Steps for Nursing Research Utilization?

Step 1: Preutilization. The first step in the application of nursing research to nursing practice is the recognition that some aspect of nursing practice could be done in a safer, more efficient, more beneficial, or simply a different way. This begins an exploratory phase in which nursing colleagues in the practice setting are consulted regarding their opinions about the need to find a new approach for some aspect of nursing practice. An early question should be: "Is the current practice research-based?" When current practice is research-based, the next question should be "Is the research on which the practice is based current?" (e.g., the specific details of taking temperatures with mercury thermometers became outdated when digital thermometers were used exclusively in practice).

A second phase of step 1 is consensus building, which is used to identify the specific practice to be changed. In this phase, the incorporation of the principles of change theory will increase the possibility of success. (See Chapter 10 for information about the challenges of change.) In any practice setting in which there are several nurses, a change will be more acceptable if those affected are included in the decisions related to the change. Clear communication and teamwork are essential elements of this process. Group consensus is crucial for the successful application of research findings.

The third and final phase of step 1 delineates the aspect of nursing practice that will be changed into a concise statement of the *practice problem.* This statement will answer the question, "In our current nursing practice, what do we want to change, improve, or make more efficient?"

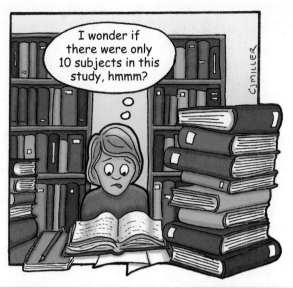

FIGURE 24-1

Nine out of ten nurses recommend …

The narrower and more specific the statement of the practice problem, the easier your task will be in Step 2.

Step 2: Assessing. The second step in research utilization is the identification and critical evaluation of published research that is related to the practice problem you have identified (Figure 24-1). Nursing literature is searched to identify those studies that deal with your practice problem. Although some studies may have explored the exact practice problem that you are examining, it is likely that most research will have approached the problem from a different point of view. Your task will be to analyze and critically evaluate the research reports to determine which findings are adaptable to your practice problem and context. Organizing and summarizing the adaptable findings into an outline format will provide you with your primary working document for the remainder of the use plan (Box 24-1). Box 24-2 contains suggestions on reading a nursing research article.

The use of the Internet and electronic databases has made a thorough search of the current literature easier. However, the enormous volume of materials now available also increases the complexity of a review of literature. For example, the keywords used in a search can either return no articles or hundreds of articles. When you are conducting an electronic search, a valuable technique is to begin searching within the most recent year and then move back one year at a time until an adequate research base is identified. Limiting your searches to the use of nursing-oriented database may also help you find pertinent literature. The Cumulative Index to Nursing and Allied Health Literature (CINAHL) is an excellent place to start your search.

There are times, however, when an electronic search is not adequate. Keep in mind that many of the classic research studies were published before electronic formats were widely used and may not be available online. Also, there may be valuable studies that are available in hard copy only. Because of these limitations of electronic sources, you may need to make a trip to the stacks in

BOX 24-1	Analyzing a Research Article for Potential Use of Findings in Nursing Practice

1a. The Purpose of the study is:

1b. The importance of this study to nursing practice is:

2. The Research Question/Hypothesis is:

(If the question/hypothesis is not stated, it could be):

3a. The Independent Variable(s) is/are:

3b. The Dependent Variable(s) is/are:

(If there are no independent and dependent variables, the Research Variable[s] is/are):

3c. Definition(s) of the variable(s) of interest to me is/are:

4. The Conceptual Model/Theoretical Framework linked with this study is:

5a. The content areas in the Review of Related Literature are:

5b. The review does/does not evaluate both supporting and nonsupporting studies:

6a. The Research Design used for the study is:

6b. The design is/is not appropriate for the research question:

6c. The control(s) used in this study is/are:

6d. The Study Setting is:

7a. The Target Population is:

7b. The Sampling Method is:

7c. The Sampling Method is/is not appropriate for the design:

7d. The criteria for participants are:

7e. The sample included _____ participants.

7f. The sample is/is not representative of the population:

8a. The Study Instrument(s) is/are:

8b. Instrument validity and reliability information are presented and are of adequate levels for confidence in using the results:

9a. The Data Collection Method(s) is/are:

9b. The Data Collection Method(s) is/are (is not/are not) appropriate for this study:

10. Steps were taken to protect the Rights of Human Subjects:

11a. The Data Analysis Procedure(s) is/are:

11b. The Data Analysis Procedure(s) is/are appropriate for the level of data collected and the research question/hypothesis:

11c. The Research Question/Hypothesis is/is not supported:

12. The author(s) major Conclusions and/or Implications for Nursing Practice are:

the library, if you are looking for historical research. See Box 24-3 for hints on conducting a literature search.

Step 3: Planning. Planning for research utilization is accomplished in three phases. The first phase involves determining the new approach, or *innovation*, that will be used on the basis of the findings from the review of the literature. Previous research findings will be used to design the innovation in the context of your practice setting (e.g., intensive care unit, ambulatory care, home care). The expected *practice outcomes* should also be determined on the basis of the literature and may need to be adjusted according to the characteristics of your particular practice.

Phase two of planning is the establishment of a systematic method for implementing the new approach. A *specific plan* should be established and followed so that the new approach is applied appropriately. Policies and procedures for implementation may need to be written. This phase may include staff training for the new approach.

BOX 24-2   How to Read a Nursing Research Article

A research article should answer the following:

What: Read the problem statement, purpose, research question, and results/findings.	Is the content of the article related to my question?
Why: Read the problem statement or the review of literature.	Why was the research done?
When: Do more recent findings provide a better answer? Read the date of publication.	When was the study done? Is it classic, current, or outdated?
How: Read the method and design sections.	What research method was used? Is it a quantitative, qualitative, or mixed methods approach?
Who: Read the method section.	Who were the subjects? What was the sample?
Where: Read the method section.	In what setting was the research done?
So What: Read the findings and discussion.	Are the findings helpful to me and my problem?
Do Not:	Do not automatically accept what you read; critically evaluate the content. You can only evaluate what is written and reported; do not assume anything about what is not written.

What to Do When: When the statistical procedures are beyond your level of understanding:

- Read the results section, being alert for specific phrases that will tell you the answer to the research question. For example, "the hypothesis was not supported."
- Look at the tables; tables should be understandable without the narrative.
- Assume that the appropriate statistical analysis was done correctly and that the researcher has interpreted the results correctly.
- Have someone who understands the statistics read the article and get his or her opinion or get a consultant.

BOX 24-3   Hints for Conducting a Literature Search

1. Do some narrowing before you go to online databases. Think about some key terms or alternate terms for your problem. Be prepared to narrow or expand your search, depending on what you find.
2. Plan to spend time conducting your literature search, but do not waste valuable time. Query the online database "help" menu to assist you with getting started.
3. Begin by identifying the major professional nursing journals that publish nursing research. Determine if those journals are available in the database, and start your literature review with those. If your problem is in a specialty area, review specialty journals.
4. If you find an article related to your problem, look at *that* author's reference list for other articles and journals.
5. Look at the table of contents in the journal where you found a related article.
6. Know the limitations of the databases where you do your search.
7. Carefully appraise information obtained from the Internet that is not part of an established online database, such as Journals@Ovid; EBSCOhost; ProQuest, Thomson Gale PowerSearch.

The third phase of planning involves establishing a *method for evaluating* the practice outcomes, or effects, of the new approach. The outcomes are usually some specific improvements in patient care. Ideally, your evaluation will indicate both the quality and the quantity of the change in the outcome.

Step 4: Implementing. This step involves the implementation or application of the new approach, along with the collection of the evaluation data. By following the specific plan that you established in Step 3, the new approach will be introduced into practice. It is important that you begin collecting your evaluation data at the same time so that you can clearly determine the effect of the new approach.

Step 5: Evaluating. Step 5 involves the evaluation of the implementation (Step 4) to determine whether the new approach improved practice outcomes. Whether you will continue using the new approach in the practice setting may also be determined on the basis of new technology, economic considerations, or changes in staffing. If there is no change in outcomes, you may want to return to the previous practice. Or, the evaluation phase may lead to another research utilization project; for example, if the practice problem is significant and the practice outcomes were not improved, another new approach may be tried.

Research Utilization: What Is It *Not*?

Research utilization does *not* entail simply taking the findings of a single research study and using those findings in nursing practice. Research studies are replicated to rule out chance findings and to validate previous studies. Similar studies with different populations are conducted to determine the applicability of findings to different groups of people. For these reasons, research utilization encompasses the findings of many studies to develop the new approach that will be put into practice.

Data are collected in the process of research utilization. However, research utilization is not the collection of data to answer a research question, as is the case when conducting research. The data collected in research utilization are needed for evaluation to determine whether there is some advantage to the new approach in the practice setting. The data collected must be carefully considered in light of your specific setting.

Research utilization should not be confused with a review of nursing practice. Practice review involves a quality control/risk management process to evaluate the appropriate use of resources related to a specific treatment. As with research utilization, practice review use does not entail the use of nursing research findings during the process of evaluation.

When you review the nursing research literature for research utilization, as mentioned previously, there is no assurance that you will find studies that are directly applicable to your practice situation. Your specific question may not have been the topic of previous research studies. In this case, you may have to either adapt the findings from the literature, conduct your own research, or both.

RESEARCH UTILIZATION COMPARED WITH NURSING RESEARCH AND THE CONDUCT OF RESEARCH

How Is the Use of Research in Practice Different from Conducting Research?

As illustrated in Table 24-1, the major steps involved in both conducting and utilizing research are the same. Both are problem-solving processes involving critical thinking. For example, a

TABLE 24-1   Comparison of Processes: An Overview of the Nursing Process, Conducting Research, and Research Utilization

Nursing Process	Conducting Research	Research Utilization
Preprocess Establish a nurse-patient relationship	Preplanning Identify the need for a research study Determine feasibility	Peruse Identify a practice problem that needs a new approach
Scan the literature	Obtain consensus	
Assessing Gather data	Assessing Identify the problem State research purpose Begin to formulate the research question Review the literature	Assessing Identify and critically evaluate published research related to your practice problem Identify the findings that are adaptable to your problem and your context
Planning Diagnose Set goals	Planning Identify and define the variables Select a conceptual or theoretical model	Planning Determine the new approach and the desired outcomes Establish a systematic method for implementing the new approach
Prioritize Determine nursing interventions	Select research design Finalize research question Plan data analysis	Establish a method for evaluating the outcomes of the new approach
Formulate care plan Negotiate a site for data collection Complete human subjects review	Write research proposal	
Implementing Initiate the plan Train data collectors Obtain subject sample Collect the data Prepare data for analysis	Implementing Prepare questionnaires Collect data about the outcomes of the new approach	Implementing Begin using the new approach
Evaluating Determine the patient response	Evaluating Analyze the data Organize the data	Evaluation of the implementation Determine whether the practice change improved patient outcomes
Answer the research question Interpret the results Report the findings Plan next project	Decide whether to continue using the new approach	

clinical practice problem may provide the impetus to conduct and use research. However, there are differences. Conducting research taps into the "ways of knowing," whereas using research taps into the "ways of doing."

When we conduct research, whether in the clinical setting or the laboratory, the primary activity undertaken is the systematic collection of new data. Following specific steps called the protocol, we gather information that will answer a specific research question. For many nursing studies, the *research question* arises from a situation in nursing practice that needs an answer.

> The *utilization of research* involves the systematic process of integrating the findings of completed nursing research studies into clinical nursing practice.

Research utilization also entails reviewing research that has already been completed to develop a new approach to nursing practice. All three processes—research utilization, nursing research, and the nursing process—have the same five major steps. However, the specific tasks for each process are different.

What Is the Relationship Between Nursing Theory and Research Utilization?

Nursing theory used as the theoretical framework of a research study is essential for the continued development of nursing theories; new research findings will support theory or will suggest the modification of theory. In contrast, when a specific nursing theory is used as the framework for nursing practice, the focus is on the intervention. The intervention that is designed in the planning phase of research utilization must be consistent with the theory. For example, if Orem's theory of self-care requisites is used for nursing practice, a successful intervention would be one that emphasizes self-care rather than care received from others. There is a close relationship between nursing research and research utilization because of the focus of both on nursing practice.

DEFINING YOUR PRACTICE CONTEXT

Your practice context will determine to what degree you can apply the findings from nursing research to your practice problem. A *practice context* entails a blending of all those factors and systems that contribute to the delivery of nursing care. This blend includes the health, social, and cultural characteristics of the patient population served; the type of practice setting; the economic resources of the setting; the type of health care delivery system; the existing policies and procedures; the staffing pattern; and the administrative structure. Each factor or system can be either enabling or inhibiting, but it is the practice context as a whole that is evaluated to determine the applicability of nursing research findings.

What Are the Health, Social, and Cultural Characteristics of the Patient Population Being Served?

To begin defining your practice context, you will need to identify any characteristics that are specific to the group of people who will be receiving nursing care. Is there some particular health characteristic that should be considered? For example, if you teach prenatal classes, the health characteristic will be pregnancy. Are there some particular social and cultural characteristics that need consideration? If your prenatal classes are for pregnant teenagers who are single, then social characteristics need special consideration. Be as thorough and as specific as possible in identifying these characteristics.

What Are the Health Care Delivery Characteristics of Your Setting?

As you continue to define your practice context, specify the type of practice setting, the economic constraints of the setting, the type of health care delivery system, the existing policies and procedures, the staffing patterns, and the administrative structures. In other words, include all the characteristics of the care setting that will either contribute to or inhibit the process of applying research findings. If your practice setting is a hospital where there is a limit to the length of stay for a particular surgery, then a new approach that would increase that length of stay would not be an appropriate one for implementation. Furthermore, when implementing a new approach in practice, care must be taken to preserve or improve the current health care delivery standards.

What Are the Motivators and Barriers for Incorporating Nursing Research Into Your Practice?

Identify your bridges (motivators) and roadblocks (barriers) in the practice setting (Critical Thinking Box 24-1). The more individuals in the practice setting from whom you can attain consensus on the new approach to practice, the easier it will be to implement. Those who understand the need for making a change in practice will be more likely to support the change. (See Chapter 10 for information on change theory.) Those who feel they had a part in the decision making surrounding the new approach are also more likely to promote it. In both instances, these colleagues become motivators for the implementation of innovation and change.

As with any change process that involves a group of people, it is very likely that some individuals in the practice setting will be very resistant to the new approach. Those who are resistant may present barriers that prevent the full implementation of the new process. They may complain about lack of time to learn the new approach, for example, in an effort to avoid being a part of what they do not support. These colleagues, as well as budgetary and personnel constraints, are examples of barriers.

In addition, the research literature may present barriers to implementing a new approach. For example, if there are only a few research studies reported in the nursing literature that are related to your practice problem, then the lack of replication of the findings may prevent you from developing a research-based approach for your particular practice problem. Another barrier is the time lag from the completion of a research project until the project report is published. This time lag, which may be a few years, may make the research findings obsolete. For example,

CRITICAL THINKING BOX 24-1

Think about ...
    What are the barriers that might inhibit your use of research findings?
    Are these findings applicable to your practice setting?
    How would you go about minimizing the barriers?

research related to glass oral thermometers would be obsolete since your practice setting now uses electronic ear thermometers. When reviewing the literature, try to limit your search criteria to studies published within the last 5 years, unless it is a classic study that will substantiate the need for conducting research on your practice problem.

What Is Evidence-Based Practice?

Evidence-based practice is similar to research utilization in that it is *a systematic method of applying research findings to nursing practice.* Spector (2007) states, "nurses sometimes don't understand what evidence-based practice means, and some nurses are even calling it a 'fad' or a 'buzzword.'" The latter couldn't be further from the truth. Evidence-based practice is here to stay, and nurses must understand what it is" (p 1). Evidence-based practice incorporates many additional sources of data that may contribute to improved nursing care. A brief definition of evidence-based practice that is generally accepted is the integration of the best research evidence with clinical expertise and patient values (Strauss et al, 2005). Driever (2002) has developed the following working definition of evidence-based practice:

Evidence on which nursing practice is based is derived from the synthesis of knowledge from research; data analyzed from the medical record; quality improvement and risk data; infection control data; international, national, and local standards; pathophysiology; cost effectiveness analysis; benchmarking data; patient preferences; and clinical expertise. Evidence-based nursing practice involves the explicit and judicious decision making about health care delivery for individual or groups of patients based on the consensus of the most relevant and supported evidence derived from theory-derived research and data-based information to respond to consumers' preferences and societal expectations (Driever, 2002, p 593).

Evidence-based practice goes beyond nursing research in considering other sources of documentation that may improve nursing care. Research published by other disciplines is included (e.g., medical research and social research), as well as non-research data that may contribute to practice (e.g., financial data and clinical experts). This is prudent at a time in history when the complexity of health problems is increasing, and at a time when the discovery of new data is more rapid than ever before (Evidence-Based Practice Box 24-1).

The U.S. Department of Health and Human Services has established evidence-based practice centers which are available through the Internet. These centers include the most current information on completed evidence reports as well as those that are in progress (for example, see *www.ahrq.gov/clinic/epcix.htm*). However, not all aspects of practice have been evaluated to date. Therefore the decision to implement an evidence-based practice that does not have a formal report requires a dedicated commitment on the part of all those involved. The steps in applying evidence-based practice include definition of the problem; identifying, reviewing, and evaluating the data applicable to the problem; designing a practice change based on the data; and implementing the change in nursing practice.

Step 1: Define the Problem. Because the focus remains on nursing practice, identification of the *practice problem* is identical to the first step of research utilization.

Step 2: Identify, Review, and Evaluate the Data Applicable to the Problem. As with research utilization, the major source of data to be reviewed is *current nursing research*, followed by *current research from other disciplines.* Scientific research findings form the base, with

BOX 24-1   EVIDENCE-BASED PRACTICE

Wound Care

PRACTICE ISSUE

The increased acuity of patient needs, combined with advances in wound care, has the potential to create frustrating situations for the new graduate nurse. It is essential for the new graduate to provide wound care that reflects the newest advances in care and technology.

IMPLICATIONS FOR NURSING PRACTICE

- From 1993 to 2006, there was nearly an 80% increase in the number of hospitalized patients with pressure ulcers causing an $11 billion increase in hospital costs (Cantrell, 2009).
- Caring for patients with pressure ulcers can increase a nurse's workload by as much as 50% (Stillman, 2007).
- Wound care has emerged as a specialty practice for RNs (Wound Ostomy Continence Nursing Certification Board, 2007).
- Wound care needs and procedures can vary significantly across practice settings.
- New graduate RNs are more competent in patient care and less competent in clinical reasoning and recognizing limits and seeking help.
- New graduate RNs are more likely to use written information, care guidelines, and agency-specific policies to guide their practice.
- New graduate RNs are more competent with using technology to seek answers and specific information related to current patient care practices.

Considering This Information:

What can you do to keep up-to-date on wound care treatments?

References for the Evidence

Cantrell S: Performing under pressure: caring for decubitus ulcers. *Healthcare Purchasing News* 33:12-15, 2009.
Stillman R (2007): Wound care. *Emedicine* from WebMD. Retrieved from *www.emedicine.com/med/topic2754.htm.*
Wound Ostomy Continence Nursing Certification Board (2010): *About WOCNCB, 2008.* Retrieved from *www.wocncb.org/about/.*

all other data building on this base. The specific nursing practice that will be changed, in addition to the practice context, will determine the types of data included for review.

Step 3: Design a Practice Change Based on the Data. Prepare a *written plan* for the new nursing practice. The plan needs to be consistent with your practice context to be effective, and it may experience motivators and barriers to the change. For maximum benefit, the plan will also require the consensus of those who will implement it.

Step 4: Implement the Change in Nursing Practice. Move the new plan into nursing practice on a *defined schedule.* Staff in-services may be required for those involved to fully understand the change. Monitor and evaluate the implementation process.

Now let's consider using the evidence-based practice process in a hypothetical situation.

Mario works in an intensive care unit in which many of the patients require mechanical ventilation. At a recent staff meeting, Mario and his coworkers learned that their unit's rate of ventilator-associated pneumonia (VAP) was greater than rates in many other hospitals. Concerned by this, Mario volunteered to work on this project. He began with a review of the literature. Using a nursing literature database,

Mario was able to find a number of research studies conducted in the past few years that examined the same issue. Additionally, he found that multiple professional organizations had issued evidence-based guidelines to reduce the occurrence of ventilator-associated pneumonia. After reading these articles, Mario drafted a set of clinical practice guidelines based on these articles that reflected the unique needs of his unit and its patient population. Mario then presented his guidelines to the nursing staff and provided short educational in-service sessions on their application. The staff agreed to adhere to these new practice guidelines for a period of 3 months. At the end of that time, they would compare their incidence of VAP using the new clinical guidelines with the incidence of VAP using the old clinical guidelines.

At the end of the 3-month period, Mario and his coworkers were pleased to find a significant decrease in the occurrence of VAP among their patients. Working with nursing administration, Mario's proposed clinical practice guidelines became the new standard of care on his unit.

THE NATIONAL INSTITUTE OF NURSING RESEARCH

What Is Its Function?

The National Institute of Nursing Research (NINR) is a branch of the National Institutes of Health (NIH), which is under the jurisdiction of the U.S. Department of Health and Human Services. Each institute within the NIH focuses on a specific area of health care research; the NINR is a major source of federal funding for nursing research. The NINR also supports education in research methods, research career development, and excellence in nursing science.

Other functions of the NINR are to establish a National Nursing Research Agenda. This agenda is composed of priority topics for nursing research and may be related to a national health need, or they may be in an area that requires research for the development of nursing science. Many nurses have received funding to support clinical and basic research on health and illness across the lifespan. Research funded includes health promotion and disease prevention, quality of life issues, health disparities, and end-of-life care.

The NINR also has a role in President Obama's American Recovery and Reinvestment Act of 2009. The act was created to assist with the economic recovery of the country and includes measures to modernize our national infrastructure including health care. For more information, visit the NINR website *(http://ninr.nih.gov/ninr/)*.

THE AGENCY FOR HEALTH CARE RESEARCH AND QUALITY

What Is Its Function?

As part of the Omnibus Budget Reconciliation Act of 1989, the Agency for Health Care Policy and Research (later renamed the Agency for Healthcare Research and Quality [AHRQ]) was established to enhance the quality and effectiveness of health care services. The AHRQ conducts and supports general health services research, develops clinical practice guidelines, and disseminates research findings and guidelines to health care providers, policymakers, and the public. One arm of the AHRQ supports the Evidence-based Practice Centers Program (AHRQ, 2007), which develops reports about interventions that are based on published scientific studies related to health care. For more information about AHRQ, visit their website *(www.ahrq.gov/)*.

CONCLUSION

Nursing has a growing body of evidence on which we can support our practice. Nursing research has been very important in establishing a platform for the development and utilization of evidence-based practice. Whether you are a new graduate or an experienced nurse, there are ample opportunities for you to apply research in your area of clinical practice. When areas of practice need to be changed, it is important to have valid information and data to support the need for change. You can get involved in nursing research. Check out your hospital resources, establish networking and colleague support, and initiate a research project of your own.

BIBLIOGRAPHY

Agency for Healthcare Research and Quality (2007): Evidence-based Practice Centers. Synthesizing scientific evidence to improve quality and effectiveness in health care. Retrieved from *www.ahrq.gov/clinic/epc/*.

Cumulative Index to Nursing and Allied Health Literature (CINAHL): EBSCO Publishing. Birmingham, Ala, 2010, EBSCO Publishing.

Driever MJ: Are evidenced-based practice and best practice the same? *Western J Nurs Res* 24:591-597, 2002.

Newhouse R, et al: Evidence-based practice: a practical approach to implementation. *JONA* 1:35-40, 2005.

Spector N (2007): Evidence-based health care in nursing regulation. National Council State Boards of Nursing. Retrieved from *www.ncsbn.org/Evidence_based_HC_Nsg_Regulation_updated_5_07_with_name.pdf*.

Strauss S, Richardson WS, Glaziou P, et al: *Evidence-based medicine: how to practice and teach EBM*. 3 ed, London, 2005, Churchill Livingstone.

Additional resources are available online at *http://evolve.elsevier.com/Zerwekh/nsgtoday/*.

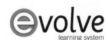

CHAPTER 25

Workplace Issues

Susan Lynne Ahrens, RN, PhD

> *Fear is the father of courage and the mother of safety.*
> —Henry H. Tweedy

> *The safety of the people is the supreme law. (Salus populi suprema lex.)*
> —Cicero (106-143 BC)

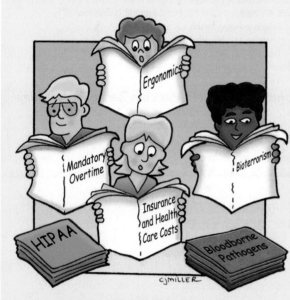

Workplace issues.

After completing this chapter, you should be able to:

- Determine your risk for encountering a workplace issue that can affect your health or well-being.

- Understand ergonomics and ways to safeguard your musculoskeletal system.

- Understand the experience of making an error and strategize how to manage your experience and do the right thing.

- Discuss the importance of personal protective devices.

- Understand the risk for violence at work and how to reduce your risk.

- Understand workplace bullying and harassment.

- Identify useful Internet sites to keep up to date with potential workplace issues (e.g., OSHA, CDC, ANA).

hospital, nursing center, clinic, or physician's office can be hazardous to your future health and well-being. *This is especially true if you are not informed.* Many nurses are aware of the risk of exposure to infection, but they are not aware of other hazards that exist in health care organizations. Nurses in a health care organization are exposed to the risk for injury, toxic chemicals, bioterrorism, and violence. How well a health care organization plans and protects workers from occupational hazards is a measure of how safe you will be and what risks you may encounter as you work. This chapter addresses workplace issues that could potentially affect your health and explains what you need to do to avoid injury, occupational exposure, and illness.

QUESTIONS TO ASK WHEN STARTING A NEW POSITION

As a nurse, when you are preparing to start a new position, ask your new employer to answer the following questions to enable you to evaluate the impact workplace issues will have on your health and well-being:

- Is the hospital latex-free? If not, what latex will I be exposed to?
- What ergonomic devices exist to protect me from harm? How much will I be lifting, pulling, and tugging? Are there lift teams? Are there lift devices?
- How much moving of furniture, stretchers, or equipment will I be doing?
- Will I be using a computer?
- What is the injury rate for the unit I will be working on?
- Does the organization have an antiviolence program? How are bullying behaviors and other hostile work situations such as sexual harassment being addressed by the organization?
- Is the organization needleless? If not, what is my exposure risk?
- What is the organization's policy for exposure to infectious agents? Does it include testing, medication, counseling, and follow-up? What is the process for this?
- What is the organization's tuberculosis (TB) prevention plan? Does the plan adhere to Occupational Safety and Health Administration (OSHA) regulations? How often will I be tested?
- Does the organization have an influenza prevention plan? Does it follow the Centers for Disease Control and Prevention (CDC) guidelines?
- Is there a plan for handling potentially toxic or infectious substances such as blood, chemoprophylaxis, and suction canisters? What is my potential exposure? Will I receive training in correct handling? Will annual refreshers be offered?
- Where will I park? Is the area well-lit? Is it patrolled? What is my risk?
- What is the workmen's compensation program? Would I be able to return to work in a light-duty capacity if I am injured? For how long?
- Does the organization provide vaccinations for infections I might be exposed to, such as influenza, chickenpox, and hepatitis B?
- Does the hospital have a surveillance plan for multidrug resistant organisms (MRSA, VRE)? Does it follow current CDC guidelines?
- How often will I be expected to work "off shift" (shifts other than what I normally work), on-call, or mandatory overtime?
- How often will I need to work on a unit other than my assigned unit? How will I be oriented?

ERGONOMIC HAZARDS FOR HEALTH CARE WORKERS

According to the American Nurses Association (ANA), ergonomic hazards have become a major safety concern among health care workers (ANA, 2008), and nurses are considered to be in a profession that puts them at risk for serious musculoskeletal injuries. The most common problems tend to be back and shoulder injuries. Unfortunately, these types of injuries are the most debilitating of all. Imagine if you cannot raise your arms or reach for things without severe pain. What would happen if every step you took resulted in pain in your back and down your leg? What if sitting or lying down does not relieve your distress? These problems can be yours if you do not take the risk seriously.

Back Injury

So, what is your risk? That is somewhat unclear, since studies investigating work-related injuries in nursing are sporadic. However, it has been reported that more than 50% of nurses complain of chronic back pain. In addition, nurses in one study reported transferring to a different unit, position, or employment because of a back injury, and many of those who remained in their position said they had considered leaving nursing altogether because of back pain (Owen, 1989). More than one-third of nurses have had back injuries severe enough that they were required to take a leave from work (Owen, 2000). In other words, 4 out of every 10 nurses will, at one time or another, have a back injury severe enough that they need to take a leave from work. Back-related injuries reduce the already short supply of nurses, and because there are fewer nurses, the risk for back-related and other musculoskeletal injuries increases.

Why are these injuries so common in nursing? It is simply the nature of the work that nurses do. Patient-handling tasks are repetitive and are usually done manually with very little mechanical support. Lifting, transferring, repositioning, and reaching are the actions that are associated with injuries. Often the configuration of the patient's room and the placement of furniture, monitors, blood pressure cuffs, thermometers, and other hanging devices contribute to injury because nurses are required to reach and stretch in nonergonomic positions to perform tasks.

Until recently, it was believed that good body mechanics with proper lifting techniques could prevent back and shoulder injuries. However, according to the ANA (2008), the idea that there is a safe way to manually lift or turn a physically dependent patient is no longer valid. These studies of body mechanics were not useful for nursing because they used *static objects* for lifting, and this does not reflect the environment in which most nurses work. Many of the situations in which nurses are injured involve sudden, quick changes in position and human beings rather than static objects; therefore, proper body mechanics are not enough, because the nurse cannot adjust in a way that fully protects the back. *Teaching nurses to use proper body mechanics to lift and turn patients does not result in fewer injuries* (ANA, 2008). Therefore the current recommendations by the ANA include the use of assistive patient-handling devices for lifting, transferring, and turning patients.

It is important that nurses take good care of their backs, even when they are young, flexible, and strong, because aging contributes to the risk for a career-ending injury. Repetitive stress on the structures of the spine, shoulders, and hips can cause small, repeated damage that could manifest in serious, debilitating injury. The ANA has sponsored a program called "Handle with Care®" to raise awareness, promote the use of ergonomic equipment and assistive devices, and encourage health care organizations to invest in a safe patient-handling program. In addition, by reducing work-related injuries to nurses, safe patient-handling programs can reduce some of the hidden costs of health care organizations and improve patient care (ANA, 2008).

"Prompted by ANA's Handle with Care Campaign®, which began in 2003 nine states have enacted 'safe patient handling' legislation: Illinois Maryland, Minnesota, New Jersey, New York, Ohio, Rhode Island, Texas, and Washington, with a resolution from Hawaii. California, Connecticut, Florida, Hawaii, Kansas, Maryland, Minnesota, Missouri, and New York introduced legislation in 2008 seeking health care worker programs restricting or eliminating manual lifting of patients" (ANA, 2010, para 1).

What can the nurse do to reduce the risk for a serious back injury? First, be aware of the potential risk by assessing each patient's dependency needs and abilities when deciding what assistive devices to use. Do not move, lift, or turn a dependent person without an appropriate assistive device or help. Next, know what assistive devices are available to you and learn how to properly use them. If your organization does not have devices readily available, become an advocate for a safe patient-handling program. It is also important to keep yourself fit and do not ever "tough it out" when you suffer an injury. Make sure you report your injury and follow the advice of your health care provider so that your body can properly heal. For more information on ways to promote safe patient handling and prevent work-related injuries, see the following websites: *www.patientsafetycenter.com* and *www.nursingworld.org/handlewithcare*. At the ANA site, *www.anasafepatienthandling.org/Main-Menu/ANA-Actions/State-Legislation.aspx,* you can join the team to fight for legislation to enact laws protecting nurses from harm. Finally, it has been suggested that nurses consider developing a practice for "warming up" and stretching before they start their workday. This is to be followed up by stretching again at the end of a day. Another strategy to maintain a limber, flexible body core is to enroll in a yoga or Pilates program.

Repetitive Motion Disorders (RMD)

Many of today's jobs are performed at a computer work area, often in a "shared" area. This is the case in a hospital setting, where nurses, physicians, and ancillary caregivers all use the nursing station 24 hours a day. There may be dozens of workers trying to use the same computer workstation almost constantly. Change, variation, and adjustment to fit an individual worker are basic to the well-being of each worker. Workstations should accommodate users of many different heights, weights, and individual needs. Computer vendors must keep in mind that the "typical" nurse is in his or her mid-40s, and letter size and font as well as proper lighting and the avoidance of shadows are vitally important to aid in viewing computer screens.

The successful ergonomic design of an office workstation depends on several interrelated parts. The task, the posture, and the work activities all interact. The three activities alone can be difficult to deal with, but these activities also must interact properly with existing furniture, equipment, and the environment. The combination makes the picture more complicated. Important parts of the workstation are the chair, the desk, and the placement of the computer (CPU), keyboard, and monitor.

The chair should be padded appropriately, easily adjustable, and have strong lumbar supports. Usually, wheels allow easy movement and armrests may or may not be used, because they sometimes cause more problems, depending on the individual needs of the user.

| **CRITICAL THINKING** BOX 25-1 | What is your workplace environment like? What lift equipment do you have? Have ergonomics been considered? How could you make it better? |

The desk must be wide and deep enough to accommodate the computer's monitor, keyboard, and mouse, with ample space around the machine to write, use the phone conveniently, and perform all other desktop activities. Keep the area clear of clutter and crowding.

Ideally, the placement of the monitor, keyboard, and mouse would be adjustable for every worker, but because this is rarely possible, the monitor height should be approximately 18 to 22 inches above the desk surface, causing most users to view the screen with slightly lowered eyes. The keyboard should be placed directly in front of the user and the mouse on the user's dominant-hand side of the machine. Some nursing stations designate certain machines as left-handed mouse machines so that the mouse will not need to be switched numerous times during a shift. Be sure to use a mouse pad to ensure traction, lessening the frustration and continual long movements of the mouse (Critical Thinking Box 25-1).

Poor workplace design is often the major source for repetitive motion disorders (RMDs) or cumulative trauma disorders (CTDs). RMDs have been associated with users who work for long periods of time at poorly constructed or poorly arranged workstations.

Ergonomic design of work tasks can reduce or remove some of the risks. Other solutions may include:

- Information and training to workers about body positions that eliminate the opportunity for repetitive stress injuries to occur
- Frequent switching between standing and sitting positions, reducing net stress on any specific muscle or skeletal group
- Routine stretching of the shoulders, neck, arms, hands, and fingers

Having a good understanding of ergonomic principles can help prevent injuries.

WORKPLACE VIOLENCE: A GROWING CONCERN IN HEALTH CARE

Witnessing the aftermath of a violent attack on a nurse colleague is a powerful realization that the potential for being harmed by another person at work is very real. As a nurse, you are at risk for harm from coworkers, patients, and families. No matter what the occupation, workplace violence is a growing risk and the second leading cause of occupational death in the United States. The nature of health care workers' jobs puts them at risk for workplace violence, which can result in injury or death (Henry, 2002).

Studies on nurses and workplace violence show that 80% or more nurses have experienced some sort of violence in their career. Workplace violence is defined as violent acts, including physical assaults and threats of assault, directed at individuals at work or on duty. Violence is the intentional use of physical force that has a high likelihood or results in injury or death (Henry, 2002). This can include verbal abuse, threats, unwanted sexual advances, physical assault, and murder.

Nurses often fail to report acts of violence because of a lack of understanding or a belief that "nothing will be done" (Henry, 2002). This has the risk of escalating the situation until physical harm occurs. Many times nurses have never encountered a hostile person before and do not understand how to recognize and de-escalate the situation.

Recently, a nurse in a large urban hospital was working with a young man who had been hospitalized with chest pain. He had denied any drug use; however, it was found that he habitually used cocaine and also consumed large amounts of alcohol on a regular basis. Once the physician discharged him, the patient grew increasingly agitated waiting for the paperwork for his discharge. He wanted to leave the facility to resume his drug-related behaviors.

The nurse had been working on the unit less than a year after graduation and did not recognize the patient's increasing agitation. He used the call light to repeatedly summon the nurse to the room to find out when he could leave. When she entered the room in response to his fifth call and told him it would be another 30 minutes before she could complete the paper work for his discharge, he attacked her. Before she was able to summon help, she was assaulted. The nurse recovered physically but was not able to return to her chosen profession because of posttraumatic stress syndrome. A huge emotional toll was also seen in the rest of the nurses on staff, who were fearful of another similar event happening.

In response to incidents such as this, along with other events occurring in local industry, the hospital administration developed a crisis intervention program. This program taught nursing staff how to recognize signs of escalating anger that could result in an attack and strategies to de-escalate the situation. Nurses were also taught how to protect themselves during an attack. Knowing how to recognize an escalating situation and how to defend against an attacker helped these nurses believe they could deal with future situations that put them at risk for harm.

Additionally, the hospital instituted a "code white" program. It was explained that a "code white" stood for a potentially violent situation, which anyone could initiate if *any* person became loud or abusive, made threats, or started throwing objects. A code white ensured that resources were available to help de-escalate the situation and that no nurse would be alone with someone who was "acting out." Trained volunteers and other staff from the hospital, including security, would respond to a code white, which would be announced over the PA system. It was stressed to nursing staff members that any time they felt unsafe, a code white should be called. The code could be implemented by using the phone system or by pushing a strategically placed alarm button. After instituting the program, there were no further incidents in which nurses were harmed.

So what do you need to do when you start your first job? First of all, be familiar with your organization's policies regarding workplace violence. Next, take a crisis intervention course to become familiar with the signs of escalating violence such as pacing, using foul language, raising one's fist, or using threats. Learn strategies to de-escalate anger. Finally, do not ever try to handle a potentially violent person on your own. Use whatever procedures your organization has put in place to defuse situations; for example, call security or call a "code white" (Figure 25-1).

Horizontal Violence (Bullying) and Other Forms of Workplace Harassment

Judy was excited to start work in the critical care department. She was pleased that the manager had selected her to start there because she understood the criteria for working there as a new graduate were very strict. She had chosen a preceptor from the nurses she knew.

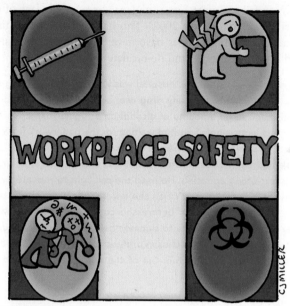

FIGURE 25-1

Workplace safety is important.

Soon, she found herself to be totally stressed out by work. Always an optimistic, carefree person, she was now nervous and had an onset of migraine headaches. She sometimes had to vomit on her way to work. She was not sleeping or eating normally. Her family was very concerned.

At the request of her family, Judy went to see a counselor at the Employee Assistance Program. The counselor helped her identify that she was being bullied by other nurses on the unit. The bullying was causing her great anxiety. For example, during shift report, if she asked a question, the nurses at the report table would put down their pens and glare at her or roll their eyes. If she asked for help lifting a patient, everyone would ignore her. The nurse who was the center of the bullying would yell at her in front of everyone for minor transgressions (if she dropped a pill or forgot to write her blood glucose readings on the report board). If Judy made a mistake, everyone would know about it and the story of the event would grow as it was passed on to others. The anxiety caused by knowing she would be treated this way every day was impairing Judy's ability to grow and develop as a new nurse. It was also having a negative effect on her patient care and on her own health.

Judy needed to understand better what was happening to her so that she could recognize the signs if she was ever the victim of a bully again. She also needed to develop a plan to deal with her current situation. She found a website called the Workplace Bullying Institute.org (*www.bullyinstitute.org*) that provides a wide array of helpful information and assistance, including coaching and current legislation. With the help of her counselor, Judy developed an action plan to address her situation. After time off to contemplate her work life, Judy found another job in a local hospital and started a new position once she realized that the bullying behavior would not be addressed at her current place of employment.

At her new place, Judy found a wonderful mentor and was soon growing as a nurse. Her physical health improved, and with help from her counselor and coach, she was once again a mentally healthy person. Judy had learned from her experience and was determined never to allow a bully to have this level of impact on her again.

As a nurse and individual, it is easy to recognize overt violence. Most hospitals have procedures and policies to deal with violent events. Less common, especially in the United States, is recognition and action related to *horizontal violence*, which is often called *bullying* in the workplace. Most of us believe that the backyard bullies of our childhood will disappear in adulthood. Unfortunately, recent evidence has proven otherwise. Our bullies of childhood tend to grow into the bullies of our adulthood.

You may hear after starting your first position that, "nurses eat their young." Mild forms of hazing activity are common in many professions and can usually be overcome. Although it has not been researched per se in nursing, new nurses often need to prove that they can be counted on to provide safe care for their patients. They may find that their work ethic and skills are being "tested" by other nurses. This type of activity usually lasts for the first weeks of a new position and gradually improves as a new nurse becomes integrated into the work life of the unit.

Horizontal violence, on the other hand, goes beyond this initial struggle and has serious physical and psychological consequences for the victim, which has been documented in the non-nursing research literature (Lutgen-Sandvik et al, 2007). Horizontal violence is a systematic health-harming mistreatment of one or more individuals (targets) by one or more perpetrators that can be verbal, behavioral, and sabotage. The purpose of the bullying is to control the target. Horizontal violence or bullying is initiated by the perpetrator, not by the target or victim (Namie & Namie, 2003). Bullying is not a single event—it occurs over time.

Horizontal violence can occur in any workplace setting. Health care environments are particularly situated to foster bullies because they are hierarchical in nature and tend to involve a great deal of change. In addition, the underlying culture of health care has tended to foster the idea that there are certain rites of passage that must be endured by all new staff. Many of our health care organizations are fear-driven and feel pressured to raise productivity standards higher and higher to improve profits. According to the Workplace Bullying Institute, these factors can create a culture that fosters bullying *(www.bullyinginstitute.org)*. You can be bullied by a manager, supervisor, physician, or coworker. The signs that you may be experiencing being bullied are identified by individuals who had been targets at the workplace (Box 25-1).

For most nurses, the idea that another person would deliberately target them for horizontal violence or bullying is difficult to comprehend. As a result, the person being bullied can experience a multitude of psychological and physical reactions. Most often, the target of horizontal violence believes that the bullying is his or her fault. In the hypothetical situation above, Judy, as a new nurse, believed that she was not doing a good job, and as the bullying continued, she even decided that she should find another profession to work. Her migraine headaches were a direct result of the bullying she was receiving.

Research has indicated that many psychological and physical effects can result from horizontal violence. Bullying creates anxiety, fear, and anger in most adults. As horizontal violence is unrelenting and often severe in nature, the individual has a heightened stimulation of the sympathetic nervous system. As a result, if you are the target of a bully, you can develop anxiety disorders, chest pain, abdominal pain, vomiting, and pains. Depending on the bullying situation, you can

| BOX 25-1 | Signs of Being Bullied |

Being falsely accused of errors

Regularly being stared at or glared at or receiving any other intimidating nonverbal behavior, such as eye-rolling and sighing while you're speaking

Ideas or thoughts being discounted

Being given the "silent treatment"

Dealing with a person who has uncontrollable mood swings

Dealing with a person who makes up rules on the fly

Having satisfactory or exemplary work quality disregarded

Experiencing harsh and constant criticism

Dealing with a person who starts or fails to stop spreading rumors about you

Dealing with a person who encourages others to bully you

Being singled out and isolated from others

Dealing with displays of gross but not illegal behavior

Being yelled at, screamed at, or having someone throw a temper tantrum in front of others that is humiliating to you

Having someone systematically steal credit for your work

Having someone lie about your performance in evaluation process

Being called insubordinate when not true

Having someone use confidential information to publicly humiliate you

Experiencing retaliation

Experiencing verbal put-downs

Being given undesirable assignments as punishment

Being assigned undoable demands

Experiencing sabotage of your work, plans, progression

From Workplace Bullying Institute *(www.bullyinginstitute.org)*.

also develop the signs and symptoms of posttraumatic stress disorder (Matthiesen & Einarsen, 2004).

Because most of us are totally unprepared to deal with a bully, it is very difficult to determine what to do. The Workplace Bullying Institute (2010) website *(www.workplacebullying.org/targets/solution/three-step-method.html)* has an excellent plan to follow. Drs. Namie and Namie suggest that you take the following three steps if you are the target of a bully:

1. *First of all, name it.* Say, "I am being bullied!" "I have a bully at work!" "Jackie is a backyard bully." Other ways to validate it for yourself is to say, "I did not ask for this! I was targeted by Jackie to bully." This type of self-talk will help validate your experience and that it is not your fault.

2. *Seek respite.* From their work, Drs. Ruth and Gary Namie believe that if you are being bullied, you need to take time off work to "BullyProof" yourself. During time off work you need to accomplish five things: (a) check your mental health, (b) check your physical health, (c) research state and federal legal options, (d) gather data regarding the economic impact the bully has had on your unit, and finally, (e) start a job search for a new position because this will give you more options as you address your current work situation.

3. *Expose the bully.* Most people who are being bullied are not willing to expose the bully. However, for your mental and physical health, you need to give your employer an opportunity to address the situation (Workplace Bullying Institute, 2010).

BOX 25-2	Facts About Needlestick Injuries

- Health care workers (HCWs) suffer between 600,000 and 1,000,000 injuries from conventional needles and sharps annually. These exposures can lead to hepatitis B, hepatitis C, and human immunodeficiency virus (HIV), the virus that causes AIDS.
- At least 1000 HCWs are estimated to contract serious infections annually from needlestick and sharps injuries.
- Registered nurses working at the bedside sustain an overwhelming majority of these exposures.
- Needlestick injuries are preventable. More than 80% of needlestick injuries could be prevented with the use of safer needle devices.
- Less than 15% of U.S. hospitals use safer needle devices and systems.
- In 1992, the Food and Drug Administration issued an alert to all health care facilities to use needleless IV systems whenever possible. This alert is merely a recommendation, not a mandate. Therefore, health care facilities are under no legal obligation to comply.
- The first safe needle designs were patented in the 1970s and the FDA has approved more than 250 devices for marketing as safety devices.
- More than 20 other infections can be transmitted through needlesticks, including tuberculosis, syphilis, malaria, and herpes.

Adapted from American Nurses Association (2008): *Needlestick injury fact sheet.* Retrieved from *www.nursingworld.org/ MainMenuCategories/OccupationalandEnvironmental/occupationalhealth/SafeNeedles/NeedlestickInjuryFacts.aspx.*

Often organizations do not understand the tremendous costs in turnover, workmen's compensation, absenteeism, and decreased productivity incurred by allowing a bully to continue working. When you expose the bully, make the business case that the bullying individual is simply too expensive for the organization to continue to have working. In other words, do not go into a huge discussion about *your* experience. Rather, point out the recent turnover, sick calls, workmen's compensation, and decreased productivity that the bully has cost the organization. Give your employer this opportunity to correct the situation. If the employer does not take positive action to correct the situation, then you may need to consider finding another job.

At this point in the United States, there are not many states that have legislation to control horizontal violence in the workplace. The major strategy at the time is to take care of yourself first by protecting your health and well-being. Depending on your situation, there are other ways to address workplace issues. You can also find advice online *(www.bullyinstitute.org)* or you can pay to receive coaching services.

OTHER WORKPLACE ISSUES

Needlestick and Sharps Safety

In addition to the workplace issues already identified, latex allergy, SARS, HIV, tuberculosis exposure, and needlestick injuries are issues that can affect your health if you are not aware of how to prevent exposure and injury (Box 25-2). OSHA has established guidelines that organizations must follow to protect workers. The Needlestick Safety and Prevention Act (P.L. 106-430), which became law on November 6, 2000, provides important protections for health care workers regarding needlestick injuries. Advocating for workplace safety, the ANA was very instrumental in having this piece of federal legislation passed. This act amends the Blood-Borne Pathogen

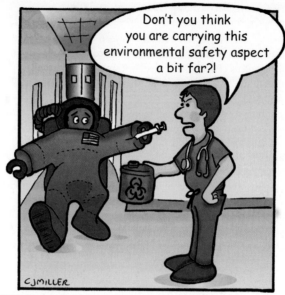

FIGURE 25-2

Nurses must be aware of potential threats to their health.

Standard (administered by OSHA) to require the use of safer devices to protect from sharps injuries. It also requires that employers solicit the input of nonmanagerial employees who are responsible for direct patient care regarding the identification, evaluation, and selection of effective engineering and work-practice controls (Figure 25-2).

In addition, the act requires employers to maintain a sharps injury log to document, at a minimum, the type and brand of device involved in each incident, the department or work area in which the exposure occurred, and an explanation of how the incident happened. The information is to be recorded and maintained in a way that protects the confidentiality of injured employees. The log serves as an important source of data to help determine the relative effectiveness and safety of currently used devices and to guide the development of future products. You need to be familiar with these requirements, as well as any additional guidelines that have been established by your local or state health departments. In some states, the guidelines established by health departments are more strict than those established by OSHA.

Dealing with Staffing Shortages

The shortage of experienced nurses has created many challenges and changes in the health care environments in which we work. Many of these changes are just beginning. We will see many more in the years to come as nurses become scarcer and the need for nursing grows. As a nurse, you need to understand these issues, how to find the best place to work, and how to cope with situations like high nurse-to-patient ratios and mandatory overtime.

An organization (hospital, clinic, nursing center) that provides an environment that is conducive to good nursing care is the best place to be. It does not need to be the newest, most sparkling, or technologically advanced hospital in a large city. For instance:

One of the most spectacular places to practice nursing may be a modest nurse-managed clinic that meets the needs of indigent people in a rural county. The salaries may not be the best, and the clinic will always need something, but the environment is great in that it allows nurses to care for patients and make a difference in the lives of the people they serve.

Finding a good place to work can be difficult. For many years, health care organizations have ignored the needs of nursing (Duclos-Miller, 2002). To attract nurses, many health care organizations use incentives rather than making substantial changes to the environment for nursing (workloads, autonomy). Of course, the lure of higher salaries, benefits, sign-on bonuses, and tuition repayment programs can be highly appealing for new nurses; however, these incentives can distract new nurses from investigating other issues that will have a greater effect on long-term job satisfaction. As a new nurse looking for a position, it may be challenging to find the best fit for you. Fortunately, there are research-based criteria that can help you determine whether an organization provides a good environment for nursing.

In the early 1980s, the American Academy of Nursing (AAN) commissioned a study to determine what characteristics of hospitals attracted nurses. It was interesting to learn that things such as nursing autonomy, low nurse-patient ratios, and collaborative relationships with physicians were some of the draws. From this work, Magnet® hospitals were identified that embodied these essential characteristics that promoted nursing. Today, in our current nursing shortage, hospitals actively seek "Magnet" status to attract nurses. In addition, Magnet® hospitals are known to have better patient outcomes. The American Nurses Credentialing Center (ANCC) is responsible for judging whether hospitals achieve this status. A hospital awarded as a Magnet Recognition Program® would be a good place to work for most nurses (Critical Thinking Box 25-2).

In today's world, no matter where you work, you may need to cope with a situation in which the number of patients under your care and their needs for nursing may be greater than what you are able to provide. What should you do?

First of all, it is important to understand the chain of command for your organization. In other words, to whom should you report your concerns, and what are your next steps if you are not satisfied with the response you receive? Next, remain calm and use your great assessment skills to determine the exact nature of your situation. Here are some things to consider:

- How many patients do you have? What is going on with each of them? What nursing tasks do you need to accomplish? What are your priorities (safety issues)? What tasks would be "nice to do?"
- What are your resources? Do you have someone to whom you can delegate tasks? What support do you have from patient's families (for example, to keep an eye on a confused patient)?
- Are you aware of a nurse colleague who might be able to come and help (perhaps someone who was not considered by those who worked on staffing)?

CRITICAL THINKING
BOX 25-2

To find out more about the characteristics of the Magnet® model, see *www.nursingworld.org/ancc/magnet/*. Determine whether your clinical practice site has a Magnet Recognition Program.®

- Is there any other way to deliver care? For example, working together as a team to take care of patients can be a more efficient way to function for a particular shift, rather than not meet your patient needs.
- What are your hospital policies for high census or high patient load situations?

Gather your facts and present your concerns to the next person in authority—a charge nurse or a supervisor. Do not threaten to leave or make rash statements; just present your facts. Ask for whatever assistance is available. Tell this person what your concerns are and what you can and/or cannot accomplish in your shift based on the high patient load.

Document Your Concerns. If the support you receive is not appropriate, then you need to calmly tell your charge nurse or supervisor that you are going to report your concerns to the next person in charge. Again, do not threaten. If the situation is continuous rather than intermittent, use the notes you have documented to figure out the pattern of what is happening.

Remember that difficult situations tend to be in the forefront of your mind, whereas reality might be different. This is human nature.

Consider the following example.

Some nurses told their nurse manager that they were always getting patients from surgery who did not meet criteria to be discharged from the recovery room. The examples that they gave were very disturbing to the new manager, so she asked them to keep a log of patients who were unstable when they reached the unit. In the next month, instead of a large number of patients coming back from the recovery room unstable, they found only two. In both situations, the patients became hypotensive and required a significant amount of care to stabilize their condition. What the staff and the manager realized after looking at the data was that those two situations were so stressful that they "forgot" the 50 patients who came back without a problem. This is why documentation of events is so important.

If your notes tell you that poor staffing occurs more often than not and you are not able to get your patient care done, then you need to work with your manager to determine the reasons. Is your unit understaffed for the needs of your patients? Does your unit have many vacancies? Does your unit have a lot of sick calls? Are assignments being done correctly? Are nurses doing frequent non-nursing functions such as phlebotomy, running errands, or transcribing orders? Does your unit need someone to help with nonessential nursing duties such as bathing or feeding patients? Many organizations involve staff nurses in helping to solve these problems. Volunteer to work with a group to make changes. If your organization or unit is not willing to work with you to make the workload easier, then you may need to consider a job change.

Mandatory overtime is another way that hospitals deal with poor staffing. Mandatory overtime creates a loss of control for the nurse over the ability to schedule non-work activities, including essential family functions. Mandatory overtime may also put safe patient care at risk because of nurse fatigue and subsequent loss of the ability to concentrate and make good decisions. Although many other professional groups have worked to decrease the incidence of mandatory overtime in cases where fatigue can jeopardize the public's safety, 67% of nurses report that they worked some sort of mandatory or unplanned overtime per month (Bosek, 2001). Mandating overtime is a major concern of our professional associations.

Although it is our professional duty to ensure that our services are continued for our patients until transferred to another nurse, our duty to ensure that patients receive safe treatment may be in conflict if mandatory overtime results in fatigue and the possibility of a serious error occurring. According to Duclos-Miller (2002), we all need to recognize that by accepting a nursing position, we have made a commitment to the institution to provide nursing care at specified intervals. Once we accept responsibility for a patient assignment, we have that responsibility until either our services are no longer needed or we transfer the responsibility to someone else. Does this mean we need to work beyond our capacity?

Many states have enacted legislation prohibiting mandatory overtime. Is your state one of them? You can go to the ANA website to find out whether your state has mandatory overtime legislation.

Legislation that is opposed to mandatory overtime is a priority of the ANA. Legislating overtime of nurses may not be the only answer. Health care organizations must be able to provide care to their patients, and legislation will not be sufficient to alleviate the workloads imposed if there are not enough nurses to take care of patients.

In addition to the previous discussion related to developing a good work environment for nursing, creative solutions can be developed by management and nursing staff to deal with shortages without resorting to mandatory overtime. Some ideas include the following:

- Develop an on-call system that provides one or two extra nurses per shift.
- Develop policies that limit mandatory overtime and ensure rotation among all staff.
- Provide incentives to encourage part-time nursing staff to pick up extra time.
- Develop creative shifts for high-activity, high-volume times (e.g., perhaps a special 11 AM to 2 PM shift to staff for admissions and transfers and reduce the workload for the rest of the staff).
- Develop processes to identify shortages with enough time to arrange coverage.
- Reward nurses who do put forth extra effort for the organization. For example, one hospital provides a bonus of $100 for every 100 hours of on-call time (in which an individual agrees to be available to come in if needed).

What should you do if you are mandated to stay over your scheduled shift because of a staffing shortage? First, you should be familiar with your organization policies regarding mandatory overtime *before* this happens. If the policy is unacceptable to your life circumstances, you probably should not be working in the facility. If you find yourself in a situation in which you believe you are too fatigued to stay over your shift, you need to follow the chain of command in asking for assistance with your situation. Again, you need to assess your situation and provide the charge nurse, supervisor, or manager with the facts of your situation. You need to document your concerns and follow-up as needed after the event. If you believe your organization policy regarding mandatory overtime can be improved or eliminated, work with your manager and others to change it.

Most causes of medical errors relate to system problems:

1. Communication problems
2. Inadequate information flow
3. Human problems
4. Patient-related issues
5. Organizational transfer of knowledge
6. Staffing patterns/work flow
7. Technical failures
8. Inadequate policies and procedures (AHRQ, 2003)

Making a Mistake—What Do I Do Now?

Every year, thousands of medication errors are made in hospitals (Institute of Medicine, [IOM], 1999). Many of them are as benign as the case situation above, but others are very serious. In addition to medication errors, other errors compound to contribute to many serious effects on patients every year, including death. The IOM was chartered in 1970 as the advisor for the U. S. health care system regarding the quality of care *(www.iom.edu)*. In 2003, Congress mandated that the IOM carry out a comprehensive study regarding drug safety and recommendations for a systemwide change. According to the most recent IOM report on errors in health care, 44,000 to 98,000 people die every year from errors (IOM, 2006). In a study on role transition conducted by the National Council of State Boards of Nursing (NCSBN) to examine outcomes of clinical competence and safe practice, a discussion on practice errors and risks for practice breakdown was reported (Suling, 2007).

Karen was a cautious person and a *very* cautious nurse. As a new nurse, she was constantly worried that she would make a mistake! Every day, throughout her orientation, she would breathe a sigh of relief at the end of her shift that she did not make a mistake. In fact, a year went by without any event. One very busy day as she charted her last medications of the day, she had an awful realization that she gave a medication to the wrong patient! She went into the room hoping that somehow the medication (an intravenous piggyback) had not gone through the pump. Unfortunately, the patient had received a dose of medication that she was not ordered to receive!

Karen quickly checked the patient's allergies; then she went about assessing the patient for any untoward effects. Fortunately, the patient did not have any problems at this point. Through checking, Karen determined that the medication did not have any interaction with any other drug the patient was receiving. The medication was rather benign (Pepcid), and a case could be made that the patient would benefit from the medication, even though it was not ordered.

Now Karen must decide what to do. She had been touted as the "perfect" new graduate. She had not made a mistake in the year since she had been out of school. What would happen to her image with her colleagues? What about her manager, who had just last week praised Karen for her "careful attention to detail." Now she thought, "Could I be fired?"

Fortunately for Karen, her patient did not suffer adverse effects from the medication; however, the fact that a very cautious nurse made such an error demonstrates a gap in medication safety. What might have contributed to this event? The only way that this event can contribute to the understanding of what happened is if Karen reports her event. Karen did not necessarily realize this because she was thinking mainly of the implications for the patient and her practice of nursing.

In order to meet regulatory agency standards, hospitals need to have a process for reporting and analyzing errors. Karen remembered that she was shown the process for reporting medication and other errors or events (including injury to herself). She also remembered that there was a policy for how to do this and how to document the event. She went to the policy book online and looked it up.

As she read the policy, Karen learned that she needed to complete the online report for medication error, which included all aspects of what happened. The form also asked her to report her feelings regarding the event because her hospital was trying to understand what it was like to experience an event and what kept nurses from reporting. She learned from reading the policy that the leadership of the hospital appreciated her taking time to complete the form and for reporting the event. She also learned that unless she was deliberately harming the patient, she would not receive disciplinary action; however, the event would be reviewed by her peers to determine what she could have done to prevent it.

Another step in the process was for Karen to notify the charge nurse, supervisor (or her manager), and the physician. Just what she did not want to do! However, being the cautious and conscientious nurse she was, Karen followed through on completing these steps of the process. To her surprise, the physician, charge nurse, and supervisor were all understanding and kind to her when she notified them of the event.

Karen's manager thoroughly discussed the medication error with her the following day. Karen was glad she had taken notes and thought through what had happened because this enabled her to provide her manager with a lot of detail about what had happened. Her manager was very matter of fact about the situation and did not berate or otherwise demean Karen in any way. She also suggested (strongly) that Karen see a counselor at the employee assistance program because she assumed that Karen would have a lot of feelings about what had happened and it could potentially affect her self-confidence. Karen followed through on this advice as well. She was glad that she did because she eventually realized that her medication error, although minor, had indeed shaken her confidence and was affecting her ability to care for her patients (Evidence-Based Practice Box 25-1).

Floating—What Do I Do Now?

One interesting phenomenon about health care is that it has a cyclic nature to some extent. What this means is that during certain times of the year, there may be fewer or greater numbers of patients needing any one service at any given time. Thus sometimes you may have more and sometimes fewer patients. It would be great to have a break when your patient volumes are lower; however, it does not work this way in most situations. For both economic and logistical reasons (another unit is very busy), nurses who are less busy are often instructed to work on a unit that is not their "home unit." The question becomes, "What will I do if this happens?" Consider the following situation and imagine what you might do.

BOX 25-1 EVIDENCE-BASED PRACTICE

Medication and Practice Errors

PRACTICE ISSUE

As the care of patients becomes more complex, the delivery of medications also becomes more complex. Today, nurses are frequently faced with interruptions during the delivery of medications. The problem is that at a time when the reporting of all errors is extremely important, not all are reported (Ulanimo et al, 2006). Nurses fear retribution or disciplinary action, despite the fact that most organizations do not punish nurses in any way for errors that occur (unless they are committed deliberately).

IMPLICATIONS FOR NURSING

- Nurses need to be aware of potential errors by examining the complexity of their workflow and report-ing near misses.
- Nurses need to follow standards of care and avoid shortcuts to care.
- During the delivery of medications, nurses must take steps to avoid interruptions (e.g., don't page a physician, don't start a procedure, don't start a conversation with another person, don't answer the phone unless it is absolutely necessary).
- Nurses need to know their hospital policy and procedure for dealing with and reporting errors.
- If an error occurs that a nurse is involved in, that nurse should seriously consider counseling to deal with the strong feelings that result from making a mistake in a nurse-patient relationship. Nurses often experience posttraumatic stress disorder following an event in which an error is made.
- Nurses should be actively involved in finding solutions to prevent errors in the future. This might include participating in a quality initiative such as Lean or Six Sigma.

Considering This Information:

Knowing that you could be involved in an error someday, how can you prepare yourself to prevent this from happening and to be able to deal with an error if it does happen?

References for the Evidence

Baker H: Rules outside the rules for administration of medication: a study in South Wales, Australia. *Image J Nurs Sch* 29:155-158, 1997.

Institute of Medicine: *To err is human: building a safer health system.* Washington, DC, 1999, National Academy Press. Retrieved from *www.iom.edu/?id=12735.*

Ulanimo V, O'Leary C, Connolly P: Nurses' perceptions of causes of medication errors and barriers to reporting. *J Nurs Care Qual* 12:28-33, 2006.

Denise was done with her orientation and had been working on her own for approximately 6 months. She had been told about the floating policy on her unit—how everyone "took turns." The unit had been very busy since she had started working, so she did not often think of the issue of floating until this evening. When she came to work, the unit was very quiet and she was told to report to the surgi-cal unit. Since Denise normally worked on a medical unit, she was naturally anxious about this assign-ment. The nurses on her unit were sympathetic, but they reminded her of the floating policy and said that it was her turn to go to another unit.

When Denise arrived on the surgical unit, she was given an assignment of eight patients with a variety of surgical problems (gallbladders to colon resections). Most of her patients had tubes, dress-ings, and a variety of comorbidities such as diabetes and hypertension that complicated their recovery. Two hours into her shift, she was completely overwhelmed. The nurses she was working with were very kind, but they were also busy and Denise did not want to bother them with ongoing questions about the location of items and the policies for dressing changes and management of nasogastric tubes. Denise managed to get through the night without any mishaps; however, she was charting until 5 AM (she was off duty at 3 AM).

Denise continued to be angry and upset about the floating for many days. She was hostile toward the leadership for making her do this. Since her unit did not get busy right away, she worried about the same situation recurring. She felt she could handle it maybe once a year, but not repeatedly. She began to think about leaving. Denise's manager Joyce approached her after several days and asked to discuss the situation. Joyce said she had some thoughts and ideas that might help. Denise reluctantly went to see her manager.

Issues surrounding floating are some of the most hotly debated and intensely felt by nurses, managers, and administrators. Some journal articles and nursing newsletters tell nurses to agree to float and always take an assignment. Others advise nurses to agree to go but to only do basic nursing care and not to take an assignment. The ethical issue involved in floating is that if you are not on your assigned unit, there will be a disproportionately high number of patients to nurses, which increases errors, or there is the risk of having a less skilled nurse on a unit, which can also lead to problems. Studies have not demonstrated that the risk of a less skilled nurse has really contributed to patient harm, whereas studies of nursing workload have indicated that the greater the workload, the greater the risk for harm to patients (Kane-Urrabazo, 2006).

Data are available to tell us that the more patients a nurse has, the more likely an error will occur (Kane-Urrabazo, 2006); however, there are no data that tell us as nurses how many—if any—patients are harmed by floating nurses. Although many nurses passionately believe that if they go to another unit, the likelihood of error occurring is very high, there are no data to support this contention.

Therefore some argue that it is unethical for a nurse to refuse an assignment if it is reasonable. Refusing an assignment to float could result in harm to a patient because of unreasonable workloads on the other unit. On the other hand, the organization owes its nurses orientation to all the units that they may be assigned. This notion is based on the ideas of distributive justice (Kane-Urrabazo, 2006). Many states, such as Iowa and Texas, have written guidelines or position statements on floating, as have many nursing organizations such as the American Association of Colleges of Nursing (AACN) and the American Organization of Nurse Executives (AONE). Regulatory agencies such as The Joint Commission (TJC) have stated that leaders in organizations must define the qualifications and competencies necessary to provide patient care. Hospitals need to have floating policies and plans to orient staff to units they may be assigned. Again, what should conscientious nurses do to ensure the safety of their patients and to protect their ability to practice?

As Denise met with her manager, she first was given thanks for floating and not making a big deal about it at the time. Her manager acknowledged that floating was very unsettling, and she asked Denise what would have made the change in assignment better. Denise told her manager that she was glad to have been able to help on the unit because it was very busy, and she did not know what they would have done had she not been there. However, Denise felt that it would have been better if she had been given orientation to that unit and surgical patients before being asked to float there. She added that it would have helped to know where supplies were located and to know what patient care standards were used to help them recover from surgery.

As a result of Denise's conversation with the manager, an orientation program was developed to help nurses who were floating to another unfamiliar unit. In order to make this successful, the hospital was divided into "pods" of similar units. Nurses would only float within their pod. A support system was built into floating situations by assigning a manager or supervisor "buddy" to check on the floating nurse periodically throughout the shift to see whether there were any issues. A debriefing session was held with each nurse who floated to determine ways to make the experience better.

Several months later, Denise was pulled to another unit to help out. Although she did not like being off her normal unit, she tolerated the experience much better than she did the first time. She made sure she had a resource person to help her with problems and questions. She was able to leave at her normal time. Overall, she felt good about helping out another unit.

If you are given an assignment to float, don't panic! It is also important to remember first that you are going to help out another unit that does not have enough staff to care for their patients. Think of the other unit and consider what types of patients are on the unit. When you arrive, ask for any "overflow" patients who might have needs similar to patients on your normal unit (e.g., any overflow medical patients if you have a medical background). Ask for a quick tour of the unit and the unit standards of care (e.g., how to manage care of the postoperative mastectomy patient). Ask to be assigned to patients who are less complex since you will be learning as you go along. Ask for help as you need it. Ask whether a nursing assistant can be assigned with you.

If you arrive to the assigned unit and things do not go well, report the experience to your next chain of command person as soon as possible. Document your conversations. As much as possible, try to enjoy your patients and appreciate what you have learned during your shift. Use the Internet to investigate unfamiliar patient care issues (if you have it available). Remember, regardless of your experience, you are doing what is best for the patient.

CONCLUSION

As you stand at the door, your new license in hand, the greatest human adventure awaits you. Nursing is one of the hardest and most awesome professions that exist. As a nurse, you have the opportunity to be part of and witness the most intimate moments of the lives of individuals and families. You have the ability to change people and be changed forever.

Nurses in the hospital need to become more involved in the design, management, and environment of their unit. Too often, nurses give over their responsibility and power to the nurse manager and lose out on this opportunity. Nurses need to speak up in non-motional (but passionate) voices to correct situations that put them and their patients at harm. There are solutions to mandatory overtime, floating, back injuries, and workplace violence. We need to be at the forefront of developing demonstration projects and research on ways to improve the work and healing environment. With all the wonderful critical thinking and problem-solving skills nurses have, together we can make a difference.

In the meantime …

However grand the profession, it is not without risk, and workplace issues exist that require your vigilance. Make sure that you wash your hands often, stay current about workplace issues, maintain standard precautions, ask for what you need to be safe, take care of your back, and most of all, work hard, but not too much!

BIBLIOGRAPHY

AHRQ's Patient Safety Initiative: Building Foundations, Reducing Risk. Interim Report to the Senate Committee on Appropriations. AHRQ Publication No. 04-RG005, December 2003. Agency for Healthcare Research and Quality, Rockville, MD.

American Nurses Association (2010): *Enacted safe patient handling (SPH) legislation*. Retrieved from *www.nursingworld.org/MainMenuCategories/ANAPoliticalPower/State/StateLegislativeAgenda/SPHM/Enacted-Legistation.aspx.*

American Nurses Association (2008): *Safe patient handling and movement*. Retrieved from *www.nursingworld.org/MainMenuCategories/ANAPoliticalPower/State/StateLegislativeAgenda/SPHM.aspx.*

Bosek M: Mandatory overtime: professional duty, harm, and justice. *JONA's Healthcare Law, Ethics, Regulation* 3:99-102, 2001.

Duclos-Miller P: Mandatory overtime: is it really necessary? *Connecticut Nurs News*, March-May 2002.

Henry J: Violence prevention in healthcare organizations within a total quality management framework. *J Nurs Admin* 32:479-486, 2002.

Institute of Medicine (1999): To err is human: building a safer health system, *National Academy Press.* Retrieved from *www.iom.edu/?id=12735.*

Institute of Medicine (2006): Identifying and preventing medication errors, Washington, DC, *IOM.* Retrieved from *www.iom.edu/CMS/3809/22526.aspx.*

Kane-Urrabazo C: Management's role in shaping organizational culture. *J Nurs Manag* 14:188-194, 2006.

Lutgen-Sandvik P, Tracy S, Alberts J: Burned by bullying in the American workplace: prevalence, perceptions, degree and impact. *J Manag Studies* September 2007.

Matthiesen SB, Einarsen S: Psychiatric distress and symptoms of PTSD among victims of bullying at work. *Br J Guid Couns* 32:335-356, 2004.

Namie G, Namie R: *The bully at work: what you can do to stop the hurt and reclaim your dignity on the job.* Naperville, Ill: 2003, Sourcebooks.

Owen BD: The magnitude of low-back problem in nursing. *Western J Nurs Res* 11:234-242, 1989.

Owen BD: Preventing injuries using an ergonomic approach. *AORN J* 72:1031-1036, 2000.

Suling Li (2007): Assessing clinical competence and practice errors of newly licensed registered nurses. *National Council State Boards of Nursing.* Retrieved from *www.ncsbn.org/ICN_competence_for_Dawn.pdf.*

Workplace Bullying Institute (2010): *What bullied targets can do.* Retrieved from *www.workplacebullying.org/targets/solution/three-step-method.html.*

Additional resources are available online at *http://evolve.elsevier.com/Zerwekh/nsgtoday/.*

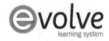

CHAPTER 26

Emergency Preparedness

Tyler Zerwekh, MPH, DrPH, and JoAnn Zerwekh, MSN, EdD, RN

> *We're in a new world. We're in a world in which the possibility of terrorism, married up with technology, could make us very, very sorry that we didn't act.*
> —CONDOLEEZZA RICE, FORMER U.S. SECRETARY OF STATE, 2008

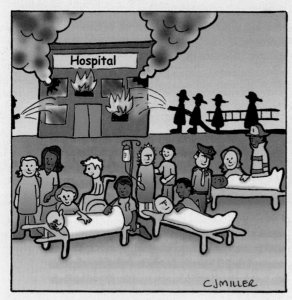

We are prepared.

After completing this chapter, you should be able to:

- Identify various public health threats the medical community is susceptible to.

- Identify regulatory initiatives undertaken to prevent future emergencies.

- Discuss what constitutes an all-hazards plan.

- Discuss the variety of diseases that are likely to be involved in a bioterrorism attack and what to look for.

- Discuss the importance of personal protective devices and how to use them.

errorism alarms millions of people every year. It is a violent and deadly form of intimidation with the intent to debilitate governmental function and create a climate of hysteria. Terrorists take advantage of people's panic to achieve their goals. To the terrorist, an event that results in mass fatalities, disruption, and overconsumption of vital resources is a profitable outcome. Since the events of September, 2001 and subsequent anthrax mail attacks, terrorism on U.S. soil is now a reality. Preparation for responding to acts of terrorism and to natural disasters has increased immensely, both in the community and on health care fronts. Community health nurses and clinical nurses have been assigned new responsibilities and roles in the wake of massive federal, state, and local efforts to prepare for public health emergencies. This chapter will highlight the various public health threats the medical community is susceptible to, regulatory initiatives undertaken to prevent future emergencies, and recent public health preparedness efforts bestowed to the nursing profession as the shift to an all-hazards plan is integrated throughout the medical and nursing community.

WHAT IS PUBLIC HEALTH PREPAREDNESS?

Public health preparedness, as it relates to the nurse, can be divided into two major categories: (1) clinical preparedness and (2) community-based approaches. The clinical aspects of public health preparedness will focus on agent identification and education for the various threats, administrative and regulatory efforts to increase preparedness, and epidemiological clues that may indicate a public health event has occurred.

The basis for public health preparedness has focused on the concept of preparing for chemical, biological, radiological, nuclear, and explosive threats—or CBRNE events. The term *CBRNE* originates from previous military and emergency response organizations such as the U.S. Marine Corps, the U.S. Army, and the Canadian Military Services (U.S. Army, 2008). Although not covered in detail in this chapter (because emphasis will be placed upon individual radioactive isotopes and "dirty bombs"), additional information about nuclear weapons and preparedness can be found at the Nuclear Regulatory Commission website *(www.nrc.org)*. The first section of this chapter focuses primarily on chemical, biological, and radiological events as they relate to the preparedness and response measures necessary for the licensed nurse to provide efficient and expedient care.

CLINICAL PREPAREDNESS

What Are Biological Agents?

Given the importance of responding rapidly to a bioterrorism-related outbreak, nurses need to be able to recognize the major syndromes associated with high-risk agents. Anthrax, botulism, plague, and smallpox are considered the four top agents for potential bioterrorism because plague and smallpox can be spread person-to-person and botulism and anthrax can be disseminated to a population via airborne release (they are not spread person-to-person). Table 26-1 discusses the etiology, signs/symptoms, transmission, and isolation/prevention of these agents. For more information on diagnostic and medical management of biological agents, visit the University of Alabama at Birmingham's website on bioterrorism agents *(www.bioterrorism-uab.ahrq.gov/)*.

What Are Chemical Agents?

The use of chemical weapons poses an array of problems for the clinical nurse, including contamination, decontamination, and personal protection within the health care facility. Chemical agents can be divided into major classifications based on the makeup of the chemical agent and its clinical presentation. The following section focuses on the primary chemical agents most likely to be used in a terrorist event, along with their symptoms, diagnosis, and treatment options.

Of all the chemical agents of concern for the registered nurse, whether in the clinical or public health sector, the nerve agents present the greatest challenge in recognition, treatment, and

TABLE 26-1   Bioterrorism Agents

Agent	Etiology	Signs and Symptoms	Transmission	Isolation/Prevention

Anthrax	*B. anthracis*	*Pulmonary:*
		 Flu-like
		 Respiratory failure
		 Hemodynamic collapse
		 Usually fatal
		 Cutaneous:
		 Local skin—head,
		   forearms, hands
		
		 Localized itching
		   followed by a papular
		   lesion that turns
		   vesicular and *develops*
		   a black eschar in 2-6
		   days
		 Responds well to
		   antibiotics
		 Gastrointestinal:
		 Abdominal pain, nausea,
		   vomiting, fever
		 Bloody diarrhea, emesis
		 Usually fatal
			Anthrax is a
			   durable spore
			   that lives in the
			   soil; transmission
			   by inhalation of
			   the spore, contact
			   with the spore,
			   and the ingestion
			   of contaminated
			   food
				Vaccine is available. (This
				   vaccine is not traditionally
				   given to health care
				   workers.)
				 Standard isolation
				   precautions; however, once
				   the patient is sick, there is
				   no person-person
				   transmission.

Botulism	*Clostridium*
	 botulinum—
	 produces a
	 neurotoxin
		Responsive, no fever
		 Drooping eyelids,
		   weakened jaw clench,
		   difficulty swallowing
		   or speaking
		 Blurred vision and
		   double vision
		 Arm paralysis followed by
		   respiratory and leg
		   paralysis
		 Respiratory depression
			Ingestion of
			   toxin-
			   contaminated
			   food; the toxin
			   can be made into
			   an aerosol and
			   inhaled
			   (manmade)
				Vaccine is available.
				 Pentavalent vaccine is
				   effective only for the toxin
				   that the person was
				   vaccinated for (A-type
				   vaccine protects only
				   against type A botulism).
				 Supportive care only. No
				   isolation precautions
				   implemented.

Plague	*Yersina pestis*	Fever, cough, chest pain
		 Bloody sputum
		 Sputum can be thick
		   and very purulent or
		   watery with gram-
		   negative rods
		 Bronchopneumonia
			In a bioterrorist
			   event, most likely
			   to be aerosolized
				There is no proven vaccine
				   for the pneumonic plague,
				   which is the most likely
				   version in a bioterrorist
				   event.
				 Droplet isolation
				   precautions.

Smallpox	*Variola virus*	Prodrome of fever,
		   myalgia
		 Vesicles on the distal
		   limbs (hands, feet) as
		   opposed to truncated
		   vesicles with
		   chickenpox
				Vaccine created in late 1700s.
				   Routine vaccination
				   ceased with eradication of
				   smallpox in 1979.
				 Droplet precautions
				   recommended, especially
				   if pocks develop inside the
				   buccal cavity.

response to a public health event. The nerve agents, also known as organophosphate esters, are the most severe, most incapacitating, and most likely to be implemented of all chemical agents (Wetter et al, 2001). Sarin, soman, tabun, and VX gases are the major chemicals in this group that inhibit acetylcholinesterase. These agents are liquid at room temperature, but in vapor form they penetrate the cornea, dermis, and respiratory tract. VX gas presents a unique threat because of its markedly greater toxicity and lower volatility, which translates into greater concern for secondary contamination among stricken patients. The effects of these agents are due to unopposed action of acetylcholine at muscarinic and nicotinic receptors. Initial effects are related to the muscarinic effects, including rhinorrhea, salivation, miosis, and headache. With severe poisoning, nicotinic effects can be observed. The muscarinic and nicotinic effects are manifested by bronchospasm, vomiting, incontinence, muscle fasciculation, convulsions, respiratory failure, and death (Wetter et al, 2001). The antidotes for nerve agent poisoning include atropine at fairly high doses—several milligrams to hundreds of milligrams in some cases—and pralidoxime (2-PAM), up to 8 mg.

The choking, or pulmonary, chemical agents are similar to the blister agents; however, in the choking agents the mechanism of action takes place primarily in the respiratory system. The agents of note in this category are chlorine gas and phosgene (Wetter et al, 2001).

In chlorine gas, the majority of exposures occur by inhalation and lead to symptoms of ocular, nasal, and respiratory irritation. Common signs and symptoms of exposure can include eye redness and lacrimation, nose and throat irritation, cough, and suffocation. For cutaneous exposures, burning and blistering of the dermal layer are possible. Currently, there is no biological marker for chlorine exposure available (CDC, 2008).

Another choking chemical agent, phosgene gas, has often been described as smelling like fresh-cut grass. The majority of exposures to phosgene occur by inhalation. Phosgene exposure has clinical presentation/symptom patterns similar to those of chlorine gas (CDC, 2008). See Critical Thinking Box 26-1.

What Are Radiological/Radioactive Agents?

Another concept the clinical or emergency department (ED) nurse is aware of is the potential for patients entering the hospital exposed with radiation. The concept of "dirty bombs" is relatively new to the field of emergency preparedness, coming to prominence after the 9/11 World Trade Center attacks. A dirty bomb is a radiological dispersal device (RDD) that combines an explosive such as dynamite with a radioactive material. In the field the explosion itself would be of greater concern in terms of damage to property and human life; however, the concern in the hospital ED would be the arrival of patients contaminated with radioactive material. The extent of local contamination would depend on a number of factors, including the size of the explosive, the amount and type of radioactive material used, the means of dispersal, and weather conditions. Those closest to the RDD would be the most likely to sustain injuries due to the explosion. As radioactive material spreads, it becomes less concentrated and less harmful (U.S. Nuclear

CRITICAL THINKING BOX 26-1	What personal protective equipment is available to you at your clinical facility? How does your facility deal with exposure to hazardous or toxic material (e.g., blood, bacteria, radioactive)?

CRITICAL THINKING BOX 26-2

What is your organization's policy for dealing with CBRNE events? Who is the designated safety officer? Where is a copy of the organization safety plan and emergency situation's response plan?

Regulatory Commission, 2007). Acute radiation syndrome (ARS) is an acute illness caused by irradiation of the entire body (or most of the body) by a high dose of penetrating radiation in a very short period of time (usually a matter of minutes). The major cause of this syndrome is depletion of immature parenchymal stem cells in specific tissues (CDC, 2008). See Table 26-2 for a listing of syndromes associated with ARS. An excellent website to learn more about radiation syndromes and radioactive agents can be found at *www.bt.cdc.gov/radiation/arsphysicianfactsheet.asp*. Also see Critical Thinking Box 26-2.

What Is a Pandemic?

In April 2009, public health and medical professionals around the country experienced the first wave of an influenza pandemic on U.S. soil in more than 40 years. Not since the Hong Kong pandemic flu strains of 1968-1969 had the medical and scientific community seen such a rapid and expansive surge of H1N1 influenza cases both in the United States and worldwide (CDC, 2010a).

A traditional influenza pandemic can be distinguished from regular seasonal flu epidemics in two major facets: (1) widespread, worldwide cases of the same strain, and (2) a novel strain of influenza virus unexpected or previously unidentified in the human population (CDC, 2010a). Typical influenza pandemics often work in "waves," which are periods of 6 to 8 weeks between spikes in case totals that can be attributed to primary public health prevention (vaccination), a mutation in virus strain, or a new host susceptibility.

The World Health Organization (WHO) has developed a global pandemic influenza preparedness plan, which categorizes various events of a pandemic into different phases (Figure 26-1). Each phase requires both the clinical and public health nurse to execute specific preparedness and responsive measures to mitigate the influenza pandemic threat.

For nurses, pandemic influenza planning and response presents a unique and novel approach to clinical and evidence-based practice. It can be expected during pandemic influenza operations that in the onset of mass vaccinations of the general population, the availability of influenza vaccine will be limited as vaccine manufacturers rush to create and fill vaccine orders. When this occurs, federal health authorities, such as the CDC and Department of Health and Human Services (DHHS), recommend prioritizing population groups to receive the initial limited supplies of influenza vaccine. These priority groups are identified based on individual medical fragility (i.e., immunosuppression) and susceptibility to the pandemic influenza virus. The astute nurse must be aware of the variability of influenza virus from season to season and must consider priority options when vaccinating selected populations based on these factors. The Centers for Disease Control Influenza website is an excellent source to locate current influenza vaccine priority groups *(www.cdc.gov/flu/)*.

The critical component for the community and public health nurse is the careful medical screening and identification of these priority groups to receive the pandemic influenza vaccine. Along the lines of medical screening persons for pandemic influenza vaccination, the nurse must

TABLE 26-2 Acute Radiation Syndromes

Syndrome	Dose*	Prodromal Stage	Latent Stage	Manifest Illness Stage	Recovery
Hematopoietic (bone marrow)	Above 0.7 Gy (above 70 rads) *(mild symptoms may occur as low as 0.3 Gy or 30 rads)*	• Symptoms are anorexia, nausea, and vomiting. • Onset occurs 1 hour to 2 days after exposure. • Stage lasts for minutes to days.	• Stem cells in bone marrow are dying, although patient may appear and feel well. • Stage lasts 1 to 6 weeks.	• Symptoms are anorexia, fever, and malaise. • Drop in all blood cell counts occurs for several weeks. • Primary cause of death is infection and hemorrhage. • Survival decreases with increasing dose. • Most deaths occur within a few months after exposure.	• In most cases, bone marrow cells will begin to repopulate the marrow. • Full recovery is probable for a large percentage of individuals; recovery process may last from a few weeks up to 2 years after exposure. • Death may occur in some individuals at 1.2 Gy (120 rads). • The LD50/60† is about 2.5 to 5 Gy (250 to 500 rads).
Gastrointestinal (GI)	Above 10 Gy (above 1000 rads) *(some symptoms may occur as low as 6 Gy or 600 rads)*	• Symptoms are anorexia, severe nausea, vomiting, cramps, and diarrhea. • Onset occurs within a few hours after exposure. • Stage lasts about 2 days.	• Stem cells in bone marrow and cells lining GI tract are dying, although patient may appear and feel well. • Stage lasts less than 1 week.	• Symptoms are malaise, anorexia, severe diarrhea, fever, dehydration, and electrolyte imbalance. • Death is due to infection, dehydration, and electrolyte imbalance. • Death occurs within 2 weeks of exposure.	• The LD100‡ is about 10 Gy (1000 rads).

Continued

TABLE 26-2   Acute Radiation Syndromes—cont'd

Syndrome	Dose*	Prodromal Stage	Latent Stage	Manifest Illness Stage	Recovery
Cardiovascular (CV)/central nervous system (CNS)	Above 50 Gy (5000 rads) (*some symptoms may occur as low as 20 Gy or 2000 rads*)	• Symptoms are extreme nervousness and confusion; severe nausea, vomiting, and watery diarrhea; loss of consciousness; and burning sensations of the skin. • Onset occurs within minutes of exposure. • Stage lasts for minutes to hours.	• Patient may return to partial functionality. • Stage may last for hours but often is less.	• Symptoms are return of watery diarrhea, convulsions, and coma. • Onset occurs 5 to 6 hours after exposure. • Death occurs within 3 days of exposure.	• No recovery is expected.

*The absorbed doses quoted here are "gamma equivalent" values. Neutrons or protons generally produce the same effects as gamma, beta, or x-rays but at lower doses. If the patient has been exposed to neutrons or protons, consult radiation experts on how to interpret the dose.
†The LD50/60 is the dose necessary to kill 50% of the exposed population in 60 days.
‡The LD100 is the dose necessary to kill 100% of the exposed population.
From Centers for Disease Control and Prevention (2008): *CDC Emergency Preparedness and Response.* Retrieved from *www.bt.cdc.gov.*

WHO Pandemic Influenza Phases (2009)	
Phase	**Description**
Phase 1	No animal influenza virus circulating among animals have been reported to cause infection in humans.
Phase 2	An animal influenza virus circulating in domesticated or wild animals is known to have cause infection in humans and is therefore considered a specific potential pandemic threat.
Phase 3	An animal or human-animal influenza reassortant virus has caused sporadic cases or small clusters of disease in people but has not resulted in human-to-human transmission sufficient to sustain community-level outbreaks.
Phase 4	Human-to-human transmission of an animal or human-animal influenza reassortant virus able to sustain community-level outbreaks has been verified.
Phase 5	The same identified virus has cuased sustained community-level outbreaks in two or more countries in one WHO region.
Phase 6	In addition to the criteria defined in Phase 5, the same virus has caused sustained community-level outbreaks in at least one other country in another WHO region.
Post Peak Period	Levels of pandemic influenza in most countries with adequate surveillance have dropped below peak levels.
Post Pandemic Period	Levels of influenza activity have returned to the levels seen for seasonal influenza in most countries with adequate surveillance.

FIGURE 26-1

World Health Organization pandemic phases. *(Adapted from WHO Pandemic Phase Descriptions and Main Actions by Phase. World Health Organization. Retrieved from* www.who.int/csr/disease/influenza/pandemic/en/index.html.*)*

be cognizant of different criteria that make the recipient eligible or deferred for a pandemic influenza vaccine. Many times the deferral list for pandemic influenza vaccination is similar to the same deferral groups for seasonal influenza. Some of the maladies and conditions that could defer pandemic influenza vaccination include (1) severe allergy to eggs or egg products, (2) life-threatening allergic reaction to a previous influenza vaccination dose, (3) Guillain-Barré syndrome, (4) sick or ill or symptoms of illness at the time of vaccination (CDC, 2010b).

What Is Disaster Nursing?

As witnessed by the 2005 Hurricane Katrina and Indonesian tsunami events, natural disasters are a reminder of the critical role that emergency and public health nurses play in disaster response.

Disaster nursing integrates a wide range of nursing-specific knowledge and practices that facilitate the promotion of health while minimizing health hazards and peripheral life damaging factors (Kandasamy, 2007). Disaster nursing can be further subdivided into two major components: (1) implementation of the public health levels of prevention and (2) emergency triage and response.

In community health nursing, the role of the nurse in disaster response is to effectively promote the three levels of public health prevention. In *primary public health prevention* during disasters, the community health nurse must emphasize the components and principles of preparedness (Kandasamy, 2007). Community health nurses will be required to maintain strong physical and mental health during a disaster to provide a concerted response to their patients. This includes knowledge of the disaster plans of the community and the facility, inclusive of staff and patients. Nurses also need to educate their patients in the awareness and implementation of disaster kits and family emergency response plans in anticipation of a potential natural disaster. In the next stage—*secondary public health prevention*—the nurse must emphasize the components and principles of response (Kandasamy, 2007). The response stage is one of the most important aspects of natural disasters, because it requires efficient execution of nursing practice while maintaining professionalism and mental support to the afflicted community and patients. As the scale of disaster increases, the role and responsibilities of the nurse increase proportionately.

The last stage of *public health prevention—tertiary*—integrates the community health nurse's operations after the disaster has occurred. These skills and practices are often known as recovery (Kandasamy, 2007). In the recovery stage, the nurse is confronted with unexpected or sudden loss of key personnel and patients in addition to the management of mental health issues in individuals related to the disaster.

What Are the Levels of Disasters? During small natural disasters, also known as Level I disasters, the community health nurse works in cooperation with local emergency medical systems and the community to provide medical support. Examples of Level I disasters include auto accidents and house fires. Level II disasters require the community health nurse to respond in a greater capacity using larger casualty practices in coordination with regional response agencies (such as state health and emergency management agencies). Examples of Level II disasters include train derailments, building collapses, and tornadoes. Level III disasters exhaust the most resources (including both the physical and mental resources of the community health nurse). Level III disasters consume local, state, and federal resources to the fullest extent and require an extended response time by the community health nurse that can last weeks and even months. Examples of Level III disasters include earthquakes, tsunamis, and hurricanes.

WHAT IS TRIAGE?

The core concept that ED nurses face is *triage*. Triage is a system of sorting patients according to medical need when resources are unavailable for all persons to be treated. For example, a patient presenting to the ED with chest pain will take priority in receiving intervention than a patient coming in with nausea and diarrhea. Remember, ABCs when triaging patients! While the genesis of triage has been documented in hospitals back to the mid-20th century, the concept was brought to wide attention by the California emergency medical services in response to earthquakes in the 1990s. In disaster triage, a mass casualty incident causes a surge of patients in the

ED requiring emergency assessment. In addition, disaster Patients' needs are usually categorized by the placement of printed triage cards/tags. Figure 26-2 depicts a sample triage card. The START (Simple Triage and Rapid Treatment) system is the most common type of disaster triage employed by ED personnel (Box 26-1). It can be used by lightly trained ED personnel and is not to supersede or instruct medical techniques.

Another concept of triage used at the scene of a disaster is that of advanced triage, where colors replace the common terminology. The standard colors used in advance triage have been paired with the START terminology. All advanced triage concepts are similar and can be applied to START concepts.

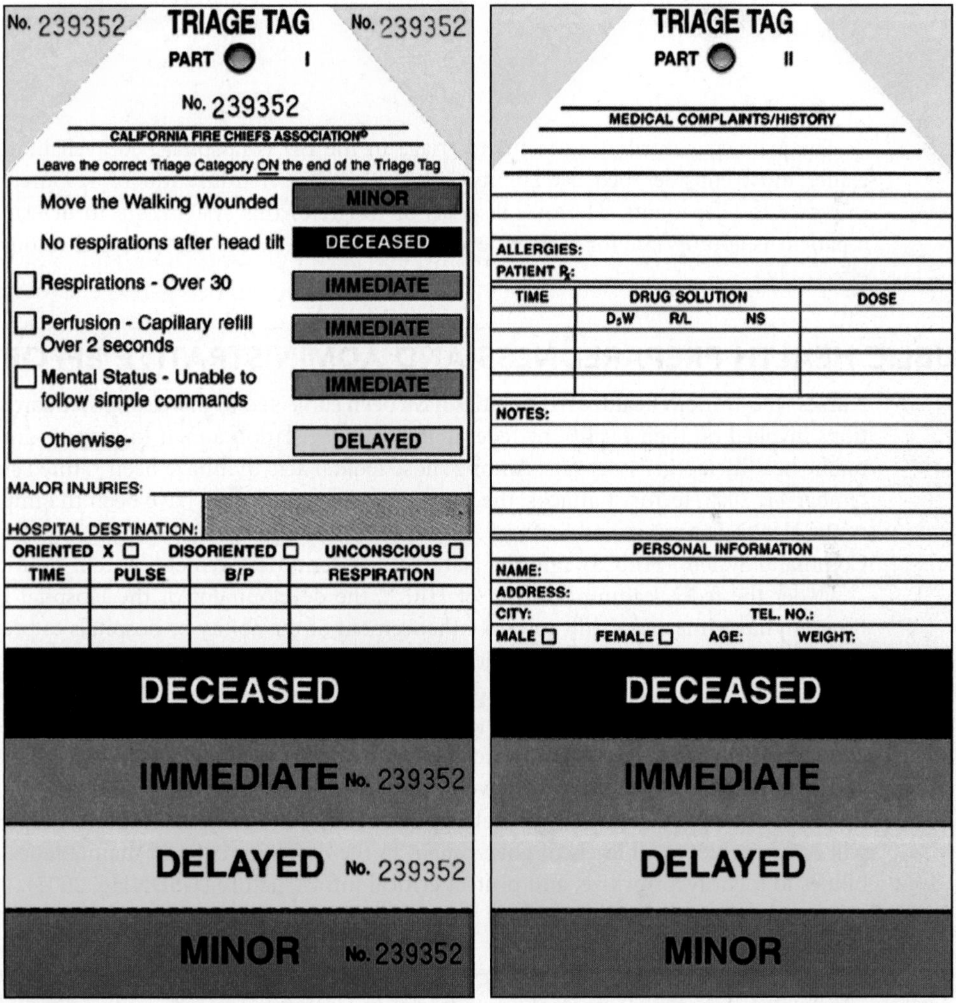

FIGURE 26-2
An example of a triage tag.

BOX 26-1   The START System of Triage

The START system divides injured personnel into four separate groups:

- Deceased (Black)—Injured persons who are beyond the scope of medical assistance. Persons are tagged "Deceased" only if they are not breathing and attempts to resuscitate have been unsuccessful.
- Immediate (Red)—Injured persons who can be assisted or their health aided by advanced medical care immediately or within 1 hour of care.
- Delayed (Yellow)—Injured persons who can be assisted after "Immediate" persons are medically cared for first. "Delayed" persons are medically stable but require medical assistance.
- Minor (Green)—Injured persons who can be assisted after "Immediate" and "Delayed" persons have been medically attended. Persons tagged "Minor" will not need medical care for at least several hours and can usually walk with assistance (usually consisting of bandages and first aid).

The primary contributing factor to triage in the ED is hospital bed availability. The triage leader must consider bed availability issues for optimal utilization of resources to provide safe care to all patients. The overall goals of triage, in this system, are to determine whether a patient is appropriate for a given level of care and to ensure that hospital resources are used effectively.

PUBLIC HEALTH PREPAREDNESS AND ADMINISTRATIVE EFFORTS

Nurses who work in health care facilities have been subjected to increasing standards and regulations invoked on their facility by federal and state legislation aimed to prepare and respond to public health emergency events. Among those federal acts that have been ratified since the September 11, 2001, terrorist attacks, the most important outcomes have been the implementation of the Health Resources and Services Administration (HRSA), the Hospital Emergency Incident Command System (HEICS), and the National Incident Management System (NIMS).

Under the federal administration of HRSA, the development of the Hospital Preparedness Program has witnessed a shift toward enhancement of the ability of hospitals to prepare for and respond to public health emergencies. Hospitals and outpatient care facilities have initiated coordination with EMS and other health care partner agencies to collaborate with local and state public health agencies in receiving funding for public health emergency preparedness (USDHHS, 2005). This funding is applied toward the National Preparedness Goal, which aims to develop and maintain the capabilities to prevent, protect against, respond to, and recover from major events, including Incidents of National Significance. Additionally, the National Preparedness Goal will assist entities at all levels of government in the development and maintenance of the capabilities to identify, prioritize, and protect critical infrastructure (USDHHS, 2005).

The National Preparedness Goal has shifted from a sole bioterrorism preparedness effort to *all-hazards preparedness* collaboration.

The key areas of focus under the National Preparedness Goal for 2007 include interoperable communications systems, bed-tracking systems (which incorporate "real-time" availability of open beds that can be accessed by hospital and emergency responder stakeholders in the event of an emergency), Emergency System for the Advance Registration of Volunteer Health Professionals (ESAR-VHP), fatality management plans, and hospital evacuation plans. Additionally, all hospitals and health care facilities must incorporate NIMS, education and preparedness training, and evaluations for corrective actions (based on preparedness training) to reach all capabilities established under the Hospital Preparedness Program (USDHHS, 2005).

As mentioned earlier, hospitals receiving HRSA and other federal preparedness funds must comply with the application of the National Incident Management System developed by the Federal Emergency Management Agency (FEMA). NIMS provides a consistent nationwide template to establish federal, state, tribal, and local governments and private sector and nongovernmental organizations to work together effectively and efficiently to prepare for, prevent, respond to, and recover from domestic incidents, regardless of cause, size, or complexity, including acts of catastrophic terrorism. NIMS benefits include a unified approach to incident management; standard command and management structures; and emphasis on preparedness, mutual aid, and resource management (FEMA, 2008).

Hospitals and health care facilities were required by The Joint Commission to be NIMS compliant by the end of calendar year 2007, to confirm successful training of hospital staff under NIMS, and to implement the HICS emergency response command structure during hospital emergency responses (The Joint Commission, 2008).

One component of NIMS is for hospitals and health care facilities to execute the Hospital Incident Command System (HICS) during hospital and public health emergencies. HICS is a comprehensive incident management system intended for use in both emergent and nonemergent situations. It provides hospitals of all sizes with tools needed to advance their emergency preparedness and response capability—individually and as members of the broader response community. HICS is designed to be implemented for all routine or planned hospital events, regardless of size or type; this helps establish a clear chain of command and standardizes response processes. This standardized response allows entities from different organizations to be integrated under one common structure that can address response issues and delegate responsibilities (California Emergency Medical Services Authority, 2007). Additional information regarding HICS can be found online at *www.emsa.ca.gov/hics/hics.asp*.

COMMUNITY HEALTH NURSE ISSUES AND PUBLIC HEALTH PREPAREDNESS

Epidemiological Aspects

The epidemiological response to a terrorist event plays a pivotal role in public health, both related and unrelated to biological terrorism. Epidemiologists and infection control nurses must recognize and act upon rapid determination that an unusual event has occurred. These nurses must be able to perform surveillance for additional case identification and tracking, and they must

BOX 26-2   Epidemiological Clues That Could Signal a Biological Event

- Large numbers of ill persons with a similar clinical presentation, disease, or syndrome
- An increase in unexplained diseases or deaths
- Unusual illness in a population
- Higher morbidity and mortality in association with a common disease or syndrome or failure of such patients to respond to regular therapy
- Single case of disease caused by an uncommon agent, such as smallpox, Machupo hemorrhagic fever, pulmonary anthrax, glanders
- Several unusual or unexplained diseases coexisting in the same patient without any other explanation
- Disease with an unusual geographic, temporal, or seasonal distribution—for instance, influenza in the summer or Ebola hemorrhagic fever in United States
- Similar disease among persons who attended the same public event or gathering
- Illness that is unusual or atypical for a given population or age group
- Unusual or atypical disease presentation
- Unusual, atypical, unidentifiable, or antiquated strain of an agent
- Unusual antibiotic resistance pattern
- Endemic disease with a sudden, unexplained increase in incidence
- Atypical disease transmission through aerosols, food, or water, which suggests deliberate sabotage
- Many ill persons who seek treatment at about the same time

prevent the spread of disease through the implementation of effective intervention methods. This component of emergency response, when executed correctly and expeditiously, can significantly reduce morbidity and mortality in exposed populations (Zerwekh and Waring, 2005).

A critical component of an effective epidemiological response to an emergency—both in the health care facility and in the community—is the acute identification and recognition of epidemiological clues that could signal a biological event. Early recognition of these clues can be achieved though surveillance (passive and active) and monitoring of patients presenting to health care facilities (Zerwekh and Waring, 2005). Two major clues that a biological terrorism event has occurred are a clear differential diagnosis and the formation of an epidemiological curve. Additional epidemiological indicators of a biological event are listed in Box 26-2.

It is possible that none of the listed clues will occur during a given bioterrorism event. However, the presence of one or more indicators on the list should tip off infection control nurses, ED nurses, or community health nurses of such an event.

Another practice in both the health care facility and public health realms at the forefront of biological terrorism early detection is the concept of *syndromic surveillance*. Syndromic surveillance applies health-related data such as trends in patient symptomology or disease presentation that precedes clinical diagnosis and can indicate a substantial probability of an outbreak that would warrant further investigation and public health response (Zerwekh and Waring, 2005). For example, investigation of ICD-9 codes, chief complaint, similar signs and symptoms exhibited by patients in the ED, and frequency of antibiotic/prophylactic therapy prescribed can all be applied and integrated into a successful syndromic surveillance network. In the public health setting, monitoring inventory of over-the-counter medications (e.g., cough/cold medicines) and identification of excessive absenteeism of students at a school or employees in the workplace setting are other trends surveyed to detect the possibility of an outbreak or bioterrorism event before clinical diagnosis has been made. Different frameworks (such as Outbreak Management System) are currently being developed to determine the most efficient approach to a successful syndromic surveillance network. The key concepts of a successful syndromic surveillance program are timeliness of reporting data, validity and quality of data, and system experience (Zerwekh and Waring, 2005).

The epidemiological response plays a pivotal role in public health emergencies. The implementation of surveillance, case identification and tracking, and early intervention methods can significantly reduce morbidity and mortality in exposed populations.

What Is the Strategic National Stockpile?

The CDC Strategic National Stockpile (SNS) program stores large quantities of medicine and medical supplies to protect the citizens of the United States during a public health emergency, including (but not limited to) a terrorist attack, pandemic outbreak, or natural disaster such as an earthquake or hurricane (CDC, 2008). This national inventory of antibiotics, chemical antidotes, antitoxins, airway maintenance supplies, and other medical equipment will support and refresh existing community resources being implemented during a public health emergency. The SNS "push-pack," once requested, will be delivered to any state or U.S. territory within 12 hours of request. Federal authorities have ensured enough medicine and equipment to supply multiple communities for an extended period during an event. In such an event, public health nurses can expect to be enlisted in assistance of the evaluation and delivery of medications and equipment to every person in the affected community (CDC, 2008).

What Is a CHEMPACK?

The Strategic National Stockpile CHEMPACK is a federal program designed to supplement the medical response in the event of a chemical nerve agent release. The scope of this program is specifically targeted for nerve agents classified as organophosphates, such as sarin and VX gases. The CHEMPACK containers, delivered to each of the 50 states and stored in geographically strategic locales, possess both EMS and hospital caches. Both caches contain such chemical antidotes as MARK-1 kits (intramuscular auto-injectors of atropine and pralidoxime [2-PAM]), atropine injectors, PAM kits, diazepam, and sterile water.

The public health nurse must be aware of the possibility of administering such medications during a chemical weapon event and must be refreshed on the proper dosage and clinical practice applications.

What Is ESAR-VHP?

The Emergency System for Advance Registration of Volunteer Health Professionals (ESAR-VHP) is a federally funded program through the HRSA that will form a national system that will allow efficient utilization of health professional volunteers in emergencies by providing verifiable, up-to-date information regarding the volunteer's identity and credentials to hospitals or other medical facilities in need of the volunteer's services. Each state's ESAR-VHP system is built to standards that will allow quick and easy exchange of health professionals with other states, thereby maximizing the size of the population able to receive services during a public health or presidential declared emergency (Critical Thinking Box 26-3).

How do you register for ESAR-VHP in your state? What organization is responsible for coordinating the process? Who should register?

Medical Reserve Corps

The Medical Reserve Corps (MRC), initiated by the U.S. Office of the Surgeon General, is another resource developed to help communities in planning for and responding to a public health or medical emergency (MRC, 2008). Community-based MRC units function as a mechanism to organize and utilize volunteers who want to donate their time and expertise to prepare for and respond to emergencies on a local scale. MRC volunteers supplement existing emergency and public health resources by including medical and public health professionals such as physicians, nurses, pharmacists, dentists, veterinarians, and epidemiologists. The primary objectives of MRC units are to improve health literacy, increase disease prevention, eliminate health disparities, and most important, improve public health preparedness (MRC, 2008). MRC units were deployed during the hurricane onslaught of 2004 and during Hurricane Katrina in 2005 to assist health assessment teams during these natural disasters and to assist in staffing special-needs shelters and community health centers and clinics.

Public health nurses need to be aware of the presence of MRC units and are encouraged to enlist in the MRC at their local jurisdiction. During times of medical emergencies, it is likely that public health nurses will be working alongside MRC units in a collaborative effort to minimize morbidity and mortality while maximizing the public health and medical response.

Disaster Medical Assistance Teams

Disaster Medical Assistance Teams (DMAT) are yet another public health preparedness and response resource a community health nurse may have interaction with during a medical emergency. These teams, supported through the National Disaster Medical System, are 35 deployable units divided by geographic region (USDHHS, 2008). The units are composed of teams of various clinical health specialties that include (but may not be limited to) communications, logistics, maintenance, and security. These teams are locally based but can be deployed federally on request. The responsibilities of DMAT teams include triage of victims at a disaster site, medical care at the site, and staging of locations outside the disaster site for transportation of patients to alternative health care facilities. DMAT teams also serve as care centers for evacuation areas, where they can set up mobile medical care facilities for injured and trauma persons evacuating a declared disaster area.

WHAT DO I NEED TO KNOW ABOUT COMMUNITY PREPAREDNESS ISSUES?

The community health nurse has a responsibility not only in promoting public health and preventing disease, but also in delivering primary prevention methodologies related to disaster and emergencies preparedness. For the community health nurse, the three critical components of preparedness include mental health preparedness, family/individual preparedness, and business preparedness. The National Response Framework (USDHS, 2008a), which aligns federal

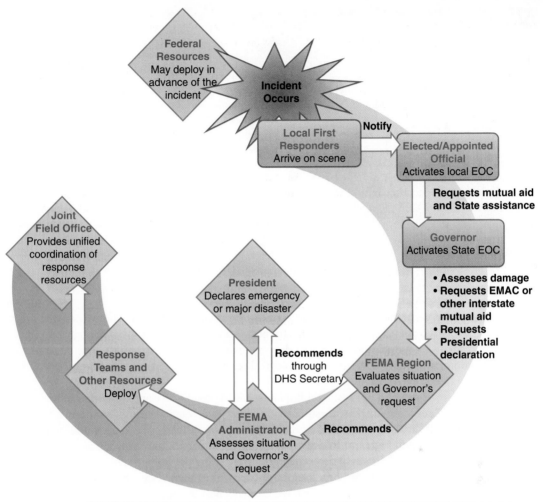

FIGURE 26-3

Overview of the Stafford Act support to states, tribal, and local governments that are affected by a major disaster or emergency. *(From U.S. Department of Homeland Security:* National response framework. *Retrieved from* www.fema.gov/pdf/emergency/nrf/nrf-stafford.pdf.*)*

coordination structures, capabilities, and resources into a unified local and community response, is presented in Figure 26-3.

WHAT DO I NEED TO KNOW ABOUT DISASTER MENTAL HEALTH?

Any type of public health or medical disaster can cause a range of psychological reactions, from acute moderate symptoms to chronic severe stress-related psychological disorders. Traumatic medical emergencies can induce an array of personal stress responses, ranging from horror,

TABLE 26-3 Common Responses to a Traumatic Event

Cognitive	Emotional	Physical	Behavioral
Poor concentration	Shock	Nausea	Suspicion
Confusion	Numbness	Lightheadedness	Irritability
Disorientation	Feeling overwhelmed	Dizziness	Arguments with friends
Indecisiveness	Depression	Gastrointestinal problems	and loved ones
Shortened attention	Feeling lost	Rapid heart rate	Withdrawal
span	Fear of harm to self	Tremors	Excessive silence
Memory loss	and/or loved ones	Headaches	Inappropriate humor
Unwanted	Feeling nothing	Grinding of teeth	Increased/decreased eating
memories	Feeling abandoned	Fatigue	Change in sexual desire or
Difficulty making	Uncertainty of feelings	Poor sleep	functioning
decisions	Volatile emotions	Pain	Increased smoking
		Hyperarousal	Increased substance use or
		Jumpiness	abuse

From Centers for Disease Control (2008): *CDC Emergency Preparedness and Response.* Retrieved from *www.bt.cdc.gov.*

helplessness, and anger to more progressive and severe reactions such as depression, substance abuse, and disconnection from society. Traumatic events affect those who witness the event, as well as survivors, rescue workers, and friends and relatives of victims. Although prevalence of immediate emotional reactions is well documented, the community health nurse must focus and be aware of the development of psychological reactions that persist from days to years after the public health event (CDC, 2008).

The first practice a nurse should implement is the cognizance and awareness of onset of psychological reactions in persons suffering from disaster mental health symptoms. When confronted with a patient suffering from such symptoms (Table 26-3), the nurse must identify concrete needs and attempt to assist—for instance, a person may ask, "How do I know if my friend is alive?" or "Are my parents OK?" or "How is my pet doing?" These concrete needs may be critical in identifying early symptom development of mental health problems.

The following guidelines have been recommended to the nurse in responding to patients after a public health emergency or disaster (CDC, 2008):

- Provide attention to patients' experience and compassion and sympathy for their emotions.
- Empathize with patients and their emotions and experiences.
- Encourage patient discussion of their experience; positive and negative.
- Speak to patients in nonmedical terms—be their friend, their confidant.
- Reinforce their emotions and reactions; these reactions are natural and tacit.

Once the community health nurse has identified psychological reactions, it is imperative to help the patient address the associated symptom progression. The following may assist the patient in coping with the emotional stressors (CDC, 2008):

- Suggest methodologies for relaxation.
- Encourage discussion of the situation or event in a calm and compassionate approach.
- Reinforce sources of support, including, but not limited to, family and friends.
- Encourage patient's communication of emotions to supportive networks.
- Advocate for a return to normal routine.

- Encourage patient to defuse day-to-day potential stress-building conflicts that might otherwise catalyze psychological stress onset.

As the medical emergency or disaster continues, the nurse's role is essential in identifying patients whose symptoms could progress to long-term mental afflictions. The following are key exposure factors in determining a potential of long-term psychological manifestations as a result of a disaster (CDC, 2008):

- Proximity to the event. Persons geographically closer to the event may be inclined to a greater psychological response.
- Previous psychological stability and history of past traumatic events. Patients who have experienced previous traumatic events or were experiencing psychological disorders prior to the event are predisposed to increased psychological reactions after the event.
- Importance and depth of the event. Patients who lose a friend or immediate family member may be inclined to greater psychological reaction development.

The nurse must be cognizant of continued progression of psychological reactions. Certain symptoms can assist the nurse in recognizing the development and onset of long-lasting psychological reactions, including the development of posttraumatic stress disorder. When such symptoms are identified, the community health nurse is recommended to do the following (CDC, 2008):

- Refer patients for follow-up with a mental health professional (specifically trained in traumatic events, if possible) to seek additional counseling and guidance.
- Provide follow-up and guidance as needed.

Individual and Family Preparedness Issues

In regular practice, the public health nurse must be cognizant of the concept of community and family emergency preparedness. Whether in mitigation of a previous event or in everyday practice, the promotion of community/family preparedness to the population is critical in minimizing morbidity and mortality and alleviating personal confusion and anxieties during a public health event. Special emphasis toward the promotion of family/community preparedness is encouraged each year during the month of September, which has been designated as National Preparedness Month (USDHS, 2008c).

Community preparedness can be further subclassified under efforts initiated at home, work, and school. Preparedness efforts undertaken at the home should focus on creating a disaster preparedness kit, establishing family emergency communication and evacuation plans, and recognizing potential disasters in the family's community. A family disaster preparedness kit should include enough essential supplies for each family member to last a minimum of 3 consecutive days; it is important for the family to replace expired supplies every 6 months (USDHS, 2008c) (Box 26-3, Figure 26-4, Critical Thinking Box 26-4).

The development of a family communications and evacuation plan will help prepare family members to share responsibilities and work together as a team during a public health event. The public health nurse should recommend family members discuss the types of probable disasters in their community and consider how members might respond to each scenario. Evacuation routes should include primary and secondary "meeting places"—it is recommended that the primary place be somewhere in the immediate vicinity around the house and that the secondary site be at a location away from the home in case family members are unable to return to the neighborhood (USDHS, 2008b). It is important that each family member know the phone

BOX 26-3	Recommended Disaster Preparedness Kit

RECOMMENDED ITEMS TO INCLUDE IN A BASIC EMERGENCY SUPPLY KIT

- Water
  - One gallon of water per person per day, for drinking and sanitation
  - Children, nursing mothers, and sick people may need more water
  - If you live in a warm weather climate, more water may be necessary
  - Store water tightly in clean plastic containers such as soft drink bottles
  - Keep *at least* a 3-day supply of water per person
- Food—at least a 3-day supply of nonperishable food
- Battery-powered or hand-crank radio and an NOAA weather radio with tone alert and extra batteries for both
- Flashlight and extra batteries
- First aid kit
- Whistle to signal for help
- Dust mask, to help filter contaminated air, and plastic sheeting and duct tape to shelter-in-place
- Moist towelettes, garbage bags, and plastic ties for personal sanitation
- Wrench or pliers to turn off utilities
- Can opener for food (if kit contains canned food)
- Local maps

ADDITIONAL ITEMS TO CONSIDER ADDING TO AN EMERGENCY SUPPLY KIT

- Prescription medications and glasses
- Infant formula and diapers
- Pet food and extra water for your pet
- Important family documents such as copies of insurance policies, identification, and bank account records in a waterproof, portable container
- Cash or traveler's checks and change
- Emergency reference material such as a first aid book or information from *www.ready.gov*
- Sleeping bag or warm blanket for each person; consider additional bedding if you live in a cold-weather climate
- Complete change of clothing including a long-sleeved shirt, long pants, and sturdy shoes; consider additional clothing if you live in a cold-weather climate
- Household chlorine bleach and medicine dropper (a solution of 9 parts water to 1 part bleach can be used as a disinfectant. Or in an emergency, you can treat water by adding 16 drops of household liquid bleach per gallon of water. Do not use scented or "color-safe" bleaches or bleaches with added cleaners).
- Fire extinguisher
- Matches in a waterproof container
- Feminine supplies and personal hygiene items
- Mess kits, paper cups, paper plates, plastic utensils, paper towels
- Paper and pencil
- Books, games, puzzles or other activities for children

Courtesy Department of Homeland Security (*www.ready.gov*).

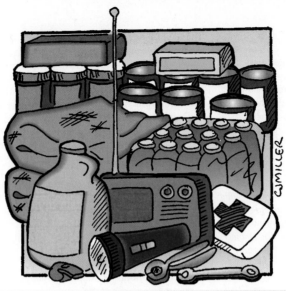

FIGURE 26-4
Disaster preparedness kit.

number and address of the secondary site. Families should also nominate an out-of-area family friend who can serve as an "emergency contact" should the scale of disaster overwhelm local communication resources and local telephone calls become more difficult. This contact will serve as the information hub for family members not only if they are separated but also for event update information. It is important to encourage family members to practice their communications and evacuation plans regularly.

CONCLUSION

Whether in the clinical or community environment, the role of the nurse in relation to emergency preparedness continues to expand and develop as local, state, and national preparedness efforts are executed. The nurse must continue to be aware and informed of evolving threats such as biological, chemical, or radioactive terrorism while maintaining up-to-date training and knowledge of effective response to public health disasters. The initiatives and programs mentioned in this chapter will ultimately aid nurses in comprehensive and efficient preparation, response, recovery, and mitigation to any public health emergency with which they may be confronted throughout their professional nursing tenure.

BIBLIOGRAPHY

California Emergency Medical Services Authority (2007): HICS overview. State of California. Retrieved from *www.emsa.ca.gov/hics.*

Centers for Disease Control (2008): *CDC Emergency Preparedness and Response.* Retrieved from *www.bt.cdc.gov.*

Centers for Disease Control (2010a): *Seasonal flu.* Retrieved from *www.cdc.gov/flu/.*

Centers for Disease Control (2010b): *Persons who should not be vaccinated.* Retrieved from *www.cdc.gov/flu/professionals/acip/shouldnot.htm.*

Federal Emergency Management Agency (2008): *The national incident management system.* Retrieved from *www.fema.gov/emergency/nrf/NIMS.htm.*

Kandasamy M: Community health nurse in disaster management. *Nurs J India* 98:227, 2007.

Medical Reserve Corps (MRC) (2008): Retrieved from *www.medicalreservecorps.gov/HomePage.*

The Joint Commission: Emergency management standards. *Hospital and Critical Access Hospital Accreditation Programs.* Oakbrook Terrace, Ill, 2008, The Joint Commission.

U.S. Army Medical Research Inustitute of Chemical Defense (2008). Retrieved from *www.chemdef.apgea.army.mil.*

U.S. Department of Health and Human Services: *Hospital Preparedness Program.* Public Law 109-417, 2005.

U.S. Department of Health and Human Services (2008): *Disaster medical assistance teams (DMAT).* Retrieved from *www.hhs.gov/aspr/opeo/ndms/teams/dmat.html.*

U.S. Department of Homeland Security (2008a): National response framework. Retrieved from *www.fema.gov/pdf/emergency/nrf/nrf-core.pdf.*

U.S. Department of Homeland Security (2008b): Ready campaign-disaster preparedness kit. Retrieved from *www.ready.gov/america/getakit/index.html.*

U.S. Department of Homeland Security (2008c): Ready campaign-national preparedness month. Retrieved from *www.ready.gov/america/npm08/intro.html.*

U.S. Nuclear Regulatory Commission (2007): *Fact sheets on dirty bombs.* Retrieved from *www.nrc.gov/reading-rm/doc-collections/fact-sheets/dirty-bombs.html.*

Wetter DC, Daniell WD, Treser CD: Hospital preparedness for victims of chemical or biological terrorism. *Am J Pub Health* 91:710-716, 2001.

Zerwekh JT, Waring SC: The epidemiology of bioterrorism. In Pilch R, Zilinskas R, editors: *The Encyclopedia of bioterrorism,* New York, 2005, Wiley and Sons.

Additional resources are available online at *http://evolve.elsevier.com/Zerwekh/nsgtoday/.*

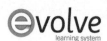

Index